Anesthesia for Ambulatory Surgery

J. B. Lippincott Company
Philadelphia

London
Mexico City
New York
St. Louis
São Paulo
Sydney

Anesthesia

for

Ambulatory Surgery

Edited by

Bernard V. Wetchler, M.D.

Director, Department of Anesthesiology
Medical Director, Ambulatory Surgery Center
The Methodist Medical Center of Illinois
Clinical Professor and Chief, Division of Anesthesia
University of Illinois
College of Medicine at Peoria
Peoria, Illinois

With 18 Contributors

Sponsoring Editor: Sanford J. Robinson
Manuscript Editor: Don Shenkle
Indexer: Barbara Littlewood
Art Director: Tracy Baldwin
Designer: Arlene Putterman
Design Coordinator: Anne O'Donnell
Production Supervisor: Kathleen P. Dunn
Production Assistant: Carol A. Florence
Compositor: McFarland Graphics & Design
Printer/Binder: R. R. Donnelley & Sons Co.

6   5   4   3   2   1

Library of Congress Cataloging in Publication Data
   Main entry under title:

Anesthesia for ambulatory surgery.

   Includes bibliographies and index.
   1. Anesthesia.   2. Surgery, Outpatient.
I. Wetchler, Bernard V. [DNLM: 1. Ambulatory Surgery.
2. Anesthesia. WO 192 A579]
RD82.A677   617'.96   84-23399
ISBN 0-397-50660-0

The authors and publisher have exerted every effort to
ensure that drug selection and dosage set forth in this text
are in accord with current recommendations and practice
at the time of publication. However, in view of ongoing
research, changes in governmental regulations, and the
constant flow of information relating to drug therapy and
drug reactions, the reader is urged to check the package
insert for each drug for any change in indications and
dosage and for added warnings and precautions. This is
particularly important when the recommended agent is a
new or infrequently employed drug.

To Jorie

always understanding

always supportive

always interested

Contributors

BENJAMIN G. COVINO, Ph.D., M.D.
Chairman, Department of Anesthesia, Brigham and Women's Hospital;
Professor of Anaesthesia, Harvard Medical School, Boston, Massachusetts

Benjamin G. Covino obtained his Ph.D. degree in Physiology from Boston University. He began his professional career as a cardiac physiologist with particular interest in the field of cardiac arrhythmias related to hypothermia. He received his M.D. degree from the University of Buffalo and took his anesthesia training at the Massachusetts General Hospital. For the past 20 years, he has been active from a research and clinical point of view in the field of regional and local anesthesia, and he is particularly interested in the role of regional anesthesia in ambulatory surgery. When he gets the chance he enjoys skiing and tennis.

ANNE FREY DEAN, R.N., B.S.N.
Consultant, Primary Resources, Inc., DeLand, Florida

Anne Dean received her nursing degrees from San Antonio College and the University of Texas Health Science Center. She was instrumental in planning, equipping, and staffing the Outpatient Surgery Center at Southwest Texas Methodist Hospital and served as its director.
Ms. Dean has spoken at many national meetings on the subject of ambulatory surgery, has authored several articles, and a book, Designing and Managing an Ambulatory Surgery Program. *She is a member of the American Academy of Medical Administrators and the American Nurses Association and is a past president of her local AORN chapter.*
A former art major, Ms. Dean spends her spare time redoing a 100-year-old Victorian estate. She enjoys fishing, hiking, reading, and music of all kinds.

BURTON S. EPSTEIN, M.D.

Professor and Chairman, Department of Anesthesiology, The George Washington University School of Medicine and Health Sciences, Washington, D.C.

Burton S. Epstein graduated from the George Washington University School of Medicine and completed a residency in anesthesiology at the Hospital of the University of Pennsylvania. He joined the faculty of George Washington University Medical Center in 1964 and was present during the time their ambulatory surgery unit opened in 1966. He has written and spoken extensively on the subject of ambulatory surgery. He lectured on outpatient anesthesia at the ASA refresher course in 1972 and his first article on the subject was published in 1973. He served as Chairman of the Department of Anesthesiology at the Children's Hospital National Medical Center, Washington, D.C., from 1974 through 1983.

He is an avid tennis player. He and wife Diane have two sons, Steve, who is in a psychiatric residency, and Jerry, who is completing law school.

WILLIAM A. FLEXNER, Dr. P.H.

President, Flexner and Associates, Inc., Minneapolis, Minnesota

William A. Flexner's background spans the two fields of health care and business. On his way to creating his management consulting firm, Mr. Flexner completed graduate work in government and health administration and in business marketing; worked in Central America in the development of urban and rural health services as part of the U.S. foreign aid program; and served on the faculty of the Center for Health Services Research at the University of Minnesota as a specialist in health care marketing.

He has written extensively and has taught numerous seminars dealing with the concepts of marketing and strategic planning in the health care industry, including ambulatory surgery.

Having recently moved to a park-like setting on the bluffs of the Mississippi River, he hopes to pursue his longtime hobby of photography and capture in pictures the deer, birds, and other wildlife that frequent the area.

JAMES LEWIS GRIFFITH, J.D.

Griffith & Burr, P.C., Philadelphia, Pennsylvania

James Lewis Griffith received his J.D. degree in 1965 from Villanova University School of Law. He has been a very active lecturer and teacher in law and medicine at several universities and has presented on a variety of subjects, including ambulatory surgery, at many national programs. He serves as an editorial consultant to Same Day Surgery, Hospital Infection Control, Peer Review, and Medical Economics. His entire professional practice has featured a combination of defending hospitals and physicians.

Mr. Griffith's other interests include sailing, canoeing, and travel. He is currently coauthoring a book on Pennsylvania Trial Practice and Procedure.

RAAFAT S. HANNALLAH, M.D.

Associate Professor of Anesthesiology, Child Health and Development, Children's Hospital National Medical Center, George Washington University, Washington, D.C.

Raafat S. Hannallah was born in Egypt and graduated in Medicine from Cairo University in 1966. Following his anesthesia training at McGill University in Montreal, he remained on the faculty at the Montreal Children's Hospital and helped develop its modern hospital-based day surgery unit. He is currently the director of the residency training program in pediatric anesthesia at Children's Hospital National Medical Center, where he is actively involved in the day-to-day functions of its busy ambulatory surgery unit. His particular interests include anesthesia induction in children and management of airway problems, and he has lectured extensively on these subjects. He is interested in classical music, traveling, and gourmet dining.

LESLIE K. LEIDER, M.H.A.

Consultant, Management Consulting Services, Ernst & Whinney, Minneapolis, Minnesota

Leslie K. Leider received a Masters of Hospital and Health Care Administration from St. Louis University. He was a hospital consultant with Robert Douglass Associates, Inc., and Assistant Vice President at St. Mary's Hospital in Minneapolis. He is a member of the American College of Hospital Administrators, an associate of the American Association of Health Consultants, and has served on the faculty of the American Hospital Association's seminar "Ambulatory Surgery: Implementing and Managing a Successful Hospital Program" since 1982. When he is not consulting, he can usually be found enjoying the theater, windsurfing during the short Minneapolis summers, or cross-country and downhill skiing during the long winters. Occasionally, he may be seen riding the thermals in a hang glider.

MONTE LICHTIGER, M.D.

Vice-Chairman, Department of Anesthesiology, and Director, Gumenick Ambulatory Surgical Facility, Mount Sinai Medical Center, Miami Beach, Florida; Clinical Professor of Anesthesiology, University of Miami School of Medicine, Miami, Florida

Monte Lichtiger graduated from Columbia College in 1961 and received his medical degree from the Albert Einstein College of Medicine in 1965. He then took internship and residency training in Miami. Upon completion of his residency, he served in the U.S. Air Force, stationed at Wilford Hall USAF Hospital in San Antonio, Texas. In 1971, he returned to Miami, Florida, to join the faculty of the University of Miami School of Medicine. He was Director of the Residency Training Program at Mt. Sinai Medical Center before assuming the directorship of its ambulatory surgical facility. He is co-author of the book Introduction to the Practice of Anesthesia.

After residing in Miami for so many years, he has become an avid boater and scuba diver. He also enjoys deep-sea fishing off the coast of Florida and in the Bahamas.

PETER M. MANNIX, M.H.A.

Director of Facility Development, Health Management Services, Syracuse, New York

Peter M. Mannix is responsible for long-range planning, building programs, and new programs and services for the eight member hospitals of Health Management Services.

Prior to joining HMS, Mr. Mannix was a hospital consultant with Robert Douglass Associates, Inc., Minneapolis, Minnesota, and Herman Smith Associates, Hinsdale, Illinois. His project experience focused on the development of long-range plans, certificates of need, and building consultations. A number of these studies are specifically related to ambulatory surgery programs. Since 1982 he has been a faculty member of the widely successful American Hospital Association seminar "Ambulatory Surgery: Implementing and Managing a Successful Hospital Program."

When not jogging he can be found backpacking, having recently completed an Alaskan trip.

SLADE H. McLAUGHLIN, J.D.

Griffith & Burr, P.C., Philadelphia, Pennsylvania

Slade H. McLaughlin was born in Philadelphia, graduated cum laude *from Ursinus College, and received his J.D. from Villanova University in 1982. His professional practice involves the defense of*

medical practitioners in malpractice cases. His other interests include scuba diving, long-distance running, and rafting.

HERBERT E. NATOF, M.D.
Medical Director, Northwest Surgicare (Medical Care International),
Arlington Heights, Illinois

Herbert E. Natof was born, raised and educated in Illinois, graduating from the University of Illinois College of Medicine in 1954 and completing his residency in anesthesiology at the University of Illinois Research and Education Hospitals in 1957. While visiting the Phoenix Surgicenter in 1971 he met Wallace Reed, and from that moment on became deeply involved in the ambulatory surgery concept. He was one of the founders of Northwest Surgicare—the fourth freestanding ambulatory surgery center in the United States.

He has served on the Board of Directors of the Freestanding Ambulatory Surgery Association; as a representative of the AMA to the Professional and Technical Advisory Board for Ambulatory Care of the Joint Commission; on the ASA Committee on Ambulatory Surgical Care; and as a surveyor for the Accreditation Association for Ambulatory Health Care.

He enjoys swimming, long walks, and suffering with the Chicago Cubs. His secret ambition is to publish a novel, and he is currently working on his second.

CYNTHIA ALEXANDER NKANA, M.D.
Associate Medical Director, Methodist Ambulatory Surgery Center, The
Methodist Medical Center of Illinois, Peoria, Illinois

Cynthia Alexander Nkana has fond memories of her childhood and early adult life in Evansville, Indiana. Her undergraduate studies were completed at Indiana State University. When she graduated from the Medical College of Wisconsin in 1979, 10% of her class went into anesthesia residency programs.

Amidst the unspoiled beauty of West Virginia she took her anesthesia training at West Virginia University. She returned to the midwest to begin her anesthesia practice at The Methodist Medical Center of Illinois in Peoria. Following her exposure to its active ambulatory surgery center she quickly realized the importance of the anesthesiologist in maintaining the efficiency of the facility and also in providing for patient safety. She currently finds working in ambulatory surgery one of the most interesting and exciting areas of her practice.

Her most precious moments are spent with her husband and two children, who are due a "thank you" for relinquishing some of their family time so that she could contribute to this book. She relaxes at the piano, playing the music of Mozart and Schubert.

PATRICK G. O'DONOVAN, M.H.S.A.
Administrative Fellow, William Beaumont Hospital, Royal Oak, Michigan

Patrick O'Donovan recently received his Master of Health Services Administration degree from the University of Michigan in Ann Arbor. He is currently serving an administrative fellowship at William Beaumont Hospital in Royal Oak, Michigan.

Mr. O'Donovan has authored a research paper entitled "The Current Status of Ambulatory Surgery in the United States." In addition, he coauthored two chapters in Ambulatory Surgery: A Guide to Perioperative Nursing Care, *edited by Brenda Cole Mauldin.*

Mr. O'Donovan's interests include travel, weight lifting, Tigers baseball, and golf.

THOMAS R. O'DONOVAN, Ph.D.

President, American Academy of Medical Administrators, Southfield, Michigan

Thomas R. O'Donovan has been President of the American Academy of Medical Administrators for the past 5 years and was administrator of Mt. Carmel Mercy Hospital for 15 years before that. He received his Ph.D. from Michigan State University and is a fellow of the American Academy of Medical Administrators and the American College of Hospital Administrators. Dr. O'Donovan was selected for inclusion in "Who's Who in Health Care" and received the AAMA Health Care Executive of the Year award in 1971. He received an honorable mention from ACHA for his article "Dynamics of Ambulatory Surgery" in Hospital Administration *and is the author of* Ambulatory Surgical Centers, *published by Aspen Systems Corporation in 1976. He was the chairman and speaker of the conference "Ambulatory Surgery: Directions for the 1980's" conducted by American Health Consultants in Atlanta, Georgia, November 3–4, 1980, and has also been the contributor of chapters in five books on ambulatory surgery.*

FREDRICK K. ORKIN, M.D., M.B.A.

Associate Professor of Anesthesia, University of California Medical Center, San Francisco, California; formerly Medical Director, Same Day Surgery, Hahnemann University Hospital; Associate Professor of Anesthesiology, Hahnemann University School of Medicine, Philadelphia, Pennsylvania

Quite by accident, Fredrick K. Orkin discovered the wisdom of Francis Weld Peabody who, decades before modern medicine, noted that new physicians "are too 'scientific' and do not know how to take care of the patients" and emphasized that "the secret of the care of the patient is in caring for the patient." An interest in returning care to the overall patient underlies Dr. Orkin's enthusiasm for ambulatory anesthesia, as well as his other professional interests. A graduate of the Wharton School's health care administration program, he has studied the geographic distribution of anesthesia providers, both privately and as chairman of the American Society of Anesthesiologists' Committee on Manpower. He is coeditor of the 1983 sourcebook Complications in Anesthesiology. *During the past year, he worked on health legislation in the U. S. Congress as a Robert Wood Johnson Health Policy Fellow. His other interests include office automation, photography, and home repair. He is married and has two teenagers.*

BEVERLY K. PHILIP, M.D.

Director, Day Surgery Unit, Brigham and Women's Hospital; Assistant Professor of Anaesthesia, Harvard Medical School, Boston, Massachusetts

Beverly Khnie Philip received her M.D. degree from Upstate Medical Center, State University of New York, and her anesthesia training at the Peter Bent Brigham Hospital, Boston, Massachusetts. Dr. Philip organized the Day Surgery Unit at the Brigham and Women's Hospital, Boston, in 1980 and remains its director. She teaches the practice of ambulatory anesthesia, showing that excellent care yields patients' appreciation. Dr. Philip has spoken to national and regional audiences on how to establish a hospital-based program and on tailoring anesthesia to fit the special needs of ambulatory surgery. She has a particular interest in ambulatory regional anesthesia and has spoken and published on that subject.

Dr. Philip is married and has two sons. She is a scuba diver with experience in underwater archeology and in marine-life collection. She is also an avid dancer and skier and is a Senior Member of the National Ski Patrol.

BERNARD V. WETCHLER, M.D.

Director, Department of Anesthesiology, Medical Director, Ambulatory Surgery Center, The Methodist Medical Center of Illinois; Clinical Professor and Chief, Division of Anesthesia, University of Illinois College of Medicine at Peoria, Peoria, Illinois

Born and raised in New York City, Dr. Wetchler graduated from New York Medical College and completed his anesthesia training at the Flower and Fifth Avenue Hospitals. Since moving to Peoria, Illinois, in 1955, he has juggled a private practice with his administrative and teaching duties. He has written and spoken extensively on the subject of ambulatory surgery anesthesia; is a member of the ASA Committee on Ambulatory Surgical Care; is Chairman of the Committee on Ambulatory Surgery, 9th World Congress of Anaesthesiologists; is President of the Society for Ambulatory Anesthesia; is a member of the Editorial Advisory Board of the Same Day Surgery Newsletter and chief consultant for the Anesthesia Up-Date column; and is a Past President of the Illinois Society of Anesthesiologists. Dr. Wetchler is a jogger who likes travel, photography, and pasta.

HARRY C. WONG, M.D.

Director, Salt Lake Surgical Center, Clinical Professor of Anesthesiology, University of Utah School of Medicine, Salt Lake City, Utah

Born of immigrant Chinese parents in Beloit, Wisconsin, he was the fifth of seven children. He received his M.D. in 1958 from the University of Wisconsin in Madison, where he also completed his anesthesiology residency. Since 1961 he has lived in Salt Lake City, Utah, and been in the private practice of anesthesiology. Dr. Wong joined with two other anesthesiologists, Drs. John Adair and Wallace Ring, to found the Salt Lake Surgical Center in 1976.

He has been a frequent speaker and contributor to the literature about ambulatory surgery care and computer applications; is Chairman of the ASA Committee on Ambulatory Surgical Care; represents the ASA on the JCAH Ambulatory Health Care Professional and Technical Advisory Committee; is an officer on the Board of the Freestanding Ambulatory Surgery Association; and has served on the Board of the Accreditation Association for Ambulatory Health Care.

Dr. Wong has commented on his "good fortune to have a lovely wife, Jean Nagahiro Wong, and four children." His leisure time is devoted to tennis, photography, and travel.

Preface

The future of anesthesia involvement in the care of the ambulatory surgery patient is now! As we approach the last decade of the 20th century, it is predicted that 40% to 60% of all surgery in the United States will be performed on an ambulatory basis. The practice patterns of anesthesiologists will have to be changed, and anesthetic techniques will have to be modified to accommodate the changes that are taking place. At The Methodist Medical Center of Illinois, where I practice, 51% of all surgical patients walk through our ambulatory surgery center doors. Surgical health care is moving away from hospitalization.

Whereas originally ambulatory surgery meant short procedures on ASA physical status 1 or 2 patients, we are currently seeing more physical status 3 patients, more geriatric patients, and, because of improved surgical techniques and instrumentation, a continually expanding list of acceptable procedures.

Hospital-affiliated ambulatory surgery programs, the Freestanding Ambulatory Surgery Association and the Society for Office Based Surgery continue to explore all aspects of ambulatory surgical care. Anesthesia services will be needed by all three groups if they are to be successful and remain competitive.

With the development and use of short-acting anesthetic and analgesic agents, anesthesia has played a major role in the growth of ambulatory surgery. The future success of any ambulatory surgery program depends on anesthesiologist participation and the quality of anesthesia provided. To maintain a position of continued involvement and leadership, anesthesiologists must understand how we arrived where we are today and what our role will be tomorrow in managing the ambulatory surgery patient.

What are the challenges to the future growth of ambulatory surgery? What are the challenges anesthesiologists may face as this "subspecialty" of anesthesia continues to grow? *Anesthesia for Ambulatory Surgery* was written to provide anesthesiologists with the information needed to understand and meet the challenges.

Many different people helped make this book a reality; I now have the opportunity to acknowledge their help. My sincere thanks to the chapter contributors, who provided excellent material and met deadlines; the members of my department, who understood the importance of what I was doing and who allowed me the time to complete this book; Trudy K. Landwirth, M.S.L.S., and her staff at the Medical Library in The Methodist Medical Center of Illinois; Kathy Lange and Skip Smith, R.N., B.S., who not only helped, but took on added office duties to allow my secretary more time to help with the book; and Pam Blayney, my secretary, to whom I owe a special "thank you"—and so do all of you who read this book.

Bernard V. Wetchler, M.D.

Contents

Anesthesia
for
Ambulatory Surgery

1

The Future Is Now

Thomas R. O'Donovan, Ph.D.

Patrick G. O'Donovan, M.H.S.A.

Definition and Scope of Ambulatory Surgery

Health care cost containment remains a national priority. Efforts are being made to reduce duplication of medical services and temper the rate of increase in costs, while at the same time to improve the overall quality of health care delivery. Ambulatory surgery is one of the major developments in this field, and it is being used increasingly in hospitals and independently operated facilities in the United States, Canada, Europe, and Latin America. For many hospitals, it has become a significant component of their strategic plan.

Ambulatory surgery refers to formal, organized programs of elective surgery in which patients arrive and are discharged on the same day. It is performed in hospitals, hospital satellites, or independently operated, freestanding facilities. Ambulatory surgery is also referred to as *outpatient surgery, come-and-go surgery, in-and-out surgery*, and *same day surgery*.

According to the American Hospital Association (AHA),[13]

> Many types of minor surgery do not require overnight hospitalization. Therefore, hospitals must plan and provide outpatient surgical facilities so that, whenever appropriate, surgery can be performed on an outpatient basis, thereby reducing costs to the patient, the hospital, and the community, and assuring optimum use of inpatient beds.

Nonemergent, noninfected patients scheduled for elective operations are typical candidates for ambulatory surgery. The majority of these procedures are performed under general anesthesia, take less than an hour, and allow the

1

patient to go home after a 2-hour stay in the postanesthesia care unit. Ambulatory surgery procedures can also be performed under local or regional anesthesia.

Our framework for ambulatory surgery does not include minor surgical procedures that are performed in hospital emergency departments or in outpatient clinics of hospitals. We will, however, discuss the increasing role of office-based surgery.

Ambulatory surgery reduces the average total cost per patient treated at the hospital because it reduces the number of inpatient days required for treatment. Health care experts contend that over 30% of all surgery performed in the United States could be performed on an ambulatory basis and that, by 1990, 50% of all surgery performed in hospitals will be on an ambulatory basis.

Hospital administrators are concerned, however, about the loss in revenue that may result from the establishment of a comprehensive ambulatory surgery program within their institutions; hospitals rely for much of their income on inpatient occupancy, and this source of revenue would be undermined by such a program.

Nevertheless, because of the significant savings to government and private-sector health care consumers that can be realized through these programs, ambulatory surgery will continue to evolve as a cost-containment tool, thus creating a substantial impact on the public and the health care system. Ambulatory surgery is one area in which enhanced quality of care and cost savings can occur simultaneously.

Historical Development of Ambulatory Surgery

Even though ambulatory surgery was being performed successfully during the first half of this century, few cases were reported in the literature. During this time, many physicians, oral surgeons, and podiatrists performed a variety of ambulatory surgical procedures. Beginning in the early 1960s, improvements in anesthesia set the stage for a substantial increase in the amount of ambulatory surgery performed. In the early 1970s, hospital medical staffs began to support ambulatory surgery in an effort to free up beds in order to accommodate patients who were more in need of inpatient care.

The practice of ambulatory surgery was first documented in 1909 when J.H. Nicoll[19] of Glasgow informed the British Medical Association that 8988 operations on ambulatory patients had been performed at the Glasgow Royal Hospital for Sick Children. The surgical results he reported were as successful for outpatients as for inpatients.

In 1916, Ralph Waters opened the Down-Town Anesthesia Clinic in Sioux City, Iowa, for dental cases and minor surgery. Within 2 years he enlarged the facility, moving into an office building in which 50 physicians and dentists had their offices. Waters[30] said,

> As to the satisfaction of my patrons, I think I can say this: There are none who have fault to find with our work. We aim to keep an abundant supply of N_2O-O and use it freely. Many patients and some doctors object to the fees, but they come back and their friends come back. Satisfactory anesthesia and too large fees work out better than bargain sale fees and unsatisfactory anesthesia. . . . People forget

the fee, but they never forget the hurt nor fail to tell their friends about it. . . . The future for such a venture, I believe, is bright.

In 1937, Gertrude Herzfeld[12] of Edinburgh reported on more than 1000 hernia repairs performed on children; many of these were done on an ambulatory basis using general anesthesia.

In the late 1950s, a shortage of hospital beds in Canada provided the impetus for expanding outpatient surgical facilities.[31] In his book *Surgery of the Ambulatory Patient* (1966), Ferguson[9] reviewed all of the advantages and disadvantages of performing surgery on ambulatory patients and concluded that, when selections are made wisely, it is safe to operate in an outpatient environment.

In the United States, papers by Cohen and Dillon[6] in 1966 and Levy and Coakley[17] in 1968 made anesthesiologists aware that anesthesia for outpatients was becoming a viable concept. At this time, Dornette[8] presented a paper at the American Society of Anesthesiologists' meeting in which he pointed out that "a safe and efficient facility for the performance of general anesthesia and minor surgical procedures need not be affiliated either administratively or geographically with the hospital."

The Dudley Street Ambulatory Surgical Center, a freestanding facility, opened in 1968 in Providence, Rhode Island. In 1970, the Phoenix Surgicenter, described as "a facility designed to provide quality surgical care to the patient whose operation is too demanding for the doctor's office, yet not of such proportion as to require hospitalization,"[10] offered a challenge to the traditional health care system. The freestanding ambulatory surgery program had officially been launched. Ambulatory surgery was rediscovered.

Early Ambulation

The basic principles behind ambulatory surgery have been researched and reported by Ted Lahti, senior attending surgeon, William Beaumont Hospital, Royal Oak, Michigan.[16] Lahti notes that the hospitalization period required following surgery has declined steadily in the last 30 years. He further concludes that

1. If a healthy person were put to bed for a week and given narcotics periodically, it would take several weeks to recover from this experience.
2. It is now possible and desirable to discharge a large proportion of surgical patients on the first or second postoperative day.
3. Most patients entering the hospital for surgery are frightened of the unknown; when they awake from the anesthetic, their fears surface and any minor discomfort becomes real pain.
4. Medication prolongs the recovery; patients who know they will be mobile the same afternoon and home the following day are relaxed and unafraid, and require much less postoperative medication than they otherwise would need.

Infants and young children have not been conditioned to being ill after surgery and, consequently, usually are not.

When patients are hesitant to go home after surgery, Lahti takes time to explain that, because of the small but definite occurrence of postoperative complications or infections caused by being inactive in the hospital setting, the patient is much better off at home. In doing so, he is causing a shift in process. Patients' fears that something might go wrong if they go home can now be changed to the idea that something might go wrong if they stay in the hospital. Although traditions and habits are difficult to overcome, the results are certainly worth the effort. The bottom line is that if patients spend a shorter time in the hospital, health care delivery resources are used more effectively, which in turn can help stabilize escalating hospital costs.

The Pros and Cons of Ambulatory Surgery

As with most newer practices, ambulatory surgery has its distinct advantages and disadvantages. However, based on the significant upward trend in the number of ambulatory surgical procedures performed in the past 10 years, it appears that the benefits far outweigh the drawbacks.

ADVANTAGES

As previously mentioned, one of the most significant features of ambulatory surgery is reduced costs. For a given procedure, more laboratory tests are ordered and pharmacy items prescribed for inpatients than for ambulatory surgical patients. Outpatients tend to receive less medication both pre-operatively and postoperatively, than inpatients, because they are under medical supervision for a shorter period of time. There is a definite difference in the scope of medical management between inpatients and ambulatory surgical patients. The physician's time is used more efficiently; there is no need for a preoperative visit the night before surgery or for postoperative hospital visits.

Another advantage of ambulatory surgery is that it can reduce bed congestion in busy hospitals. More rooms become available for more seriously ill patients, and this will reduce or delay the need to provide additional inpatient beds in a community.

Ambulatory surgery can be described as patient care tailored to meet the needs of the "nonsick." Putting such patients in the hospital for 1 to 3 days makes them a part of the hospital's typical inpatient pattern. It separates them from the family unit, increases their susceptibility to nosocomial infections, and results in a slower return to normal activities. Furthermore, ambulatory surgery reduces the psychological stress associated with hospitalization, especially in children who have an easier and more agreeable recovery in the home.

Another advantage that can accrue from more efficient use of anesthesia and operating room services is attraction and retention of highly qualified anesthesiologists.

DISADVANTAGES

One of the alleged problems with ambulatory surgery is lack of patient and physician acceptance. In certain areas ambulatory surgery is still a relatively new practice, so it is not uncommon to hear such comments as, "My friends were always hospitalized for a D&C—why shouldn't I be?" "My hospitalization insurance policy pays for inpatient care, and I want all that is coming to me," or "It must be safer to be hospitalized because my doctor never uses the ambulatory surgery program of the hospital."

Such statements encourage physician resistance, which stems from force of habit, lack of general community acceptance, and concern about a lack of immediate availability of care should sudden complications arise. Physicians are also concerned about a potential increase in malpractice litigation, a phenomenon that depends on area practice because courts give great weight to what is considered common usage.

A physician in a community where ambulatory surgery does not routinely occur is more likely to take a conservative view of what may be considered experimentation. Reduced income is anticipated by some physicians, from loss of inpatient follow-up care.

It should be noted, however, that patients and physicians are becoming more receptive to the concept of ambulatory surgery as quality care. To illustrate, a recent survey of 100 physicians in Iowa revealed that 81 supported ambulatory surgery, 5 did not, and 14 had no opinion.

Statistics on Ambulatory Surgery

In 1980, the AHA expanded its annual survey to collect data about hospital ambulatory surgery programs; in Burns's words,[4] "data was collected from general hospitals in the United States. These statistics comprised the first and most comprehensive nationwide data on hospital ambulatory surgery programs." The results of this survey indicated that 66.4% of the hospitals in the United States provided ambulatory surgery services. For hospitals with over 100 beds, approximately 16% of all their surgery was on an ambulatory basis. In 1980 approximately 19.6 million surgical procedures took place, and 16.4% of these were performed on ambulatory surgery patients.

In 1981 the AHA published *Hospital Statistics,*[5] which provided information on the status of ambulatory surgery in the United States. "The purpose of the survey was to determine which hospitals were offering ambulatory surgery services, the volume of procedures performed, and the type of facility used. Analysts aimed to gain perspective on hospital involvement in ambulatory surgery."

All nonfederal hospitals in the 134 largest U.S. standard metropolitan statistical areas were mailed this survey. Out of a possible 2955 hospitals, 2137 responded. Among the hospitals that responded, 70% offer ambulatory surgical services, but only 54% have organized ambulatory surgery programs. The tendency is that the larger the hospital, the greater is the likelihood of a formal program in ambulatory surgery, although 43% of the hospitals having between 100 and 199 beds do have an organized ambulatory surgery program.

In 1983, 78% of all reporting hospitals in the United States provided ambulatory surgery services, and of those that are nonfederal short-term general hospitals 88% were involved in ambulatory surgical care. For hospitals with over 100 beds, ambulatory surgery has increased to 23.8%. Of the 20.8 million surgical procedures that took place in 1983, 23.9% were performed on ambulatory surgery patients.

The Orkand Study showed that in the greater Phoenix area approximately

25% of all the surgery performed is done on an ambulatory basis.[22] In individual hospitals this figure is reaching close to 50%. Historically, the level of ambulatory surgery has been increasing. It will probably continue to do so, at least within the next few years, because of all the cost pressures that have been placed on hospitals and physicians from insurance companies and the public. We believe that by 1990 approximately 50% of all surgery performed in the United States will be done on an ambulatory basis.

The bottom line is that ambulatory surgery can lower hospital costs, and hence the cost of community health care delivery, only if there is a corresponding reduction in staffing requirements. In other words, if a community hospital removes beds from use because of ambulatory surgery, and reduces its nursing and general staff at the same time, then this cost avoidance translates into a real savings. Since reduction in beds and staffing doesn't often occur, one should be very careful in trying to document how much money can be saved by performing 20% to 40% of surgical procedures on an outpatient basis. Multiplying the cost per patient day by the number of inpatient days saved is not an accurate reflection of the amount of savings in dollars.

Types of Ambulatory Surgery Centers

Ambulatory surgery occurs in a variety of settings:

Integrated
Separated
Satellite
Freestanding

The most common location is the hospital, but there are at least three different types of hospital-affiliated ambulatory surgical centers. In one often used model, the *integrated* facility, the hospital establishes a formal ambulatory surgery program by incorporating it into its existing inpatient surgical program. Construction of more operating rooms is not required, and ambulatory surgery patients use the same admitting, preoperative, and postoperative areas as do the inpatients.

The second hospital model, the *separated* facility, is a facility within the hospital or on the grounds of the hospital usually connected by a tunnel, bridge, or other structure to the hospital. It is constructed especially for ambulatory surgery.

Variations of these two hospital models include the partially integrated system, wherein at least one of the following is common for both inpatients and outpatients: preoperative holding room, operating rooms, and postoperative recovery rooms. Registration and waiting areas may be shared or discrete. At times, ambulatory surgery is performed in hospital emergency departments. Phalen notes that when ambulatory surgical services are provided within the emergency room, the same operating room that is used for minor emergency procedures is also used for minor elective procedures.[23] Continuous staff coverage and nonduplication of facilities and equipment are the key advantages of this arrangement. A disadvantage is that patients may not receive the individualized attention they may expect. Personnel are likely to shift attention from the elective D&C patient (and probably keep her waiting) to attend the unscheduled accident patient with multiple lacerations. The tense emergency room environment, along with the unpredictable activity levels and concomitant allocation of personnel resources, often results in a poorly functioning ambulatory surgery facility.

Some hospitals, such as suburban hospitals in Bethesda, Maryland, have transformed their former obstetric unit into an ambulatory surgical facility in recent years as a declining U.S. birthrate has rendered the units unnecessary.

A third hospital model, the *satellite* facility, is a separate ambulatory facility located some distance from the hospital.

The fourth setting is a nonhospital model: an independently operated, *freestanding* ambulatory surgical center. The freestanding facilities have generally been owned and managed by physicians, but we are seeing an increasing trend of ownership by profit-oriented hospital and health care corporations (American Medical International, Medical Care International).

Although in the past we became familiar with two distinct modes of ownership (affiliation with a hospital and independent operation), the future may bring changes in the ownership and operation of the different models of ambulatory surgery facilities. Independent ownership and operation, once restricted to the freestanding facility, may become the way of the separated or satellite facility. For example, a group of anesthesiologists may undertake a contract with the hospital to organize and staff the ambulatory surgery program that is presently on the grounds of the hospital. They would do separate billing and perhaps even hire all the employees used in the program.

THE HOSPITAL-INTEGRATED UNIT

ADVANTAGES
The hospital-integrated model by using existing facilities allows the hospital to embark on an ambulatory surgery program without making a large capital investment. In some cases additional personnel may be necessary, depending on how busy the unit is, but it is often possible to begin offering ambulatory services without adding nurses or admitting clerks. In this way, greater economies of scale are realized because the new subunit is incorporated into the overall system. Furthermore, the basic inpatient facilities already exist, thus eliminating construction time.

This arrangement also affords the hospital great flexibility. If the medical staff does not choose to use the ambulatory surgery program, there has been no great outlay of funds. If a brand new unit were built but not efficiently used, serious financial difficulties might occur.

Finally, the hospital integrated model allows the surgeon to perform more complex surgical procedures, which can encourage use of the ambulatory surgical program. If the pathology report on a breast biopsy indicates cancer, for example, more definite surgery can be performed immediately rather than waiting until the patient is transferred to the hospital's inpatient area.

DISADVANTAGES
The hospital is basically established for, and oriented toward, inpatient care, and problems can ensue when ambulatory surgery is superimposed on the existing inpatient system. Ambulatory patients are often looked upon as "second-class

citizens" by some hospital personnel. This can adversely affect the respect with which these patients are treated. It often starts in the admitting office, where preoccupation with inpatients results in ambulatory surgery patients having to wait a long time for registration and subsequent treatment. Outpatients scheduled for surgery may be displaced by emergency cases that require the use of the operating room. Inpatient surgery often takes precedence over ambulatory surgery. Failure to resolve these problems may prevent the unit from reaching its full potential.

Since the preoperative holding areas and postanesthesia care units are designed for inpatients, healthy outpatients, who are not under sedation, must be accommodated in the same areas as inpatients, many of whom may be seriously ill. Thus, the outpatients may be subjected to additional psychological stress.

In addition, separate private waiting rooms for families of ambulatory surgery patients may not be available in hospital-integrated facilities. Comingling the families of inpatients and outpatients can have an adverse psychological effect on families of outpatients. Furthermore, operating room personnel may be accustomed to dealing only with inpatients, and as such may not be familiar with the special needs of ambulatory surgery patients.

There may be greater potential for nosocomial infection occurring in hospital-integrated facilities than in satellite or freestanding centers.

Finally, an excessively detailed inpatient medical record is often used for the outpatient, causing additional and sometimes unnecessary recordkeeping for both nursing staff and physicians.

THE HOSPITAL-SEPARATED UNIT

The hospital-separated model is located within the hospital or adjacent to it on hospital grounds. It is a newly constructed or remodeled facility custom made for ambulatory surgery.

ADVANTAGES
The most significant benefit realized through this model is that it offsets many of the disadvantages identified in the hospital-integrated ambulatory surgery model. It is important to note, however, that good management techniques can also counteract many of the disadvantages attributed to the integrated model.

In regard to physical facilities, an area specifically established for ambulatory surgery can promote the best patient care. Scheduling is easier, and there is no competition for operating rooms: a ruptured aneurysm does not take precedence over a laparoscopy. There is a higher degree of satisfaction on the part of patients, physicians, nurses, and other personnel. If the hospital chooses to remodel rather than newly construct, care should be taken when selecting a site. In an attempt to start a program quickly, too little space may be designated for ambulatory surgery, and this may limit growth potential.

From a community standpoint, a separated facility can also attract a large share of the ambulatory surgery market, particularly if it is convenient for physicians who are not presently members of the hospital staff.

DISADVANTAGES
The basic problem with the hospital-separated model is high cost. There is also duplication of staff and equipment. Some degree of flexibility is sacrificed in this

approach because, if the unit is not successful, it is unlikely that the space can be efficiently used for other hospital purposes without additional capital investment.

THE SATELLITE

A satellite ambulatory facility is freestanding and located some distance from the hospital. It is under the direction of the hospital and is specifically designed for ambulatory surgical care. Hospitals have also opened satellite ambulatory care health facilities without the central thrust being ambulatory surgery.

ADVANTAGES
The advantages of this model are similar to those outlined in the hospital-separated model; that is, the facility is specifically designed to serve ambulatory surgical patients. Furthermore, the health care needs of a specific geographic area can be uniquely addressed. In addition, the hospital-affiliated satellite can serve as a point of departure for a possible future satellite hospital, or perhaps for the relocation of the mother facility. It can also be used as a marketing tool to refer patients to the main hospital.

DISADVANTAGES
The disadvantages of this model are also similar to those of the hospital-separated model; namely, it can be expensive and flexibility is lost. In addition, such an arrangement may increase the overall cost of comprehensive health care to the community.

THE FREESTANDING CENTER

An independently operated freestanding ambulatory surgery center (FASC) is a facility that performs ambulatory surgery but is not affiliated with any hospital. This approach to ambulatory surgery gained national attention in 1970 when two anesthesiologists, Wallace Reed and John Ford, opened their Surgicenter in Phoenix, Arizona. This was a landmark accomplishment, a true flagship of the freestanding ambulatory surgery movement, and earned the developers the Lambert Award for outstanding contributions to medical care in the United States.

From 1970 to 1975, the number of such facilities grew to 55 throughout the United States, and 7 years later over 100 were in operation. As of 1985, the number is probably close to 350. One of the major characteristics of the independent centers is that governance, management, and overall decision making are simpler than those of hospitals. Part of the reason for this is their small scale in comparison to hospitals.

Reed has indicated that screening tests are quite simple and rely on examinations and clinical judgments designed to determine whether or not the patient is ready for ambulatory surgery.[25] The screening procedure he recommends is as follows:

A registered nurse measures or checks

    Temperature
    Pulse
    Blood pressure

Hemoglobin
Urine (by reagent strip)
Bleeding and clotting time

An anesthesiologist performs

Medical history
Examination of heart
Examination of lungs

ADVANTAGES

If a community has no reasonable access to ambulatory surgery facilities or if existing outpatient facilities are insufficient, a freestanding unit can fill the void by making ambulatory surgery available in that area.

Fees are usually lower in the independent freestanding units than in hospital-affiliated centers. There is also a tendency for patients and physicians to be more satisfied because much of the bureaucratic red tape commonly associated with hospitals can be avoided. The freestanding units have capitalized on this advantage, and the results have been highly favorable.

Because the freestanding facilities are small and close knit, their administrators claim that employee morale is higher. Operators of independent facilities are noted for using a team approach. They believe that patients receive a high degree of personal attention, which often does not occur in the hospital setting.

Another advantage is that the patient's family is not subject to the hospital's rules and inconveniences when visiting (for example, limitations on visitation time and inadequate parking facilities).

The advantages described in the two previous paragraphs also apply to the hospital satellite facility.

DISADVANTAGES

One disadvantage of the freestanding facility is that there is a potential increase in net community cost, often caused by duplication of facilities. This is an important issue that needs to be researched.

There is also a greater distance from hospital emergency backup facilities (as with the hospital-affiliated satellite), although the independent operators argue that this does not threaten patient safety.

Herbert Notkin observed in Business Week that "skimming off low-risk, no-overhead surgery from hospitals will simply increase the cost of those operations that must be performed in hospitals."[2] Business Week goes on to say that same day surgery could improve, or possibly destroy, the present health care system. Independent facilities thus present a challenge to hospitals that deliver similar care.

ACCREDITATION

Reed has described the process of accreditation for independently operated FASCs.[25] These facilities formed an organization called the Society for Advancement of Freestanding Ambulatory Surgical Care (FASA) in 1974. One of their goals was to develop an accreditation procedure. Several freestanding units were accredited from 1975 to 1978. About the same time, the Accreditation Council for Ambulatory Health Care of the Joint Commission on

Accreditation of Hospitals (JCAH) was developing special standards common to a variety of organizations involved in ambulatory care. This was dissolved in 1978, and the function was taken over by a new agency called the Accreditation Association for Ambulatory Health Care (AAAHC). Founded in 1979, it has the support of the six founding members, (American College Health Association, American Group Practice Association, Group Health Association of America, Medical Group Management Association, and National Association of Community Health Centers), including the group that makes up FASA. One of the tenets of AAAHC is that surveys be performed by peers. It should be noted, however, that JCAH can also accredit FASCs that are not governed by hospitals. The JCAH operates an ambulatory health care accreditation program in addition to a hospital accreditation program. Freestanding facilities must meet the guidelines set forth in the JCAH Accreditation Manual for Ambulatory Health Care.

In 1982, there were about 100 independently operated freestanding ambulatory surgery facilities in the United States, of which 25 were approved by the AAAHC.[29] As of 1982, about half of all of the freestanding surgery centers in the United States were located in California, Texas, Illinois, and Florida, whereas the greatest concentration of hospital-based ambulatory surgery was found to be in Massachusetts and Rhode Island.

OTHER HOSPITAL COMPARISONS

FASCs may perform a more limited range of operative procedures than most hospital-integrated units, where support services are more readily available. A review of 13,433 patients treated at one freestanding ambulatory surgery center in suburban Chicago revealed that almost 50 percent of the patients were younger than 20 years and only 3 percent were over 60. Ninety-seven percent of the patients were considered in good health while only 3 percent showed evidence of serious systemic disease.[18] Freestanding centers screen their patients carefully for evidence of serious systemic disease in order to weed out potential complications from surgery as well as to reduce their exposure to professional liability. Careful screening is important for all ambulatory surgery facilities.

It is interesting to note what effect creating an FASC might have on the provision of ambulatory surgery in hospitals. "The presence of the Phoenix Surgicenter and the establishment of freestanding hospital sponsored satellites has stimulated 66.6 percent of Arizona hospitals to develop organized ambulatory surgery programs as well as compete with the freestandings on the basis of service and price."[28]

In the freestanding centers the most frequently performed procedures are those relating to gynecologic surgery. These include dilatation and curettage (D&C), pregnancy termination, and tubal ligation.

FACTORS THAT INFLUENCE THE FUTURE GROWTH
OF FREESTANDING SURGERY CENTERS

The growth of freestanding ambulatory surgery centers has generally been slow. Although growth will continue in the future, it probably will not be rapid.

> Under current federal health planning law, new health care facilities cannot be built unless a need for additional beds or service capacity can be demonstrated on the local level; in other words, the legislation favors the status quo and limits the

competitive impact of new delivery modes. As a result, health insurers, planners, and state regulatory agencies have allowed the scale to remain tipped in favor of the hospitals, thereby discouraging the development of FASC's.[29]

In recent years, hospitals have significantly expanded their ambulatory surgery activity, increasing competition for the independent entrepreneur who wishes to establish such a unit. Only a careful feasibility study would indicate those geographic areas where there is a high potential for success of an independently operated freestanding ambulatory surgery unit. There is no substitute for doing all the required homework.

It is interesting to compare the growth of freestanding ambulatory centers with emergicenters and urgent care centers. The latter two modes of health care delivery are relatively recent, having been started, like the first FASC, in the early 1970s. The growth of the urgent care centers has been quite remarkable, over 1000 being in operation as of 1985. This number will triple in the next few years, whereas the outlook for the number of independently operated FASCs is not likely to go much beyond 450 or 550 during the same time period.

Urgent care centers place heavy emphasis on marketing. Advertising seeking to persuade the health care consumer to use these facilities appears in newspapers and other media nationwide. This is not the case, generally speaking, for freestanding ambulatory surgery, in which physicians, rather than patients, make the referrals. Many surgeons, for example, have long-standing loyalties to hospitals and, because of inertia and other reasons, may continue to use the hospitals rather than the FASCs.

THE ORKAND STUDY
In 1977 the Orkand Corporation, led by Donald S. Orkand, conducted a federally contracted 3-year study that examined 11 surgical procedures (myringotomy, tonsillectomy, D&C, laparoscopy with tubal cautery, breast mass excision, ganglionectomy, inguinal herniorrhaphy, vasectomy-circumcision, augmentation mammoplasty, eye muscle repair, and excision of lipoma or sebaceous cyst).[22] A sample of 900 eligible ambulatory surgical procedures in the Phoenix area were followed, and the costs of the procedures were compared in alternate settings:

The independently operated freestanding Phoenix Surgicenter
A hospital in which an inpatient stays overnight
A hospital in which surgery is performed on an outpatient in the regular operating rooms
Hospital satellite ambulatory surgical units with their own staff and operating rooms
Physician's offices

Teams of nurses followed patients throughout their surgical stays in order to keep track of material used and labor hours expended. The fees of the independently operated freestanding ambulatory surgery facilities were compared with those of the hospital-affiliated facilities and found to be significantly lower.

In commenting on the data, Orkand points out that only part of the reason for hospital inpatient charges being so much higher than those of the independent unit was the cost of an overnight stay. He states that there tends to be a greater use of laboratory tests and ancillary services when the patient is an inpatient in the hospital than with the independent facility and concludes that if an independent facility adopted the full spectrum of testing done in hospitals, the cost differential between the two facilities would be reduced significantly.

In regard to quality of care, one of the major conclusions of the Orkand study was that the independent freestanding setting was at least as good as alternative settings. They found no surgical deaths and no major differences in patient satisfaction. Physicians ranked the independent unit highest in terms of their own satisfaction.

In evaluating the impact on the health care system, Orkand indicates that in 1967 only 8% of the surgery done in Maricopa County, where Phoenix is located, was done on an ambulatory basis. In 1977, only 7 years after the Surgicenter opened, 25% to 28% of all surgery in Maricopa County was done on an ambulatory basis. By 1985 this figure exceeded 35%.

In an editorial on the challenge of the Orkand study the following conclusion was presented:[26]

> to bring the concept of ambulatory surgery to its full national and international fruition will require the active participation of hospitals, which provide in most communities, the major proportion of surgical care. The challenge of the Orkand Study, then, is to hospitals: to leave behind the preoccupation with the so called threat from a small number of independent clinics and to get on with the job of providing a modern, streamlined, ambulatory surgery service for their patients.

The major impact of the Orkand study was to present confirmed evidence of the value of independently operated FASCs, prompting the federal government to provide a facility fee for Medicare patients.

This may make it more attractive for physicians to develop independently operated ambulatory surgery centers that will directly compete with hospitals for the future ambulatory surgery caseload.

COMPETITION BETWEEN HOSPITAL-AFFILIATED AND INDEPENDENTLY OPERATED FASCS

The proliferation of independently operated FASCs has prompted some traditionally conservative hospitals to develop their own ambulatory facilities aggressively.

Implementation of an ambulatory surgery program by the hospital, however, does not ensure immunity from the competitive effects of the freestanding centers. For one thing, hospitals are under community pressure to treat all patients with limited regard for their ability to pay, and this is not always the case among the independently operated facilities. Hospital administrators worry that the independents will woo paying patients away from them. This concern is well founded in both ambulatory surgery and minor emergency treatment markets. The problems for hospitals may be further intensified by the federal government's commitment to increased competition throughout the health care industry. Competition between and among the hospital-affiliated and independently operated facilities is particularly intense in the Des Moines, Iowa, area. In November 1983, the 246-bed Des Moines General Hospital lowered its ambulatory surgery rates 30% to compete with the outpatient rates at other area hospitals and the Surgery Center of Des Moines—Des Moines' only freestanding surgical center. Iowa Methodist Hospital followed suit by cutting prices for 42 common ambulatory surgical procedures by an average of 33%. The action prompted Mercy Hospital to develop its own outpatient package for 51 common operations.[14] Welcome to the world of competition for the health care dollar.

Experts in the field do not agree on the issue. Some believe hospitals should be an umbrella of community care, while others contend that independent competition with hospitals benefits community health care and reduces costs. Bruce Flashner, who owns several facilities called Doctors Emergency Office Centers, openly acknowledges that many hospitals will suffer and some may even be forced to close because of competition with the independents. He points out, however, that competition will create a more efficient and cost-effective health care network. "Competition," he believes, "may achieve better patient care, the ultimate goal of any health care system."[21]

Furthermore, hospitals generally charge more for similar ambulatory surgical procedures than the independently operated facilities. There is no valid reason why this should be so. In fact, a nonprofit hospital should enjoy an advantage, since the operating suites are already there, the life-saving support equipment is available, and property tax requirements in an independent facility can be eliminated. In regard to minor emergency care, Lee Hone, administrator of the Newark (Delaware) Emergency Room, a privately sponsored freestanding facility, observes that "no institution has more potential for delivering this mode of service than do hospitals. They already have the existing personnel, accounting, auditing, and management skills needed to effectively operate these types of facilities."[21]

Unfortunately, the hospital can be placed at a disadvantage by the very agencies (government and Blue Cross) that should display the most interest in encouraging the existing facilities to be competitive and in eliminating the duplication of services, since such duplication can only result in higher community health care costs. This disadvantage stems from the cost reimbursement mandated by some of the third-party payers, which requires allocation of costs for medical records, housekeeping maintenance, and so on. This allocation may be completely disproportionate to the realities of the added costs incurred, but the system often requires this allocation. The end result is that the so-called costs force hospitals to charge more for procedures than freestanding facilities. Much of this will likely change under "prospective payment."

Some third-party payers, on the other hand, cover ambulatory procedures performed under the auspices of the hospital, but not by a freestanding center. A FASC in Iowa, for example, has filed a petition in district court requesting a review of the state insurance commissioner's decision that Blue Cross of Iowa cannot provide coverage for services performed at the Surgery Center of Des Moines. In his ruling, the insurance commissioner reasoned that since state law permits Blue Cross to contract for hospital services only with hospitals, it has no right to contract with an independent facility. In its petition, the Surgery Center asked the court to expand the definition of the term "hospital" to encompass freestanding centers.

Certificate of need is another issue that both hospitals and independents have to face. In the future, proposed new construction of independently operated ambulatory surgery facilities may have increased certificate of need rejections as hospitals continue their efforts to meet community needs.

Similarly, the increase in ambulatory surgery among hospitals will come more from hospital-integrated units than from hospital satellite units because facilities in many urban centers are presently underused, resulting in relative difficulty in obtaining a certificate of need for new facility construction. Hospitals will also experience problems in obtaining capital for these kinds of facilities.

To date, the following views are held by various groups. The AHA favors the performance of ambulatory surgery in general acute hospitals as opposed to independently operated facilities. In contrast, the American Medical Association (AMA) apparently favors independently operated ambulatory surgical centers over those controlled and operated within hospitals. Although the federal government has not taken an official stand, it favors a system that will generate the lowest possible costs.

The JCAH has adopted guidelines that may soon become standards for ambulatory surgery. These guidelines state that in order to minimize duplication of services, the objectives and plans of the ambulatory surgery center should be coordinated with those of other health service providers and planning agencies in the community. The main emphasis of JCAH is on quality care, in sharp contrast to the policy advocated by the federal government and other sources that tend to emphasize cost containment.

Notwithstanding these concerns, hospitals should implement a program of ambulatory surgery if it is feasible to do so. As previously mentioned, general acute hospitals in the United States that have a surgical suite are the best candidates for such a program. The development of the program should be accompanied by an extensive marketing effort, primarily aimed at educating the physician, physician's office staff, and public about the facility. In addition to a widely publicized open house, tours for community physicians and their staff as well as physicians and nurses from area industries should be arranged.

Freestanding Birthing Centers

A new trend has been emerging in the freestanding arena. Short-stay birthing centers are cropping up in hospitals and freestanding centers. About 5% of all the births in the United States now take place in these centers, and the portion will grow to 40% by 1990, according to an excellent article[15] that features the results of an interview with John S. Short, Executive Vice President of Health Resources Corporation of America, a multihospital system based in Houston. Some of the major conclusions included in this article are as follows:

> The present number of 100 birthing centers will rise in a few years to between 300 and 400.
> By 1990, 40% of the present 3.5 million yearly births that now take place in 3600 hospital delivery rooms will be in birthing centers.
> There are many economic similarities between birthing centers and FASCs.
> Freestanding birthing centers are attractive because births in these facilities cost significantly less than in hospitals (hospital costs range from $2200

to \$5000, vs. \$1000 for birthing centers, including the obstetrician's professional fee).

A large number of health insurers, particularly Medicaid, have a strong interest in "drumming up business" for birthing centers in order to reduce costs.

Costs can be reduced in birthing centers by "eliminating unneeded tests that hospitals routinely require," Short said. "Most hospitals require fetal monitors, intravenous solution set-ups, batteries of tests upon admission and other procedures, none of which are needed."

In the literature, we have seen some questions about the increasing amount of cesarean sections that are occurring in many parts of the country. Birthing centers cut costs by closely monitoring the need for cesarean deliveries.

"A freestanding birthing center pulls in gross profits of between 25 percent and 40 percent of revenues and eventually will earn 100 percent a year on capital invested."

There are still many questions that remain, such as whether prospective mothers really accept the concept of the birthing center. Since the present level is 5%, it remains to be seen whether this number will multiply eightfold in less than 6 years. It also remains to be seen what affect birthing centers will have on the practice patterns of anesthesiologists.

Office-Based Surgery

Historically, the surgeon's office has always been a setting for "minor surgery." However, as the mid-1980s approached, surgeons performed fewer office procedures because of the following reasons:

The availability of organized ambulatory surgery programs in hospitals and freestanding surgery centers

The fear of malpractice suits

Savings on cost of equipment and related supplies

The reluctance of insurance companies to pay facility fees for procedures done in the office

As the pendulum continues its swing toward cost containment, we would expect to see more of the minor procedures, particularly those done under local anesthesia, being performed in the physician's office. In addition, reimbursement incentives are being offered to physicians if they perform surgery in an office setting.

Of importance to anesthesiologists is the number of surgical procedures being performed in offices under general anesthesia. Many surgeons would like to do more but have not been able to obtain anesthesiologists' coverage. Office-based surgery was pioneered by oral surgeons and plastic surgeons; this has now spread to other specialties, including otolaryngology, ophthalmology, gynecology, and orthopedics.

The American Association of Accreditation of Ambulatory Plastic Surgery Facilities (AAAAPSF), founded in 1980, began reviewing office practices and plastic surgeon centers in 1981. The Society for Office Based Surgery (SFOBS)

was established in 1979. It has over 200 members nationwide and is growing. The Society requires Board certification as well as verification of hospital admission privileges before membership is approved.

Table 1-1 identifies the three levels of anesthesia capability, along with equipment recommendations for each level. Note that there appears to be little difference between a freestanding ambulatory surgery center and Level 3 office-based surgery. Some authors call the distinctions arbitrary. Having surgical suites in private offices certainly requires less capital investment and avoids the "certificate of need" process as well as state licensure. There have been instances in which a group of physicians would attempt to obtain a certificate of need and, after being rejected, built an office surgery center instead.

Currently, reimbursement for a facility fee is rarely made. Blue Shield of California now allows a facility charge of approximately $200 for approved office-based procedures, and several other insurers have paid similar claims in the United States. This trend will probably increase in the near future, making Level 3 office-based surgery more attractive. According to Trainer et al, "Blue Cross/Blue Shield of Arizona developed a different approach and now grants a bonus to surgeons using office based facilities. The Arizona plan has identified 17 procedures that can be performed safely in an office setting and is paying 25 percent above usual and customary surgical fees."[29] There is also an experimental program, started in early 1984 at Ford Motor Company and Chrysler Corporation, which will motivate physicians to perform ambulatory

□ **Table 1-1 Equipment Recommendations for Office-Based Suites**

Anesthesia Capability	Examples of Appropriate Operations	Equipment Needed	Room Size	Probable Costs
Level 1: local anesthesia with light sedation	Myringotomy with tubes (adult) D&C Bartholin cyst Small biopsy	Crash cart IV stand Ambu-Bag Airway tube O₂ tank with valve Suction machine Appropriate light	7'–10' × 10'–14'	$2,000–$10,000
Level 2: local anesthesia with heavy sedation	Septoplasty Cosmetic surgery Minilap tubal Breast biopsy Open laparoscopy	Add: Operating table Cardiac monitor Defibrillator Bovie unit	10'–12' × 12'–20'	$15,000–$35,000
Level 3: general anesthesia (same as Freestanding Surgical Center)	Hernia repair Hemorrhoids Closed laparoscopy Vaginal tubal Myringotomy with tubes (pediatrics)	Add: Anesthesia machine Autoclave	12'–15' × 15'–20'	$35,000–$50,000 or more

(Based on Society for Office Based Surgery: Same Day Surg 7(4):43, April 1983)

surgery in their own offices by offering them 125% of their fee. The same procedure performed in the hospital would result in a 75% payment (unless medical indications warrant).

William Porterfield and Lewis Franklin are strong advocates of Level 3 office-based surgery. "Our experiences constitute 16 years of office outpatient surgery procedures. Over this time we have performed 13,000 procedures under local anesthesia with or without sedation and 5,038 procedures under general anesthesia. There is a significant cost saving in these outpatient procedures."[24] They state that

> if general anesthesia is to be used in an outpatient [office] facility, the services of a trained, competent and compassionate anesthesiologist should be enlisted. This person must be delegated the responsibility for final selection of patients, including a veto power over the surgeons' selection. Only in this manner can a safe and effective environment exist for the benefit of the patients.

Their conclusion is that

> the availability of general anesthesia for surgery in the office facility offers the following advantages:
>   1. Patient satisfaction
>   2. Broadens the scope of procedures to be performed in the office facility
>   3. Provides cost savings to the patient or insurance carrier
>   4. Provides convenience to the surgeon
> The disadvantages are:
>   1. Increased start up cost of the office facility
>   2. Increased responsibility of the surgeon and the office staff.[22]

As the surgical caseload moves from inpatient facilities to outpatient facilities to physicians' offices, anesthesia practice patterns may have to change in order for the anesthesiologist to maintain a share of the available caseload. Before providing anesthesia coverage in an office-based surgical procedure, the prudent anesthesiologist should check the equipment provided, its preventive maintenance program, and whether the office has been accredited to perform surgery.

Short-Stay Surgery

There is an emerging trend that may intensify in the months and years ahead. The success of ambulatory surgery in providing safe, cost-effective care to satisfied patients and their physicians is prompting hospitals to explore variations of the ambulatory model. As hospitals provide increased services to patients and better serve the needs of physicians and all other components of the health care system, their efforts will be directed toward:

Limiting hospital stay
Lowering hospital charges
Expanding self-care areas
Increasing consumer satisfaction

Attempts to shorten length of inpatient stay derive their impetus from presurgery testing and screening procedures developed by ambulatory surgery facilities. Traditionally, elective surgical inpatients are hospitalized the day before scheduled surgery. By using presurgery screening programs, one night of hospitalization can be eliminated, generating enormous cost savings to the health care system. We are currently seeing short-stay patients admitted on the evening before their procedure and discharged following surgery, or admitted on the morning of surgery and discharged the following day. In addition, more healthy elective inpatients are admitted on the morning of their procedures, undergo their procedures (cholecystectomy, hysterectomy), and then remain in the hospital for however many days are needed for appropriate recovery.

In 1982, the American Society of Anesthesiologists passed a resolution supporting the concept of same-day admission of elective surgical patients whenever appropriate in terms of cost containment and provided quality of patient care is maintained. As these changes surface, anesthesiologists must be certain appropriate preanesthesia interviews continue to be conducted in advance of surgery. Patterns of practice are changing, and anesthesiologists must be involved with fellow physicians and hospital administrators to effect changes that do not affect the quality of care provided. An example of such an application has taken place at St. Joseph's hospital in Tucson, Arizona, where the ambulatory surgery department is handling morning admissions, not only for its own patients, but also for selected inpatient cases scheduled for surgery that day. The hospital calls its program "A.M. Admit."[27]

As a result of contraction of health care services nationwide, hospitals have empty beds. Use of operating rooms has decreased. Space is becoming available, and with this availability of space has come the creation of self-care units. In these units, nurse staffing would be minimal or even unnecessary if adequate patient surveillance could be provided.

Patients who live a great distance from the hospital could be better served by coming in the night before ambulatory surgery and staying in a self-care unit. Distance from the hospital might no longer influence a patient's acceptability into an ambulatory surgery program. Depending on the decision of the anesthesiologist or the attending surgeon, the patient could either be discharged on the day of surgery or stay in the self-care unit and be discharged the following day. Costs for the use of a self-care unit would be far less than the charges for overnight hospitalization. According to Ellen Barron,

> A seven room self-care suite pilot program was started in 1983 at The Methodist Medical Center of Illinois, Peoria, Illinois. This has now been expanded to a twelve room unit that the Medical Center calls the Hospitality Inn and that serves patients for ambulatory surgery, presurgery testing, radiation oncology, and families of hospitalized patients who reside a distance from the hospital and wish to stay over night. Costs are covered by voluntary contributions from either the patient or family members.*

Such a unit should generally be as close as possible to the ambulatory surgery area and should have access to cafeteria facilities. If we go back 10 or 20 years, there was often mention of the advantages of having motel-like services available either in the hospital or, for patients who didn't need full nursing care before or after certain periods of hospitalization, near the hospital. Partly because the need was not clearly identified, and partly because third-party

*Barron EV: Personal communication, 1984

payers were not farsighted enough to see the potential cost savings, this concept never gained acceptance.

Hospitals need to be creative. By providing additional services that can attract a larger number of ambulatory surgery patients, the hospital's financial position can be improved. This same self-care unit can serve other areas of the hospital in addition to ambulatory surgery (presurgery testing, transfusion, or chemotherapy treatment). Administrative questions that need answering are: What is the start up cost? What are the legal implications? What are staffing needs? What should the charges be?

We are not advocating hospital self-care units, but it is one option to be considered in seeking ways to better serve our patients.

We will now briefly describe an example of how one hospital developed an 18-bed short-stay medical-surgical unit. This is a state funded and authorized alternative-care experiment involving a hospital that expanded its same day surgery unit to serve overnight medical and surgical patients as well. The program was developed in 1979 by Freehold (New Jersey) Area Hospital and was first described in the literature in 1981.[7]

The hospital's present program of ambulatory surgery was expanded from a 12-stretcher unit to accommodate 18 patients overnight. There were two sections. One was staffed 12 hours per day, the other had 24-hour staffing and provided care for a wide variety of medical-surgical patients who had to be held overnight. Many administrators may feel that this defeats the purpose of ambulatory surgery, but we hasten to say that this is one more way to serve surgical patients.

One of the major effects of this experiment was to reduce the average length of hospital stay from 3 or 4 days to 1 or 2 days. It is also interesting to note that this experiment took place in New Jersey while a new reimbursement program—diagnosis-related group (DRG) program—was being established there. This program paid hospitals on the basis of resources needed to treat specific diagnoses rather than on the basis of how many days patients were hospitalized. Note that the federal government now pays hospitals for all Medicare inpatient hospitalization on this basis.

The operation of the unit was governed by strict protocol under agreement with the New Jersey Department of Health: "the new unit attempts to provide essential care on the first day; to discharge the patient within 24 hours, when possible; and to allow further testing and follow up to be accomplished on an outpatient basis."[7]

The results for 1979 showed that there were 1471 ambulatory surgery patients cared for in the facility; the number of overnight surgical patients cared for was 464; and the overnight medical patients cared for was 726. Of the 1190 patients that were held overnight, 65% were discharged within 24 hours, and the remainder required a transfer to regular inpatient facilities because further treatment was necessary, their conditions changed, or complications arose. In most other hospitals in the United States, we would never see such a high percentage of patients admitted to the inpatient facility from the hospital's ambulatory surgery unit. This shows that the program at Freehold Area Hospital is unique and indicates that a broader range of patients are selected for admission, which may not be the case in most other hospitals.

The article concludes that "public policy aimed at limiting hospitals growth and containing health care costs is currently being invoked. Nonetheless, patient demand for health services inevitably will grow. Creative alternatives must be found to help institutions relieve overcrowding, and short stay medical-surgical units may become increasingly important as such an alternative."[7] We should note, however, that "overcrowding" is not common among our nation's institutions in the 1980s, but perhaps examples such as those described herein may warrant further looking into.

Reasons for Hospital Involvement in Ambulatory Surgery

Several factors motivate hospitals to establish or expand available ambulatory services. The changing demand for health services is shifting preferences toward substitute ambulatory care and away from inpatient care. An additional factor that contributes to the trend toward ambulatory care is competition.

Demand for health care refers to the willingness and the ability of consumers to purchase health services. This should be distinguished from need. *Need* is based on clinical determination and cannot necessarily be equated with the patient's ability and willingness to pay for services. Factors that increase demand for ambulatory services include the expansion of coverage by insurance companies and other third-party payers, particularly Blue Cross.[5] They are beginning to require that specified procedures be performed on an ambulatory surgery basis if they are to pay fees. The Blue Cross State of Illinois Employee Insurance Program, for example, has issued a list of surgical procedures for which no benefits will be provided when performed on an inpatient basis, except in certain isolated incidences. Other Blue Cross plans are following suit.

With the increased rates of state Medicaid programs, selected states are formulating lists of surgical procedures that must be performed on an ambulatory basis in order to be reimbursed by Medicaid.

According to Linda Burns, former director of the Division of Ambulatory Care for the American Hospital Association, "ambulatory care benefits have expanded through the development of health maintenance organizations and selected private insurance plans. For example, from 1970 to 1976, the proportion of the population under age 65 with insurance coverage for physicians' office and home visits grew from 35.2 percent to 62.2 percent."[5]

Employers will also support ambulatory surgery because it will lower the health care premiums they are required to pay for their employees. In addition, employees are able to return to work sooner than if they had been hospitalized.[32]

Medicare's new prospective payment system should also stimulate growth of ambulatory surgery. Under this system, patient diagnoses are divided into some 487 DRGs. The hospital receives a fixed price for each DRG treated. Although the impact of DRGs will be indirect, it should result in a higher volume of ambulatory patients. According to Daniel J. Sullivan, of Amherst Associates, a medical consulting firm,[1]

> The current Medicare prospective payment system will only be applied to inpatient stays, not to outpatient services. You will still have 100 percent cost reimbursement for outpatient services; so to the extent that you can move your costs out of inpatient to outpatient, you can get more money back from the government. One

of the reasons why many hospitals around the country are looking at ambulatory surgery programs is because the inpatient environment is getting so heavily regulated and so constrained by reimbursement.

However, it should be noted that the federal government is currently investigating methods by which outpatient care can be included in the DRG scenario. One such case-mix methodology is called the ambulatory visit group (AVG).[11] Such a system would benefit the freestanding ambulatory surgery centers because their price is often lower than hospital-affiliated facilities.

When considering the development of a formal ambulatory surgery program, hospital boards, administrators, and other health care leaders encounter an interesting dilemma. Ambulatory surgery reduces the number of inpatient beds used. This will reduce revenue for the hospital unless there is a large patient waiting list for admission or unless the number of ambulatory surgical procedures performed can offset the effects of reduced inpatient occupancy. Why, then, should a hospital embark upon a program that very likely will reduce its inpatient occupancy and quite possibly its revenue?

Hospital administrators with a strong philosophic commitment to patient needs can be seen throughout the United States. This is reflected not only in the great increases in ambulatory surgery programs, but also in many other attempts to provide cost-effective quality health care. In other words, these administrators are facing their responsibility, meeting the challenge, and successfully reaching their objectives. Hospitals must also compete with the freestanding movement and office-based surgery, as well as respond to pressures by third-party payers, industry, government, and patients. These are the challenges of the 1980s.

Ambulatory Surgery Facility Design

In order for an ambulatory surgical center to be successful, it is essential that it be designed and laid out properly.

The design must reflect a detailed knowledge of the way the unit functions. Flexibility is important to permit variations in surgical practice. Most importantly, it must allow the staff to maintain a level of care that equals or surpasses that available to inpatients. Medical staff involvement throughout the planning process is crucial for success. Facility planning will be covered in great detail in Chapter 10.

Size of the unit is measured in terms of number of operating theaters. Besides the initial construction costs and restrictions imposed by available space, there are other major factors that influence size—patient population, medical attitudes, and economic pressures.

PATIENT POPULATION

The number of patients who require minor or intermediate elective surgery is directly proportional to the size and demographic characteristics of the population in the hospital service area. An average figure is approximately 550 patients per year for every 10,000 population. For surgical, anesthetic, or social reasons, up to 10% of these patients will be treated on an inpatient basis, leaving about 500 ambulatory surgery candidates yearly.[3] For the hospital, its planning department can be helpful in identifying the relevant ambulatory surgical market.

MEDICAL ATTITUDES

The number of patients who are obviously inappropriate for ambulatory surgery notwithstanding, the percentage of the remaining patients actually selected for outpatient treatment depends in part on the surgeons' ability and enthusiasm. The overall movement away from traditional practices of requiring patients to remain in the hospital routinely after an operation and toward earlier postoperative ambulation has resulted in a more rational management of patients undergoing minor and intermediate surgery. As surgeons gain experience in ambulatory surgery, they are becoming more ambitious in the types of procedures they are prepared to perform on an outpatient basis (including, but certainly not limited to, menisectomy, cholecystectomy cervical sympathectomy, and many extensive plastic surgical procedures). In a like manner, the anesthesiologist can eliminate the need to manage some patients on an inpatient basis by using special techniques designed to relieve significant postoperative pain (for example, supplement inhalation anesthesia with regional block.)

ECONOMIC PRESSURES

Despite the inherent medical, psychological, social, and other benefits associated with ambulatory surgery, the major impetus behind its development has been economic. As health care costs continue to rise, ambulatory surgery is likely to become the only affordable method of providing surgical treatment of minor and intermediate conditions. Therefore, since the size and number of ambulatory units is likely to expand significantly in the future, such units should be designed to accommodate a future increase in workload or be flexible enough to allow for expansion as required.

Illustrations of Ambulatory Surgery Programs

PRESBYTERIAN HOSPITAL, DALLAS

Presbyterian Hospital of Dallas has raised the quality of care, reduced the duplication of services, and lowered costs through their ambulatory surgery program. Because of the high occupancy rate in their existing inpatient facility, a seven-bed trial ambulatory surgery unit was built in a 1200-square-foot area in the lower level of the hospital. It was about 75 feet from the entrance to the main operating room and recovery area, suitable for transporting patients and close to backup emergency services. Policies and procedures were developed governing patient flow and delineating the roles of all departments involved.

The program is directed by the hospital administration and the nursing service, with medical direction coming from the staff operating room committee. Patients are admitted in the morning, have the required surgical procedures, and return home that afternoon.

Because of the overwhelming success of the pilot seven-bed unit, a 20-bed unit was subsequently opened 3 years later. Each double room in the unit is equipped with air, oxygen, vacuum, television, a nurse-call system, and a toilet facility. The unit also has a consultation room for the completion of preadmission work, a small specimen collection area, a small pantry area for convenient meals, a large nurses' station, and a family waiting room.

The total number of surgical procedures performed each year at Presbyterian Hospital has steadily increased. Before the ambulatory surgery unit opened, however, there were long waiting periods for elective surgery; patients scheduled for ENT, dental, or plastic surgery had to wait 2 to 3 weeks, and gynecologic patients had to wait nearly 5 weeks.

Increasing the number of operating rooms from nine to 17 reduced the waiting period and redistributed all types of cases; it even brought back some surgeons who had been taking their patients to hospitals with shorter waiting periods. At the same time, physicians at Presbyterian Hospital became convinced that operations that routinely kept patients in the hospital for 2 to 3 days could now be done in 1 day with more convenience and patient satisfaction.

VIRGINIA MASON HOSPITAL, SEATTLE

Virginia Mason Hospital is a 300-bed general surgical hospital located in the middle of metropolitan Seattle. Among other operations, open heart surgery, major neurosurgical procedures, and organ transplants are performed there. It is directly adjacent to a large multispecialty clinic of about 100 physicians.

The reason for establishing an ambulatory surgery unit in the hospital was a shortage of hospital beds. The community health planning agency would not permit additional beds to be added because other nearby hospitals were not routinely filled. Physicians were waiting 2 to 3 weeks to schedule elective procedures, but the operating room suite was operating at only 50% of capacity. The establishment of ambulatory surgery was the obvious answer to the problem.

The key elements for a functioning ambulatory surgery unit include an admitting area with a receptionist; a laboratory; an interview, scheduling, and examination area; a waiting room for both patients and family or friends accompanying them; a dressing area; an operating area; and a postanesthesia care unit. All of these areas, although widely dispersed, were generally available in the hospital. Hence, the short-stay surgical services of the Virginia Mason Hospital commenced as a hospital-integrated unit. The reception and interview areas were in vacant emergency room space on the first floor south; the admitting area was housed on the first floor center (in the hospital regular admission area); waiting and additional interview areas were located in the hospital's main entrance waiting room on the first floor center; the laboratory was on the second floor of the west wing; and the operating room and postanesthesia care unit were on the second floor of the east wing. An additional receptionist and advance scheduling area were located on the seventh floor of the adjacent clinic building. There were often delays in the operating room schedule; patients and physicians were inconvenienced; laboratory workup and operating room charges were the same. For the program to be successful, changes had to be made not only in the physical plant but in the areas of patient and physician satisfaction and costs.

The hospital encouraged the implementation of a "package charge" for the most commonly performed operations, such as D&Cs and cystoscopies. This was based on a relevant laboratory workup determined by the surgeon and the anesthesiologist, and a man-minute charge for surgery based on the personnel, equipment, and operating room time required. In order to reduce delays in the surgery schedule, written instruction sheets, informational brochures, and a specially designed reception area were developed.

Soon, use of the surgical suite increased to more than 80% and the postanesthesia care unit was too small to handle the additional surgical volume. More recovery space and another operating room were needed. In planning and designing the construction for this additional space, the amount of surgery was taken into consideration, and the newly constructed facilities were coordinated to serve the ambulatory surgery patients in a more personal and expeditious manner. The new area was comparable to a freestanding ambulatory surgery unit in its convenience to patients and physicians.

The new facilities were constructed immediately adjacent to the existing operating suite and postanesthesia care unit. It offered flexibility of use of vacant operating rooms and the contiguous postanesthesia care area. In addition, personnel who are not used in one unit can be used in the other unit if the surgical volume of either is increased. The plan allows either area to contract or expand depending on the inpatient or the ambulatory surgery volume. If new operations or federal cost standards should change the ratio of inpatients to ambulatory surgery patients, the necessary redistribution of resources could easily be managed without the construction of new facilities.

The result of 6 years' experience with a hospital-integrated ambulatory surgery unit indicates it can provide facilities for the surgical outpatient as conveniently and efficiently as a specialized freestanding or hospital satellite unit can, without the additional cost resulting from duplicate construction costs for facilities or personnel. This assumes, however, that the hospital realizes that ambulatory surgery is a special service that requires individualization of admitting procedures; proper laboratory requirements; conveniently located waiting room, interview, and dressing facilities; special operating room handling; and special charges for all of these procedures. Personnel working in these areas as well as the postanesthesia care unit must be specially trained to be sensitive to the special needs of ambulatory surgery patients. Success or failure of an ambulatory surgery unit can be more a function of dedication and interest on the part of personnel than on the actual type of unit.

MT. CARMEL MERCY HOSPITAL, DETROIT

At Mt. Carmel Mercy Hospital in Detroit, ambulatory surgery was first initiated in an investigative way and quickly gained full-fledged acceptance. As more and more physicians used the program and its facilities in the new north tower surgical suite, it became apparent how the patient, the physician, and the hospital benefited. The hospital gained by freeing more beds for the care of acutely ill patients, and the physician benefited by being able to schedule more time for the more seriously ill.

When Mt. Carmel first began an ambulatory surgery program in 1974, 117 patients were scheduled for this 1-day procedure. In the following year, that number increased to 1246 patients, and to over 4000 during 1983.

Much of the remainder of this illustration is taken from an interview with Willard S. Holt, Chairman of Mt. Carmel's Ambulatory Surgery Department:

> At Mt. Carmel, we haven't jumped right in. We have taken time to know what we want and how to go about it. We are now averaging 25 ambulatory surgeries a day, and I feel we should be doing twice that. There are institutions that are doing more, although many of them are doing procedures that we as a Catholic hospital would not do. But we are fortunate to have an administration and a chief of surgery who believe in the value of this kind of service, believe in exploring all dimensions of the best way for us, and have cooperated completely as we have been feeling our way.[20]

As Holt explains, beginning an ambulatory surgery program is not just as simple as deciding, "We're going to have one. Let's get started." Many other issues are involved—changing laboratory procedures, streamlining the admitting process, educating the medical staff to the benefits of the service, educating patients to the concept, learning to carefully identify appropriate candidates for this type of surgery.

A good ambulatory surgery program must be carefully planned and efficiently structured to pull other affected departments into the total process of getting the patient in and out in one day, while rendering to that patient the same quality care he or she would receive as an inpatient.

All hospitals, and most patients, are aware of the high cost of health care today. Newspaper articles, television commentators, and magazines all cover it. A comparison of costs of ambulatory surgery with those of a 2- or 3-day hospital stay—a dollar and cent view—is one way to convey the benefits to all concerned.

> A housewife with a family, for instance, can be back home in the same afternoon after a procedure such as a breast biopsy. She doesn't have to find a babysitter to care for the children, at least not for more than a few hours. Nor does her husband have to take more than a day off from work—and not even that if she is accompanied to the hospital by another family member. She's back in her own home, in her own bed, and the psychological boon to quick recovery is much greater than if she were separated from her family and worrying about them.
>
> At the hospital a bed is reserved and available for a more acutely ill patient, one who might be on our medically urgent admitting list who is waiting for that bed.
>
> And it has one very important advantage. Ambulatory surgery certainly cuts down apprehension for the patient. They don't have time to be too afraid. The very fact that they come and go in a day is a tension-reliever. It is unfortunate, but so many patients get so much bad information about surgery. A short stay minimizes fear.
>
> As an added benefit, we hope this type of program will bring down insurance premiums, for the patient and for the hospital.

Setting Up an Ambulatory Surgery Program

How does a hospital go about establishing a sound program of ambulatory surgery? The answer is, "very carefully." We examined this issue in a number of hospitals that had already established a successful ambulatory surgery program. In virtually every case, a medical committee of some kind had been formed in order to launch the project. Initial support must come from the hospital administration, the board of trustees, or the medical staff, although the motivation can come from more than one source. The hospital administrator must ensure that the process is properly managed and that input is obtained from all key areas (anesthesiologists, surgeons, nurses, etc.).

A committee charged with examining the implications of ambulatory surgery with a possible view to establishing a program must have medical staff representation (particularly anesthesiology, general surgery, orthopedic surgery, otolaryngolic surgery, plastic surgery, and gynecologic surgery—the physicians who are going to use the facility). Many other surgical specialities will eventually be interested in the program, but their membership on the original committee, though valuable, is not necessary. Other representation should include administration, nursing, and the controller's office.

In some hospitals, one of the early questions is whether a formal ambulatory surgery program should be created. At other hospitals, that objective is assumed, and the question is what steps should be taken to create such a program. Every effort should be made to avoid having the issue become a political concern within the medical staff. Hospitals have enough political problems without deliberately creating additional ones. Ambulatory surgery should be a perfect example of a "safe" issue that can generate cooperation among the medical staff, administration, and nursing staff.

Does the size of the hospital (number of beds) enter into decision making? Does it determine whether the hospital has need for a formal ambulatory surgery program in addition to its regular surgery program for inpatients? Probably not. All hospitals with an active surgery program whose schedule includes operations that can be done on an outpatient basis should make a formal ambulatory surgery program available to the surgeons and the potential patients in the community.

Before the program becomes a reality, the optimum level of ambulatory surgery that could be performed should be determined. This is essential for projecting space requirements. By retrospectively reviewing the operating room schedule for a number of months and comparing each surgical procedure with the patient's admission profile, the hospital's potential ambulatory caseload can be determined with reasonable accuracy.[33] Information to be obtained includes the patient's age, the distance he or she lives from the hospital, procedures already performed on an ambulatory basis, and procedures with the potential to be done on an ambulatory basis. In a retrospective review, the patient's physical status may be unobtainable. Information about the patient's willingness to have the procedure performed on an outpatient basis and whether there is responsible home care available is impossible to obtain. There is a difference between a 25-year-old healthy woman and a 93-year-old with uterine bleeding, each undergoing a D&C. The results of the survey will provide a solid general estimate for committee review.

There is a health systems agency (HSA) in the Midwest with a technical advisory committee that examines how area hospitals establish their criteria for ambulatory surgery. During one of their meetings, the HSA presented a surgery "use rate" for the area, which would help determine, in part, how much ambulatory surgery should be performed. The physician members became quite upset that surgery "use rates" were being imposed on the community by the HSA.

The HSA's rationale was interesting. If we know what the total amount of surgery should be, and if we assume that 30% of it should be done on an ambulatory basis, then we can project the total of the ambulatory surgery caseload. Calculations were not projected from the actual surgical activity at any one hospital. HSAs all over the United States have been looking at ambulatory surgery criteria for some years now, and will continue to track trends. An HSA projection can provide information, but each hospital should determine an institution-specific number derived from an internal surgical assessment.

The assessment can be carried one step further. The medical records department should obtain comparable surgical assessment records from as many other area hospitals as possible. It will be useful to see the different procedures performed at each hospital and what percentage of these procedures are done on an ambulatory surgery basis. Data obtained will depend on the type of hospital (community, pediatric, tertiary care). At a hospital in Miami Beach, Florida, that has a large percentage of Medicare patients, the percentage of ambulatory surgery will be rightfully lower than that at a typical hospital in Peoria, Illinois. The local situation must be taken into consideration.

Once the decision is made to establish a formal ambulatory surgery program, other major issues need to be resolved. A subcommittee can be formed to handle the details of location, construction, and finance (for example, whether a given program is a separate custom-made unit or uses the existing inpatient system). Physicians should concentrate on the professional aspects; without their support, the program will stagnate. Anesthesia is also a key issue; many programs have been ineffective because of an insufficient number of anesthesiologists or a lack of interest by the anesthesiologists. That should no longer be the case. If projections hold true that 50% of surgery will soon be performed on an ambulatory surgical basis, then anesthesiologists should lead, not follow, in developing a formal program at their hospital or in their community.

Even after a hospital has established a solid program of ambulatory surgery, there will still be occasions when certain staff members refuse to accept it. A case in point: an anesthesiologist involved in the direction of an active ambulatory surgery program in a large hospital was very pleased one day when a prestigious surgeon admitted an adult to the program for a hernia operation. This surgeon had never before used the ambulatory surgery program of the hospital. A few weeks later, these two physicians were discussing the case in the hallway, and the surgeon who had handled the case mentioned that he never realized what an excellent approach to medical care this was until he had actually experienced it first hand. The anesthesiologist was elated because he knew that other "slow movers" would follow this surgeon's example. In effect, the surgeon would act as a catalyst and stimulate other surgeons to use the unit.

It is also important to realize that no particular group, (anesthesiologists, physicians, nurses, etc.) is the most important in the development or maintenance of an ambulatory program. In this chapter emphasis has been given to the role of the physician because the active participation of surgeons and anesthesiologists is an essential ingredient to any successful facility. In fact, ambulatory surgery centers might also be looked upon as "ambulatory anesthesia centers" because the key to an effective come-and-go surgery facility is the availability of anesthesiologists and the quality of anesthesia they provide.

It is a definite plus for the facility when anesthesia coverage is available throughout the day.

Itemization of Charges vs. a Single Price Structure

One of the important early decisions to be made is whether the health care facility should establish a single price for each procedure on the patient's bill.

Although hospitals generally cannot charge different amounts for the same tests or procedures for different patients (because of Blue Cross and Medicare regulations), certain justified modifications can be made. For example, if a hospital charges $200 for the first hour of surgery for a typical inpatient procedure, it may establish a price of $100 for an ambulatory procedure because it can be shown that most ambulatory procedures are shorter than many inpatient procedures and require fewer instruments and personnel. We need to determine whether or not it is justifiable to charge a different price for similar inpatient and outpatient procedures. If a D&C, for example, is surgically the same for the inpatient as it is for the ambulatory patient, can two different prices for the operation be justified?

Use of itemization or a single price structure tends to vary among hospital-affiliated and independently operated freestanding facilities. To compare hospital bills from two locales, one must know what the local practice is. If certain required procedures and tests are performed on all patients in one locale and on no patients in another, there is no basis for comparison. In certain institutions, for example, it is common practice for ambulatory patients to receive a preoperative chest radiograph and an electrocardiograph; in others, only a hemoglobin and hematocrit are required.

The independently operated freestanding units tend to charge a single fee for each ambulatory surgery procedure, rather than itemizing all services rendered. This practice varies widely among hospitals. There is no way to identify the best system. Some hospitals defend itemizing each service, and others defend the single blanket charge for the complete procedure. The objective is to have the *price match the service performed*, so that patients are treated individually. Accounting departments in many hospitals must itemize because third-party payers require a complete list of charges. Every possibility should be explored in order to simplify billing procedures.

Hospitals are aware of allegations that they overprice certain services and procedures in order to help underwrite the cost incurred for other procedures. This practice is known as cross subsidization or cost shifting. For example, a common public statement is that hospitals charge too much for ambulatory surgery in order to cover the cost of highly sophisticated inpatient procedures.

It is recommended that hospitals charge for each service separately. If a patient has had an ambulatory surgery procedure performed, he or she should receive either an itemized bill showing individual charges for each item or, alternatively, a single blanket price for the particular procedure that would be an accurate reflection of itemized costs. Itemizing charges for both surgery and anesthesia supplies requires significant cost analysis, both in establishing the original charge and in maintaining an up-to-date profile. An argument often advanced in favor of blanket billings for ambulatory surgery procedures is that these procedures are quite simple and frequently do not require radiography, central supply charges, or unusual pharmacy charges. Both hospital-affiliated and freestanding centers should address the issue of charges for services rendered. What has been the common practice in the past should not be the only influencing factor in what can be done to simplify billing procedures for the future.

New Medicare reimbursement regulations under the Tax Equity and Fiscal Responsibility Act of 1982 (TEFRA) will soon have major fiscal effects on hospitals. We predict that within 1 to 2 years Medicare will mandate which operative procedures must be performed on an ambulatory surgery basis. Although exceptions will be allowed with physician justification, the net effect will be to drive up the national current rate of ambulatory surgeries as a percentage of total surgery within 5 years from 24% to nearly 50%. Pressures for the increase will also come from Blue Cross/Blue Shield, commercial insurance companies, preferred provider organizations (PPOs), HMOs, and business coalitions.

Directions for the Future

There have been few major research studies on the subject of ambulatory surgery in hospitals in the United States reported in the literature. One reason for this may be that it has only been in recent years that we have seen a significant level of attention being given to ambulatory surgery by hospital administrators and physicians. There has been an increase in the number of formal programs of ambulatory surgery in hospitals, primarily because of developments in anesthesia that promote greater patient safety, earlier discharge of patients, and the motivation of hospital administrators and physicians to free up beds that were in short supply a few years ago.

However, times are changing and beds are no longer in short supply; in fact, there is an excess supply in many urban areas. Trends in utilization review, professional standards review organizations, HMOs, PPOs, and other social forces are freeing up our nation's hospital beds, especially in urban areas.

Many hospitals have seen a decline in surgery as T&As are performed with much less frequency. Operating rooms that used to be fully scheduled now have schedule times available.

There is some evidence that over 30% of all surgical procedures performed in most hospitals can be done on an ambulatory basis. Communities with hospitals that operate at a level less than this have an obligation to examine their situation. Hospitals being faced now with new payment systems will use existing health care resources to the optimum capacity. There is the ever-present possibility of independent freestanding ambulatory surgery facilities coming forth to fill needs that may be found. The freestanding organization can provide a good deal of competition for hospitals, especially in urban centers. A void will be created if hospitals do not begin to serve the reasonable and proper level of needs of patients for ambulatory surgery. There is no question that this void may be filled in the years ahead by independently operated surgical centers.

Statistical studies must continually assess the extent of ambulatory surgery performed in the United States. Regional data should be generated comparing the number and types of ambulatory procedures performed in hospital-affiliated programs, FASCs, and office-based surgery programs. Only by evaluating past and present trends can we make reasonably accurate projections for the future.

References

1. Ambulatory surgery units will increase volume with DRGs. Same Day Surg, p 77, July 1983
2. An answer to soaring hospital costs. Business Week; p 62, July 7, 1976
3. Burn J: Facility design for outpatient surgery and anesthesia. In Woo SW (ed): Ambulatory Anesthesia Care, pp 135-151. Boston, Little, Brown, & Co, 1982
4. Burns LA: Ambulatory Surgery, pp 4-9. Rockville, Maryland, Aspen Systems Corporation, 1984
5. Burns LA: Ambulatory surgery growing at a rapid pace. AORN J 35(2):263, February 1982
6. Cohen D, Dillon JB: Anesthesia for outpatient surgery. JAMA 196:1114, 1966
7. DeCerse J, Reiss JB: Shortstay unit serves overnight medical and surgical patients. Hospitals, pp 140-143, September 16, 1981
8. Dornette W: Planning Tomorrow's Hospital Today. Presented at the American Society of Anesthesiologists' meeting, Washington, DC, 1968
9. Ferguson LK: Surgery of the Ambulatory Patient. Philadelphia, JB Lippincott, 1966
10. Ford JL, Reed WA: The surgicenter—an innovation in the delivery and cost of medical care. Ariz Med 26:801, 1969
11. Freestanding centers, clinics could benefit in case mix reimbursement. Same Day Surg 7(10):121, October 1983
12. Herzfeld G: Clinical recollections and reflections: Abdominal surgery in infancy and childhood. Edinburgh Med J 2:753, 1909
13. Hospitals. JAHA, p 132, August 1, 1973
14. Iowa hospitals compete fiercely for Des Moines area Patients. Hosp Week 20(17):3 April 1984
15. Johnson DEL: Forty percent of births in hospitals could be born by birthing centers. Mod Healthcare 13(12):124, 1983
16. Lahti PT: Early postoperative discharge of patients from the hospital. Surgery 63:410-415, 1968
17. Levy ML, Coakley CS: Survey of in and out surgery-first year. South Med J 61:995, 1968
18. Natof HE: Complications Associated with Ambulatory Surgery. JAMA 244:1116-1118, September 5, 1980
19. Nicoll JH: The surgery of infancy. Br Med J 2:753, 1909
20. O'Donovan TR: Ambulatory Surgical Centers: Development and Management, pp 230-233. Aspen Systems Corporation, 1976
21. O'Donovan TR, O'Donovan PG: Emergicenters: The next wave. Health Serv Manager, p 2, January 1982
22. Orkand Corporation: Comparative Evaluations of Costs, Quality, and System Effects of Ambulatory Surgery Performed in Alternative Settings. Washington, DC, U.S. Department of Health, Education and Welfare, Health Care Financing Administration, December 1977
23. Phalen JF: Planning a hospital based outpatient surgery program. Hosp Prog 57(6):65, June 1976
24. Porterfield HW, Franklin LT: The use of general anesthesia in the office surgery facility. Clin Plast Surg 10(2):292, April 1983
25. Reed WA: Freestanding surgical care facilities. Int Anesthesiol Clin 20(1):110, Spring 1982
26. Same Day Surg, 1(8,9)102, November 1977
27. Same Day Surg 4(1):1, January 1980
28. Trauner JB et al, p 104, In addition, this study quoted the following reference in regard to this issue: Orkand DS, Jagger FM, Hurwitz E: Comparative Evaluation of Cost, Quality, and System Effects of Ambulatory Surgery Performed in Alternative Settings, Final Report, Chap 5, pp 127-129. U.S. Department of Health, Education, and Welfare, Health Care Financing Administration, Office of Policy, Planning and Research, December 1977

29. Trauner JB, Luft HS, Robinson JO: Entrepreneurial Trends in Health Care Delivery, p 96. Federal Trade Commission Report, Institute for Health Policies Study, University of California, San Francisco, July 1982
30. Waters RM: The Down-Town Anesthesia Clinic. Am J Surg Anesth Suppl 33(7):71, 1919
31. Webb E, Graves H: Anesthesia for the Ambulant Patient. Philadelphia, JB Lippincott, 1966
32. Wetchler BV, Batstone R, Barron E: Back to work sooner: Another way ambulatory surgery cuts costs. Methodist Med Center J 3:13, 1984
33. Wetchler BV: Development of a successful ambulatory surgery program. In Jackson J, Roach C, Myers M, Norins LC (eds): Development of a Successful Ambulatory Surgery Program. Atlanta, American Health Consultants, 1981

2
Legal Implications

James Lewis Griffith, J.D.

Slade H. McLaughlin, J.D.

In any discussion today of anesthesia and the risks of anesthesia, there must be a consideration of the legal climate that prevails in this country. There is a tremendous preoccupation with the legal risks associated with the practice of medicine, and particularly a specialty such as anesthesiology that deals with the control of the basic cardiopulmonary functions of the body during surgical procedures and the control of sensations by use of topical, local, or regional anesthetic blocks. The purpose of this discussion is not to give specific legal advice but rather to suggest an approach in the form of risk management to prevent, to the extent possible, future litigation. Obviously, any specific case has its own particular facts and circumstances, and the laws in various states may also be materially different. It should be understood that each case must be considered on its own merits and that specific legal advice should be sought on each such occasion. It should also be understood that the discussion in this chapter is not intended to state what the law is, but rather to provide a standard that may, in fact, be higher than the minimal requirements that have been developed through the caselaw to date. It is hoped that, by adhering to these elevated standards, the risk of harm to patients and, accordingly, the risk of legal involvement on the part of anesthesiologists and ambulatory care centers will be materially reduced.

General Considerations

TERMS

Ambulatory care centers are diverse in their nature and function. Each may have its own merits, safety considerations, or risks. Generally, throughout this chapter recognition has been given to two principal categories: the hospital unit and the freestanding unit. Within the category of the hospital unit there are a number of subcategories, including integrated, separated, and satellite units. Unless specifically stated otherwise, a reference to a *hospital unit* is meant to include all three subcategories, and the material presented is meant to apply to all of these units. The term *freestanding unit* refers to an independent, freestanding ambulatory center and does not include the hospital unit or any of its subcategories. The terms *ambulatory surgical center, ambulatory center,* and *center* have been used interchangeably throughout the text and are intended to include both hospital and freestanding units.

SURGEON SELECTION

As a practical matter, surgeon selection may have many diverse and important ramifications for any ambulatory surgical center. A center must be careful to choose surgeons who strive to provide first-rate surgical services under maximum safety conditions. Today, many states hold ambulatory surgical centers to the same standard of care as hospitals. Since virtually all hospitals have established criteria to assess the propriety of allowing a particular surgeon to practice at their facility, it is essential that all ambulatory surgical centers develop and adopt standards as to the qualifications that a surgeon must meet and as to minimum safety guidelines that he or she must follow in using the center's facilities.

The standards developed by the Accreditation Association for Ambulatory Health Care (AAAHC)* provide that surgical procedures should be

> performed only by health care practitioners who are licensed to perform such procedures within the state in which the organization is located and who have been granted privileges to perform those procedures by the governing body of the organization, upon the recommendation of qualified medical personnel and after medical review of the practitioner's documented education, training, experience, and current competence.

Clearly, any ambulatory treatment center that allows a surgeon to practice at its facility without a prior review of the physician's education, training, experience, and current competence is leaving itself open to the possibility of being held jointly liable for any negligence committed by that surgeon. To prevent this risk, an ambulatory center should perform an initial screening of all surgeon applicants using guidelines and standards similar to those employed by established hospitals. In a hospital ambulatory care unit, the problem is simplified by the fact that privileges in the unit are ordinarily limited to surgeons who have been reviewed and granted privileges by the hospital to operate in the inpatient facility. With respect to freestanding units, no surgeon should be permitted to do any procedure that he or she does not have privileges to do in the inpatient operating suite. Unqualified or underqualified applicants should be denied privileges at the facility. Additionally, peer review on a regular

---

*Copies of these standards may be obtained by writing directly to the Accreditation Association for Ambulatory Health Care, Inc., Westmoreland Building, Old Orchard Road, Skokie, IL 60077 or calling (312) 676-9610. In addition, the Joint Commission on Accreditation of Hospitals publishes an Accreditation Manual for Ambulatory Health Care that applies to freestanding facilities only. This manual can be obtained by writing to JCAH, 875 N. Michigan Avenue, Chicago, IL 60611 or calling (312) 642-6061.

basis, as well as thorough investigation and evaluation of any maloccurrence, is required to ensure the continued competence of the surgeons practicing at the facility. Institution of the aforementioned procedures will, unquestionably, reduce the number of lawsuits against the center and will assure that the facility's patients receive an appropriate level of medical care.

Under no circumstances should a freestanding unit be turned into a "retreat" for surgeons who are unable to obtain surgical privileges at other institutions. It is advisable to select only surgeons with demonstrated competence whose judgment and ability are respected and who currently have privileges at other reputable institutions.

A final word of caution is in order. Once standards and guidelines are established, they must be enforced. Otherwise, they can be used as a basis of liability against the center by a skillful plaintiff's attorney in a malpractice action. For example, the ambulatory center may establish guidelines requiring that certain preoperative diagnostic studies be performed on patients. If a surgeon routinely fails to order these tests, and a complication and resultant injury occur as the result of the surgeon's failure to order the diagnostic studies, the center may be held jointly liable with the surgeon for failing to enforce the medical standards it has established. Clearly, this type of vicarious liability can be prevented with a modicum of effort by enforcement of the standards and regulations established by the facility.

PROCEDURE SELECTION

The range of treatment that may be provided in an ambulatory surgical setting is quite wide and often encompasses procedures as simple as the removal of a mole and as extensive as breast reconstruction. The complexity of the procedures attempted at an ambulatory surgical center should be circumscribed by the type of unit (i.e., hospital-affiliated facility or independent freestanding ambulatory surgical unit).

The hospital-affiliated unit is usually connected to, or in physical proximity with, a hospital. Such hospital adjunct centers have the advantage of easy access to many of the hospital's ancillary services and facilities such as pathology and radiology. In addition, the hospital can provide the convenience of timely consultation with specialists in the event of an emergency. The hospital setting provides an extra margin of safety that may not be available at some freestanding units. For this reason, a greater range and complexity of procedures may be authorized in this setting than might be appropriate at a nonhospital-affiliated facility.

The primary consideration of a freestanding ambulatory surgical unit in determining what procedures it will permit is the availability of extensive and in-depth emergency care for a sudden and unexpected maloccurrence. Surgeons at these freestanding facilities must not be allowed to become too ambitious in the procedures they undertake. Any operation that poses a substantial threat to a patient's life is best performed on an inpatient basis.

Some reasonable judgment must be made as to what types of procedures the freestanding surgical unit should handle. This determination should be made only after considering the adequacy of the unit's facilities, the qualifications of its personnel, and the proximity of the center to the nearest hospital. The experience of other centers may also be taken into consideration, assuming the units are comparable to the facility in question.

PATIENT SELECTION

Physicians practicing at an ambulatory surgical center should select their patients with a number of considerations in mind. First, the capabilities of the facility should never be overestimated. A patient who is scheduled to undergo an extremely difficult and intricate operation that poses a significant risk of complications is not a proper candidate for outpatient treatment. This patient should be hospitalized so that if an emergency does develop, all of the hospital's extensive resources may be brought to bear on the patient's problem. Treatment of a patient in a setting that is neither equipped nor staffed to handle untoward events is medically inappropriate and an invitation to legal disaster.

Second, physicians must be attuned to the needs and wants of their patients. For example, the hypercritical patient who is obviously unhappy and apprehensive that his or her procedure is being performed in an outpatient clinic should be admitted to an inpatient facility instead. This patient is a lawsuit waiting to happen. Ambulatory surgery procedures should be attempted only on patients who, after appropriate exploration, have no objection to undergoing "same day" surgery that will involve recovery in a home environment.

The final, and perhaps most important, consideration in determining whether a patient is an acceptable candidate for ambulatory surgery is whether that person's past medical history or present state of health would place him or her at an unreasonable degree of risk by performance of the procedure in an outpatient setting. Evaluation of every patient should include a careful and detailed history, with particular emphasis on prior surgical experience and problems. For example, patients with a history of massive bleeding during surgery or patients who have previously experienced a severe reaction to anesthesia are poor candidates for ambulatory surgical care. Any history or physical examination that raises the possibility that the surgical facility may be confronted with a sudden, catastrophic emergency or prolonged postoperative recovery excludes consideration of ambulatory surgery. It is foolish to proceed in an outpatient setting under such circumstances, since it is then likely the physician will be sued for undertaking the procedure in a facility that is ill-equipped to handle a complication that might have been anticipated.

Where there is any indication, from past medical history, present state of health, or otherwise, that the patient is at risk of developing a complication the surgical center may not be able to handle as efficiently as a hospital, the procedure should be performed in an inpatient setting. Again, it must be stressed that a physician will be able to isolate patients with a predisposition to development of complications only if appropriate presurgical diagnostic procedures are performed and if careful present and past medical histories are obtained.

Anesthesia Management of the Ambulatory Patient

The anesthesia management of the patient is the responsibility of the person who administers the anesthetic agent. If that person is a nurse anesthetist, ultimate responsibility for his or her acts or omissions may also rest upon the surgeon, the director of the anesthesia service, or the ambulatory center that employs the nurse anesthetist. It is, therefore, imperative that there be strict adherence, not only to the rules and regulations of the ambulatory surgical center, but also to the various licensing, regulatory, or reviewing agencies.

Some of the guidelines that have been published are discussed later in this section, but a word of caution is necessary at the outset. Strict adherence to the standards established by an industry or profession may be essential to proving that one acted in accordance with accepted standards of care. However, that alone is not a guarantee that one is out of the legal briarpatch. No profession or industry can ever isolate itself from legal liability simply by adopting a standard of care and then proving that it followed the standard. The courts have repeatedly stated that, in each case, it is for the jury to determine whether the standard itself was inadequate or unsafe. Likewise, no matter how appropriate the standard may be generally, it is for a jury to determine whether, for other reasons, it was inappropriate or even negligent for the anesthesiologist to have acted in a certain manner for a given patient under a particular set of circumstances. Accordingly, such guidelines, suggestions, or regulations should be known and adhered to in a general sense, but should not be followed unbendingly. The physician is always responsible for treating the patient in the safest possible manner and must act quickly and appropriately to protect the patient in the event of an emergency or other misadventure.

HOSPITAL UNITS

Hospital-affiliated ambulatory surgical centers are required to have published regulations that pertain to most situations and procedures. There must be a departmental chain of command and formalized supervision. These and other similar procedures are specifically required by the *Accreditation Manual for Hospitals*, a publication issued by the Joint Commission on Accreditation of Hospitals (JCAH).* The materials promulgated by the JCAH are published as "standards." Each standard is followed by an "interpretation" section that further defines the scope of required action implicit in the standard. A great amount of time and effort was devoted to getting the JCAH to adopt a term other than "standard," but to no avail.

Is it any wonder then that judges and juries regard these materials as standards by which the administration of anesthesia services to patients is to be judged? If the hospital unit has submitted to a JCAH survey and is "accredited," it is understood that the unit has agreed to comply with the JCAH standards. The patients are deemed to be, in effect, the beneficiaries of these standards to the extent that they pertain to patient safety during the administration of anesthesia.

It would be valuable for all anesthesia personnel to observe a trial to see how these materials are used in questioning by a plaintiff's attorney. Since it is unlikely that such an opportunity will be available, the following is an abbreviated hypothetical version of a case involving patient injury in a hospital relating to problems with the anesthesia apparatus:

Q: Doctor, is your hospital accredited by the JCAH?
A: Yes.

---

*This publication, which applies only to hospitals and hospital-affiliated ambulatory units, may be obtained by writing to the Joint Commission on Accreditation of Hospitals, 875 N. Michigan Avenue, Chicago, IL 60611 or calling (312) 642-6061.

Q: Are you familiar with the accreditation process?

A: Yes.

Q: Have you reviewed the JCAH standards for accreditation as they relate to anesthesia services?

A: Yes. (If the answer is "No," the witness becomes vulnerable for not having ever read what is supposed to be an applicable standard in the hospital.)

Q: Does your hospital have regulations for anesthesia safety?

A(1): Yes. (At this point the witness can be examined as to whether there was compliance with the hospital's own regulations or about the inadequacy of those regulations.)

A(2): No. (The witness is then vulnerable because under a number of the standards, the director is responsible for developing such regulations.)

Q: Does your department have a program for continuing education?

A: No. (Another violation of JCAH standards.)

Q: In this specific case, what inspection of the apparatus that was to be used did you carry out?

A: None. I assumed it was working properly, since it had been used the day before without problems.

Q: Doctor, was there a written regulation in your hospital that required you to inspect all of the equipment before it was used?

A: No. (A violation of JCAH standards.)

Q: Doctor, if there had been such a regulation would you have complied with it?

A: Yes. (Now the failure to comply with the standard may be argued as the cause of the injury if such a preprocedure check would have found the defect or leak in the delivery system.)

Q: After the incident in the operating room, were there any specific problems that this patient had?

A: Yes. We were concerned that the patient might have an increase in secretions, and it was very important that the patient be suctioned at frequent intervals.

Q: How frequently did you intend to do so?

A: At least once every half hour and more frequently if necessary.

Q: What specific instructions did you give to the recovery room personnel?

A: None—they are well trained. (A violation of JCAH requirements.)

Q: Well, Doctor, were the personnel in the recovery room informed of the event in the OR?

A: Not by me.

Q: By anyone?

A: I do not know.

Q: Well then, how were the recovery room personnel supposed to know about this specific problem?

A: I do not know.

Q: Why didn't you tell them?

A: I was getting ready to do another case.

Q: Do you know that the patient became obstructed in the recovery room, became cyanotic and, as a result, suffered cerebral anoxia, resulting in brain damage?

A: I know that now.

Q: If the recovery room personnel had been told by you of the particular problem you encountered during the procedure and had been instructed by you to aspirate as frequently as you had previously indicated, would that not have significantly reduced the risk of airway obstruction?

A: Yes.

Q: And this brain death or injury could have been prevented if you had given such instructions and they had been carried out?

A: I suppose so. (At this point, get out the check book.)

Q: By the way, Doctor, where in the anesthesia record does it describe the fact that the patient's drop in blood pressure was caused by the leak you found in the delivery system?

A: It is not written there. (A violation of JCAH standards and a basis for arguing fraudulent concealment of the problem to prevent a lawsuit.)

This is not an Alice in Wonderland dialogue. It is a synopsis of what any experienced malpractice trial lawyer has heard on more than a few occasions, and it illustrates the accreditations trap. It is important for a facility to be accredited, but accreditation is not an honor—it is an ongoing responsibility to comply with the very standards (there's that word again) that you agreed would govern the anesthesia services performed in your institution.

The failure to achieve accreditation is equally hazardous if the facility or the director admits that an accreditation survey was conducted and the anesthesia service was cited for numerous inadequacies when accreditation was denied. You can be certain that if a patient injury can be linked with any one of the inadequacies found by the accreditation survey team, the case is lost.

FREESTANDING CENTER

What has been stated above is equally applicable to the freestanding center. An examination of the text of the accreditation standards published by the AAAHC shows no rational distinction that can be made between these standards and those of the JCAH. There is, likewise, no dispute as to the fact that one of the primary purposes of all such standards is the delivery of anesthesia to patients under conditions that are as safe as possible. Because patient safety is the keystone of these accreditation programs, their suggestions, guidelines, instructions, and standards become the proverbial sword of Damocles. One must comply to become accredited but once accredited, full compliance is mandated not only to keep the accreditation but also to ensure that patient safety is preserved. In the event of a mishap, those same standards then take on the role of the yardstick by which your conduct will be measured.

One additional point needs to be stressed. From a legal standpoint, there is no justification for a difference in standards of anesthesia management in an ambulatory surgical center from those provided to inpatients at a hospital. In the context of patient safety, the criteria for anesthesia management must be the same. If an ambulatory center's medical director or anesthesiologist involved in a malpractice action were to argue that there is a reasonable basis for a lower level of patient safety in their facility, the first question that will be asked is:

Q: Doctor, you have argued here that because of the nature of the ambulatory center and in an effort to provide a lower cost for your procedures, you are not able to provide the same level of patient safety in your anesthesia services as that provided by hospitals. Is that correct?

A: Yes.

Q: Now Doctor, before you gave this patient anesthesia, did you tell the patient that there was a risk of death, anoxia, hypoxia, brain damage, and other potential morbidities associated with general anesthesia, even if you do everything as best you know how?

A: Yes.

Q: But Doctor, did you tell the patient that his risks were greater if he had the procedure done in your ambulatory surgical center because you, in an effort to lower costs, were not maintaining the same levels of patient safety in your center as would be available in a hospital?

A: No.

Q: Would you then agree, Doctor, that this man did not know of that risk (because you didn't tell him) when he agreed to be anesthetized in your center?

A: Yes.

So much for informed consent! There is an admitted failure to inform a patient of a risk factor.

Is it possible to overcome the informed consent problem? Sure—if you want to announce publicly that it is less safe to have anesthesia in your ambulatory surgical center than it is in a hospital. Why don't you just close the front door and sell the building now before the word gets out! The conclusion is obvious that there should not be and cannot defensibly be two disparate levels of patient care, management, and safety between the ambulatory center and the hospital inpatient administration of anesthesia services.

OFFICE-BASED SURGERY

Recently, third-party payers have been giving financial encouragement to surgeons to perform certain procedures in their offices by agreeing to a higher level of reimbursement. To the extent that a particular surgeon is highly judicious in the selection of patients and of the procedures he or she will perform in that setting, this monetary incentive may be appropriate. To the extent that it affords some semblance of propriety to such surgical locations for all surgeons and all procedures, it may ultimately be a disaster in terms of patient safety.

There is no doubt that a number of physicians are marginally safe when they are supervised and made to comply with standards and regulations in a hospital or ambulatory center. There may be surgical residents or other staff physicians to help them or to suggest that the patient might be better served if referred to a more senior or capable surgeon. The fear of losing one's privileges if one attempts procedures beyond one's competence is a sanction that may serve to protect the patient. But who supervises the physician in his or her own office? Who says what procedures he or she can or cannot do? Who determines whether a given patient has been properly evaluated in accordance with some predetermined preoperative criteria? Are these problems peculiar to the surgeon? What about the anesthesiologist who goes into that office to participate in the procedure? What responsibility does the anesthesiologist bear? What about the JCAH or AAAHC safety standards in that setting? Are they no longer applicable? Are the Quality of Surgical Care Recommendations* promulgated by the Society for Office Based Surgery (SFOBS) comprehensive and thorough enough to ensure optimal patient care? These are just a sampling

*This pamphlet, which applies only to office-based procedures, may be obtained by writing to the Society for Office Based Surgery, PO Box 9494, San Diego, CA 92109 or calling (619) 692-9115.

of the many and diverse issues that confront practitioners involved in the performance of office-based procedures.

The obligations imposed upon the anesthesiologist in the office-based setting may, in fact, be greater and involve a greater risk of being sued. In an office setting, the anesthesiologist does not have all of the support personnel to assist in an emergency and, consequently, the risk of harm in the event of an anesthesia emergency may be greater. What about resuscitation equipment, medications, monitoring equipment, and the like? Is it not the responsibility of the anesthesiologist to adequately monitor the patient during the procedure and to treat the patient if respiratory function ceases or another emergency arises? What about transport arrangements and access to hospital facilities? Suppose the surgeon is not on the staff of any hospital in town.

The anesthesiologist has to protect the patients as well as his or her own stake. The patients have to be carefully evaluated and all pertinent medical factors weighed and considered. The anesthesiologist should not accept any patient who is at greater risk in the office setting than he or she would be in an inpatient facility. If all of the procedures are minor and the patients are all in excellent health, there may be less risk of having to *use* resuscitation equipment, but is that an acceptable basis for *having* less emergency equipment? If the patients are not all young and healthy, and the procedures are not all quick and innocuous, the need increases to have all of the requisite equipment and personnel to promote the interests of safety. If the patient gets into anesthesia-related trouble, remember that it will be the surgeon who will testify that he or she relied upon the anesthesia expert—you—to clear the patient for the procedure and to determine what, if any, equipment was necessary. With a straight face the surgeon will tell the jury that if you had mentioned that you did not think it was safe, he or she would never have operated in the first place.

You cannot stop a surgeon from doing any procedure in his or her own office, but you do not have to participate. Carefully assess all of the personnel, equipment, supplies, medications, and so forth, and if you find them inadequate, refuse to participate in any procedure until the deficiencies have been corrected. That is probably the biggest favor you will ever do for a patient—and yourself. Since the risks associated with anesthesia are the same regardless of whether the patient is admitted to a hospital or operated on in an office, the standards must be the same.

WAYS TO AVOID LEGAL HAZARDS

The preceding paragraphs have addressed this issue in part. Basically, a starting point has to be to sit down and read the accreditation standards (see footnotes on pp 34, 37, and 40). Careful consideration of your practices and procedures in the context of these documents should be undertaken. Do you, in fact, have the written policies and regulations they require? Weigh all such procedures and regulations in the context of patient safety. Are they as current and appropriate as they should be? Can they be improved? When was the last time they were reviewed with the anesthesiologists and nurse-anesthetists who work in the ambulatory center? Is your equipment given regular inspections and maintenance checks? To whom do you report suspected problems? If you suspect an equipment problem, do you take the device out of service until the suspected problem can be checked?

There is no magic formula to avoid legal risks—certainly not a mechanical adherence to a lawyer's checklist. Patient care and the safe management of anesthesia service for ambulatory surgery, wherever it is performed, must become a method of thinking. A major part of the problem has already been overcome if your foremost concern centers on the question, "what is safe for this patient?" Once the importance of this perspective is recognized, the rest is detail. It then becomes the yardstick by which you evaluate your ambulatory center, your equipment, your personnel, and the surgeons whom you have approved to use your facility. It becomes the touchstone by which you evaluate what procedures should or should not be attempted in your facility. Lastly, and perhaps most importantly, it becomes the litmus paper by which you decide whether each patient has been appropriately selected, tested, and informed before the procedure is undertaken. If any of those factors, when weighed against the overriding factor of patient safety, tips the scale in such a way that the patient being given anesthesia is placed at greater risk in an ambulatory center than in an inpatient facility, then don't administer the anesthesia. Resolve all such doubts in favor of the patient's safety. Transfer to an inpatient facility.

Finally, all conduct by health care providers is evaluated in court in terms of its degree of consistency with applicable prevailing standards of conduct at the time the treatment was rendered. There may be many physicians who are willing to testify as expert witnesses that ambulatory centers or physicians' offices are not as safe as inpatient facilities. It does not matter whether such testimony is biased, based on ignorance of ambulatory surgery, or even inaccurate. It will still be heard by the jury because the judge is not medically qualified to the point where he or she can substitute his or her opinion for that of the physician-witness. It is, therefore, urgent that in the ambulatory center there be as little difference as possible in the level of patient care and that, in all respects, the anesthesia management of the patient be as good as or better than its inpatient counterpart.

Preanesthesia Visit

DEFINITION AND PURPOSE

The preanesthesia visit, or patient interview as it is commonly called, serves as a vehicle to facilitate the exchange of information between the anesthesiologist and the patient. In essence, there are two objectives the physician should seek to accomplish during this meeting with the patient. First, this initial interview is the appropriate forum to elicit relevant information from the patient about his or her present state of health, past medical history, prior reactions to any anesthetic agent, and any other information that may be pertinent to the form of anesthesia contemplated. Second, the anesthesiologist should educate the patient during the patient interview about all of the relevant information that is necessary in order for the patient to give a truly *informed* consent (the specifics of this issue are addressed later in this chapter).

As illustrated above, the anesthesiologist should strive to impart as well as to extract information during the patient interview. In this fashion, he or she will be apprised as to the likely difficulties and problems that may be encountered with this individual, and the patient will have a genuine awareness and understanding of the anesthesia aspect of the procedure he or she is about to undergo. Proper use of the patient interview will, in many instances, forestall litigation, not only by averting anticipated complications through advance preparation, but also by removing liability for medical risks by making the patient aware of what might occur.

WHEN AND WHERE

Unquestionably, every patient deserves an ample amount of time to consider and reflect on the risks, benefits, and alternatives associated with the planned anesthetic agent as well as with the method by which it is to be administered. Similarly, the anesthesiologist needs time to analyze, evaluate, and deliberate about the information received from the patient. Depending on the data that have been elicited, ordering past medical records or contacting prior treating physicians may be indicated.

The benefits hoped to be gained through use of the preanesthesia visit can be brought to fruition only if sufficient time for contemplation and deliberation is afforded both the patient and the physician. For inpatients, who are generally the higher risk patients, the preanesthesia conferences frequently occur on the evening before surgery. It is not surprising, therefore, that in ambulatory surgical centers, the preanesthesia visit normally occurs on the day of the procedure. But this visit should be conducted as soon as the patient arrives so that as much time as possible is gained for thought and reflection. A good surgeon who really knows the patient and who is concerned about that patient's welfare should clearly notify the anesthesiologist far in advance of the upcoming procedure. This may allow the anesthesiologist to call the patient several days before the procedure to review the relevant information or to retrieve the patient's records. This prior notice of suspected problems may avert last-minute postponements and consequent patient displeasure.

Quite clearly, a meeting with the patient in the operating room itself just before the surgical procedure is unacceptable. These are a few of the many problems with this practice:

A meaningful exchange of information is rendered more difficult owing to the patient's anxiety about the imminent surgical procedure.

The anesthesiologist has foreclosed the opportunity for investigation of significant risk factors that might have been elicited during the interview.

A truly informed consent may not be obtainable since the anesthesiologist has not had sufficient time to adequately analyze the risks, benefits, and alternatives associated with the planned anesthesia management, and, perhaps more importantly, the patient has not had an opportunity to make any meaningful choice as to whether the contemplated anesthesia plan is acceptable.

All of these problems can be obviated if the patient interview is conducted in advance of the surgical procedure. There is no question that this will involve additional time, effort, and planning. However, in the long run, it may save the time, energy, and expense associated with litigation of a malpractice suit.

There is no one right answer to the question of where and how the preanesthesia interview should be held. The optimal encounter would involve a face-to-face meeting between the anesthesiologist and the patient in either the physician's office or in some other private space at the surgical center. This has the advantage of allowing the two to meet in a relaxed atmosphere and develop some sort of rapport before the anesthesia is administered. In addition, there is a greater opportunity for follow-up questions by both parties about the information exchanged.

In situations where a face-to-face meeting is not possible, either because of space restrictions or scheduling problems, a telephone conference may be substituted. Again, the telephone interview should take place either before the patient comes to the center or upon arrival, as long before the scheduled surgical procedure as possible, and should involve a comprehensive exchange of information between the anesthesiologist and the patient.

Some type of direct contact between the patient and the anesthesiologist should take place before surgery. Some institutions, as a time-saving measure, have resorted to preprinted forms and questionnaires to obtain informed consent and pertinent medical history from patients. These are appropriate measures, but should always be personally reviewed with the patient on the day of the procedure. Such an approach promotes a meaningful exchange of information between the physician and the patient. The use of forms alone should never be used in lieu of a complete preanesthesia interview by the anesthesiologist as described above.

Finally, the physician should carefully record on the patient's chart the significant aspects of the history and physical examination. It is extremely important to record what the patient admits as well as what he or she denies. A simple note "Denies S.O.B., allergies, asthma, or other respiratory problems" may save the day if the patient subsequently claims to have advised the physician of such a problem and the procedure went forward—with untoward consequences. The note should clearly reflect that there was also a detailed discussion of the risks of anesthesia and that the patient understood the discussion and consented. A listing of the most critical risks is particularly helpful: "Death, respiratory arrest, infection, hemorrhage, etc." The point is simple. Let's assume Mrs. Lange sustains a pulmonary problem that requires medication, postprocedure radiography and follow-up, and perhaps even a prolonged admission. The patient claims she was never told of this remote and unusual risk and that she would not have undergone the procedure had she been so advised. If the anesthesiologist can then present a signed consent stating that patient was willing to run the serious risk of hemorrhage and even death, it is much easier to convince the jury that a person who is willing to risk death would have accepted the risk of a relatively benign complication that might have occurred. Getting the patient to sign the note as well as a written consent form is highly recommended.

Appropriate Preanesthesia Laboratory Tests

The use of preordained, mandatory, preoperative or preanesthesia laboratory tests is meeting with increasing disfavor. The cost of these tests outweighs their limited usefulness and the information they provide. Certainly the federal program of prospective payment (DRG) takes away the incentive to do any test that is not absolutely essential for the inpatient.

The ambulatory center, by defining its purpose, procedures, and personnel, is in a positive position to specify its preprocedure tests. The center has the responsibility to state what tests it will require to be done before the patient undergoes a given procedure. It must be emphasized, however, that these requirements are minimums. At no time should the ambulatory center appear to be inhibiting a physician from doing any further testing he or she believes is medically indicated. This caveat is based on the simple fact that, in certain cases in which physicians did not perform indicated tests, they have sometimes sought to extricate themselves by arguing that the hospital or other facility had dissuaded them from doing the tests because of the institution's financial status. They have even gone so far as to suggest that they were in fear of losing staff privileges if they performed more than the minimum specified tests. Defendents in lawsuits take strange positions when trying to defend their professional reputations and their assets. They are not above distorting sound restrictions into total bans. It is, therefore, important to state unequivocally in the written regulations of the center that the required preoperative and preanesthesia tests are minimums and that the ultimate responsibility for the medical judgment as to what additional tests are required for a particular patient remains with the attending surgeon and anesthesiologist.

HOSPITAL UNITS

With that preamble, there are potential legal pitfalls in the event of variations in treatment between hospital inpatients and patients undergoing the same procedures in hospital ambulatory centers. The public at large remains relatively ignorant of the important distinctions between hospital inpatient units and hospital ambulatory centers. Hospitals are still the major teaching institutions and may, therefore, permit or encourage the performance of numerous preoperative procedures or tests on their inpatients as part of the teaching process.

Thus, there are good reasons why a hospital, for its anticipated inpatient population, may specify a much more intensive program of preoperative testing. Likewise, hospital inpatient surgical services are not able to screen their patients in the same way as ambulatory surgical centers. In fact, any patient of whatever age who represents an inordinate risk is going to be admitted for their procedure to a hospital's inpatient surgical service and not to its ambulatory center. There are many operative procedures that cannot and should not be performed in an ambulatory center.

It is the responsibility of the surgical and anesthesia staff in the hospital to specify their preprocedure requirements. In so doing, however, the temptation to become dogmatic must be avoided. It is this tendency to say, "This is how we do it in the inpatient service and therefore this is the way it *must* be done," that creates legal risks for the hospital ambulatory center.

It is, therefore, very important in a hospital ambulatory surgical center that the staff of both the inpatient unit and the ambulatory unit carefully review, procedure by procedure, their recommendations as to presurgical testing. If a real difference between the patients receiving the same procedure does not generally exist, there should not be a lesser standard of preprocedure testing in the hospital ambulatory unit. On the other hand, if the patients who are chosen to go to the ambulatory unit are materially different from their inpatient counterparts in terms of age, health, or other relevant criteria, then there may be a rational, medically justified basis for a less intense testing protocol. However, protocols should never be followed blindly. Again, they are minimums and not a prohibition for aggressively testing a patient whose signs, symptoms, history, and so forth suggest that greater caution is indicated.

FREESTANDING AMBULATORY CENTERS

The ability of a center to screen its patients and surgeons may justify a freestanding center in adopting a less intensive program of mandatory preprocedure testing. In so doing, however, it exposes itself to the argument that the center practices "inferior medicine" because it did not work-up the patient with the same level of care as the patient would have received if treated as an inpatient at the hospital just four blocks away. The plaintiff will moan that if he or she had been told the tests were not going to be performed in the same careful manner as inpatients can expect at the hospital, he or she would never have agreed to go to the center. Then comes the critical testimony of the professional witness or, worse yet, the surgeon or anesthesiologist from a competing hospital, and the stage is set for a potentially costly loss. The loss is not just a monetary one; it is also a setback for a center's attempts to reduce costs and unnecessary procedures and will undoubtedly have an adverse impact on the center's reputation.

It is with reluctance, therefore, but with legal survival paramount in mind, that each freestanding center will have to measure the legal climate in its community in determining whether its preoperative and preanesthesia testing can vary from that of the inpatient surgical service at nearby hospitals or even hospital-based ambulatory surgical centers with which it is comparable in terms of procedure and patient selection. If the inpatient hospital surgical services and physicians are supportive of the center and its approach to the delivery of quality medical services, then a variance is possible without a severe increase in the legal risks. It may be advisable, to the extent possible, to have some of the hospital-based physicians review, in an advisory role, the proposed testing protocols for the freestanding center if for no other reason than such an approach might neutralize any criticism from them in the event of a maloccurrence.

The specific enumeration of tests that should be done by an ambulatory center or those that can or should be dispensed with is not a legal question but rather a medical one and, thus, is not pertinent or appropriate for this discussion. Other chapters in this text deal with the medical aspects of this issue. Medical practitioners will continue to develop guidelines as to specific test procedures, and these guidelines will be further modified in accordance with future clinical experience.

OFFICE-BASED SURGERY

Because the risk of harm in the event of a severe complication during a surgical procedure is potentially greater in a physician's office than in other facilities, greater caution in patient evaluation and selection is mandatory. This, by definition, may require additional testing. However, unlike the ambulatory center, which can mandate certain tests as a prerequisite for doing the procedure, the physician is free to decide in his or her own office what will or will not be done. The physician makes this election at his or her own risk. However, what about the anesthesiologist who, sight unseen, is now asked to anesthetize the patient?

In view of the foregoing, the anesthesiologist is strongly urged to develop his or her own preanesthesia minimal testing protocol. This protocol should be no less intensive than that of the ambulatory surgical center for the same operative procedure, and there may be justification for making it even more intensive, depending on the anesthesiologist's experience with each particular surgeon. The more cautious and careful the surgeon is in the selection and preprocedure workup, the easier the burden on the anesthesiologist. But clearly, this situation demands a closer working dialogue between the two physicians. A continuous reassessment of working protocols is required, and each patient must be strictly followed in accordance with those protocols. If the surgeon is unwilling to adhere to the suggested protocol, the anesthesiologist is advised to terminate the relationship with that surgeon's office.

CONCLUSION

The one element of legal risk that is common to the hospital-affiliated ambulatory center, the freestanding center, and the physician who operates in an office is the failure to adhere religiously to whatever protocol of testing and evaluation has been adopted. If you, yourself, have said that a particular combination of tests, at a minimum, are necessary for a safe and adequate evaluation of a patient, then how do you justify going forward with a procedure without performing them?

Make up your mind to follow a "no-exceptions" policy. Specify how soon before the procedure the tests must be done *and* the results must be available. Doing the tests but then going forward with surgery without the results being on the chart is the equivalent, from both a legal and a common-sense point of view, of not doing the tests at all. If the results aren't there, cancel the procedure! Let the surgeon who delayed doing the tests or did not order them at all explain the cancellation to the patient. Remember, the accreditation standards mandate that the facility is responsible for its regulations and procedures and must enforce what it has adopted! If the parent of a minor scheduled for surgery did not sign the operative permit, you would not operate. Likewise, if other preanesthesia requirements are not met, cancel the procedure. Preoperative and preanesthesia testing is no less legally significant than consent. If you want to gamble with the patient's safety and your facility's reputation and liability, then go ahead—lots of your colleagues do, and the ever-increasing number of new malpractice cases proves it.

Informed Consent

BACKGROUND AND PHILOSOPHY

A patient's consent to medical treatment has been a legal requirement for centuries. However, the consent required in the 1800s differs substantially from that required today. Formerly, a physician was required only to obtain the patient's "authorization" to treat. The only explanation that was required involved providing information about the nature of the treatment (i.e., the type of procedure to be performed). Today, however, it is incumbent upon a physician to explain to a patient not only the nature of the proposed treatment, but also the risks, benefits, and alternatives associated with it. Standards developed by the AAAHC specifically provide that "the informed consent of the patient or, if applicable, of the patient's representative [be] obtained before an operation is performed." Many physicians are unaware of this modern standard of care, and it is for this reason that informed consent is rapidly becoming the most popular theory of liability used against physicians in malpractice actions.

In today's society, the patient is given an important role in the medical decision-making process. Many recent court opinions have stressed that the patient's individual right to self-determination of treatment includes his or her right to refuse treatment, even if such refusal will have deleterious effects upon his or her physical well-being. The law has created an innate conflict between the patient's right to decide on a course of treatment and the physician's right to treat the patient in the manner he or she feels is most appropriate. Such a conflict is difficult, if not impossible, to resolve without a cooperative working relationship between the physician and the patient.

HOW TO OBTAIN AN INFORMED CONSENT

Inherent in the concept of patient determination of treatment is the assumption that physicians will give patients the requisite information necessary to make an informed decision. This is the touchstone by which all informed consent cases are judged.

Generally, a physician risks civil action by withholding any facts that are necessary for the patient to form an intelligent decision as to whether or not to undergo the proposed treatment. Such a disclosure involves a discussion of the risks, benefits, and alternatives associated with the contemplated treatment. In the context of anesthesia, the following checklist details the proper procedure for obtaining a patient's informed consent:

1. Provide a simple and concise explanation of the type of anesthesia to be administered, as well as the method of its administration.
2. Explain why you think the anesthetic agent and its method of administration are the most appropriate in this instance.
3. Provide a thorough explanation of alternative types of anesthesia and methods of administration that might be appropriate.
4. Disclose any material risks associated with the anesthetic agent or its method of administration.
5. Disclose and discuss any material risks relevant to the particular patient's past or present medical history, signs, symptoms, clinical findings, radiograms, or other diagnostic tests.
6. Answer any questions the patient has about the proposed anesthesia management.

In the vast majority of cases, litigation arises out of the failure to discuss the risks associated with the anesthetic agent or its method of administration. Obviously, a patient does not ordinarily sue his or her anesthesiologist unless a maloccurrence has come to pass. In many instances, this maloccurrence falls within a risk category that was associated with the use of a particular anesthetic agent or its method of administration. If the anesthesiologist has failed to inform the patient of this risk before administration of anesthesia, it is going to be very difficult to convince the members of a jury that they should not find the physician liable for proceeding without the patient's informed consent.

The law does not require an anesthesiologist to disclose all risks no matter how minute or remote. The only risks that must be disclosed are those that a reasonable anesthesiologist would have disclosed (i.e., material and probable risks). In addition to warning about the general category of risks to which all patients are susceptible, the anesthesiologist has a duty to warn a patient of any additional risks to which that patient might be particularly susceptible. Examples include risks associated with administration of anesthesia to the anemic patient, the obese patient, the patient with respiratory or coronary impairments, the pregnant patient, and the patient with abnormal blood study results. An anesthesiologist can be apprised of such patient peculiarities only if the proper studies and lab work are performed before surgery. For this reason, it is absolutely essential that an appropriate preoperative workup be undertaken for every patient. Only then can the anesthesiologist explain the probable and material risks to the patient and be assured that a truly informed consent has been obtained.

The phraseology and semantics of an informed consent conference with the patient are extremely important. Simple, plain, layman language must be used. Even a signed consent form is not going to provide a defense if a patient with a third-grade education tells a jury that every word you spoke had ten syllables and that he or she had no understanding of the medical terminology you used. If indicated, use an illustrative diagram to demonstrate where problems might be encountered with intubation or where other complications might arise. Above all, use plain English (e.g., say "swelling" rather than "edema"; say "numbness" rather than "paresthesia").

DOCUMENTATION OF INFORMED CONSENT

Even the most thorough and comprehensive informed consent discussion with a patient will not be of any benefit to you years down the road when litigation has been instituted unless you can demonstrate that it actually occurred. Many patients conveniently "forget" that the discussion ever took place, and others genuinely do not have a present recollection of the event years after the fact. In any case, the more facts you have to substantiate that an informed consent conference did take place, the better your chances of achieving a favorable verdict in the litigation forum.

It is advisable to have a member of your staff (RN, CRNA, etc.) sit in on the patient conference. Also, if the patient has brought a family member or friend along, encourage that person to attend the meeting. In this way, you have a number of witnesses to attest that the patient was given information about the risks and alternatives associated with the contemplated anesthesia treatment. After conferring, have the patient sign an informed consent form on which you have listed all significant risks and alternatives about which the patient was informed. Also, make sure the form is dated.

Finally, document in the patient's chart that an informed consent conference was held, that there were witnesses (note their names), and that the patient gave his or her written consent to proceed with the proposed anesthesia plan. In addition, if a patient was advised of susceptibility to certain peculiar risks, note these risks on the chart. It is also advisable to have the patient sign this chart notation.

These measures often deter a plaintiff's attorney from proceeding against an anesthesiologist on an informed consent theory, since any hope for recovery is slim in view of the documented preanesthesia interview with the patient.

TIME CONSIDERATIONS

As discussed above under Preanesthesia Interview, the timing of the informed consent discussion between the physician and the patient is crucial. Bear in mind that an ambulatory surgical center is an unfamiliar setting for most patients and frequently evokes feelings of fear, uncertainty, and anxiety. All of these emotions are intensified on the day of the procedure when surgery is imminent. For this reason, an informed consent discussion should be held in the most relaxed setting the facilities at the unit permit. Obviously, it should be held outside of the operating suite itself. It must be held before the patient is premedicated with any sedative. If the patient is elderly, retarded, or a minor or if he or she appears confused, the discussion must be held with a spouse, parent, or guardian present. The atmosphere should be relaxed, but there should be no attempt to downplay the seriousness of this discussion by jokes, overinformality, or an attempt to brush this aside by saying, "the lawyers make me do this, so don't worry about it." Such a comment has been held by one court to destroy the consent. Always record who was present during the discussion. Document their presence and consent by asking them to sign the consent form along with the patient's signature.

Inherent in the concept of informed consent is the assumption that the patient will have an informative, noncoercive discussion with the physician about the proposed treatment and, thereafter, will have the opportunity to make a decision, without pressure, as to whether he or she wishes to proceed in view of the explanation of risks and alternatives.

The caselaw in this country is replete with examples of patients who have been awarded damages under a theory of lack of informed consent in which the alleged "informed" consent was obtained by the physician in the operating room immediately before the operation. A patient already in a gown, lying on a litter, who has been premedicated, and who is scheduled to undergo surgery in the next few minutes is not in any condition to make decisions that involve potential loss of life or limb. Because of the tension and anxiety associated with the impending surgical procedure, the patient's reasoning process may be temporarily impaired, and he or she may be unable to assimilate much of the medical information that has been communicated to him or her. Such a state of mind is not conducive to making calm and reasoned decisions. Unless a patient is given adequate time for contemplation and deliberation, a physician can, at best, hope to obtain a mere "authorization" to treat and not the informed consent required by law.

All of the aforementioned problems can be eradicated by adoption of a simple technique: *conduct informed consent conferences as far in advance of the surgery as time and circumstances permit.* The extra time and effort required to implement this scheduling procedure is a small price to pay for the confidence that you have obtained a truly informed consent.

Some patients or even their surgeons may request a conference before the day of the procedure. This request should be accommodated. If the patient is that concerned, there may be some problem they want to specifically discuss. This may lead to the disclosure of problems that may cause the procedure to be cancelled. If that is going to happen, it is better to know it in advance and thus not lose valuable operating time on the schedule. For example, suppose this conference discloses an extremely frightened patient who has a past medical history that requires a very prolonged discussion to allay his or her fears and to explain all of the risks. If the anesthesiologist was confronted by such a patient on the morning of the procedure, the entire schedule for that day could be delayed. On the other hand, the anesthesiologist, as a result of seeing the patient a few days before the surgery, may decide this patient belongs on an inpatient service. Clearly, everyone has benefited in this situation. A good informed consent discussion can disclose all of the reasonably foreseeable risks and yet be done in such a manner as not to frighten the patient, and it can also help to allay unreasonable fears. However, if the patient's fears are not allayed and he or she decides the next day not to undergo the procedure or opts to be admitted to an inpatient facility, then the extra time for this preprocedure visit was well spent indeed!

Discharge from an Ambulatory Surgical Center

While in the center, a patient is subject to your direction and control, but after the patient leaves, you are at his or her mercy. This is true because once the patient is discharged, usually within a few hours after the procedure, he or she must be relied on to monitor signs, symptoms, or complications. To be able to do that, the patient needs very careful instructions and predetermined lines of communication and immediate access, if necessary, to alternative medical centers. Perhaps discharge is not even feasible, and an immediate admission or transfer is in order. These are critical decisions, and various people must play important roles in making them. The wrong people should not be asked to serve inappropriate roles.

STANDARDS FOR DISCHARGE

The ultimate standard is whether it is medically appropriate to discharge a patient. The JCAH anesthesia standards suggest that it may be appropriate to develop discharge criteria approved by the medical staff to ensure the same standard of care for all patients. If it is deemed appropriate to develop such criteria for inpatient hospital-affiliated anesthesia services, it is certainly appropriate to do so in the ambulatory center. The bottom line, however, is that if such criteria are developed, they must be rigidly enforced. Departures from established criteria are just invitations to the courthouse.

STATUS OF THE PATIENT

Discharge decisions must be based on the status of the patient at the time the decision to discharge is made. The decision should not be made hours in advance because the patient's status may have deteriorated during the interim. It is, therefore, important to evaluate the patient just before the patient leaves the facility. The patient's status must meet all of the discharge criteria. Unexplained symptoms, fluctuations in blood pressure, temperature elevations, sensations of dizziness, or other significant findings should not be ignored or downplayed. Sometimes there is nothing more suspicious than the fact that the patient "looks funny." Keeping the patient a little longer for observation may be the best medicine you have practiced all day. If the patient doesn't improve, you have time to start alternative planning, including transfer to an inpatient facility. Admission to such a facility is a lot safer, legally, than gambling on a discharge under questionable clinical conditions.

PATIENT'S EDUCATIONAL LEVEL

The patient's level of education may be an important variable in the discharge equation. It may affect the patient's ability to comprehend what is happening. It will determine the level of instructions to be given to the patient. If the patient is unable to understand detailed and vital instructions, the risk is too great that he or she will not follow them. In order to protect the patient, that risk should not be undertaken, and admission should be considered. If a responsible adult is present and indicates that they understand and are capable of carrying out the instructions for the patient, then the decision may be resolved in favor of discharge. Discharge evaluation and instructions as to outpatient care and monitoring of symptoms play an important role in patient discharge. It is the physician's responsibility both to evaluate and to instruct the patient in a timely and appropriate fashion. The instructions must be tailored to the patient's educational level. It may be necessary to give a simple set of general written instructions. The telephone numbers of the physicians and of the center should be included if the patient seems in any way confused or uncertain. In the case of a freestanding center, the telephone number of a transfer hospital should be supplied. It is also important to note that centers that treat patients who are not proficient in the English language have a duty to ensure that these patients are given discharge instructions in their own language so that they understand how to proceed after surgery. Centers that cater to a large foreign-speaking population should have an interpreter as a member of their staff and should have written discharge instructions printed in the native language of their patients.

ACCESSIBILITY TO EMERGENCY FACILITIES

Another factor to be weighed is the patient's ability to gain access to emergency facilities. Measuring this factor correctly requires knowledge of the transportation facilities available, including public emergency transportation, as well as the time and distance necessary to reach them. These factors are too varied and too important to leave to the last 5 minutes before the patient goes home. These and all discharge-related procedures should be discussed and explained before the patient ever arrives at the center. Preadmission discharge planning may eliminate most problems. Clearly, the presence of a responsible adult to assist the patient home, to review the discharge instructions, and to be ready to summon aid if an emergency develops is indispensable. If it appears that in the event of a foreseeable emergency, there is a significant risk that the patient could not reach the emergency facility, then discharge is not indicated. This, of course, involves weighing the patient's status against the risk that the patient could not reach an emergency facility if a complication developed. The ultimate decision to discharge must involve considerations of the procedure the patient underwent, the patient's general health, risk factors disclosed by the patient's preprocedure testing, the patient's present status, and the accessibility of emergency facilities in the event of a complication.

INPATIENT ADMISSION

A great part of the discussion of legal risks has been devoted to the prevention of harm by opting for the course of conduct that is safest for the patient. Specific rules have been avoided in an attempt to reinforce and teach a methodology of thinking. If one gets in the habit of resolving troubling conflicts, doubts, or risks by doing that which has the highest probability of patient safety, a significant amount of patient harm and legal culpability can be avoided. In this context, the difficult issue of discharge vs. inpatient admission must be resolved. In most cases, there is no contraindication to discharge, and the decision is easy and appropriate. There will be cases, however, in which a minor concern about the patient's status is resolved in favor of discharge because of ready access to the center or other emergency care facility and because the patient is sufficiently intelligent to know how to respond. If, however, the patient's status suggests a significant possibility of a postoperative complication that no degree of ready access to emergency facilities is going to prevent, the patient must not be discharged. In terms of the cost of malpractice cases, safe medicine can be best described by the lawyers' adage: "the trouble you don't get into is the trouble you don't have to pay me to get you out of." An overnight admission may turn out to be an unnecessary precaution or it may save the patient's life. Patients do not sue you for taking great precautions to protect them—they sue you for not taking those precautions when reasonably indicated. When in doubt, admit! You and the patient may both sleep more peacefully that night.

JCAH AND AAAHC STANDARDS

The role of the physician in making the postanesthesia discharge decision is clearly stated in both the JCAH and AAAHC standards. The purpose of the postanesthesia visit is defined and, significantly, the standards speak of delaying the discharge decision until the patient is fully recovered from the anesthetic agent. The patient's anticipated recovery is not the criterion; rather, it is the status of the patient after he or she is fully reacted that determines whether discharge is appropriate. Documentation of the patient's condition is mandated, and the identity of the physician responsible for the discharge decision should also be clearly noted.

RESPONSIBILITY FOR PATIENT DISCHARGE

WHO SHOULD EXAMINE AND DISCHARGE?

The answer to this question is unequivocal—a physician. The discharge decision that must be made only a brief time after the procedure is fraught with danger and legal pitfalls. Only a physician is medically qualified to assess all aspects of the patient's status. No patient should ever be allowed to leave until the physician makes the final examination and gives clearance for the patient to be discharged. It is not appropriate to impose this final clearance decision on the nursing personnel, and the ambulatory center should promulgate explicit guidelines to prevent its nurses from being put into this position. Many physicians write such orders as, "OK to discharge when stable." "Stable," in an ambulatory center, should be clearly stated to be a medical decision to be made by a physician only. If the nurse were to discharge when the patient was medically not ready for discharge, the nurse might be culpable, but so, too, would be the center that employs the nurse and the physician who wrote the order. Why? Because when the nurse was so instructed by the physician, he or she became the physician's agent for that purpose. Similarly, the nurse is the agent of the center by virtue of being employed there. If the nurse acted negligently as an agent, then the principal of that agent is also liable under the theory of respondeat superior. Since the physician is going to be culpable for a negligent decision, he or she should at least make the decision alone. If further incentives are necessary, consider the fact that only the physician discussed the patient's history, symptoms, preprocedure consent, discharge planning, risks, benefits, and medical follow-up with the patient, and discharge involves a weighing of all those factors.

The more interesting question is "Which physician should discharge?" More often than not the surgical criteria for discharge may be met upon the completion of the procedure. The surgeon may, thereafter, leave the center or may be involved in another procedure when the decision as to discharge has to be made. It is, therefore, much more likely that the discharge evaluation will be made by the anesthesiologist. The discharge decision generally does not involve a decision as to whether or not the patient is surgically recuperated. That process may take days or even weeks, in some instances. Therefore, what is really being assessed in an ambulatory center is whether the patient has recovered from the anesthesia sufficiently to be able to return home to continue with his or her surgical recovery and to respond intelligently if a delayed complication of the surgery or anesthesia should develop.

Anesthesiologists are, therefore, most qualified to make the discharge decision. This may also involve discharge instructions to the patient about return visits to the surgeon, medication, home care, and so forth. This discharge conference is extremely crucial and can be legally very important for the center. Apart from performing an integral part of patient care for the center's legal protection, the anesthesiologist's discharge decision also involves the important function of ensuring patient safety. From a proprietary standpoint, it should also be noted that anesthesiologists often own the freestanding centers and certainly, in terms of job security, have a much greater interest in the financial survival of the center than does a single surgeon. In no way are we implying that surgeons are not qualified to perform a discharge examination and make a discharge decision; they certainly are qualified in this area. Finally, being involved in the discharge decision serves to reinforce the role of the anesthesiologist as a physician in the broader sense. The anesthesiologist's role is too often limited in the minds of both laymen and other physicians. Anesthesiologists are not "time passers" or the "gas guys," as many think. The more responsibility for patient care and safety they assume, the more they enhance their own medical image.

JCAH AND AAAHC REQUIREMENTS

The requirements of both the JCAH and the AAAHC are consistent with the guidelines discussed above. The JCAH provides that "the basis for decision to discharge a patient from any postanesthesia care unit shall be made only by a physician . . . and not by nursing service personnel. . . . When discharge criteria are used, they shall be comprehensive, approved by the medical staff to assure the same standard of care for all patients, and rigidly enforced." Similarly, the AAAHC requirements mandate that "patients who have received general anesthesia [be] examined by a physician after recovery from anesthesia, prior to discharge."

MANNER OF DISCHARGE

The written policy of the ambulatory center about discharge should be adhered to in all respects. The requirements specified in that policy should be reviewed before the procedure so that there is no doubt that full compliance can be assured. The policy should specify the decisions to be made by the surgeon and those that are to be made by the anesthesiologist. The center's director has the overall responsibility to make certain these written requirements are, in fact, being complied with. Physicians who do not properly brief their patients in advance of admission about the discharge procedures and requirements should be identified and counseled about the importance of these procedures. Noncompliance should not be condoned.

Discharge by Written Policy. The policy should state what discharge orders must be written and should particularly insist on clear identification of who will follow the patient on what date and where. The policy may insist that the information be given to the patient in written form. Medication instructions should be given by the physician who prescribes the medication. However, in many instances, the discharging physician may not be the prescribing physician, and in those instances the discharging physician should verify that the patient has been instructed and *understands* the instructions about the medication. Particular procedures may lend themselves to a checklist of signs and symptoms to watch for and, if reduced to written instructions, the center may direct, in its discharge regulations, that such materials be given to the patient. The patient, as a matter of policy, should be encouraged to report to the surgeon, the anesthesiologist, or the center any changes in his or her status after discharge.

Nurses in ambulatory centers should not be given any greater role in the discharge instruction process than would be given to their inpatient counterparts. Many inpatient facilities do not permit nurses to give medication, decide dosages, or give instructions about side-effects and contraindications. Nurses may be permitted to remind the patient to follow the physician's instructions or to remind the patient that the particular medication should be taken with or without food, without dairy products, and so forth. However, the nursing role should not be expanded in the ambulatory center for the sake of expediency or to save costs. Putting physician duties on the shoulders of the nursing personnel may enhance the nurses' sense of professional pride, but watch how fast they pass the baton back to the physician when they get sued.

Discharge by Phone Order. This practice should not be encouraged. It should be a rare exception if it is permitted at all. If the surgeon or the anesthesiologist is unable, because of an emergency, to examine the patient, another physician should be contacted to come and actually see the patient. Nurses should not be asked to report the patient's signs and symptoms to a physician over the phone and then receive a verbal order to discharge. This makes the center, as well as the physician, potentially liable if the nurse has incorrectly ascertained the patient's status. The decision to discharge should be an on-the-spot medical decision made by a physician. The foregoing discussion is completely in accordance with the standards set forth in the JCAH Accreditation Manual for Ambulatory Health Care, as well as those established by the AAAHC. These mandates may sound drastic, but the single most frequently cited reason for patients suing their physicians, ambulatory centers, and everyone else in sight is the patient's perception that once the operation is over, a doctor is never around. In short, the patient feels abandoned, and when something adverse occurs, he or she blames it on that lack of attention.

If the anesthesiologist accepts the important role as the discharge physician, which we advocate, these patient fears are allayed in most instances. The patient is grateful for the fine professional attention and remembers the doctor who came to "see them off." If the patient later develops a surgical complication and decides to sue, it may be the final impression the patient formed of the anesthesiologist and the center that keeps these parties from also being named as defendants in the suit against the surgeon.

No Physician Available. The question is frequently asked as to, "What policies can be established to protect the nursing personnel and the facility in the event of a discharge when no physician is available?" The response is to adopt regulations that guarantee, to the extent humanly possible, that this situation will never arise. This responsibility starts with the burden on the admitting physician and the anesthesiologist and proceeds down to the center's administration itself. The center should adopt regulations so that at least one of its anesthesiologists will remain on site until the last patient of the day has departed. There should always be a physician on the premises in the event of a medical emergency. The regulations should further state that before any discharge is made in the absence of the admitting physician or the anesthesiologist, contact should be established with one of the center's other physicians, and the appropriateness of the discharge, as well as that of the discharge instructions, should be reviewed. Finally, emergency care facilities should be identified.

At a recent seminar, one of the attendees cited an instance in which the admitting surgeon scheduled a number of procedures and, with at least four patients still on the premises, signed out to a physician in another community some miles distant and left for the weekend. The surgeon on call was busy operating on his own patients and could not even come to the phone when one of his colleague's patients began to experience problems. There was no way he could assist the patient. The center's director, who was not a physician, refused to allow the discharge of any of the recalcitrant physician's patients under these circumstances, and ordered that they all be admitted to the transfer hospital. As the reader can imagine, this stirred up quite a row with the patients and the surgeon. The patients refused to pay for their hospital admissions since it was caused by their surgeon going sailing and, ultimately, it cost the surgeon over $1000 in patient hospital bills and a lot of bad publicity in the community. He now discharges all of his patients in person.

An important point to note is that the surgeon was not the only one who received adverse publicity. The patients were also critical of the center for allowing this situation to occur. There were several qualified anesthesiologists on staff and present in the center who were just as capable as the surgeon to have made the discharge decision—had they been asked. Likewise, in units that are directed by a physician, the director should be prepared, when necessary, to perform the discharge evaluation. It is one thing for the surgeon to drop the ball, but the idea is not to compound the error. The center has an equal responsibility with the surgeon for the quality of all aspects of the medical care of its patients. It also has an interest in creating a favorable impression among patients and should encourage its staff to become deeply involved in patient care. The anesthesiologist is the most likely candidate for this role and should welcome the additional patient contact.

Physician Attendance. As stated in the preceding paragraph, there should always be at least one physician in attendance until the last patient has left the facility. In a hospital unit, the patients are generally given the telephone number of the physician on call as well as that of the hospital emergency room. Patients are told that, if for any reason, they need to be seen, then they should come to the emergency room. It is a good idea for the hospital unit to give the emergency room staff a list of that day's patients and their procedures so that the emergency room has access to their charts in the event they are needed.

In the freestanding unit, the discharge instructions should advise the patient of his or her surgeon's telephone number. It is important also to advise the patient that in the event of an acute problem, he or she should go to the nearest hospital emergency room. Since all freestanding units should have arrangements with a transfer hospital, that facility should also be identified by name, address, and telephone number. The transfer hospital should always have a list of the physicians who are on call for each date. If a patient should sustain a delayed reaction and no physician was available to attend to that patient, it would be very difficult to convince a jury that the center was providing an acceptable level of medical care.

WRITTEN DISCHARGE INSTRUCTIONS

The three most recurrent excuses for patient delay in responding to a significant postdischarge change of symptoms are that the patient:

Did not know what to look for
Did not know the significance of what he or she subsequently found
Did not know what he or she was supposed to do or whom to contact

With medications, the claim is that the patient did not know when to take it, when not to take it, and when to stop taking it. The great "nobody ever told me" defense is particularly troubling. The patient is one of many, and the attending physician may not be able specifically to recall the discussion several years later. The physician is then forced to rely upon what he or she "usually" tells patients. The plaintiff invariably contends that although the doctor may "usually" give patients those instructions, I did not receive them and, furthermore, had I received the "usual" instructions, I would have followed them and would not have been harmed. Many plaintiffs' lawyers believe that any time they can reduce a case to a credibility question and get the jury to weigh the absolute denial by the plaintiff against the defendant's qualified "I usually tell my patients," the odds are overwhelmingly in favor of the plaintiff. In that context, the use of written discharge instructions is strongly recommended. The center should retain a copy of what was given to the patient, and the patient should sign the center's copy acknowledging receipt of the instructions.

Some centers are now using a two-part form with carbon inserts. The top part contains general information such as emergency numbers or who to call. The bottom part contains general cautions about possible side-effects, symptoms to watch for and to report, and so forth. There is a space for the discharging physician to write in specific warnings and to detail discharge instructions about follow-up care and the use of prescribed medications. Some centers have developed separate instruction sheets tailored for each procedure done in the center, which are then attached to these general forms.

It is important that these discharge instructions, in whatever form they may be used, are written in a concise, clear manner. Obviously, they should be dated and the time of discharge noted. Even if this type of form is not used, the same information should be imparted to the patient, and this process should be memorialized by an appropriate entry in the patient's chart and signed by the patient acknowledging that these instructions were actually received and understood.

FOLLOW-UP PHONE CALL

There is no case that states that a follow-up phone call is legally required. However, the patient response to such a call is so great and its cost in time and dollars so small that the justification for the call is self-evident. The mere fact that somebody calls the patient just to see how he or she is recovering is a very positive statement about the center and its approach to medicine. It is not, however, just a great marketing and public relations scheme. The call should be documented on the chart. The recorder should note the patient's statement that "everything is fine" or "I'm doing great." On the other hand, if the patient is having some problem and has been reluctant or embarrassed to call, this affirmative reaching-out to the patient may elicit the problem and prompt potentially life-saving activity. Even if the nurse who may make the call simply reports the problem to the physician or puts the physician on the line to discuss the problem with the patient directly, serious harm can be avoided and you have a great record of concern to submit to a jury if you are ever sued thereafter. Such a call may keep you out of the suit altogether simply because the patient feels, as a result of that call, that the center, if not its surgeon, really cared about them.

The postdischarge call is a very human, considerate step that will pay dividends in a lot of ways. However, it must be done correctly. In other words, if the patient does relate a sign or symptom, it must be accurately recorded, reported to the surgeon or the anesthesiologist, and *acted upon*. Once you receive potentially adverse information, there is a corresponding duty to act upon it in a timely fashion. It may be advisable to have one physician, with no other duty assignment, available for a half-hour or so each day to discuss any positive feedback as it is elicited from the patients by the center personnel who are placing the calls. It would not take much time to call the patients from the previous day and check out their condition. The overwhelming majority will be doing great. They require little of the caller's time and none of the physician's. The few who may be having a problem warrant the additional time of the caller, and their complaints should be brought to the attention of a physician. Sometimes it is the little personal touches that bring patients back, encourage them to recommend the center to their friends, and help prevent a lawsuit. If your center does not now have a routine postdischarge call policy, think seriously about implementing one. By the way, get your friendliest, cheeriest people to make the calls, and tell them the importance of what they are doing.

Some centers use a postcard system of follow-up. This is not as legally helpful as the phone call. The phone call is instant and can be verified and noted in the chart. When you mail a postcard, there is no proof that it was ever received. Most mail surveys indicate that the response rate, whether it be for a sale, a donation, a cocktail party, or whatever, is very low. Assuming the patient got the postcard, an effective follow-up requires the patient either to initiate a call or to mail the card back. Many patients will be inclined to do neither. Follow-up by the patient in response to the postcard may require further time and expense.

Some institutions give the patient a postcard at the time of discharge. It is self-addressed and, of course, postage is prepaid. It lists several questions about the patient's health and recovery and about the overall performance of the center. This has increased the response rate and overcomes the argument that the patient never received the follow-up inquiry. It is critical, however, that all such returned cards be carefully reviewed and follow-up initiated where indicated.

Many anesthesiologists are secure about their expertise in providing anesthesia services to patients during inpatient sugical procedures. Ambulatory surgical centers, on the other hand, are a fairly recent innovation and present an entirely new environment and experience to most anesthesiologists. For this reason, it is extremely important to stress that all anesthesiologists who intend to practice in an ambulatory setting are responsible for acquiring an awareness of the medical and legal considerations involved in providing anesthesia services outside of an accredited hospital facility. An insightful comment by the editor of this book, Bernard V. Wetchler, aptly describes this responsibility: "As we [practicing anesthesiologists] spread our wings, we don't want them clipped."

The legal commentary that follows comprises twenty questions that were submitted by practicing anesthesiologists throughout the country. In this question-and-answer section, the authors have attempted to put the principles contained in the foregoing chapter into perspective and to demonstrate how these principles may be practically applied to everyday situations that commonly confront the practicing anesthesiologist.

Legal Commentary: 20 Questions

1   *We do not premedicate our patients. Some of our anesthesiologists insist on performing their preanesthesia interview after the patient is in the operating room on the table. Is this appropriate?*

☐   This procedure is not advisable for two reasons. The purpose of the preanesthesia interview is to obtain the information necessary to determine whether the patient is able to tolerate the anesthesia, to get a relevant past medical history of potential risks or complication factors, and to obtain an anesthesia-related informed consent. The dangers of the approach are that (1) there are too many diagnoses involved for the proper exercise of care and (2) the patient's consent may not be truly informed.

In considering the first danger, the patient is at the center, is psychologically geared to the procedure, the surgeon is standing near, ready to go, and all of the pressures of the situation on both you and the patient are to go ahead no matter what is elicited in the interview. The overwhelming tendency is to downplay any risk factor that might otherwise cause you, in a less-committed moment, to postpone the procedure. It may be infinitely easier to tell a patient in the waiting room while fully dressed that you are concerned about his or her history and want to get prior medical records and review them than to try to explain that to someone who has gone through the mental stress of getting undressed and being wheeled into the operating room. At this point, the patient just wants to get the procedure over with and go home. Just knowing that may induce you to forget about getting the prior chart or trying to track down the treating physician in another community. It is at this point that you start rolling the dice that the potential problem won't occur, but you are gambling with the patient's life, your reputation, and the center's financial survival. Give yourself and the patient a real opportunity—do not put either of you so far down the road that it becomes almost impossible to turn back. Let's get the interviews done outside the operating room as far in advance of surgery as is practically possible.

The second danger concerns the issue of consent. If you do not have the opportunity to even investigate the significant risk factors elicited during the interview, how can you give the patient a meaningful assessment of his or her particular risks in proceeding or not proceeding, benefits, alternatives, and so forth? Or, suppose you tell the patient that you are concerned about some risk-related aspect of his or her history. This inappropriately drops the decision to "go" or "no go" in the patient's lap. Many the plaintiff who has told the jury that when they went into that operating room they were so scared they didn't know who they talked to, who talked to them, what was said, or what it all meant. They were confused and disoriented and couldn't remember their name. Now, you try to tell the jury that you had a meaningful discussion, without pressure or coercion, with that patient and they made a calm, rational decision about the potential risks of losing their life or limb! Do you still want to do the interviews with the patient in the operating room lying on the table? No, you don't.

2   *What are our alternatives when Mr. Bradley insists on being admitted after an ambulatory surgery procedure?*

☐   If you have tried by persuasion and reassurance to get the patient to go home and he refuses, you have, practically speaking, no alternatives. You can't abandon the patient or ask the police to evict him as a trespasser. If anything should happen to that patient in the immediate postoperative period, you can imagine the patient's anger as he tells his lawyer that he insisted there was something wrong and that he needed to be admitted while you ignored him. The problem is that if you do admit him, how do you get him out of the hospital? This question highlights the necessity of educating patients in advance about ambulatory surgery. If the patient balks at the idea of coming in and going home the same afternoon, that patient shouldn't be treated in the ambulatory center. You are just asking for trouble by forcing that patient to have the surgery in a setting that he already views with hostility. That patient is a lawsuit waiting to happen—to you.

3a   *We require a responsible adult to accompany a patient home after general or regional anesthesia. One responsible adult came to get a patient after surgery and our recovery room nurse was sure he was drunk. What do we do?*

☐ To highlight this basic problem, let us assume the adult *was* drunk and causes an accident en route to the patient's home, thereby injuring the patient, or perhaps gets the patient home, passes out, and is unresponsive when the patient is seriously harmed as a result of a significant delay in getting needed medical attention. The first question a lawyer is going to put to you will be "what was the reason for insisting that a responsible adult come for the patient in the first place?" Your response has to be that after surgery, because of pain or the effects of the anesthesia or medication, patients are often unable to properly drive or otherwise care for themselves en route home. Also, you will state that it is advisable to have someone observe a patient to make certain there is no delayed complication, such as a hemorrhage or embolism. A third reason is that if such a complication should arise, this adult could expedite the patient's return to the hospital or center or call emergency services to the patient's assistance. If you analyze those responses (and others equally valid that you might add), how can you entrust an impaired patient to a drunk? Would you let such a person drive your children home in a school bus? You have a duty of due care for a patient's safety until he or she reaches home and is fully recovered (intellectually and functionally) from the procedure.

Placate the "drunk" as best you can, but get some other adult to come for the patient. If there is an adult at home who is rational, coherent, and cooperative but doesn't drive or can't come for the patient, then send the patient home in a cab or get some other family who lives nearby to drop the patient off on their way home. In some communities the local police force is willing to assist patients in getting to and from a hospital, and their assistance can be particularly helpful not only in getting the patient home but also in getting the drunk out of your center and to his own home.

We have been addressing the problem of an intoxicated person, but clearly the situation would be the same regardless of the cause of the mental or physical impairment.

3b *The responsible adult turned out to be a 17 year old. In our state, she would be considered a minor. Could she qualify as a responsible adult?*

☐ The term "responsible adult" has been used not so much to specify an age, but to indicate the requisite level of maturity and ability to care for the patient. There are many 17 year olds of both sexes who are more calm, caring, and intelligent than persons twice their chronological age. Statistically, however, judgment and maturity are correlated with advancing years and so, obviously, in doing one's preadmission planning, emphasis should be placed on finding a person over the age of 18. However, if no such person is available and the only one available to help the patient is a 17 year old who is capable, then there is no legal impairment to releasing the patient to the care of such a person. In many states, young people are granted drivers' licenses at 16 or 17 years of age. Many people at that age hold responsible positions in their schools or jobs. Many young women are married at that age and may have children of their own. It is, therefore, an individual judgment that should be made by the physician who knows the family or is persuaded by the parent that the teenager is capable of driving him or her home and is able to comprehend and carry out the discharge instructions. In that regard, the discharge instructions should be tailored to the degree of comprehension demonstrated by the young adult.

Obviously, the next question is, "If you accept an occasional 17 year old, then how about 16 or 15 or 14?" The line has to be drawn somewhere and, arbitrarily, we have drawn it at the age a particular state grants an unlimited driver's license. In that way, there is a driver who can get the patient home and has met certain tests of maturity and judgment. However, the mere fact that a person has a driver's license is not enough. There must be some additional evidence that the young person is capable of understanding the medical realities and is going to be present to assist the patient for the initial period following surgery.

4   *What are the legal implications of obtaining a pregnancy test on women of childbearing age scheduled for general anesthesia?*

☐   The implications cut both ways—that is, doing or not doing the test. If you do the test, there is the legal requisite that it be done early and accurately and that the patient be told of the significance of the test, particularly if it is positive for pregnancy. Obviously, greater care must be exercised for the safety of the fetus, particularly in the choice of anesthesia methods and the selection of preoperative or postoperative medications. This is especially true with respect to certain anesthetic agents administered during the first 3 months of pregnancy that can pass through the placental barrier and may have an effect on fetal development.

In elective cases, the choices may include not doing the procedure at all. The problem is, of course, easier when the female patient is an adult and can make the choice for herself. However, when the patient is a 14-year-old girl, the parent is still the legal guardian, and the parent cannot give an informed consent if there is any attempt to conceal the pregnancy from the parent. There are many physicians who believe there is no legal obligation to inform the parent in this situation, but that is simply not true in virtually all of the states, and the physician is placing his or her neck in the proverbial legal noose by participating in an operation on a pregnant teenager without notifying the parents of all the relevant facts. If a complication associated with the pregnancy occurs, there is no legal defense. The child is a minor incapable of consent, and the physician has committed a concealment from the parents. What do you think the attitude of the other parents who may be on the jury will be? Do you really believe that parents think it is acceptable for a physician to substitute his or her judgment for theirs as to what is best for their child?

What about not doing the pregnancy test? Is ignorance bliss? It never really is. Does that mean that every female patient between the ages of 13 and 55 has to have a pregnancy test? Clearly not. What is needed is to develop a protocol based on the nature of the proposed procedure and the type of anesthesia that is contemplated. For example, if an 18-year-old girl comes in to have a mole removed from her back under local anesthesia and is otherwise asymptomatic, it seems unnecessary to do a routine pregnancy test. On the other hand, if a woman in her 30s wants a tubal ligation and has been having some vague pelvic problems and has a slightly enlarged uterus, no one who is thinking clearly is going to operate or anesthetize that patient without first checking to see if she is pregnant. It comes down to the patient's history and symptoms, the proposed procedure, and whether it involves local, spinal, caudal, or general anesthesia. The worst possible case would be a procedure done under general anesthesia on a woman with an undiscovered pregnancy, and as a result of a complication associated with the pregnancy, the mother and child are both lost. How many expert witnesses could the plaintiff find to testify that you never submit a woman of childbearing age to that procedure under general anesthesia without first determining whether she is or is not pregnant? Can you think of one responsible physician who would testify on your behalf that there is no deviation from accepted standards in operating on or administering anesthesia to a pregnant woman when you didn't even endeavor to determine that factor in assessing this patient preoperatively?

5   *We require a pregnancy test on women of childbearing age (12–50) scheduled for general anesthesia. A 16-year-old girl is having a breast biopsy. Her mother is furious that we are going to do the test and refuses to have the test done. What do we do?*

☐   Nobody adopts rules in a rational society for the sake of rule-making alone. Obviously, if the center decides, upon due reflection, that the risk of pregnancy is sufficiently serious that all women should be evaluated before receiving anesthesia, then there is a valid reason for the rule. Once you admit that the risk justified the adoption of the rule, then how do you explain not following your own rules?

Patients are notorious for urging their physicians to accommodate them. They do not want to come back as frequently as they should be seen. They want renewable prescriptions so they do not have to make return visits. They do not want certain tests, but they want the surgery. Whose neck are they asking to be put in the noose? Not theirs! It is always the physician or the ambulatory center's staff that will ultimately be put in the position of trying to explain why they deviated from a rule they insisted upon enacting for the safety of their own patients.

Since there is no reason to have a rule and then ignore it or bend it to suit every patient, the solution is simple. Explain to the parent that the reason for the test is patient safety and you are not going to practice in what you consider to be an inappropriate manner. In short, if local anesthesia cannot be agreed upon as a satisfactory substitute for general anesthesia, then they either agree to the test or take themselves and their potential lawsuits to your competitor.

6   *A 6-year-old scheduled for a scar revision was accompanied by mother and grandmother. The mother signed the consent and left for work. Is a preanesthesia interview with grandmother and patient appropriate?*

☐   The key to this question is the second sentence. The mother apparently came into the facility and was given a preprinted form with no discussion and with no informed consent as that term is intended. An informed consent is not synonymous with signing a piece of paper. The written piece of paper is important only to the extent that it memorializes a discussion with the responsible person, in this case a parent, as to the relevant risks, alternatives, and benefits of the procedure, and indeed, with regard to the administration of anesthesia itself. Since there was no discussion with the mother, what good is the written paper?

If the subsequent discussion, which is entitled a preanesthesia interview, is intended to imply a meaningful discussion about the risks, alternatives, and benefits, then the question arises whether the grandmother is able to fully supply an accurate medical history and current health status about the child sufficient to enable the physician who is going to obtain the anesthesia consent to assess properly what the risks, benefits, and alternatives may be. If the grandmother indicates that she is not really certain about the child's health, medications the child is taking, past surgical history, the response of the child to prior anesthestic agents, and so forth, there is no way that a realistic evaluation of these factors can be undertaken.

Let's assume, however, that the grandmother is a terrific historian and gives very accurate information but then says, "I don't think that I should be the one to make the decision whether to go forward or not because of the risks that you have just outlined to me." In that situation, the parent is the one who must be notified and, thereafter, give consent. If the grandmother gives consent and an unfortunate event should occur, the facility may not be protected because the mother is going to state that she was the one who signed the consent form and that signifies that the facility understood that she was the one who had the right to consent or not to consent. Since the facility chose to obtain her signature without really giving her the explanation, it is at risk of the mother indicating after the tragic event that, had she been told of these risks, she would never have given consent. She will, no doubt, testify under those circumstances that the grandmother was left simply so someone could accompany the child home after the procedure and be with the child while awaiting the start of the procedure. She may indicate that she never gave permission for the grandmother to consent, nor did she indicate that the grandmother was an appropriate person for such an important discussion.

All of this points out the need to have meaningful discussions with the parent or parents of a minor in advance of the scheduled procedure so that you don't have situations like the one described here.

7   *What are the legal precedents regarding preoperative workup for an outpatient who is about to undergo a general anesthesia?*

☐   There are no general legal precedents that would serve as an adequate response to this question. It must be remembered that individual cases decide only the issues that pertain to the patient at hand. In short, each malpractice case stands for the proposition that under the particular circumstances existing at that time, applicable to that patient, and to that proposed procedure and anesthetic administration, certain acts or omissions were or were not negligent. However, as a result of an analysis of those cases, certain general guidelines have been developed.

Those general guidelines state that, for each individual patient, it is incumbent upon the surgeon who is going to operate on the patient and the anesthesiologist who is going to administer the anesthesia to conduct a thorough and appropriate physical examination germane to their specialty and to elicit a comprehensive medical history. They are also charged with the responsibility of conducting such inquiries, tests, studies, and so forth that are necessary to provide them with the information needed to fully assess the propriety of the proposed procedure and the propriety of administering a particular form of anesthesia or particular anesthetic agents to that patient. Obviously, those tests may differ from patient to patient. For example, a patient scheduled for a gynecologic procedure who has given a history of heavy menstrual bleeding may require hemoglobin and hematocrit tests. Another patient may disclose under occupational history that he or she works in an asbestos plant. That patient would be a candidate for a chest film. A patient who has history of tuberculosis may require not only a chest film, but also a skin patch test, in order to determine whether he or she is still suffering from active tuberculosis before exposing other patients and the operating room staff to the risk of contracting the disease. A pregnancy test may be appropriate for women of a certain age, but not those beyond the childbearing years. A history of an earache may require an ENT consultation. Complaints of burning urine would require a urinalysis and perhaps a culture. A history that disclosed the use of certain medications might indicate that it is not wise to use general anesthesia, and that the procedure should be done under either local or spinal anesthesia, or perhaps the procedure should be postponed for some additional period of time. An asthma history may be relevant for the purpose of determining whether certain additional tests should be carried out or whether the patient should simply be given anesthesia by mask rather than being intubated.

The usual reaction of most physicians to this approach is the suggestion that lawyers and judges are dictating the practice of medicine and mandating defensive medicine by imposing a burden to test, test, test, and test some more. The fallacy of this rebuttal is that it is not the lawyers or the judges who are getting sued when something happens to patients. If a particular test is suggested, and the physician chooses to gamble on what the tests might have disclosed by not ordering them, then that physician runs the risk of losing the gamble. The physician loses if he or she does not do the test and some injury occurs to the patient that could have been avoided if the tests had been done and the condition found. The physician elected to gamble not only with the patient's safety, but also with the physician's own legal safety by exposing himself or herself to a risk. The more you choose to play with fire, the greater the likelihood that you will be burned. If you are burned, it is because a patient has sustained a harm that could have been avoided if you had ordered the test for the patient. It is recognized and admitted that this adds to the cost of medical care in this country. However, if the patient sustains harm because, without consulting the patient, you elected not to undertake a particular test and the patient sustains a severe injury as a result thereof, do you really think the patient, in retrospect, is going to concur with your decision because you saved him or her $7.00 on a blood test? More likely than not, the patient will say, "If the doctor had told me that this risk could have been determined before the procedure by doing a simple $7.00 blood test, I would have paid for 50 such tests rather than have happen to me what did happen." Since the physicians don't pay for the tests, there is little likelihood that a jury observing a severely injured patient is going to have much regard for the physician who tried to save $7.00 by not doing a test when the patient is now stuck with a lifetime of medical expenses and pain and suffering. Applying a risk-vs.-benefit analysis to this situation yields the following result: the physician gambles by not doing the appropriate tests and gains nothing for himself or the patient if he wins, but on the other hand, if he loses, he has not only hurt the patient, but has also put himself and his own assets at risk.

The conclusion is, therefore, that if the patient's history, physical examination, or other data suggest that it may be appropriate to conduct a certain test in order to assess the risks, benefits, and alternatives for that patient fully and completely, then the tests should be ordered regardless of the fact that it may result in a temporary postponement of the procedure or an increase in the patient's overall cost of medical care.

8   *If something goes wrong after the patient leaves the unit, who is liable—the anesthesiologist who examined and signed the patient out, the unit, or the surgeon?*

☐   The answer to this question depends on what goes wrong. If the maloccurrence is related to failure to detect or observe signs or symptoms that would have warranted further evaluation of the patient rather than discharge, the anesthesiologist who examined and signed the patient out is responsible. If the anesthesiologist is an employee of the surgical center, the center is also responsible under an agency theory of liability. On the other hand, if the patient's complication results directly from some aspect of the surgeon's care (e.g., improper technique), the surgeon is solely liable (assuming he or she is not an employee of the surgical center), as long as the anesthesiologist who discharged the patient could not reasonably have been expected to detect the problem that eventually caused the patient's complication.

A few examples should serve to clarify this point further. A 35-year-old woman undergoes a surgical procedure involving the use of internal sutures. Shortly after the operation, she is lucid and her vital signs are recorded as normal. She is discharged by the examining anesthesiologist and returns home accompanied by a neighbor. Shortly after returning home, a number of the patient's internal sutures come loose, causing massive hemorrhaging. Who is liable? Any injury caused by loosening of the patient's sutures cannot be attributed to the anesthesiologist who discharged the patient, since he or she had no reason to know of the condition of internal sutures. Similarly, the surgical center is not liable, since none of its employees were responsible for the patient's harm. The surgeon, however, may be found liable for the woman's injuries if the sutures are shown to have come loose because he or she used improper technique in applying them.

A 40-year-old woman undergoes extensive oral surgery under general anesthesia at an ambulatory clinic. The woman tells the examining anesthesiologist that she feels "fine" and, based upon this representation, the physician discharges the patient in spite of her elevated blood pressure level and rapid pulse rate. The woman suffers a stroke later that evening. Who is liable? In this case, the anesthesiologist should not have discharged the patient without performing additional tests to determine the cause of the woman's rapid pulse and elevated blood pressure level. The anesthesiologist will be liable for the woman's injuries if it can be shown that failure to obtain additional tests in view of the woman's symptoms increased the risk that the patient would suffer a stroke. The surgical center will be held vicariously liable on an agency theory if the anesthesiologist is an employee of the center. The oral surgeon will incur no liability unless it can be shown that the operative procedure caused or contributed in some way to the woman's stroke.

9   *A patient has no one to escort her home and stay with her after surgery and general anesthesia. She insists on taking public transportation. Our policy requires that a responsible adult escort a patient home. What do we do? What are our options and our liabilities?*

☐   Before administering any anesthetic agent or performing any surgical procedure, the surgical center must ensure that the patient intends to meet all of the facility's preoperative and postoperative requirements. If a patient cannot assure the discharging physician that she is prepared to comply with the unit's discharge criteria, as in the example above, no treatment should be rendered.

The intention behind the requirement that a responsible adult accompany a patient home involves considerations of safety. A person's physical and mental capabilities are markedly reduced immediately after surgery under general anesthesia. The center's policy is obviously designed to ensure that a patient has available assistance, if needed, in traveling from the clinic to home, and to ensure that there is a responsible person on hand to alert medical authorities in the event that a complication should occur.

If a patient lies and says that a responsible adult will be present after the surgery to provide the required supervision, and no one shows up, the center is in a quandary. Every attempt should be made to induce the patient to call some responsible adult to accompany her home (e.g., relative, neighbor, friend). Failing this, the question arises whether the patient should be discharged on her own recognizance and, if so, whether the patient should be permitted to take public transportation home.

As a practical matter, when the patient is young and healthy, the surgery minor, and the postoperative course (vital signs, etc.) exemplary, such a discharge might be acceptable. However, this would be the exception rather than the rule. If a patient shows any questionable signs or symptoms, or if the patient is at risk of developing complications, admission to an inpatient facility is indicated. If the patient refuses admission and insists upon leaving the center without accompaniment, the person should be discharged only after signing out "against medical advice."

It is certainly unwise to allow an unescorted patient to take public transportation home after a surgical procedure under general anesthesia. If a complication should arise while the patient is on a public bus or subway, there would be no one available who would know that the person had just undergone surgery and who could communicate this information to medical personnel once they arrived on the scene. Consequently, much valuable time might be lost as the medical team attempted to ascertain what was wrong with the patient. Another major concern is the utter indifference of many individuals, especially in large cities, to the plight of others. Many people simply don't want to get involved and are unwilling even to summon medical aid for one obviously in need. Such conduct could easily result in the loss of valuable time in treating the patient's complication. These problems can be averted if the patient is escorted home by a responsible adult. Obviously, it is not the type of transportation the patient takes home that creates potential legal hazards; rather, it is the patient's returning home unescorted, regardless of what mode of transportation is used.

Surgical centers that routinely allow patients to leave unaccompanied, contrary to their own expressed regulations, are inviting trouble. In a malpractice action against such a surgical center, there is very little that can be raised to rebut the contention that the center's conduct was negligent since the patient was discharged without accompaniment, in direct contravention of the unit's own rules and regulations. Consequently, it is imperative that the facility abide by the guidelines it has established.

10 *A family practitioner who has no surgical privileges at our local hospital wants privileges in our freestanding unit to perform D&C and lump and bump removals. What are the legal hazards of the situation? Is there a difference if this is a hospital satellite unit or a proprietary freestanding unit?*

☐ Although there will be some dispute about this answer, the response is that a physician should not be permitted to do in a hospital satellite or a proprietary freestanding unit any procedure that he or she does not have privileges to do in a hospital. If the reputation, utility, and quality of ambulatory surgery are to be preserved, one of the first lines of defense has to be physician selection. If a physician does not have privileges to do a particular procedure at a hospital, then he or she should not be afforded such privileges in an ambulatory center. Ambulatory units require physicians of great skill and not second class physicians.

If privileges were given to the family practitioner, and during the course of a D&C procedure, the physician's technique produced a massive hemorrhage that he or she was not qualified to treat, or the hemorrhage required the performance of an emergency hysterectomy in order to save the patient's life and the physician was not trained in that procedure, a great tragedy could occur to the patient, and a lawsuit would undoubtedly be brought against the physician and the center. If the plaintiff was able to prove that the physician had been refused privileges at a number of hospitals because of inadequate skills, training, or education, but that the ambulatory center had granted privileges, there is then a strong likelihood that the center would be held liable for placing that physician in a position in which he or she could undertake such procedures on patients. From a legal standpoint, the safest course always has to be that only those physicians who have been found qualified to do procedures in a hospital setting should ever be given privileges to do them in an ambulatory center. Taking that equation one step further, we do not recommend giving a physician any greater privileges in terms of the complexity of procedures in the ambulatory center than that physician is authorized to do in the inpatient setting.

11   *Some physicians see their patients immediately postoperatively in the recovery room. They sign the patient out at that time and write a discharge when stable order. What liabilities can be incurred by the nurse who eventually discharges the patient? What liabilities can be incurred by the ambulatory surgical facility or institution? What liabilities can be incurred by the physician?*

☐   This procedure demonstrates poor medical practice and will, in almost all cases, serve as a basis for liability if the patient suffers harm. The nurse is put in the position of having to make a medical judgment as to whether or not the patient is stable. Many nurses do not have the requisite knowledge, training, and experience to make such a crucial determination. The responsibility for determining when a patient is stable is one that should be shouldered by the physician who has the ultimate responsibility for the patient's well-being.

In almost any case in which this practice results in harm to the patient, liability will be imposed on the surgical center for allowing the physician who uses the facility to adopt and implement such procedures. The center has tacitly given its approval to the practice by not putting a stop to it. Similarly, the surgeon will be liable for any harm to the patient caused by the nurse's decision to discharge. The surgeon has made the nurse his or her agent and has by implication condoned and acquiesced in any determination of the patient's stability that the nurse ultimately makes. The nurse may or may not be personally liable for harm suffered by the patient resulting from having made a decision to discharge. If the nurse determines the patient to be stable, and that judgment is in accordance with that of a "reasonable" nurse, then he or she is not liable for any harm the patient may have suffered. This situation might arise when the complication is one that would have been discerned by a physician but not necessarily by a nurse, since nurses do not have the advanced degree of education and training that physicians do. However, if the nurse discharged the patient and a "reasonable" nurse would not have, then the nurse would be personally liable for his or her own negligence, and the surgical center would also be liable on an agency theory since the nurse is its employee.

12 *In a freestanding unit (without a transfer agreement with a hospital), the responsible party leaves while the patient is in the recovery area. At discharge time, no one can be found to take the patient home. The patient now wants to leave unescorted. What are our alternatives?*

☐ The unit's policy of requiring all of its patients to be accompanied home by a responsible adult is a sound one. In fact, standards promulgated by the AAAHC provide that "patients [should be] discharged in the company of a responsible adult, except when they have not received anesthesia or when they have received unsupplemented local anesthesia." You can never be certain which patients will develop complications or how serious those complications might be. Although the responsible adult may not be able to render appropriate medical treatment to palliate the patient's complication, appropriate medical aid can be summoned immediately. If the patient were alone, no one would be available to summon such aid.

This discussion demonstrates that safety considerations underlie the patient accompaniment rule. It is clear that, in many cases, it is unsafe to release a patient without someone to escort him or her home. If a patient's escort has disappeared, an attempt should be made to obtain a substitute (e.g., friend, neighbor, relative, family member). If no substitute can be found, the patient should be examined very carefully, preferably by the operating surgeon. If the examining physician finds even the slightest untoward sign or symptom, the patient should be admitted to an inpatient facility.

If the patient objects to inpatient admission, there is no way that he or she can legally be forced to stay. However, if a patient insists upon leaving, the patient should be made to sign out "against medical advice." Before discharge, the risks involved in leaving under such circumstances should be fully explained to the patient, and the patient's chart should reflect this discussion. In instances such as this where the patient discharges himself or herself, the patient has assumed responsibility if complications later develop, and the physician and surgical center have insulated themselves from liability.

Even if the patient does agree to admission to an inpatient facility, there may be a problem, since the facts of this question indicate that the ambulatory center does not have a transfer agreement with a hospital. Since this is not an emergency case, there exists the possibility that the patient might have difficulty in gaining admission to a local hospital if it were nearing its patient capacity limit. Situations such as this should not be left to chance. It is recommended that all freestanding ambulatory facilities provide for implementation of a transfer agreement with a local hospital to ensure that their patients will have ready access to an inpatient facility if the need arises.

13 *During the preanesthesia interview, the anesthesiologist discovers that the patient has no idea of the nature of the anticipated surgical procedure, its risks, benefits, or alternatives. Is there any legal risk to the unit or the anesthesiologist in going forward with the procedure?*

☐ Yes. A physician does not have any right to touch a patient unless that patient has given an informed consent to being touched. Informed consent means that the patient has been fully briefed and understands the nature of the anticipated surgical procedure, its risks, benefits, and alternatives. As a necessary adjunct of surgery, the patient must be given anesthesia. In order to understand the anesthesia risks, the patient has to relate them to the surgical risks and vice versa. Once the anesthesiologist becomes aware that the patient has not given an informed consent, then he or she should refuse to go forward with the procedure until the patient has been so informed.

In a nonemergency situation, the procedure should be postponed in order to give the surgeon an opportunity to hold an informed consent conference with the patient. If there is an emergency, the informed consent discussion may have to be held with the patient as soon as possible. If the emergency is such that no delay is possible, then the consent is deemed to be waived by virtue of the emergency and, obviously, in order to protect the patient, the procedure should be accomplished as soon as possible. However, in the case of nonemergency, elective surgery, the anesthesiologist is best advised to report the situation to the surgeon and to decline to administer anesthesia to the patient until a truly informed consent has been obtained.

14 *While assisting one of our patients to get ready for surgery, the nurse observed the patient take some medication and return the container to her purse. When she questioned the patient, the patient assured her that it was just a "nerve pill," and refused to disclose what it was or who had prescribed it. The nurse reported this information to the anesthesiologist. The anesthesiologist said we were legally protected in accepting the patient's description of the medication and ordered the procedure to go forward. Were we legally protected under these circumstances?*

☐ No. This patient is about to undergo a surgical procedure under anesthesia. The purpose of obtaining an informed consent from both the surgical standpoint and the anesthesiology standpoint is to fully assess all of the risks, benefits, and alternatives associated with the surgical and anesthetic procedures to be undertaken. Those risks may be directly affected by whatever medication the patient just put into her mouth. If that medication is contraindicated with one of the anesthetic agents, there may be a severe allergic response or the effect of either one of those drugs may be potentiated by the other. If the drug the patient just took has an effect on cardiac output or may otherwise depress respiratory functions, then that drug may pose a significant risk attendant to the procedure. Therefore, without knowing the nature of the drug, its dosage, and how many more such "nerve pills" the patient took in the last 2 or 3 hours, how can one say that there has been an accurate assessment of the risks?

Suppose the pill was, in fact, nitroglycerin and the patient was suffering from angina that had not heretofore been disclosed. This may be a very relevant piece of information that the physician should know before undertaking either to operate on or to anesthetize that patient. Indeed, one of the first questions that should be asked of all patients who come to the ambulatory center is, "What medications, if any, have you taken in the last two weeks?" If the patient is unsure, then the name of the physician who prescribed the medication should be obtained and contact established with that physician. If the physician indicates that he or she has not seen the patient in a substantial period of time and was unaware that the patient was even taking that medication, then further caution has to be exercised, and it may necessitate putting the procedure off until such time as the patient makes a complete disclosure and the actual medications are reviewed and assessed.

If you need horror stories, the following case may be appropriate. A dentist who had substantial experience in extracting impacted wisdom teeth under sedation and nitrous oxide was performing such a procedure. Shortly after the extraction was begun all of the patient's respiratory functions ceased. Attempts to revive the patient were unsuccessful, and the patient was pronounced dead on arrival. At autopsy, the toxicology report indicated that the patient had taken enough sedatives to put eight insomniacs to sleep for at least 48 hours. When that medication was superimposed upon the effects of the other anesthetic agents administered in the dentist's office, the result was predictable and fatal. The award that was entered against the dentist was in seven figures simply because, before anesthetizing the patient, neither the dentist nor the nurse-anesthetist had ever questioned the patient about any other medications that might have been taken.

15 *Our freestanding surgical center does not presently have a transfer agreement with a hospital. However, all of our surgeons have admitting privileges at local hospitals, and we have never encountered any problems with the admission of our patients to the emergency room of a local hospital when an emergency has developed. Do you think we need a transfer agreement in this situation?*

☐ Yes. Even in this situation, a transfer agreement is necessary. The emergency cases aren't usually going to present a problem. In an emergency, such as cardiac arrest or respiratory failure, the emergency room of any hospital will always take the patient in.

However, suppose a patient wakes up after an operation and has a flaccid paralysis of an extremity. Clearly, this person is going to require observation, monitoring, intensive care, and possibly rehabilitation therapy. An ambulatory surgical center is not equipped to provide these services. The patient requires admission to a hospital to be properly treated and cared for. A surgical center must have some type of agreement with an inpatient facility so that patients who do not require immediate emergency care but still need observation, monitoring, and treatment can be admitted. Although the surgeons at the ambulatory center may have admitting privileges at a nearby hospital, in a nonemergency situation, the hospital can elect to reject admission of the patient. This situation will never develop if the center and the hospital have a preexisting transfer agreement.

A brief example should serve to clarify this discussion. Suppose a patient undergoes afternoon surgery and is admitted to the recovery room. Upon observation, it is noted that his or her blood pressure remains low. Very possibly, this patient is going to be fine. However, the patient's situation requires cardiac monitoring for several hours. The surgical center closes at 5:00 P.M., so the patient can't remain there. The center, in this situation, requires the use of a facility where he or she can be monitored and observed until recuperation. A transfer agreement with a local hospital is the perfect solution. Since it's worked out in advance, no time is spent worrying about which hospital the patient should be taken to, who's going to take care of the patient, and whether or not he or she will even be admitted. The transfer agreement provides an extra margin of safety for both the patient and the center and is indicated from both a medical and legal standpoint.

16 *One of our surgeons insists on using her own instruments and her own scrub nurse. We do not know the nurse's qualifications or the method of sterilization used by the doctor for her instruments. If it can be documented that these are not the center's equipment or personnel, are we legally protected?*

☐ You may or may not be. However, before worrying about whether or not you are legally protected, note that as we have repeatedly emphasized, all accrediting organizations insist that ambulatory surgical centers develop their own criteria, regulations, personnel qualifications, and so forth. It is the center's right, duty, and obligation to make certain that no one comes onto its premises to do anything that has not been previously reviewed and approved by the center. Under the circumstances suggested by this question, it is the center's prerogative and obligation to advise the surgeon that she will either provide proof of her scrub nurse's qualifications or perform procedures without her. If the center is satisfied by virtue of the nurse's background, qualifications, and experience that she is qualified, they are still entitled to a probationary period during which she can be observed by one of the center's scrub nurses in order to make certain that she is currently qualified. Once that has been accomplished, then it may be appropriate to permit this physician to use her own scrub nurse.

The same is true of her instruments. If the physician can document to the center's satisfaction that the method of sterilizing instruments meets their standards, then it may be appropriate for the physician to sterilize and use her own instruments during the procedures. However, this matter should be documented. In other words, a letter should be sent to the surgeon indicating that she has represented and warranted to the hospital that she will sterilize instruments in a certain manner, and that she assumes full responsibility for those instruments and their sterilization. The letter should also indicate that if the center is sued because it is determined that her instruments were not appropriately sterilized, the center will seek indemnification for any sums it is compelled to pay.

17 *Mr. Anderson was scheduled for an early morning procedure in our ambulatory surgical unit and was told to stay NPO from midnight on. On the morning of the procedure, the patient disclosed that he had not done so. What are our options? Would your answer be any different if the patient had traveled 40 or 50 miles to the center for the procedure?*

☐ Initially, it should be stressed that all patients who have been instructed to stay NPO must be carefully questioned in order to determine whether they have followed these instructions. Many patients do not realize the importance of remaining NPO (often because it has not been stressed by the surgeon or anesthesiologist), and will have a bite to eat or something to drink on the morning of the procedure. These same patients are often reticent to volunteer to the anesthesiologist that they have had something to eat or drink because they don't want to be chastised for failing to follow instructions. In many cases, it is only through careful questioning that individuals who have failed to follow NPO instructions are identified. Keep in mind that unless these individuals *are* identified, this significant risk factor can't even be taken into account in deciding whether or not to go forward with the procedure.

Throughout this chapter, we have stressed the necessity of closely following the procedures and regulations that have been adopted by the center to ensure patient safety. It is these procedures and regulations that will be the standard by which the anesthesiologist is judged. The policy of NPO from midnight on has obviously been implemented to prevent regurgitation and subsequent aspiration during the procedure. If Mr. Anderson discloses that he has failed to remain NPO from midnight, and the anesthesiologist proceeds in spite of this, what justification does he or she have if, during the procedure, Mr. Anderson suffers a sudden airway obstruction and subsequent injury as a result of regurgitation of the stomach contents?

There is no hard and fast rule that can be applied to every situation. In each instance, various factors must be weighed and balanced before deciding whether to go through with the procedure as scheduled. What is the patient's present state of health? Is the contemplated procedure major or relatively minor? Is regional or general anesthesia to be administered? How do patients normally react to the anesthetic agent that is to be administered? Will the patient be intubated? Is the procedure elective? What did the patient ingest? Was it a trickle of water after brushing his teeth, a sip of coffee, a glass of orange juice, a donut, or an entire breakfast of bacon and eggs with toast? When was the food or liquid ingested?

Once an assessment of all of these factors (as well as other equally valid factors you might add) is undertaken, an intelligent and reasoned medical determination can be made of the propriety of proceeding with the surgery. If there is any lingering doubt about whether complications might develop (e.g., the patient is elderly and in poor health, the patient consumed a large breakfast 1 hour before the scheduled surgery) cancel the procedure. It is far better to cause the patient the minor inconvenience of returning for the surgery on another day than to subject him or her to the possibility of permanent injury and yourself to the possibility of entanglement in a web of legal woes.

The answer to this question would not be any different even if Mr. Anderson traveled 50 miles to get to the ambulatory surgical center. This factor should have no bearing whatsoever on the decision of whether or not to go through with the procedure. A patient who has traveled 2 hours to the center should be evaluated in the same fashion as the one who has had to travel only 2 minutes. Inconvenience to the patient in cancelling a scheduled procedure is simply not a relevant consideration in the medical decision-making process of whether or not a surgical procedure can be safely performed.

18 *Recently, we had an intraoperative episode of severe hypotension and the patient is currently in an intensive care unit with signs of residual neurologic damage. The nurses in the ICU have told us the explanation that was given to the family, and it does not comply with the facts. Is there any obligation on the part of the nurses, anesthesiologists, or the administration to contradict the surgeon and to provide more accurate information? Can they legally bypass the surgeon and go to the family directly?*

☐ There are relatively few cases that deal with this issue because it is not often that an attending surgeon would withhold information from a patient's close relatives about the cause of that patient's medical complications. However, the courts that have reviewed this type of situation have held that a duty of disclosure is mandated based upon the fiduciary relationship between the health care provider and the patient.

From the standpoint of the nurses and the anesthesiologist, how should this difficult situation be approached? Clearly, a scenario should never develop where a number of different people approach the patient's family and give them discrepant versions as to how the injury to their relative actually occurred. While there is no legal barrier preventing the patient's health care providers from bypassing the surgeon and making this disclosure to the relatives, it is probably not the best solution to the problem. The family is likely to be overly distraught and upset and will, undoubtedly, want to sue everyone in sight. It would be much more prudent for the treating nurses or physicians to confront the surgeon with the facts and give him or her the opportunity to meet with the family again to explain what really happened. If the surgeon rejects this option, the administration should be informed, and it is then incumbent upon them to meet with the family to apprise them of all the relevant facts.

Under no circumstances should the anesthesiologist or treating nurses cooperate with the surgeon in the cover up. Aside from the legal ramifications of incurring joint liability with the surgeon, ethical considerations mandate disclosure of the facts to the administration.

19 *We recently terminated the operating privileges of a surgeon at our center because, on repeated occasions, he arrived in an impaired condition. We know from his application that he has operating privileges at several local hospitals. We have no legal or financial relationship with those hospitals. We also have no information of any improper conduct at those hospitals. I am an anesthesiologist and medical director of our center. Do I have a legal obligation to communicate our experience with those hospitals? Am I protected from a civil suit if I do so? On the other hand, can we be compelled to give our records to other institutions if we decide not to voluntarily turn this data over to them? What are my obligations or liabilities? What are the center's liabilities and obligations?*

☐ The accreditation agencies mandate that there be ongoing peer review in the ambulatory center. The center, in that sense, is no different than a hospital and bears a responsibility to make certain that the patients who come to that center receive quality medical care from competent physicians. When the center determined that this surgeon was not competent and therefore not entitled to operating privileges at the center, it was carrying out a peer review function that is protected in many states by statutes that give the peer review personnel and the center not only confidentiality as to their records, but also a qualified exemption from being sued. Those protections, however, must be kept in the context of the center that is exercising them. If the center acts to protect its patients in this way, the protections given to it under the peer review statutes have been properly invoked. However, there is nothing in these statutes that compels an institution to take on a prosecutorial role against the physician because he may be practicing at some other institution. Accordingly, a director of the ambulatory center should not voluntarily undertake to contact those other hospitals. This answer would be modified in a situation in which the ambulatory center was a satellite unit of a hospital that had a common staff and a common peer review program.

The situation would be altered, however, in the event that the medical director of the center is subsequently contacted by a peer review coordinator at the other hospital. The medical director would be protected in that event if he or she were to attend a regularly scheduled peer review committee meeting at the other hospital and in the course of that meeting respond fairly, accurately, and without malice about the ambulatory unit's experience with the surgeon. If the medical director of the center undertakes to conceal the surgeon's problems, he or she may then be creating liability for the center if that surgeon's privileges are preserved as a result of the concealment, and some patient is subsequently injured by this impaired surgeon. The point is, however, that the communication expressed by the medical director of the center should be an integral part of the peer review program at the institution that is raising the issue. The information communicated should be factual and objectively supported. Rumor or innuendo is fair neither to the surgeon nor to the investigating hospital.

There is no justification for turning over any records of your facility that may pertain to your patients. The patients have a right to their privacy, and even though these records may be requested because of a peer review investigation at another institution, it is not appropriate, without the consent of the patient, to turn those records over. If the request for records pertains to the activities of your peer review program and its investigations and findings about the impaired surgeon, it would be appropriate to turn those records over, but again, only as part of a regularly scheduled peer review meeting and only after the center is satisfied that these records are objective, complete, and factual. It would be important, however, to ask the hospital that is requesting your records whether they have any provision in their bylaws or whether they have any specific authorization from the surgeon that gives them the right to contact other institutions to determine the physician's competence. It may be that the hospital does have a specific regulation whereby a physician, in consideration of being given staff privileges, gives an authorization to the hospital to make such investigations from whatever sources it may deem appropriate. In that instance, the center should request a copy of such bylaw or authorization and would then be protected by the physician's authorization in turning over its materials.

Another aspect of this question is, of course, the nature of the impairment and whether there is any legally imposed obligation of disclosure. For example, there may be some regulations that would require a disclosure depending upon the nature of the impairment. If the physician is impaired as a result of the use of narcotics he has misappropriated from the center, the federal drug authorities may require disclosure of this information. Similarly, if the physician is impaired as a result of epilepsy and is driving an automobile, there is a requirement, in many states, that a disclosure be made to the state department of motor vehicles in order that they may terminate the person's driving privileges. Generally, however, the safest rule is that, in the absence of a mandated disclosure, the hospital or the center should complete its own peer review and take such actions as it deems appropriate based on its data. It should not volunteer the data to others absent an obligation of disclosure, but, if contacted and appropriately requested, it should participate, by making available under the circumstances set forth in this response, whatever data it has about the physician's ability to treat patients appropriately and safely.

Note the use of the phrase "absent an obligation of disclosure" in the preceding sentence. Some medical societies at a state or local level have imposed an ethical obligation on their members to act affirmatively to identify suspected impaired physicians. Some state licensing boards are considering obligatory reporting of suspected impaired physicians, but the legality of such requirements, unless they specifically afford legal immunity from suit to the reporting physician, is questionable. The requirements in your community, whether imposed by ethical considerations or by regulations, should be ascertained and followed.

20 *One of our surgeons refuses to have his patients sign a written consent form. He claims that he heard a "lawyer/commentator" state that they are not worth the paper they are written on in a court of law. Do you agree? What makes a written consent form enforceable?*

☐ If the only consent in a case consists of handing a patient a written consent form with the instructions that they sign it and date it, then the legal commentator made a valid point. The purpose of the written consent form is to document that there has, in fact, been a discussion with the patient and that certain specific areas were discussed with the patient as evidenced in the written consent form. The patient's signature is intended to document not only that they participated in a discussion, but also that there was an opportunity to read and review the contents of the written consent form, which may very well supplement and further highlight what took place in the discussion with the patient. The written consent form is, therefore, not the informed consent, but rather the evidence of the informed consent.

The written consent form should identify the physician who had the discussion and provide an opportunity for that physician to record some of the principal risks, alternatives, and benefits that were discussed. Many institutions require the nurse to witness the signature. If the point of this policy is to verify that it was this particular patient who signed the consent form, there is no objection to that procedure. On the other hand, giving a pad of written consent forms to a nurse and instructing him or her to have every patient sign them is utterly meaningless. The nurse, no matter how competent, is not deemed under the law to be an appropriate person to obtain an informed consent. It is the surgeon or other physician who is going to do the procedure or to administer the anesthesia who has the obligation, by virtue of superior knowledge and training in that particular specialty, to inform the patient of the risks, benefits, and alternatives and to respond to the patient's inquiries about those areas and to then make certain that, when the patient agrees to proceed with surgery, the consent is voluntarily and knowingly made.

The direct response to the last question is that the discussion of the physician with the patient as capsulized or memorialized in the written consent form is what makes the consent form meaningful and therefore enforceable in an action that may thereafter be brought by the patient.

3
Selection

Fredrick K. Orkin, M.D., M.B.A.

Everything has been thought of before, Goethe suggested, but the problem is to think of it again. And so it is with anesthesia for ambulatory surgery. However, only relatively recently have we come to recognize the importance of the selection of appropriate surgical procedures, patients, patient preparation, and equipment, among other considerations, in the ambulatory setting. This chapter surveys this important but illusive and evolving aspect of ambulatory anesthesia care, in what now constitutes the newest and most rapidly developing subspecialty in clinical anesthesiology. Rather than present a series of static lists relating to the various selection decisions, this chapter emphasizes approaches that will enable the reader to respond to the challenges of adapting his or her own practice to the ambulatory setting as it evolves. Selection decisions in the choice of anesthetic techniques and drugs, personnel, and facility design are discussed in greater detail throughout the rest of this book.

Selection and the Evolution of Ambulatory Anesthesia

FROM ANTIQUITY TO 1900

Well before the first surgical procedures were undertaken, rudimentary ambulatory anesthesia was practiced. The Ancients knew that alcohol and opium derivatives could produce unconsciousness as well as pain relief. Physical methods of producing anesthesia, such as strangulation and a blow to the head, were used routinely in biblical Egypt prior to circumcision, one of the earliest surgical procedures. These primitive anesthetics and the first applications of ether anesthesia by Crawford Long in 1842 and William Morton in 1846 all involved *ambulatory* patients.[73] Necessarily, the emergent nature of most of the surgery and ignorance about pathophysiology and the pharmacology of anesthetics precluded consideration of selection in any aspect of the ambulatory surgical experience. With the introduction of aseptic surgical techniques in the last quarter of the 19th century, modern surgery began to develop and, simultaneously, to become an activity for which patients would be hospitalized for recuperation as well as for the surgery itself.

TWENTIETH-CENTURY PIONEERS

Yet, even as modern surgery developed during the past hundred years, several courageous physicians laid the foundations for ambulatory surgery and, quite remarkably, offered some insight on the importance of selection of appropriate patients and facilities.

Against a tide of peer criticism, James Nicoll, a pediatric surgeon in Glasgow, noted in 1909 that the successful completion of 8988 ambulatory procedures during the preceding decade had convinced him that "the treatment of a large number of the cases at present treated indoor constitutes a waste of the resources" and "we keep similar cases in adults too long in bed." He advised that infants and young children be operated on preferentially in the ambulatory setting because, "with their wounds closed by collodion or rubber plaster, [they] are easily carried home in their mothers' arms, and rest there more quietly." Decades ahead of his time, he stressed that "sucklings and young infants should remain with their mothers after operation." As a corollary, he continued, "no children's hospital can be considered complete which has not, in the hospital itself or hard by, accommodation for a certain number of nursing mothers whose infants require operation"; he provided "a small house" nearby for postoperative nursing.[101]

Only 7 years later, Ralph Waters, then an itinerant anesthesiologist, opened the Down-Town Anesthesia Clinic in Sioux City, Iowa, the prototype of the modern independent freestanding surgical facility. Following a morning of "hospital work," he provided anesthesia services and surgical facilities to suit local dentists and patients who "objected to going to the hospital because of the time and expense involved," as well as surgeons who were "also anxious to establish extra hospital clinical facilities." He made "careful physical examination on all suspicious risks," noting that a "sphygmomanometer and stethoscope are constantly present and frequently used." In particular, he noted that "the well trained and alert assistant is useful [for she] often warns me that the next patient is short of breath or shows some other evidence of needing careful examination."[134]

AMBULATORY SURGICAL CARE IS REDISCOVERED

Despite these favorable early experiences, ambulatory surgery remained largely dormant until the mid-1960s, when specialized units were established at the University of California Medical Center in Los Angeles[24] and George Washington University Medical Center in Washington, D.C.[79] In the late 1960s, the concept of the independent freestanding surgery center was reborn with the establishment of the Dudley Street Ambulatory Surgical Center in Providence, Rhode Island, and the Surgicenter in Phoenix, Arizona. The latter facility has distinguished itself by having treated almost 100,000 patients without a death, providing a stimulus for the establishment of some 237 other freestanding centers by the end of 1983, where 371,513 procedures have been completed.[44] The most recent complete national survey on ambulatory surgery (American Hospital Association, 1980) revealed that 70% of hospitals in metropolitan areas were performing ambulatory surgery, although not necessarily within an organized program. In all, the ambulatory surgery in these hospitals accounted for about one-sixth of the 19 million surgical procedures performed in this country.[7] Currently, 88% of all nonfederal short-term general hospitals provide ambulatory services, and about one-quarter of surgery in the United States is undertaken on an ambulatory basis.

Equally dramatic developments account for the recent rediscovery and growth of ambulatory surgery. These include improved anesthetic drugs, growing public interest in participating in personal health care, growing acceptance by surgeons, endorsement and encouragement by industry and health insurers, and the demonstrated safety of surgery in the ambulatory environment. In turn, a most important ingredient in ensuring patient safety and overall quality of care in ambulatory surgery is careful selection of the patient and surgical procedure.

General Considerations

SELECTION DECISIONS AS A PROBLEM IN MEDICAL DECISION MAKING

The often elegant basic medical sciences are frequently found wanting in the more complex, less structured clinical setting. Moreover, medical knowledge pertaining to a particular patient management problem is usually incomplete. Yet, decisions must be made. The physician necessarily makes medical decisions by blending the available information with clinical judgment and even some degree of intuition. Once decisions are made, however, the clinical outcomes of those decisions are rarely evaluated formally, and the opportunity to improve similar decision making in the future is lost. As a result, much dogma is carried along in medical practice, codified in authoritative statements that are based either on clinical suspicion, anecdotes, or poorly designed studies.

As in other aspects of health care, dogma exists in ambulatory anesthesia care but, through careful analysis of clinical experience, can be replaced by more rational methods of making decisions. For example, consider postoperative nausea and vomiting, certainly one of the more common minor problems associated with surgery and anesthesia, but one that can delay the patient's discharge home and sometimes prompt inpatient admission.[12,99] Dogma would suggest that even small doses of droperidol, a long-acting, major tranquilizer that also happens to be an antiemetic, are contraindicated in the ambulatory setting because its long-lasting sedation would synergize with that from general anesthesia and delay the patient's return home. Yet, careful clinical trials document that droperidol in low dosage not only treats nausea and vomiting effectively either without materially delaying discharge[2] or actually enabling earlier discharge of the patient.[137] Similarly, ketamine, another long-acting drug that dogma would suggest is contraindicated, has been shown to be satisfactory (although hardly ideal) for ambulatory anesthesia care when given by well-monitored infusion.[138] These studies suggest generally that *how* we do things, rather than *what* we do, is critically important in ambulatory anesthesia. Until more careful analysis of actual clinical practice is undertaken, most of what we do will continue to be dogma.

SELECTION AND COST-EFFECTIVE PRACTICE

Achieving more cost-effective practice has been one of the potent stimuli in the development of ambulatory surgery. Apart from the obvious and considerable savings in the hotel component of hospital care, a night or two in the hospital, little attention has been paid to the cost effectiveness of this mode of care to society at large. Surely, on an individual case basis, it is less expensive to perform a given procedure in the ambulatory setting. However, unless the hospital bed that the given patient would have used is left empty, the health care system as a whole experiences *greater* costs because the system has effectively been enlarged. That is, in tandem with the remarkable growth in ambulatory surgery, the per capita rate of surgery in the United States has increased, resulting in a greater overall number of surgical procedures (and medical care cost to the society).[115] Thus, true savings from ambulatory surgery can come only from a global effort to contain, if not shrink, the health care system. Some appropriate initiatives include a commensurate reduction in inpatient surgical caseloads through bed closures, conversion of some acute-care beds for chronic care, and moratorium on, or at least reduction in, future facility expansion.[38] Nonetheless, instead of waiting for what may be slow to occur, it is incumbent upon each of us to make selection decisions that put as much surgery as possible in the ambulatory setting without compromising quality of care.

SELECTION DECISIONS AND ACCREDITATION STANDARDS

The delivery of quality care in the ambulatory surgery setting imposes the need for various selection decisions that are embodied in the unit's policies and procedures, which are discussed in this and succeeding chapters. The policies and procedures, like those relating to other institutional services, must meet the requirements of external agencies that accredit the institution. Standard III of the accreditation program for hospital-affiliated ambulatory surgical services set forth by the Joint Commission on Accreditation of Hospitals (JCAH) specifically addresses selection decisions relating to surgical procedures, anesthesia care, and postoperative recovery care, as follows:[65]

Surgical procedures
   Types that may be performed
   Locations where they may be performed
Anesthesia care
   Types of anesthesia services provided
   Locations where they may be provided

Transportation
  Preoperative and postoperative transportation
Preoperative patient evaluation and preparation
  Definition of appropriate history, physical examination, and required
    laboratory and x-ray evaluation
  Method of intervention when designated evaluation and preparation is
    incomplete
Postoperative care
  Guidelines for postanesthesia recovery care
  Role of family members in care
  Discharge criteria
  Responsible adult to accompany patient home
  Written instructions for follow-up care and emergency physician contact

Similar JCAH accreditation requirements have been promulgated for independent freestanding ambulatory surgery centers.[64] Voluntary accreditation standards for both freestanding and hospital-affiliated ambulatory surgical programs have also been prepared by the Accreditation Association for Ambulatory Health Care (AAAHC).

EQUIVALENCE OF AMBULATORY AND INPATIENT POLICIES
The JCAH leaves to the discretion of the institution's medical staff and administration how each requirement will be met. However, the policies and procedures set forth for a hospital-affiliated ambulatory surgery program must be consistent with those applicable to inpatients undergoing the same procedures in the given facility.

LOCAL DEFINITION OF APPROPRIATENESS
Regardless of the type of ambulatory unit and accreditation sought, the underlying goal of the policies and procedures is the maintenance of patient safety and quality of care. Apart from the general principle that ambulatory surgical care be equivalent to its inpatient counterpart (if any exists), the accreditation process generally leaves the explicit requirements to the facility's professional staff. Thus, each facility is given the freedom to define the laboratory evaluation, among other aspects of the ambulatory surgical care, that is "appropriate" to the planned surgical procedure and anesthetic for a patient in a given state of health.

Other, more specific aspects of accreditation standards are discussed in this chapter (e.g., evaluating medical staff credentials, utilization review, quality assurance) and in subsequent chapters that discuss anesthesia care of adults and children, and postanesthesia care unit management (e.g., postoperative care, role of the family, discharge criteria).

Surgical Procedures

Lists of surgical procedures appropriate to the ambulatory unit abound. Typically, each year the lists grow as we continue to discover that we have not yet reached the boundaries of acceptability. The current one-quarter of total surgery that is presently undertaken in the ambulatory setting is expected to swell to 40% by the end of this decade.[25,32,34] As remarkable as this prediction seems, that fraction of surgery is *already* performed on an ambulatory basis in some localities, for example, Salt Lake City*. Moreover, for specified procedures and groups of procedures (e.g., dilatation and curettage, breast biopsy), a far greater fraction is undertaken without the traditional overnight hospital stay.

GENERAL CHARACTERISTICS OF ACCEPTABLE PROCEDURES

Given the rapid evolution of ambulatory surgical care, setting forth even the characteristics of acceptable procedures is hazardous. Any set of specific characteristics is likely to seem as "conservative" in a few years as those established by the then-pioneers only a decade ago. Nonetheless, recognizing that today's characterization of acceptability is likely to be short-lived, we may note that the most appropriate procedures are *generally* those that are accompanied by minimal blood loss and physiologic derangements and are associated with minimal, or at least readily controlled, postoperative pain, nausea and vomiting, and other postoperative complications. Prohibitions relating to durations of surgery (e.g., performing only procedures lasting less than 60–90 minutes) no longer appear warranted, particularly because the relationship between anesthesia time and recovery time is weak.[87] Moreover, in an efficient ambulatory unit, procedures generally do not lend themselves to lengthy teaching or performance by trainees.

It must be recognized, however, that the actual list of "acceptable" procedures in a given ambulatory unit is established in an evolutionary process, with accretion of procedures often in a "trial and error" fashion. On a daily basis, the medical director of the unit must decide which procedures (and which patients) are "appropriate" for the unit, given its equipment, staff and their capabilities, ability and reliability of the given surgeon, and medical condition of the particular patient. Over the long term, the medical director, in consultation with the administrative body to which he or she reports (e.g., ambulatory unit advisory committee, operating room committee), can modify the spectrum of permissible surgery, on the basis of periodic quality assurance studies and other mechanisms (see the section at the end of this chapter).

CLASSIFICATION OF SURGICAL PROCEDURES

In the past, surgical procedures have been categorized simply as major or minor. Although subjective, this classification is no longer useful in classifying the diversity of surgery that is currently undertaken in a variety of settings. A *functional* classification and terminology of ambulatory surgical settings is presented in Chapter 1. A similar functional classification of surgical procedures is needed. At the outset, one must recognize that procedures cannot be categorized according to the anesthetic technique used or whether the patient is ambulatory or an inpatient, because such categorizations are also not useful inasmuch as they overlook critically important factors such as patient condition and other highly individual factors.

Recognizing these classification inadequacies, Davis and Detmer suggested in 1972 that *ambulatory surgery* be defined as "surgery of an uncomplicated nature

*Wong HC: Personal communication, 1984.

that traditionally has been done on an inpatient basis but which can be done with equal efficiency and safety without hospital admission."[32] Their intention was to describe an intermediate level of surgical care that would fit between the more demanding surgery undertaken on inpatients and the less demanding, often "minor" procedures performed in a surgeon's private office or perhaps in an emergency room. Unfortunately, ambulatory surgery has been used synonymously with outpatient surgery (and similar terms) to describe procedures often of different complexities and requirements. More recently, they have further defined the topology of surgical care (Fig. 3–1).[31,35] Note that, in accordance with their earlier definition, ambulatory surgery ("intermediate surgery" in Fig. 3-1) lies between minor surgery that is properly performed in the surgeon's office and major surgery that truly requires hospital supportive services and postoperative hospital care. The overlapping regions emphasize the need for judgment and flexibility; that is, depending on the patient and other factors, a given procedure may be appropriate for either of two settings. As an example, consider a dental extraction: if the patient is a healthy adult, this procedure is appropriately performed in the oral surgeon's or dentist's office; however, if the patient is moderately mentally retarded, the same procedure is more appropriately undertaken in the ambulatory surgery unit where more comprehensive anesthesia care is available. A diagnostic laparoscopy that might reasonably lead to immediate laparotomy (e.g., ectopic pregnancy) is more appropriately performed in an inpatient environment than an ambulatory unit regardless of the patient's general state of health. Similarly, another patient having an inguinal herniorrhaphy but whose social situation does not permit ambulatory care would have his or her surgery as an inpatient. Alternatively, given the incentives to decrease hospital stay, the patient might arrive at the hospital on the morning of the procedure ("A.M. admission"), have the procedure possibly in the hospital's ambulatory unit, and then be admitted to a hospital room. Finally, hospital-affiliated ambulatory units can err on the liberal side in their selection decisions when uncertain whether a given procedure (or

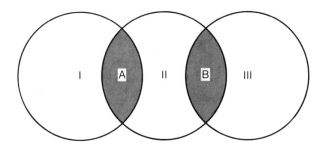

FIG. 3–1 A proposed classification of levels of surgical care. Class I comprises *minor surgery*, or procedures appropriate for the surgeon's office; Class II is *intermediate surgery* that is appropriate for an ambulatory surgery unit; and Class III consists of *major surgery* that is undertaken on an inpatient basis. Subclasses A and B include procedures appropriate for either of their immediately adjacent classes, depending on the circumstances of the particular case. (Detmer DE, Buchanan-Davidson DJ: Ambulatory surgery. Surg Clin NA 62:685, 1982)

patient) is appropriate for the ambulatory setting, because of the ease with which they can admit the patient to a hospital room if it becomes advisable.

CURRENT SPECTRUM OF AMBULATORY SURGERY

THE PROCEDURE

Below is a list of procedures currently undertaken on an ambulatory basis. The list is organized by surgical subspecialties but in no way is meant to delineate what may be performed by a given discipline, for there are many procedures that overlap specialties. Surgical complications may require additional, unlisted procedures (e.g., exploratory laparotomy to suture uterine perforation incurred during therapeutic abortion).

Dental surgery
  Closed reduction of jaw fracture
    (arch bar application)
  Intraoral biopsy
  Multiple extractions
  Multiple fillings
  Odontectomy
  Open and closed reduction of
    zygomatic fracture
  Total extractions
General surgery
  Breast biopsy
  Debridement
  Fistulectomy
  Ganglionectomy
  Hemorrhoidectomy
  Hydrocelectomy
  Hypoglossal duct cystectomy
  Incision and drainage, superficial
    abscess
  Ingrown toenail excision
  Inguinal herniorrhaphy
  Lymph-node biopsy
  Pilonidal cystectomy
  Rectal biopsy
  Small-lesion excision
  Umbilical herniorrhaphy
  Umbilical sinus excision
  Varicose vein ligation
  Varicocelectomy
  Ventral/femoral herniorrhaphy
Gynecology
  Bartholin cystectomy
  Breast biopsy
  Cervical cone biopsy
  Cervical polypectomy
  Culdoscopy

Dilatation and curettage (D&C)
  D&C with diagnostic
    laparoscopy
  D&C with laparoscopic tubal
    ligation
  D&C with suction curettage
  Exam under anesthesia
  Hymenotomy
  Hysteroscopy
  Vaginoplasty
  Tubal ligation by means of
    laparoscopy or
    minilaparotomy
  Tubal ligation transvaginally
Neurosurgery
  Intercostal neurectomy
  Median nerve decompression
  Ulnar nerve transfer
Ophthalmology
  Cataract extraction, with or
    without lens implant
  Conjunctival or corneal biopsy
  Cryotherapy
  Enucleation
  Exam under anesthesia
  Eyelid lesion excision
    (entropion, ectropion)
  Fasanella procedure of lid
  Incision and biopsy of chalazion
  Iridectomy
  Keratotomy
  Lacrimal duct probing
  Mebelene sling to frontalis
    muscle
  Recession resection of eye
    muscles
Orthopedics

Arthroscopic debridement
Arthroscopic lateral release
Arthroscopic menisectomy
Arthroscopic shelf release
Bone-spur excision
Bunionectomy
Carpal tunnel release
Cast change, with or without
   manipulation
Closed reduction
Cyst removal (e.g., Baker's cyst)
Debridement
Diagnostic arthroscopy
Epidural steroid injection
Excision and removal of foreign
   body
Excision of exostosis
Excision of ganglion
Excision of lesion
Fasciectomy (finger, palm)
Finger-joint replacement
Finger amputation and revision
Flexor tendon sheath release
Hammer-toe correction
Joint manipulation
Median nerve decompression
Muscle biopsy
Olecranon bursectomy
Olecranon-spur excision
Open reduction/internal fixation
   of fingers
Prepatellar bursectomy
Release of Dequervains hand
Release of Dupuytrens
   contracture
Release of trigger thumb
Removal of foreign body
Removal of nails, pins, plates,
   screws, wires
Simple tendon repair
Syndactylization of toes
Synovectomy
Tendon exploration
Ulnar nerve transfer
Z plasty
Otolaryngology
   Adenoidectomy, with or
      without myringotomy
   Closed reduction of nasal
      fracture

Ethmoidectomy
Foreign body removal (ear)
Laryngoscopy, with or without
   polypectomy
Mastoidectomy
Myringotomy, with or without
   tubes
Nasal polypectomy
Pharyngoscopy
Rhinoplasty
Rhytidoplasty
Rhytidectomy with
   blepharoplasty
Septorhinoplasty
Stapedectomy
Submucous resection
Tonsillectomy, with or without
   adenoidectomy or
   myringotomy
Tympanoplasty
Pediatric surgery
   Circumcision
   Excision of lesions
   Frenulectomy
   Inguinal herniorrhaphy
   Meatotomy
   Orchiopexy
   Suture of laceration
   Umbilical herniorrhaphy
   Urethral dilatation
Plastic surgery
   Augmentation mammoplasty
   Basal cell carcinoma excision
   Blepharoplasty
   Cleft lip repair
   Contracture release
   Correction of prominent ears
   Fasciectomy
   Ganglionectomy
   Gynecomastia excision
   Laceration repair
   Otoplasty
   Pedical flap transfer
   Preauricular cyst excision
   Rhytidectomy
   Scar revision
   Skin flap revision
   Skin graft
   Tendon repair
   Trigger-finger release

Vermillionectomy
Thoracic Surgery
   Esophageal dilatation
   Pacemaker battery replacement
Urology
   Biopsy and/or fulguration of
      bladder tumor
   Circumcision

Fulguration of bladder neck
Lithopexy
Orchiectomy
Prostate biopsy
Meatotomy
Testicular biopsy
Testicular prosthesis insertion
Vasectomy

Surveying all hospitals in the United States, six procedures appropriate to the ambulatory setting are among the ten most frequently performed:[95]

Procedure	Percentage of U.S. Surgery
Biopsy	5.5
Dilatation and curettage	3.3
Excision of skin	2.8
Tubal ligation	2.5
Cataract extraction	2.1
Inguinal herniorrhaphy	2.0

Thus, these six procedures account for one-sixth of U.S. surgery. Among freestanding surgery centers, the mix of cases is as follows:[44]

Procedure	Percentage of Surgery in Freestanding Units
Dilatation and curettage	21.4
Laparoscopy (including tubal ligation)	15.7
Myringotomy	14.1
Miscellaneous orthopedics	13.7
Excision of skin lesion	10.6
Tonsillectomy or adenoidectomy	5.4
Miscellaneous plastic surgery	5.1
Other procedures	14.0

Thus, gynecologic procedures represent three-eighths of the caseload in freestanding units, followed by otolaryngologic, orthopedic, and plastic surgery. Ambulatory surgery statistics are similar in Canada.[119]

THE MORE COMMON PROCEDURES
Among the many procedures that are commonly undertaken in the ambulatory setting a handful are mentioned here to highlight some of the underlying clinical considerations and possible problems. Some comments on anesthetic administration are unavoidable; more detailed coverage of anesthesia care is found throughout the rest of this text.

Oral Surgery. Historically, ambulatory anesthesia has been closely linked to oral surgery, and the association continues, the majority of procedures being performed in dental operatory units rather than either hospital-affiliated or freestanding ambulatory surgery units. The largest group of patients who require general anesthesia are those who have great fear of dental procedures; others require extensive or lengthy procedures that can be accomplished during one general anesthetic rather than several procedures under local anesthesia; and the remaining patients include those who have allergies to local anesthetics, hyperactive gag reflex, mental retardation precluding reasonable patient cooperation, or spastic neuromuscular disorders. Although the patients may be reasonably healthy, the full spectrum of anesthetic-related morbidity and mortality occurs in ambulatory oral surgery, including malignant hyperthermia (see Temperature Monitoring near the end of this chapter), muscle pains and prolonged apnea following succinylcholine, protracted nausea and vomiting, and sore throat.[72] Among the particularly common intraoperative problems are cardiac arrhythmias, even in the young and healthy patient, regardless whether a halogenated agent or narcotic technique is used.[57,140]

Tonsillectomy and Adenoidectomy. Tonsillectomy and adenoidectomy (T&A), with and without myringotomy, constitutes the majority of cases that an otolaryngologist might undertake in the ambulatory setting.[11] Yet, T&As in the ambulatory surgery unit remain highly controversial, because of the potential for large, often unrecognized blood loss.[67] Nonetheless, series of more than 40,000 T&As have been completed without mortality.[22] Advocates of ambulatory surgery T&As place great emphasis on careful selection and, in particular, preoperative medical evaluation. Inappropriate patients for an ambulatory surgery T&A include those with a history of hemophilia, leukemia, other blood dyscrasias, and sickle-cell anemia, as well as those who take aspirin chronically. Since clinical experience indicates that inflamed tissue is associated with increased bleeding, patients acutely suffering from allergic disorders or those who have had an acute attack of tonsillitis within the past month or a "cold" within a week are also not candidates for the procedure on an ambulatory basis. Although coagulation studies (e.g., bleeding, clotting, prothrombin, and thrombin times; platelet count) have been recommended to screen for those likely to experience postoperative bleeding, careful analysis of clinical experience indicates that such testing is warranted only to *confirm* a suspected bleeding tendency that is identified when taking the history (e.g., "Do you bruise or bleed easily?") and performing the brief physical examination (e.g., ecchymoses). Similarly, many have urged routine chest radiography to avoid undertaking the procedure in a patient with, say, a resolving bronchopneumonia, whereas such radiography is cost effective only to evaluate or confirm abnormalities noted in the history or during auscultation.[22] The clinical value of laboratory testing is discussed later in this chapter.

Therapeutic Abortion. Although the majority of voluntary interruptions of pregnancy in the first trimester are undertaken with sedation and local anesthesia, a substantial number of these therapeutic abortions are performed with general anesthesia, particularly when the uterus is larger and the risk of perforation is thereby greater. The common halogenated anesthetics (i.e., halothane, enflurane, isoflurane) offer a more stable depth of anesthesia and a lower incidence of nausea and vomiting than fentanyl supplementation of nitrous oxide, but risk a greater blood loss consequent to their dose-related uterine relaxation unless low inspired concentrations (less than 0.6 MAC value) are used.[29,56,121] The use of oxytocic agents is associated with diminished bleeding as well as with a higher incidence of nausea and vomiting. This is more true of ergonovine than of oxytocin.[48] Women undergoing a late midtrimester abortion, especially involving a technically difficult extraction, appear to be at increased risk for the development of disseminated intravascular coagulation and, thus, should be observed postoperatively for a minimum of 2 hours, with prompt evaluation of coagulation factors should increased bleeding occur.[139] Compared to a general anesthesia with a halogenated agent and nitrous oxide, following fentanyl and methohexital, a totally intravenous technique consisting of fentanyl (1.5 μg/kg) and methohexital (1.5 mg/kg) during oxygen supplementation seems to offer a prompter awakening, with fewer minor side effects, although memory for new facts is equally impaired.[103]

Pelvic Laparoscopy. Laparoscopy is an increasingly common procedure that is performed principally to facilitate tubal sterilization but also to assist in the diagnosis of pelvic pain and infertility. Tubal ligation is now the most frequently performed procedure in women of reproductive age, approximately 30% of these procedures are performed by means of laparoscopy.[21] The popularity and apparent simplicity of the procedure belie the numerous and diverse, potentially serious problems that may accompany it: pneumothorax,[33] bowel burns with electrocauterization (especially if nitrous oxide is the insufflating gas),[100] hypercarbia (especially during inadequate pulmonary ventilation), hypoxemia (especially in the obese and with an inadequately oxygen-enriched inspiratory mixture),[36] and gastric,[113] intestinal, and vascular perforation. Controversy exists whether to undertake tracheal intubation in the majority of cases in which general anesthesia is used.[107] Anesthesiologists in freestanding settings argue that patient comfort dictates that intubation be undertaken only when airway management is difficult whereas representatives from hospital-affiliated units respond that a mild sore throat is a small price for an adequate airway, particularly in view of the impaired oxygenation associated with a steep Trendelenburg position, elevated diaphragms, and collapsed lower lobes. Undoubtedly, lean patients *may* be safely anesthetized without a tracheal tube during brief procedures; however, considerable expertise in airway management is required with the majority of patients. It is sobering to recognize that during the period 1977 through 1981, 29 deaths occurring during laparoscopic tubal ligations were reported to the Centers for Disease Control; 11 of these deaths were related to complications of general anesthesia with six attributable to hypoventilation, which is generally preventable with tracheal intubation.[20]

Breast Biopsy. Breast biopsy under local anesthesia in the ambulatory setting has been advocated for almost 20 years.[2,90,125] Apart from the general benefits of ambulatory surgical care, its many advantages include a reduced need to confront the majority of patients (who may have benign disease) with possible mastectomy and time for additional evaluation and planning should further surgery be necessary. There has never been documentation supporting a detrimental effect of several days' delay of definitive therapy.[62,108]

Arthroscopy. Among the more recent, and now increasingly popular, additions to the ambulatory surgery caseload are arthroscopic procedures of the knee. The majority of patients who undergo these procedures are young and healthy, if not athletic, with a localized problem, who are highly motivated to recover rapidly to normal functioning; in short, the ambulatory setting is ideal for these patients.[88] But, the advantages of ambulatory care are also well suited to the carefully selected patient with rheumatoid arthritis who is having arthroscopy or finger-joint replacement (or a nonorthopedic procedure) and wishes to cope with his or her deformities in the privacy of his or her own home and family.[16] Although local anesthesia has been used preferentially,[74] especially with a small needlescope, general anesthesia and even regional anesthesia are now increasingly used.[43,88,114] A particular concern with regional anesthesia for knee arthroscopy is that, with the use of the tourniquet, the block must be fairly high (at least at midthoracic level) to reasonably avoid tourniquet pain. The resulting extensive sympathetic block may delay the patient in tolerating ambulation, particularly with spinal anesthesia, in which the level of the sympathetic block is always several dermatomes higher than the sensory level,[54] as opposed to epidural anesthesia, which also offers greater flexibility in the duration of the anesthetic through the continuous (catheter) technique, but which requires more time before the patient is ready for the incision.

Inguinal Herniorrhaphy. An accepted procedure in infants and small children for decades,[58,105] inguinal herniorrhaphy in ambulatory adults is now becoming increasingly more common. Ambulatory herniorrhaphy in adults is not new, however, for Harvey Cushing described hernia repairs under cocaine infiltration half a century ago, and the Shouldice Clinic has performed more than 100,000 repairs under local anesthesia during the past 40 years. Rather, ambulatory herniorrhaphy in adults is receiving renewed interest as a result of its inherent potential for particularly large cost savings (*several* hospital days), the availability of a superior anesthetic technique, professional encouragement, and improved acceptance by both patient and surgeon.[45,46,50,77,124] In the current version of the Shouldice technique, the unmedicated patient walks to the operating room and has his or her hernia repair under a field block anesthetic with a large volume of bupivacaine, 0.25%, ensuring many hours' postoperative comfort which, in turn, permits relatively pain-free immediate ambulation.[109] Depending on social supports, the patient departs for home or a convalescence unit near the hospital. Hernia recurrence rates are comparable to or better than those of inpatient procedures, although surgical experience is an important determinant of the actual rate.[1,75] The favorable experience with long-acting local anesthetics has prompted others to infiltrate wound margins in other surgical procedures and, where appropriate, subcostal nerves, with bupivacaine.[60] Still others have documented several days' analgesia from freezing the ilioinguinal nerve (cryoanalgesia) during inguinal herniorrhaphy, with improved appetite and mobility during recovery.[142]

Cataract Extraction. Among the procedures particularly well suited to the ambulatory surgery setting and one of the most common performed in the elderly population, cataract extraction offers its own peculiar clinical challenges. Since the patients are generally elderly, one encounters a variety of important coexisting diseases, especially those affecting the cardiovascular and respiratory systems. Hence, regardless of the anesthetic technique chosen, one must be prepared to deal with acute episodes related to coronary artery disease, hypertension, and chronic obstructive lung disease, among other disorders. Of particular significance is that when matched according to age and gender with patients undergoing other procedures, cataract patients are found to experience a mortality rate (within 90 days of the procedure) that is about twice that of the reference patients; this suggests that the senile cataract represents a systemic phenomenon rather than merely a local disease.[59] Moreover, in addition to the various cardiovascular and other drugs these patients are taking, with which the anesthesiologist is often very familiar, these patients usually also take "eye drops." This seemingly localized therapy poses systemic problems as a result of interactions with drugs, particularly anesthetic drugs and adjuvants, they may receive in association with their ambulatory surgery.[5] These ophthalmic drugs include timolol, a nonspecific β-adrenergic blocking agent that aggravates bronchospasm in susceptible patients, echothiophate, a long-acting anticholinesterase drug that has been associated with prolonged apnea following the use of succinylcholine, and atropine and scopolamine drops, which have been implicated in episodes of confusion, hallucination, restlessness, dysarthria, and, particularly in children, hyperthermia and coma. In addition, eye drops containing epinephrine and phenylephrine administered immediately before or during the procedure can enter the systemic circulation (by way of the conjunctival capillaries) and cause hypertension and coronary artery spasm.[5,19,123] Similarly, intraocular injection of acetylcholine in a patient receiving antihypertensive therapy that included β-adrenergic blockade can precipitate bronchospasm.[112]

NON-SURGICAL PROCEDURES

There are growing pressures to perform a variety of nonsurgical procedures, usually on an ambulatory basis, in hospital-affiliated ambulatory surgery units, solely because there is no other option in most hospitals. In addition, many of these "ancillary procedures" are viewed as important sources of additional revenue in all types of units. These diverse procedures include

Aspiration of breast mass
Bladder irrigation
Blood transfusion
Bone marrow aspiration[41]
Bronchoscopy (fiberoptic)[4]
Cardiac arteriography and catheterization[17,49]
Cardioversion
Chemotherapy, antineoplastic and antibacterial[110]
Colonoscopy
Cystoscopy
Dressing change
Electroconvulsive therapy
Esophageal variceal sclerotherapy
Esophagoscopy
Examination under anesthesia (gynecologic, ophthalmic, orthopedic)
Gastroscopy
Intercostal tube drainage for spontaneous pneumothorax[86]
Intervertebral disk injection (chemonucleolysis)

Liver biopsy, percutaneous
Lumbar puncture, diagnostic
Nerve block, diagnostic or therapeutic
Ophthalmic examination
Ophthalmic procedures with yttrium-aluminum-garnet (YAG) laser[144]
Paracentesis
Psychotherapy
Renal biopsy
Sigmoidoscopy
Thoracentesis

In general, the limiting factor in meeting this demand is the availability of appropriate staffing and equipment, as well as a clean, but not necessarily sterile, minor procedure room. However, vigilance must not be suspended, for many of these "minor" procedures entail substantial risks to the patient, either during surgery or for several hours afterwards.

NONSURGICAL PROCEDURES THAT INVOLVE ANESTHESIA PERSONNEL

Anesthesia personnel may be requested to monitor and possibly administer sedation during many of these nonsurgical procedures and to be available for resuscitation. Two examples involving anesthesia personnel are presented here to highlight the clinical challenges posed by these seemingly minor cases.

Electroconvulsive Therapy. Increasingly used in the therapy of affective disorders and schizophrenia, electroconvulsive therapy (ECT) is accompanied by major disturbances in autonomic, cardiovascular, pulmonary, and neuro-muscular function. Brief sinus bradycardia and hypotension are followed in succession by rapid sinus tachycardia and hypertension, apnea, hypoventilation, the desired cerebral stimulation with major motor seizure, and brief postictal coma. These disturbances are superimposed on what is necessarily a light general anesthetic—methohexital with succinylcholine—that is given principally to prevent dental injuries and compression fractures of the spine, as well as diminish the cardiovascular stress. In addition, since depression is more prevalent at advanced age, ECT is particularly likely to be performed in patients with clinically significant hypertension and cardiovascular disease. Thus, this short and seemingly minor procedure poses a disproportionately great risk for a variety of acute medical problems, such as arrhythmias, severe hypertension, and myocardial ischemia and failure. These patients require thorough medical evaluation before the procedure to ensure that they are in optimal condition.[40]

Intervertebral Disk Injection (Chemonucleolysis). Chemonucleolysis is an alternative to laminectomy recently approved by the Food and Drug Administration in patients who have demonstrable compression of a spinal nerve root due to lumbar disk protrusion and whose symptoms have not responded to conservative therapy.[23] Chymopapain, a proteolytic enzyme, is injected into the protruding disk, under fluoroscopic control, while the patient lies in a lateral position. Within minutes, hydrolysis of the disk's proteoglycans occurs, with diffusion of the hydrolyzed proteoglycans and enzyme protein into the plasma. Since papain is present as an additive in some foods, beer, contact lens solutions, and cosmetics, many persons have been sensitized to this foreign protein. As a result, anaphylaxis has occurred in 0.8% of the more than 23,000 injections administered through the end of 1983. It is much more common in women than men (1.4% vs. 0.4%) and during general rather than local anesthesia (1% vs. 0.4%).[122] In addition to the airway obstruction and severe hypotension, less severe allergic reactions include itching, urticaria, bronchospasm, and laryngeal edema. Attacks can be extremely variable in their presentations, however, with severe hypotension occurring in the absence of bronchospasm.[14] Prevention includes pretreatment with histamine H_1 and H_2 antagonists (e.g., diphenhydramine, 50 mg q6h, and cimetidine, 300 mg q6h, respectively) and steroids (e.g., hydrocortisone, 100 mg q6h), beginning the afternoon before the procedure. Patients who are sensitive to papaya or papain derivatives should not receive chymopapain. An elevated sedimentation rate is found in about half of those who suffer anaphylaxis. Although the patient often presents on an ambulatory basis for this procedure, the prevailing opinion is that he or she should remain in the hospital for at least 24 hours following the injection. Regardless of what anesthesia technique is used, anesthesia personnel are likely to be involved in the monitoring of the patients and, of course, in the resuscitation that may be required within minutes of the injection. Resuscitative drugs and equipment must be immediately available in the operating room suite (see Resuscitation Equipment near the end of this chapter). The standard therapy for anaphylaxis, including intravenous epinephrine (0.1 mg–0.3 mg) in conjunction with generous intravascular volume expansion, has terminated the syndrome in all patients who received antihistamine pretreatment.[93]

The Patient

As was the case with acceptable surgical procedures, there have been numerous lists of essential characteristics of patients who are appropriate candidates for ambulatory surgery. When ambulatory surgery was reborn 20 years ago, when there was a need to gain credibility with both the medical community and the insurance industry, only the healthiest patients were deemed appropriate candidates. With the passage of time and the accrual of experience, however, the selection criteria have become increasingly liberal, so that we are no longer restricting this mode of care to only physical status 1 and 2 patients (Table 3-1). In fact, many in physical status 3—with insulin-dependent diabetes, coronary artery disease, asthma, moderate hypertension—are increasingly found appropriate. Yet, the price paid for relaxing selection criteria is an increased rate of unplanned hospital admissions (or transfers, in the case of the freestanding units), from 0.02% to 0.6%[42,63,111,135,136] for physical status 1 and 2 patients to 0.5% to 1.5%[63,135,136] when some of the physical status 3 patients are selected. Even with the inclusion of sicker patients, however, the hospital admission rate should be below 2%.[42,135]

GENERAL CHARACTERISTICS OF ACCEPTABLE PATIENTS

Above all, the patient should be in reasonably good health. If the patient has systemic disease that places him or her in physical status 3 (see Table 3-1), the

□ **Table 3-1** **The American Society of Anesthesiologists' Physical Status Classification**

Classification	Description
Class 1	A healthy patient *Example:* inguinal hernia in an otherwise healthy patient
Class 2	A patient with mild systemic disease *Examples:* chronic bronchitis; moderate obesity; diet-controlled diabetes mellitus; old myocardial infarction; mild hypertension
Class 3	A patient with severe systemic disease that is not incapacitating *Examples:* coronary artery disease with angina; insulin-dependent diabetes mellitus; morbid obesity; moderate to severe pulmonary insufficiency
Class 4	A patient with incapacitating systemic disease that is a constant threat to life *Examples:* organic heart disease with marked cardiac insufficiency, persisting angina, intractable arrhythmia; advanced pulmonary, renal, hepatic, or endocrine insufficiency
Class 5	A moribund patient not expected to survive for 24 hours with or without operation *Example:* Ruptured abdominal aneurysm with profound shock
Emergency (E)	The suffix E is used to denote the presumed poorer physical status of any patient in one of these categories who is operated on as an emergency (e.g., 2E).

essential consideration is how stable his or her condition is. Hospital-affiliated units (integrated, separated) can often afford to accept a somewhat sicker patient than the freestanding facility because of the relative ease with which hospital admission can be arranged.

In addition to being in reasonably good health, the patient must truly accept, if not want, to have the procedure performed on an ambulatory basis; necessarily, the patient must understand the process fully. Since postoperative care will not be supervised and provided as it would be to an inpatient, the patient must also be able to understand and follow the instructions that are provided for postoperative care (see Chap. 7). Similarly, because even expertly administered sedation and general anesthesia impair mental acuity for much of the rest of the day, the patient must be accompanied by a responsible person who will transport the patient home and supervise his or her first day and night of home care. This person must be truly responsible enough to know when, how, and where to seek emergency postoperative treatment, if necessary, in accordance with the postoperative instructions. Thus, it is essential that this person be intellectually as well as physical capable.[136] Until very recently, the term responsible person was synonymous with adult; however, with emancipated minors and 16-year-old licensed drivers, one must take a broader, more functional perspective. Under no circumstances should a patient who has received sedation or general anesthesia be permitted to leave the ambulatory unit unaccompanied (see Chapter 2). Finally, the patient must live reasonably close to the ambulatory unit so that the trip home is not unduly long (individual facilities may wish to establish distance criteria based on local circumstances); traveling time to another medical facility for emergency care after hours should also be reasonably short.

THE MORE COMMON "PROBLEM PATIENTS"

Only some of the more common patient selection problems in the ambulatory setting are considered here. The specific issues posed in each situation are different, each within a given type of problem, and often must be evaluated on an individual basis. Nonetheless, with most of these problems, one should ask, whether the patient's problem is in optimal control. If not, what can be reasonably done to improve his or her health status and thereby decrease the patient's risk of suffering a complication or aggravation?

The Physical Status 3 Patient. Operative mortality increases geometrically with advanced physical status; not unexpectedly, although less studied, morbidity also increases dramatically with deterioration of health status.[51,81,84,118,129] A spate of recent books in the 'medical care for the surgical patient' genre is testimony to the growing appreciation of the importance in identifying, monitoring, and improving the patient's other health problems perioperatively.[52,68,71,92,126,130,133] Generally, physical status 3 patients are appropriate candidates for ambulatory surgery only when their health problems are well controlled, plans have been made for the postoperative monitoring and treatment of those problems, and, of course, their home situation can accommodate their postoperative needs.

The Emergency Patient. Although almost all of the procedures undertaken in the ambulatory surgery unit are both scheduled and elective, there are circumstances in which emergency procedures are entirely appropriate. These include dilatation and evacuation of the uterus following incomplete abortion, debridement and suturing of a hand laceration, and incision and drainage of a superficial abscess. Necessarily, the patient appears with little advance notice and must be evaluated without delay. Yet, unless the problem is truly urgent (e.g., moderate ongoing blood loss with the incomplete abortion) and the planned schedule must be interrupted for the patient, there is sufficient time for the anesthesiologist to perform an adequate evaluation while waiting for a space in the schedule.

The Elderly. The advantages the ambulatory surgery unit offers the elderly include a lower anxiety level, maintenance of their familiar family unit, and less disruption in their routines such as diet, medication, and sleep. Chronologic age should not be part of the selection criteria, for there are healthy old people and sick young people. Indeed, in the single study that has evaluated the relationship between age and the rate of complications, the relationship was weak.[87] Instead, the emphasis must be placed on *physiologic* age, including *functional* state. That is, can the patient undertake all of the activities appropriate to his or her age? If not, what is the nature of the limitation? Is there anything that can reasonably be done to improve the patient's health status prior to elective surgery? Particular attention must be directed toward learning all of the many medications the elderly patient may be taking, because, with a greater number of drugs, there is an increased risk for drug interactions. A greater effort must be made also to make certain that the patient and his or her responsible person understand fully what to expect, before and after the procedure. (Geriatric patients will be discussed in greater detail in Chapter 5.)

The Very Young. Infants should not be denied required ambulatory surgery solely because of their age, if the anesthesiologist and other personnel feel comfortable. However, infants with a history of respiratory distress syndrome, particularly those born prematurely (i.e., less than 46 weeks conceptual age), are at greater risk of developing life-threatening perioperative apnea; their procedures should be postponed until they have reached a more appropriate age and level of maturity.[83] Patients considered at risk are those with anemia, a history of prematurity, or apnea or aspiration with feeding. (These patients are discussed further in Chapter 4.)

The Insulin-Dependent Diabetic. Insulin-dependent diabetes spans a broad spectrum of disease severity: At one extreme is the juvenile diabetic, whose control is often brittle, with premature vascular disease affecting major organ systems. At the other extreme is the elderly patient who may have developed relatively mild diabetes only late in life but who is likely to have clinically important coexisting diseases such as hypertension, coronary artery disease, and chronic obstructive pulmonary disease. Although the latter patient would be a suitable candidate for an ambulatory surgical experience if his or her diabetes and other disorders have been well controlled, the former is likely to drift out of control during the ambulatory surgical visit, if not just before arrival, due to the effect of the increased stress, unless unusual efforts are made. Efforts necessary to maintain these patients in good control include very close collaboration between the anesthesiologist, surgeon, and internist, scheduling the procedure as the first case of the day, and monitoring the blood glucose level on arrival and frequently (e.g., every 2 hours) thereafter. Through the close collaboration among the physicians must come a plan for the *peri*operative care, including the preoperative insulin dosage, infusion of a glucose-containing fluid with supplemental potassium until the patient can resume oral intake, and postoperative surveillance and therapy to maintain control. In addition, nausea and vomiting must be treated promptly and vigorously to prevent dehydration and to ensure an early return to a normal oral caloric intake. If a given ambulatory unit cannot meet the greater requirements of the insulin-dependent diabetic, it simply should not treat the patients. Hospital-affiliated units (integrated, separated) are likely to feel more comfortable with these patients, again, because of the relative ease with which inpatient admission can be arranged.

The Obese. Some degree of obesity is common in an economically advanced society, but when is a patient too obese for ambulatory surgery? Since obese refers subjectively to excessive weight relative to the individual's height, weight and height must be standardized. One such standardizing approach is the body mass index (BMI):

$$\text{Body mass index} = \frac{\text{weight in kilograms}}{(\text{height in meters})^2}$$

One may also estimate the patient's ideal body weight, as follows:

$$\text{Ideal body weight (kg)} = \text{height (cm)} - 100$$

Patients who are modestly overweight (e.g., BMI 26–29, or weight 30% above "ideal") experience minimal increased excess mortality, whereas those more obese (e.g., BMI >30, or 35%–40% overweight) experience increased mortality following inpatient surgery.[131]

The implications of obesity are far-reaching, for it often exists as a predisposing disorder for the development of a variety of important chronic illnesses such as diabetes mellitus, cholelithiasis, cerebrovascular disease, hypertension, cirrhosis, and cardiac disease. Although its precise role is unclear, obesity appears to enable the chronic illness to begin prematurely, progress more rapidly, and become life-threatening more often.[131] Obesity stresses the cardiopulmonary systems because the increased carbon dioxide load (produced metabolically by the increased body mass) must be transported by an increased cardiac output and excreted by an increased pulmonary ventilation. When myocardial oxygen utilization exceeds supply, evidence of cardiac disease develops; similarly, those who are sufficiently overweight to be termed morbidly obese (i.e., body weight greater than twice ideal), are also close to the point of respiratory failure. These patients often become hypoxemic in the supine position because their abdominal corpulence pushes the diaphragm higher into the chest, collapsing lower lobes further and thereby producing a greater degree of shunt. Obese patients are also at greater risk for pulmonary aspiration because they tend to accumulate a larger gastric volume whose acidity is below the critical level for the development of aspiration pneumonitis.[132] In varying degrees, obese patients also present the anesthesiologist with a variety of acute problems that include difficulty in establishing intravenous access, propensity for airway obstruction and bronchospasm, and relative tolerance for anesthetics.

The pathophysiology of obesity nonwithstanding, remarkably little is known about the safety of treating these patients in an ambulatory surgery center. One study of women having pelvic laparoscopy concluded that obese patients are appropriate candidates as long as they can be classified as physical status 1 and 2. Although recovery time did not differ materially by body weight, the rate of unplanned hospital admission did: only 0.7% of patients with a BMI below 27 required admission, whereas 2% of those with a BMI of 27 to 30 and 3% of those with greater values did. Although the incidence of emesis was related to body weight, the principal reason for admitting the more obese patients was surgical (need to resort to minilaparotomy).[63] Additional studies are needed to define further what degree of obesity (and with what severity of which associated medical disorders) is appropriate for the ambulatory setting.

The Bronchospastic Patient. Despite their many differences, children and younger adults with asthma and the older city-dweller with chronic obstructive pulmonary disease share a common feature, a very reactive airway. The spectrum in disease severity is sufficiently broad that some of these patients do not require chronic medication, whereas others are taking bronchodilators daily, and still others are dependent on steroids as well as bronchodilators. Hence, it is essential that each of these patients be considered individually. The history and physical examination are the most important parts of the evaluation of these patients: Does the patient have a reasonable exercise tolerance for his or her age? Has there been a recent productive cough? How frequent are the episodes of bronchospasm, what are the precipitating factors, and how have they been treated? When was the last attack and does the patient feel fully recovered? Are there rhonchi, wheezes, or other auscultatory abnormalities? Is there any evidence of congestive heart failure? These patients should have a chest radiograph unless they appear asymptomatic and a film was normal within the past 6 months. In the end, the decision to treat these patients in an ambulatory surgery unit rests with how well controlled their bronchospasm is and how stable they have been on their therapeutic regimen. If one opts to treat them in the unit, one must collaborate closely with the patient's internist regarding optimal preoperative preparations and postoperative care; some patients may require a short preoperative course of steroids or antibiotics to treat residual bronchospasm. A halogenated agent (for bronchodilatation) should be used if general anesthesia is chosen, airway manipulations (e.g., insertion of oropharyngeal airways, tracheal tubes) must be avoided under light anesthesia, and bronchospasm must be treated promptly by deepening anesthesia or cautiously beginning an aminophylline infusion.

The Common Cold. Coryza occurs so frequently among school-age children that it is common to find that a seemingly well child has developed a "cold" in the short time since his or her ambulatory surgical care has been scheduled. Because of the more complicated social arrangements that must be made to treat children in the ambulatory surgery unit (because two adults are generally required for the trip home), the temptation is to proceed with "a little runny nose." Temptation must be resisted if symptoms are acute, for the seeming innocent "postnasal drip" often results in laryngospasm during light levels of anesthesia; although eminently treatable, this problem tends to recur throughout the anesthetic, threatening hypoxemia each time. Clearly, this risk is unwarranted for elective surgery that can be postponed until the child is well, or at least has a dry nose. (This is covered more fully in Chap. 4). Other concerns raised in connection with administering general anesthesia during an upper respiratory viral illness include the anesthetic-induced impairment (for hours) of mucociliary clearance which predisposes to spread of the disease process throughout the lungs;[47] interestingly, a recent study has suggested that enflurane is somewhat protective compared to other anesthetics.[76]

The Sickle-Cell Patient. Sickle-cell disease is actually a family of disorders in which an abnormal, genetically determined hemoglobin undergoes a change in its molecular shape, resulting, in turn, in the sickling of the red cell and secondary vaso-occlusive signs and symptoms.[94] The most serious disorder is sickle-cell anemia (hemoglobin SS disease), with a frequency in the U.S. black population of 1:625, which over time can be associated with hepatic and renal insufficiency, hemiplegia, severe infections, and congestive heart failure. Several other related hemoglobinopathies are less common and, fortunately, less severe and debilitating. Sickle-cell trait (SA disease) is present in one out of 13 black Americans but is not associated with sickling, other symptomatology, or anemia. Sickling episodes are prevented by strictly avoiding precipitating factors such as acidosis, hypoxia, hypotension, stasis, and hypothermia. Clinically, this means that the patient must be kept warm, tourniquets should be avoided, and anesthetic management must scrupulously avoid hypotension and airway obstruction. Clearly, the decision to treat a sickle-cell anemia patient in an ambulatory surgery unit must be made on an individual basis.

The Alcohol and Drug Abuser. Substance abuse is so common that we probably administer anesthesia to an occasional self-medicated patient unknowingly. Two aspects of substance abuse deserve emphasis. First, abuse patterns generally involve a combination of substances, which complicates the care of these patients (as well as precise discussion here). Second, a critical distinction must be made between acute and chronic ingestion of an abuse substance: the potential for diverse acute autonomic and cardiovascular effects is sufficiently great that elective surgery is contraindicated if recent substance abuse is reasonably likely. This is, in large part, due to the likelihood of serious drug interactions between the anesthetics and the abused substances. However, chronic abusers *may* be appropriate candidates for ambulatory surgery, but only if they are reasonably healthy and the likelihood of a withdrawal episode seems remote.

Chronic alcoholism is often associated with serious systemic disorders which adversely affect perioperative mortality (and presumably morbidity): hepatitis, cardiomyopathy, organic brain syndrome, anemia, thrombocytopenia, abnormal platelet function, prolonged prothrombin time, hypoglycemia, and lactic acidosis. Chronic abuse of illicit drugs is associated with an even more diverse set of medical problems: endocarditis, osteomyelitis, superficial infection, tetanus, septic emboli, pulmonary edema, chronic aspiration pneumonia and lung abscess, renal insufficiency, hepatitis, peripheral nerve injury, and thrombophlebitis. Although the chronic alcoholic is generally relatively tolerant of anesthetics, the response of the patient abusing other substances is more variable depending on the given substance or substances, as well as their overall health status. Narcotic addicts often require larger narcotic dosage for analgesia but reasonably normal anesthetic levels, whereas chronic amphetamine abuse is associated with reduced anesthetic requirement; barbiturate abusers tend to require greater amounts of anesthetics.

Withdrawal from chronic substance abuse is a potentially life-threatening event whose manifestations differ according to the substance. Alcoholics develop tremors and irritability within hours of their last ingestion, and seizures occur within 24 to 48 hours. The characteristic abstinence syndrome delirium tremens—which includes fever, global confusion, hallucinations, and tachycardia—occurs within 48 to 72 hours of last ingestion, but may be delayed a week or more. As might be expected, the withdrawal syndromes associated with the abuse of other substances are different, depending upon the class of substance. The barbiturate withdrawal syndrome resembles that of alcohol and can be treated acutely with short-acting barbiturates. Amphetamine withdrawal includes sleep and toxic psychosis. Narcotic withdrawal includes diverse visceral signs and symptoms that begin with yawning, diaphoresis, lacrimation, and rhinorrhea and progress after several days to myalgias, muscle cramps, vomiting, diarrhea, tachycardia, and hypertension; the syndrome is treated acutely with narcotics.[80]

The Mentally Retarded and Disabled. But for the most severely retarded and those with other clinically important health problems (e.g., symptomatic congenital heart disease), the mentally retarded are usually most appropriately treated in the ambulatory setting, surgical or medical. The ambulatory setting causes the least interruption in their otherwise psychologically fragile existence, particularly because it involves minimal separation from a familiar family or guardian. Similarly, with the exception of the most severely affected, the disabled should also be preferentially treated in the ambulatory setting, which affords them greater privacy and a more rapid return to familiar, supportive surroundings.

The Physicians

The ambulatory surgery unit is clearly a dynamic setting that represents much more than the transplantation of traditional approaches. Indeed, the success of the freestanding units is due, at least in part, to their innovation and to their ability to involve personnel of different types into the development of the facility and thereby provide high-quality care in a cost-effective manner. In this pioneering environment, personal attributes that are important for both the success of the facility and the individual personnel include initiative, flexibility, versatility, and responsibility. In particular, a "think ambulatory" orientation on the part of all personnel is essential because what clearly differentiates this care from inpatient care is the ability to discharge the patient to his or her home safely within hours of the procedure.

Because the importance of personnel policies among other fundamentals of the successful facility is discussed in the concluding chapter, this section will focus upon selection decisions which relate to the physicians who work in the ambulatory unit and which facilitate development of the unit. First, as a way of encouraging a minimal level of quality control, accreditation bodies require that specific procedures be established for evaluating the credentials and delineating the privileges of the surgeons and anesthesiologists (also nurse-anesthetists) who work in the unit. No longer can the hospital extend "full privileges" to each practitioner, assuming that peer pressure and professional integrity will ensure that an individual does not attempt a procedure for which he or she lacks substantial proficiency. Neither can a freestanding non-hospital-affiliated ambulatory unit extend the same privileges for its facility as might be appropriate for an inpatient setting without requiring that its physicians possess equivalent privileges at a local hospital; otherwise, a freestanding unit would tend to attract surgeons whose practices had already been limited or prohibited.[120] Instead, as a safeguard to ambulatory patients, accreditation bodies require that the facility's medical staff formally delineate the scope of professional practice of each member of the medical staff in its ambulatory setting. Although peer judgment is likely to be an important determinant in the delineation of clinical privileges, utilization review and quality assurance programs (see section at the end of this chapter) are likely to be important sources of documentation upon which to modify those privileges.

THE ANESTHESIOLOGIST

With advances in clinical monitoring and development of improved anesthetics and adjuvants, the anesthesiologist has the ability to render safer care to progressively sicker patients, some not too long ago regarded as "too ill" for surgery. An unfortunate corollary of this medical progress is that many anesthesiologists no longer find it necessary to communicate with their patients; instead, they function more as technicians, knowledgeable and skillful, but nonetheless operating in a largely technical role. Yet, anesthesia for ambulatory surgery offers an unusual opportunity for anesthesiologists to relate to conscious patients and their families, become more active in their preoperative assessment, and once again function more fully as physicians. In addition, there is the increasingly important challenge of providing the same high-quality care more cost-effectively in this most rapidly developing subspecialty area in anesthesiology.

THE ANESTHESIOLOGIST AS MANAGER
Anesthesiologists *selected* for the ambulatory setting, then, should be fully capable of becoming active participants; they must not be castaways from the traditional operating rooms. Because of the anesthesiologist's constant presence in the operating room (as compared with surgeons), he or she also has a natural opportunity to assume a managerial role, usually as medical director, if the unit has such a designation. For this new role beyond the care of an individual patient, the anesthesiologist must have or develop skills that enable him or her to set specific goals and objectives that must be clear to others, evolve organizational strategies rather than act alone, become a good listener, encourage constructive suggestions, and enrich the jobs of others by delegating as much as possible without losing control.

THE ANESTHESIOLOGIST'S PREOPERATIVE EVALUATION
The ultimate success of the ambulatory surgery unit depends on its ability to provide cost-effective care without jeopardizing quality and patient safety. To accomplish this, the unit must *mesh* appropriate patients with appropriate procedures performed by cooperative surgeons who understand fully the foregoing prerequisites for these patients and procedures. Although the surgeon sees potential ambulatory surgery patients first and selects appropriate candidates, he or she necessarily uses an evaluation procedure set forth by the anesthesiologists at the ambulatory surgery unit who will be looking after the overall well-being of his or her patients. Thus, by setting forth the selection policies, in particular those relating to the patient evaluation, and by being available continuously at the unit, the anesthesiologist is truly a gatekeeper and guardian in the ambulatory surgical setting.

Obtaining the Preoperative Patient Information.   Once the surgeon has decided to undertake an ambulatory procedure in a given patient (see The Surgeon, below), the anesthesiologist must gather the requisite information that will allow him or her to assess the patient, too. In perhaps half of the ambulatory units, patients are required to make a preoperative visit several days in advance of surgery, at which time they tour the facilities, meet many of the personnel who will be caring for them, and meet the anesthesiologist. In effect, they meet the anesthesiologist in a consultative role in what has been termed an anesthesia screening clinic. Here, in a relatively unhurried session, without the anxiety of an immediately impending surgical procedure, the patient undergoes a relevant history and physical examination, learns about anesthesia care, and has an opportunity to have questions answered. In other units, the necessary information is obtained from the surgeon's office or by a telephone interview in the days before the procedure, or during an interview with the anesthesiologist on the day of the procedure.

Although the time-honored complete history and physical examination provide the necessary information, this traditional approach is inefficient in the ambulatory setting particularly, where the patients are often in good health. Instead, a more focused history is usually obtained. But what pieces of information are most relevant to the decision whether to proceed with anesthesia in a given patient? A recent British study sought to establish the minimum amount of information that permits an accurate assessment of one's fitness for anesthesia. The following are the simple questions whose answers the researchers found correlated with peer consensus of fitness for anesthesia:[141]

1. Do you feel sick?
2. Have you had any serious illnesses in the past?
3. Do you get more short of breath on exertion than others of your age?
4. Do you have a cough?
5. Do you have a wheeze?
6. Do you have any (anginal) chest pain on exertion?
7. Do you have ankle swelling?
8. Have you taken any medications in the past 3 months?
9. Have you any allergies?
10. Have you had an anesthetic in the past 2 months?
11. Have you or your relatives had any problems with anesthesia?

Note how relevant each is to the patient's functional status. Using this set of questions, they noted there was agreement among ten anesthesiologists in 96% of 200 patients that they evaluated prospectively. They concluded,

> Patients who are thought to be perfectly fit on the basis of simple questions usually prove to be so after the traditional preoperative history and investigations. This suggests that a questionnaire might be developed for use in surgical outpatients to select patients for day surgery.

This provides the rationale for the patient information questionnaires that many ambulatory surgery units are formulating. The questionnaire can be completed in the surgeon's office, in the unit, or even over the phone. Affirmative answers serve as "flags" to alert physicians to obtain additional information in areas of relevance to anesthesia care.

Role of the medical consultant. Often when faced with the sicker patient, the anesthesiologist and the surgeon will consult the patient's physician, who is most familiar with the patient's medical problems, or perhaps another internist whose expertise might benefit the patient. Unfortunately, in too many cases the request for a medical consultation is termed "clearing the patient for surgery." As if in a return to the ancient days of sorcerers and rituals, it seems that the physician is being called upon for a symbolic blessing that all will go well for the patient. However, when performed in this fashion, the patient, surgeon, and anesthesiologist lose an opportunity to gain potentially valuable help. Thus, "medical clearance" is truly outdated. What is needed is a list of the patient's medical problems, an assessment of how well each is controlled, management suggestions that might improve the patient's health status, and the availability of the consultant postoperatively.

Role of the Clinical Laboratory Evaluation. Laboratory tests may be used for two different purposes. One may search for unsuspected disease in all preoperative patients by subjecting them to a battery of laboratory tests; this is termed "screening" and its underlying rationale is that finding an abnormality will be beneficial to the patient. On the other hand, knowing or suspecting from the history and physical examination that a given patient has a particular abnormality, one may obtain a specific test to confirm that suspicion. Which approach is more rational?

Because clinical laboratory studies consume a large and growing portion of health care expenditures, excessive and inappropriate preoperative testing is being scrutinized. Unfortunately, there is no national consensus regarding preoperative testing. Such testing necessarily must reflect the incidence of disease in the population, sensitivity of the given tests, and factors related to the proposed surgery and anesthesia. Although firm preoperative recommendations are not yet available, the methods for evaluating the usefulness and cost-effectiveness of tests are at hand.[18] From the application of these methods to a variety of screening procedures have come a large number of studies with the same conclusion: abnormal test results do occasionally occur, generally much less often than we would expect; the large majority of the abnormalities identified do not lead to new diagnoses; and, even in those few in whom a new diagnosis is established, there is generally no reason to alter the agreed-upon surgical plan. Thus, using panels of tests for screening asymptomatic, preoperative patients is not cost effective and should not be undertaken.

The corollary of these studies is that the history and physical examination are the most important sources of data in the evaluation of the patient. Nonetheless, individual tests may prove helpful in selected circumstances.

Hematocrit. The determination of hematocrit (or hemoglobin) is so inexpensive, the incidence of undiagnosed anemia so relatively high, and the ability of the physical examination to detect anemia so limited that this test should be performed in all preoperative patients. However, it must be acknowledged that there is no objective basis to support the oft-quoted need for a hematocrit value of, say, 30% to enable normal postoperative wound healing. Also, with 98.7% accuracy and half of the errors being conservative, it is possible to differentiate "safe" hematocrit levels from those that are "unsafe" (e.g., less than 28%) by examination of the conjunctiva.[10]

Urinalysis. Relatively unstudied, the urinalysis continues to be found among recommendations for screening because it is also a relatively inexpensive test and the incidence of abnormalities detected is so great. For example, half of the 10% of the general population with diabetes mellitus are undiagnosed, and glycosuria is reliably detected by the urinalysis. Studies are needed to determine whether the many abnormalities that urinalysis detects alter clinical care.

Chest Radiography. Chest radiography is among the most commonly performed preoperative testing, yet its clinical usefulness for screening has only recently been questioned. For example, a large number of studies suggest that, in asymptomatic persons under 40 years of age, more than half of the "routine" radiographs reported to be abnormal are falsely positive, and few cases of unsuspected clinically important disease are detected. Even in patients between 40 and 60 years of age, the yield from preoperative screening is inadequate to justify the practice. The argument that these films offer medicolegal protection is fallacious because the total number of false-negative and false-positive results may exceed the total of the true positives. Thus, an expert panel (which included anesthesiologists, internists, surgeons and radiologists) chosen by the Federal Food and Drug Administration Center on Devices and Radiologic Health recommends that the preoperative chest film not be routinely obtained in the absence of a specific abnormality noted in the history or physical examination, or a selected population already shown to have significant yields of previously undiagnosed disease.[111a] The House of Delegates of the American Society of Anesthesiologists approved the recommendation in October 1984.

Electrocardiogram. Despite its widespread use in evaluating specific cardiac problems, the usefulness of the electrocardiogram (ECG) as a screening tool has yet to be established. It has only limited value in detecting ischemic heart disease in asymptomatic persons. Similarly, the value in obtaining a "baseline" ECG for possible subsequent comparison has never been established. Although the ECG becomes increasingly valuable with older populations, formal recommendations cannot be made without knowing the underlying prevalence of ECG abnormalities in a given population.

Liver Function Tests. Tests of hepatic function (e.g., SGOT, LDH, total bilirubin) have such a low yield that such routine testing is also apt to be unwarranted; when abnormalities are noted, many can be attributed to information already obtained from taking the patient's history. Some argue that there is a medicolegal basis for obtaining such tests prior to general anesthesia which is felt to be possibly hepatotoxic, but this point of view has yet to be evaluated objectively.

Coagulation Studies. Prothrombin time (PT) and partial thromboplastin time (PTT) have been recommended as screening tests to detect unsuspected bleeding disorders and thereby avoid hemorrhagic surgical complications; yet this clinical recommendation has never been validated. In a recent study of 750 preoperative inpatients, 139 patients (19%) were suspected of having a bleeding abnormality based upon information obtained in the history or physical examination, of whom 25 (18%) were found to have an abnormal PT or PTT result. Of the 611 patients (81%) lacking an indication of a bleeding disorder, 480 had determinations of PT or PTT, and 13 (2.7%) were found to have abnormal values; of this latter group, four were found to have normal values on repeat testing, eight were operated upon uneventfully without retesting, and only one patient experienced a hemorrhagic complication which was found at reoperation to have been caused by an unligated artery. In addition, the low yield of these tests was obscured by a larger number of false positive results. The investigators concluded that these tests are useful only in those patients previously identified as having an increased risk of bleeding.[39]

Other Tests. Although not useful for screening, a variety of other tests are valuable in specific circumstances to evaluate clinical situations that cannot be assessed by other means. For example, a blood sugar is often valuable in patients with insulin-dependent diabetes; similarly, serum electrolytes are useful in patients who are receiving chronic diuretic or digitalis therapy. Yet, routine determination of pseudocholinesterase level prior to general anesthesia has such a low yield that it is unwarranted; more rational is a careful history of the patient's past anesthetic experiences.

A Clinical Laboratory Recommendation. Given that screening with laboratory tests is not cost-effective but individual tests *may* be helpful in confirming clinical suspicion, it is clear that we must be more selective when we order tests. No longer are there "routine tests"; instead, there are specific recommendations according to the patient population and particular test. Moreover, tests should be obtained only when their results will actually be part of the decision making. Or, as aptly stated by a forgotten British physician:

> When considering whether to order a test, ask yourself what you would do if the test result were positive, and what you would do if it were negative. If the answers are the same, don't order the test.

Figure 3-2 presents clinical recommendations for the laboratory evaluation of preoperative patients, both ambulatory and inpatient, based upon current knowledge about these tests. Note that specific tests are obtained only for specific indications. Test results are acceptable for 30 days, unless the patient's underlying disease would dictate that testing be repeated closer to the scheduled procedure; chest radiographs and electrocardiograms taken within the past 6 months are acceptable if they were normal and the patient has no cardio-respiratory abnormalities. These recommendations for clinical laboratory testing should be considered optional, at the discretion of the surgeon, in the case of those patients who are scheduled to have procedures performed under local anesthesia without sedation.

EDUCATING THE SURGEON AND THE OFFICE STAFF

Since the preoperative assessment relates largely to the more global concerns of the anesthesiologist and the surgeon necessarily has first contact with the patient, it is encumbent upon the anesthesiologist to take the initiative in educating the surgeon and staff. The anesthesiologist should summarize briefly his or her approach to preoperative assessment (see preceding section) and make this information available to all surgeons (and their staffs) who are potential users of the ambulatory unit. In addition, the anesthesiologist should be available to answer questions. Recognizing that the surgeon often delegates many administrative aspects of patient preparation, representatives from the ambulatory unit should also meet with the surgeon's staff to answer their

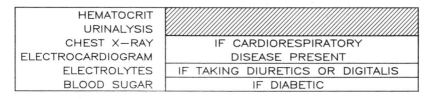

HEMATOCRIT	
URINALYSIS	
CHEST X—RAY	IF CARDIORESPIRATORY
ELECTROCARDIOGRAM	DISEASE PRESENT
ELECTROLYTES	IF TAKING DIURETICS OR DIGITALIS
BLOOD SUGAR	IF DIABETIC

FIG. 3-2 A recommended schema for minimal preoperative testing of the patient having anesthesia. The *only* tests that are recommended in all patients are the hematocrit (or hemoglobin) and urinalysis (hatched area), regardless of the patient's age. Other tests should be obtained only when specific abnormalities are present.

questions and establish rapport that can facilitate the implementation of future policy changes as the unit develops.

THE SURGEON

Given the diversity of procedures currently undertaken in the ambulatory setting, and particularly the presence of some that are clearly *non*surgical, *surgeon* must be viewed rather broadly as any physician who performs a procedure. Thus, among the "surgeons" in the ambulatory unit are the neurologist performing a lumbar puncture and the pulmonologist undertaking fiberoptic bronchoscopy. A *sine qua non* is that the surgeon have sufficient skill to perform procedures effectively and within a reasonable time. During the early development of the ambulatory unit, his or her patience (and patients!), understanding, and support will be important in launching the unit. The surgeon's investment will be amply repaid by his or her enhanced productivity, because the time previously spent in preoperative and postoperative hospital rounds will be spared, and his or her surgical schedule will move along faster and generally with greater predictability. In addition, the smallness of the ambulatory unit will be conducive to the delivery of the highest quality of care, largely because the surgeon will be working with the same small number of people, who will become familiar with his or her needs.

PREOPERATIVE ASSESSMENT IN THE SURGEON'S OFFICE

The surgeon and staff must develop an appreciation of the importance of the preoperative assessment in appropriate selection of patients in the ambulatory setting. Although very familiar, of course, with the planned procedure and his or her needs, the surgeon may not have given sufficient thought to the procedure in the given patient. Concerned about the patient's particular surgical problem, the surgical specialist is apt to overlook general aspects of the patient's health or social setting which may make him or her a poor candidate for ambulatory care. What is the patient's physical status category? What are the coexisting diseases, and are they well controlled? How far from a hospital or physician's office does the patient live? Is the patient's family capable of providing postoperative care? Does he or she live alone? What preoperative laboratory testing should be obtained? The surgeon and staff must consider each of these questions.

EDUCATING THE PATIENT IN THE SURGEON'S OFFICE

Once the decision has been made to undertake the procedure on an ambulatory basis, the surgeon and staff must explain, emphasize, and restate the importance of following the instructions that are provided in a brochure prepared by the ambulatory surgery unit for patient guidance (Fig. 3-3). The patient must be specifically told not to eat or drink after midnight, but should brush his or her teeth and take any usual medications with a sip of water unless specifically advised otherwise. Experience indicates that such patient education and, in particular, the repetition of important instructions, is invaluable in preventing unnecessary cancellations due to misunderstanding and nonadherence. The patient should also be advised about postoperative care so that, when the nurse in the postanesthesia care unit dispenses discharge instructions, the patient is more likely to understand and comply.

Your physician has scheduled your admission to the Same Day Surgery:

Name: _____

Date: _____

Day: _____

Time: _____

(This is one hour before your scheduled operating time.)

Please Be Prompt.

If you are unable to keep this appointment or have any questions please call your physician or the Same Day Surgery.
(215) 448-8190

Financial Information

It is advisable for you to contact your insurance company to determine what coverage is allowed for your scheduled procedure. Any charge not allowed by your insurance contract becomes your responsibility.

Preparation for Admission to Same Day Surgery

No food or liquid after midnight the night before surgery. YOU MUST HAVE AN EMPTY STOMACH.

Arrange to have a responsible adult accompany you home after your surgery. Two adults should accompany a child.

Wear casual clothing that can be folded and stored in a locker.

Please do not wear jewelry or bring valuables to the hospital.

Notify your physician if you have developed a cold, fever or other sign of infection.

Parking

Limited space for Parking is available in the Emergency Room parking lot of the hospital located on the south side of Vine Street. Please request a ticket from the Out Patient Registration for parking privileges.

Location

Report to the Information/Reception desk in the main lobby of the hospital one hour before your scheduled procedure.

Same Day Surgery is located on the 3rd floor of the hospital, South Tower. Take any of the elevators in the main lobby to the 3rd floor, turn left, go down several steps and follow the signs to Same Day Surgery.

After Your Procedure

You will stay in our Recovery Room until you are alert and reasonably comfortable. Should your physician decide further care is needed, an additional hospital stay may become necessary.

Please follow the written instructions that will be given to you when you are discharged from Same Day Surgery.

REMEMBER — A RESPONSIBLE ADULT (over 18) MUST ACCOMPANY YOU AT DISCHARGE.

We welcome your comments regarding the service you have received.

7c.10.83

Fig. 3-3 Information given to patients before their ambulatory surgery. (Same Day Surgery Patient Guide, Hahnemann University Hospital, Philadelphia, PA)

SCHEDULING THE PROCEDURE

Having decided that the patient is an appropriate candidate for the proposed ambulatory procedure, the surgeon or, more likely, his or her staff then calls the ambulatory unit to schedule the surgery. Although there are many administrative variations that suit local situations, the following is true of most units. Whether the unit uses "block scheduling" or schedules "as time and space is available" is largely dependent upon the maturity of the unit, with the former predominating as the unit develops. Because of the need for a minimal 2 to 3 hours' postoperative recovery period following general anesthesia, cases involving general anesthesia are scheduled preferentially early in the day, with the last case starting no later than about 1:30 P.M. Cases involving either local anesthesia administered by the surgeon, or sedation or regional anesthesia administered by anesthesia personnel may start later in the day, although they should end by midafternoon.

The patient is requested to arrive about an hour prior to the scheduled procedure, having completed preregistration (e.g., insurance forms) and having had any required laboratory testing. If the anesthesiologist has not interviewed the patient and undertaken preoperative assessment (see preceding section), he or she does so at this time; regardless, however, he or she confirms that the patient has not experienced some intercurrent illness that might warrant postponement. Also, adherence to "nothing by mouth" and the presence of a responsible person is confirmed. Many ambulatory units require the patient arriving for surgery to sign a form on which he or she certifies that he or she understands the information provided, has provided correct information, and has had nothing to eat or drink since midnight and acknowledges that he or she may not drive a car (or operate other dangerous machinery) or drink alcoholic beverages for 24 hours (see Chap. 7), must notify the physician immediately if unusual bleeding or other problems (the list often includes respiratory difficulties, acute pain) occur, and that he or she may have to be admitted to the hospital due to unforeseen circumstances.

Equipment

OPERATING ROOM EQUIPMENT

Although the risks to the patient associated with simpler, often minor surgery are generally smaller than those associated with inpatient procedures, the risks of anesthesia remain relatively constant and substantial. The same high quality of equipment is required in the ambulatory setting as in the inpatient facility; indeed, the JCAH accreditation standards (see section near beginning of chapter) require that the policies and procedures relating to the same surgical procedures be the same in both settings. This equipment includes a reasonably modern anesthesia machine capable of delivering the common anesthetic agents, a full compliment of tracheal tubes and other artificial airways and laryngoscope blades, appropriate monitoring devices and resuscitative equipment (see later in this section), suction, conventional operating table, electrocautery machine, sterilizers, and surgical instruments and ancillary operating room equipment appropriate to the type of procedures performed (e.g., operating microscope, fluoroscopy). All of this equipment must necessarily meet appropriate standards and guidelines, such as those relating to delivery and scavenging of anesthetic gases and to electrical safety.[8,9,96-98]

MONITORING EQUIPMENT

Physiologic monitoring entails the continuous observation and assessment of the patient's condition and response to anesthesia and surgery. The monitoring devices described here comprise the *essential* noninvasive equipment; additional noninvasive methods may be found elsewhere.[53,117] If more intensive, particularly invasive monitoring appears indicated for a given patient, that patient is probably not an appropriate candidate for ambulatory surgical care. In addition to the monitoring devices, personnel should maintain constant visual, verbal, and tactile contact with the anesthetized patient.

PRECORDIAL STETHOSCOPE

The most valuable—and, remarkably, least expensive—monitoring device is the precordial stethoscope which permits continuous auscultation of the heart and lungs.[37] A simple weighted stethoscope bell, or accumulator, taped to the anterior chest and connected to a monaural, molded earpiece permits moment-to-moment monitoring of both heart tones and breath sounds. For example, heart tones usually become "muffled" in the hypovolemia accompanying blood loss, whereas the extra heart sound present in the gallop rhythm signals hypervolemia or congestive heart failure. Gross alterations in cardiac rhythm, such as severe bradycardia, asystole, ventricular premature contractions, and marked tachycardia, are readily detected by their interruption of an otherwise monotonous cadence in one's ear, perhaps long before chance observation of an arrhythmia on an electrocardiogram display. Similarly, the onset of wheezing indicates bronchospasm or upper airway obstruction, and the sudden loss of respiratory sounds is often the first sign of breathing system disconnection, an important contributor to preventable morbidity and mortality in anesthesia care.[26,102] In those situations in which a precordial stethoscope is inappropriate, an esophageal stethoscope may be substituted once tracheal intubation has been accomplished.

BLOOD PRESSURE

Arterial blood pressure monitoring, particularly of the systolic pressure, is among the most reliable signs of depth of anesthesia.[30] Thus, it is not surprising that the sphygmomanometer, the prototype for indirect blood pressure monitoring, was first used during anesthesia in 1903, shortly after Riva-Rocci introduced it in 1896. Controversial, however, is the interpretation of the Korotkoff sounds that are auscultated: the American Heart Association recommends that the pressure at which a faint, clear, tapping sound is first heard be interpreted as the systolic pressure, and the pressure at which sounds disappear, the diastolic. Accurate measurement also requires that the full cuff pressure be transmitted to the brachial artery, for a cuff that is too narrow relative to the arm diameter will indicate a pressure that is higher than the true arterial pressure. Accuracy is ensured by using a cuff width that is at least 20 percent greater than the mean diameter of the arm. Appropriately proportioned cuffs can also be used on the forearm or thigh when necessary.

An alternative technique of indirect blood pressure monitoring employs oscillotonometry, originally described by von Recklinghausen in 1904. With this nonauscultatory technique, a second, pressure-sensing bladder within the cuff is connected to a pressure gauge whose needle pulsates maximally when the compression pressure has lowered to systolic pressure and ceases to pulsate when diastolic pressure is reached. A variety of automatic or semi-automatic noninvasive blood pressure monitors use oscillotonometry (e.g., Dinamap, Accutorr, Sentron), microphonic auscultation (e.g., Infrasonde), or combined oscillotonometry and microphonic auscultation (e.g., Vita-Stat). Properly used, this equipment is satisfactory for routine clinical anesthesia and postoperative care.

ELECTROCARDIOGRAM

The value of intraoperative electrocardiographic (ECG) monitoring is so well-established that no justification for its continued use is necessary. With common clinical equipment and three limb leads (right and left arms, left leg), beat-to-beat observation of the *electrical* activity of the heart is possible, including the rate, QRS configuration, repolarization, and cardiac rhythm. Hence, it is commonplace to diagnose the hyperkalemia in renal failure by observing tall, peaked T waves. Similarly, many dysrhythmias can be identified easily by their characteristic patterns during clinical anesthesia.[69]

Although observation of the cardiac rate and rhythm constitutes the principal application of ECG monitoring, understandably there has been great interest in using clinical equipment to monitor for myocardial ischemia. Unfortunately, S-T segment depression is often missed, even when ischemia is likely or otherwise known to be present. This failure is due to two factors. The standard limb leads monitor voltage changes in the frontal plane, missing acute injury occurring in anterolateral and posterior portions of the myocardium. Also, the filtering system that stabilizes the baseline, eliminates high-frequency noise, and 60 Hz interference happens to produce artifactual changes in the S-T segment and T wave configurations; fortunately, the filter can be turned off in newer equipment that has a switch labeled "monitoring" and "diagnostic." S-T segment depression can be observed with greater accuracy from a modified V_5 precordial lead.[70] For this lead to be obtained, the left leg electrode is placed at the anterior axillary line in the left fifth intercostal space, and the ECG monitor is set to lead II; the filter must be set to "diagnostic" to avoid artifactual S-T segment depression.

Exceedingly valuable as well as inexpensive, ECG monitoring does pose an often unappreciated risk of burns. In the presence of defective ECG electrodes or electrical equipment grounding, the current applied on the skin for ECG monitoring leaves the body surface by way of an alternative pathway of least resistance (macroshock situation); typically, the current exits the skin in a discrete area, concentrating its energy in a very small area, resulting in a burn. This complication is ever-present because of the multitude of electrical equipment that may also be attached to the patient, particularly the radiofrequency electrocautery (e.g., Bovie machine). A special case exists in those very uncommon circumstances in the ambulatory setting in which the patient has an externalized myocardial conductor (e.g., pacemaker insertion); here, *minute* but high current density is directed to the myocardium, causing immediate ventricular fibrillation (microshock condition). Prevention requires two programs in tandem: *safety education*, in which personnel are taught to identify potential electrical hazards (e.g., frayed insulation, cracked plugs), to operate electrical equipment safely, and how to respond when the proper function of electrical equipment is in doubt; and, *equipment control*, including the careful selection of electrical equipment in accordance with minimum safety standards, initial safety inspection before it is put into service, and preventive maintenance that includes periodic inspections.[100]

NEUROMUSCULAR FUNCTION

Neuromuscular blocking drugs have become an important component of the anesthesiologist's armamentarium. To use them most effectively and safely, the degree and type of neuromuscular blockade must be monitored.[89] Typically, a set of electrodes is placed along the course of the ulnar nerve, between the elbow and hand, and connected to a clinical peripheral nerve stimulator. The latter provides two types of stimuli: a brief stimulus ("twitch") and a sustained stimulus ("tetanus"). Observation of repetitive twitches delivered at a rate of ten stimuli per second (0.1 Hz) permits semiquantitative assessment of the degree of blockade due to a depolarizing neuromuscular blocking agent (e.g., succinylcholine infusion); stopping the administration of the drug when the twitch response disappears avoids overdosage. This is manifested as relatively long-lasting paralysis which generally cannot be antagonized (phase II block). A series of four stimuli of greater (supramaximal) intensity and longer duration (2 Hz) provides a clinically very useful method of monitoring neuromuscular function following the use of nondepolarizing relaxants. The ratio of the amplitude of the fourth response to that of the first in this "train-of-four" stimulation serves as an index of the degree of blockade. Quantifying the degree of blockade between 75% and 100% is particularly easy: when the fourth twitch in the "train-of-four" becomes undetectable, 75% blockade exists, which corresponds to adequate surgical relaxation in the presence of inhalation anesthetic agents; with abolition of the third twitch, 80%; with loss of the second, 90%, which is associated with adequate surgical relaxation during nitrous oxide-narcotic anesthetic techniques; and when all twitches disappear, 100% blockade.

TEMPERATURE MONITORING

It is also common for body temperature to change during anesthesia. Because of the high mortality and morbidity associated with malignant hyperthermia (see later in this section) and the low cost of temperature monitoring, it has become a standard of practice to monitor the body temperature of all patients having general anesthesia. The *direction* and *rate* of temperature change is of paramount concern, rather than any absolute temperature value.

Body temperature can be monitored at a variety of sites, which differ in their approximation to "core temperature" (because of differential blood flow to the monitoring site) and inherent propensity for complications. Rectal temperature monitoring is used in infants and small children, whereas the axilla or esophagus is a more common site in older children and adults. Although most closely approximating "core temperature," tympanic membrane monitoring risks tympanic membrane rupture and hemorrhage; the hazard is reduced if the probe is inserted while the patient is awake and able to vocalize discomfort. A recent comparison of accuracy and precision among potential monitoring sites compared to the tympanic membrane concluded that the nasopharyngeal and esophageal provide the optimal combination of accuracy and precision, without risking tympanic membrane trauma.[27] The typical clinical temperature probe consists of either a thermal-sensitive resistor (thermistor) or a voltage-generating circuit of two similar metals whose junction points are maintained at different temperatures (thermocouple). In either case, the temperature sensing end is generally encased in plastic and is attached to an ohmmeter or voltmeter, respectively, that has been calibrated to indicate temperature. Thermal-sensitive liquid-crystals which differentially reflect or transmit light have been sequentially arrayed and embedded in a black plastic strip that is applied to the skin for surface monitoring. Although these strips are disposable and easy to use, the measured temperature lags sufficiently behind core values to render these strips inaccurate when compared to conventional mercury/glass thermometers.[82] Yet, such strips may be useful for following trends, as in malignant hyperthermia screening.[78]

Unintentional Hypothermia. Hypothermia occurs because body heat is lost through cutaneous vasodilatation, endogenous heat production is reduced, and normal thermoregulatory mechanisms cease during general anesthesia. Despite the brevity of most ambulatory surgical procedures, hypothermia can occur in small children and infants, due to the large surface area to volume ratio of their bodies. The resultant "cold stress" is associated with increased oxygen consumption (especially if shivering is apparent), metabolic acidosis, apnea, and, in neonates, increased mortality. Hypothermia is prevented by maintaining ambient temperature above 24°C for children (above 22°C for adults), covering the patient as much as possible, and, for infants, using a heating blanket on the operating room table, warming fluids (e.g., cystoscopy irrigant), heated humidifier in the anesthesia breathing system, and a radiant heat source above the patient when possible.[116]

Malignant Hyperthermia. Much less likely, temperature elevation can also occur during general anesthesia, usually as part of a pyogenic response in septicemia (e.g., contaminated intravenous fluids).[91] However, of greater concern is the occurrence of malignant hyperthermia (MH), a hypermetabolic syndrome that occurs in 1 per 15,000 to 50,000 anesthetic exposures, depending upon the patient population. Underlying this syndrome is a rare inherited disorder of skeletal muscle in which the hypermetabolic state is triggered by common anesthetic drugs (e.g., halogenated inhalation agents, succinylcholine) and which, unrecognized or inadequately treated, is often fatal. Although the disorder occurs in all age groups, it is more prevalent in young, overtly healthy individuals with large muscle masses and those with muscular abnormalities, such as ptosis, strabismus, and kyphoscoliosis.

Detection of an MH episode is easy in the fulminant cases in which muscular rigidity and high temperature follow the administration of succinylcholine; however, most cases progress more slowly, with subtle abnormalities. Early signs can include temperature elevation of 0.5°C or more since induction of anesthesia, unexplained tachycardia, muscle rigidity (especially masseter spasm), sweating, hyper- or hypotension, hot skin, and a hot soda lime cannister. Yet, many of these early signs are variously nonspecific, secondary to sympathetic stimulation, and are not necessarily diagnostic of this disorder. A presumptive diagnosis is established during the episode by detecting an increased expired carbon dioxide concentration during constant pulmonary ventilation. Since an end-tidal carbon dioxide monitor is relatively expensive and the disorder is rare (e.g., incidence of 1 episode for every 15,000 to 50,000 general anesthetics), a more cost-effective approach in the ambulatory setting is blood gas analysis: the diagnosis is established by finding a PCO_2 greater than 55 mm Hg and a PO_2 lower than 35 mm Hg in venous blood (assuming PaO_2 is greater than 100 mm Hg and adequate pulmonary ventilation for the patient's body weight) or $PaCo_2$ greater than 60 mm Hg and a base deficit greater than 5 mEq/liter.[55]

Treatment includes the *prompt* administration of dantrolene sodium and supportive care that controls body temperature and preserves acid-base balance and renal function. The Malignant Hyperthermia Association of the United States has advanced the following therapeutic protocol:

1. Discontinue all inhalation anesthetics
2. Hyperventilate with 100% oxygen
3. Give sodium bicarbonate 1 to 2 mEq/kg IV
4. Give dantrolene sodium 2.5 mg/kg IV
5. Cool by all routes
6. Change anesthetic breathing system, including soda lime, if possible
7. Treat persisting and life-threatening arrhythmias with procainamide, 200 mg, IV
8. Give additional dantrolene, as necessary
9. Monitor urine output, serum potassium and calcium, arterial blood gases, and clotting
10. Observe patient in ICU for 24 hours
11. Monitor creatine phosphokinase (CPK), calcium, and potassium until normal
12. Obtain ECG and repeat appropriately
13. Monitor body temperature
14. Maintain urine output > 1 ml/kg/h
15. Continue dantrolene sodium (to total dose of 4 mg/kg/d) for 48 hours

During a suspected MH episode, expert assistance can be obtained at any time through the Medic Alert Foundation International (telephone 209-634-4917).

Since temperature elevation is a *result* and not a cause of the disorder, by the time it occurs, the patient's condition is already compromised. Hence, the necessity of detecting temperature elevation at the earliest possible time in all patients undergoing general anesthesia. Therapy is facilitated if, in addition to having a copy of the recommended management protocol, the following drugs, fluids, and supplies are readily available in a box clearly marked, "Malignant Hyperthermia Emergency":

Arterial blood gas sets	Mannitol
Blood specimen tubes	Methylprednisolone
Dantrolene sodium	Nasogastric tubes
Dextrose (50%)	Procainamide
Foley bladder catheter	Sodium bicarbonate
Furosemide	Sterile water
Insulin	

Prevention requires a thorough preanesthetic inquiry regarding possible prior episodes in the patient or his or her relatives. Individuals suspected of being MH susceptible should be advised to have a diagnostic muscle biopsy which affords the opportunity for *in vitro* elicitation of muscle contracture in response to triggering agents, as well as histochemical and microscopic study. Patient referral for muscle biopsy may be arranged through the Malignant Hyperthermia Association of the United States (telephone 203-655-3007). Patients diagnosed as being MH susceptible should wear a Medic Alert wrist bracelet and should be counseled regarding the anesthetic implications of the disorder for them and their children.

OXYGEN MONITORING

The ability to monitor respiratory gas exchange continuously and noninvasively in the clinical setting is rapidly approaching with the development of transcutaneous PaO_2 and $PaCO_2$ electrodes.[128] Until the technology is refined further and becomes less costly, however, the necessity of assuring adequate oxygenation during general anesthesia must continue to be met by monitoring the oxygen concentration of the inspired gas mixture. Typically, a sensor is placed within the anesthesia breathing system and connected to the oxygen analyzer whose alarm cannot be set below 21% oxygen. The analyzer is calibrated before each anesthetic by exposing the sensor to 100% oxygen and setting the analyzer to read 100%, then repeating this procedure with the sensor exposed to room air (21%). Properly calibrated, however, the oxygen analyzer monitors only the concentration of the gas mixture delivered to the patient and *not* the PaO_2, a measure of the oxygen concentration actually made available to the tissues. Thus, the analyzer warns when a hypoxic mixture is being administered but not whether tissue hypoxemia exists. The anesthesiologist must remain aware that higher concentrations of oxygen (e.g., 40%–50%) are necessary in situations in which poor pulmonary gas exchange is likely (e.g., laparoscopy in deep Trendelenburg position, moderately or morbidly obese patient).

RESUSCITATION EQUIPMENT

Even under the best of circumstances, medical emergencies will occur. The spectrum of urgent situations includes severe hypotension and hypertension, cardiac arrhythmias, bronchospasm, convulsion, respiratory arrest, and cardiopulmonary arrest. These, in turn, are caused variously by the pharmacology and toxicity of the anesthetic drugs, and interaction of anesthetic drugs and adjuvants with the patient's coexisting diseases and medications. The diversity of problems that can be encountered is so great that the reader is referred elsewhere for discussion of pathophysiology and specific treatment.[104] Overall, however, the facility must be trained and equipped to undertake cardiopulmonary resuscitation, at least at the level of basic cardiac life support, according to prescribed protocols.[6] Personnel must also be familiar with the use of the defibrillator and common drugs used in resuscitation.[61,85] Indeed, the accreditation standards promulgated by both JCAH and AAAHC require that there be an emergency cart "appropriate" to the caseload and that personnel have training in CPR.

EMERGENCY CART

The emergency cart must contain those items likely to be needed during cardiopulmonary resuscitation and other medical emergencies. Table 3-2 lists suggested drugs and initial dosages. The cart should also contain an

☐ **Table 3-2 Suggested Minimal Drugs for Emergency Cart**

Drug	Initial Dose	Route
Aminophylline	7 mg/kg over 20 min	IV infusion
Atropine sulfate	0.5–1 mg	IV
Bicarbonate, sodium	0.5–1 mEq/kg	IV
Bretylium tosylate	5–10 mg/kg	IV
Calcium chloride	5–10 mg/kg	IV or IC
Dantrolene sodium	2.5 mg/kg	IV
Dexamethasone hydrochloride	8 mg	IV
Dextrose	0.5 g/kg	IV
Diazepam	0.1 mg/kg	IV
Digoxin	0.25–0.5 mg	IV
Dopamine hydrochloride	200 mg in 500 ml	IV infusion
Ephedrine	10–25 mg	IV
Epinephrine	5–10 ml of 1:10,000 soln	IV or IC
Furosemide	10–40 mg	IV
Hydralazine	5–20 mg	IV
Hydrocortisone	100 mg	IV
Insulin, regular	10–20 units	IV
Isoproterenol hydrochloride	1 mg in 250 ml	IV infusion
Lidocaine	1 mg/kg	IV
Mannitol	0.25–1 g/kg	IV
Naloxone	0.1–0.4 mg	IV
Nitroprusside, sodium	30–50 mg in 250–500 ml	IV infusion
Procainamide	100 mg q 5 min	IV
Propranolol hydrochloride	1 mg q 5 min	IV
Succinylcholine	0.5 mg/kg	IV
Verapamil hydrochloride	0.075–0.15 mg/kg	IV

These dosages are suggested for initial therapy in cardiopulmonary resuscitation or other medical emergencies and should be individualized as the circumstances may warrant.
IV, Intravenous; IC, Intracardiac

electrocardiogram monitor, if one is unlikely to be otherwise available, a defibrillator (see next section), and appropriate sizes of the following equipment and supplies

> Nasopharyngeal and oropharyngeal airways
> Nasopharyngeal and orotracheal tubes
> Laryngoscopes with Macintosh and Miller blades
> Tracheal tube stylets
> Magill forceps
> AMBU bag and masks
> Suction catheters
> Syringes and needles (including intracardiac)
> Intravenous (including central venous) catheters
> Intravenous infusion fluids and administration sets
> Arterial blood gas sets
> Minor surgical tray (for cutdowns and tracheostomy)
> Test tubes for blood chemistry and blood bank specimens
> Adhesive tape
> Gauze sponges

Ideally, the cart should be locked and reequipped following each use; drugs should be inspected for expiration dates monthly. If the cart is not locked and its contents are available for daily use, as in a postanesthesia care unit, then the contents must be checked at the beginning of each work day.

DEFIBRILLATOR

A defibrillator is also a mandatory piece of resuscitative equipment, although a wide choice of models is available. Depending upon need, one can choose a portable unit or one that has an electrocardiogram monitor and even a strip chart recorder. An ambulatory facility that performs cardioversion may wish to economize and obtain a device that serves both functions. Regardless of these special features, however, devices delivering more than 360 joules should not be chosen. After years of argument, the American Heart Association has recently specified a recommendation for a reduced shock energy of 200 to 300 joules in adults, less than 100 in children.[6,28]

Evaluating and Modifying Selection Decisions

Conscientious ambulatory anesthesia units will seek to maintain their ability to provide high-quality, cost-effective care by modifying their selection decision according to the outcome of their care. Ideally, this process should involve continuous data collection and periodic rigorous analysis, including double-blind clinical trials of alternative drugs or other modalities of care. Realistically, however, few units can muster such an intensive evaluation process. The majority of units will find that criteria established through peer review of available literature, with adjustments to their local setting, can be modified by using the same process. Utilization review and quality assurance programs, mandated by accreditation standards, demonstrate how peer review can be used to modify selection decisions.

UTILIZATION REVIEW PROGRAMS

Utilization review (UR), another accreditation requirement, endeavors to assure appropriate allocation of the hospital's resources so that high-quality care is delivered in the most cost-effective manner.[66] UR programs specifically address overutilization, underutilization, and inefficient scheduling. In the context of ambulatory care, of course, UR programs have sought to shift the simpler, less complex elective surgery from expensive hospital operating rooms to less costly ambulatory surgery units. Among the most potent forces behind these efforts has been, not unexpectedly, the insurance industry, particularly the National Association of Blue Cross/Blue Shield (BC/BS) Plans. Some 30 BC/BS plans have successfully focused such UR programs on ambulatory surgery by using educational and financial incentive programs. These plans have cooperated in establishing lists of surgical procedures that are or could be performed on an ambulatory basis, distributed the lists to participating physicians and local hospitals, requested that the physicians perform them on an ambulatory basis unless there was a demonstrated need for hospitalization, and asked the hospitals to develop UR procedures relating to listed procedures that were being performed on an inpatient basis. The performance of listed procedures at a high rate among inpatients has prompted statewide programs to create preadmission screening criteria that assist in shifting appropriate cases to the ambulatory setting. The following preadmission screening criteria were established by the Iowa Foundation for Medical Care for the purpose of justifying hospitalization for three common surgical procedures:[127]

Preadmission Screening Criteria for Specific Surgical Procedures

 D&C or Cystoscopy
  Concomittant disease that is severe or requires intensive care
  History of severe or life-threatening systemic disease or disturbance
   (e.g., incapacitating cardiac, pulmonary, renal, or hepatic insuf-
   ficiency; diabetes mellitus with vascular complications, angina
   pectoris, or healed myocardial infarction)
  Uncontrolled diabetes mellitus or other major endocrine disorder
  Another procedure scheduled to follow D&C or cystoscopy
 Surgical dental extraction
  Concomitant systemic disease under therapy (e.g., cardiovascular
   disease, uncontrolled diabetes)
  Planned procedure is complex and may require the services of an acute
   care hospital
  General anesthesia required because of age or mental/physical handicap

A similar program in Hartford County, Connecticut, formulated criteria principally related to patient condition:[143]

Preadmission Screening Criteria Related to Patient Condition

 ASA physical status 3, 4, or 5
 Seizure disorder, insulin-dependent diabetes mellitus, coagulopathy, car-
  diovascular or pulmonary disease,
 Inability to comply with instruction and/or care for self
 Another procedure scheduled to follow
 For breast biopsy only: clinical suspicion of carcinoma, or positive
  mammogram
 For pediatric herniorrhaphy: cholinesterase deficiency, hemoglobinopathy,
  or hemoglobin less than 11.5 g/dl (or hematocrit less than 35%)

These sets of preadmission screening criteria are not designed to be standards of care or to replace good clinical judgment. Rather, they serve to assist UR personnel to evaluate whether hospitalization is warranted. Moreover, the two sets of criteria presented here are merely examples of what any peer group could establish. Undoubtedly, interest in this area will intensify.

As part of such preadmission screening programs, UR personnel certify the need for hospitalization only when at least one criterion is met; otherwise, they refer the case to a physician consultant. If the physician, through independent evaluation, cannot justify the need for hospitalization, the UR personnel notify the would-be admitting physician their belief that the admission is unnecessary and that the proposed admission is denied. The implementation of such a program has resulted in a sharp decrease in the frequency of affected procedures being performed on an inpatient basis without compromising patient care. In this way, hospital admission criteria developed through peer review effectively augment the decision making regarding patient selection in the ambulatory setting.

QUALITY ASSURANCE PROGRAMS

Ambulatory surgery centers can also assure that their selection decisions (among other aspects of their care) are maintaining patient safety and quality of care by conducting a quality assurance program. This is actually a recent addition to the JCAH accreditation requirements, as Standard VII for the hospital-affiliated program.[65] The underlying rationale for a quality assurance program is simply the improvement in patient care. The components of such a program are the identification of patient-related problems, objective assessment of such problems, implementation of meaningful solutions, monitoring the effectiveness of the solutions, and, finally, documentation of the effectiveness of the solutions.[13,15,106]

RUDIMENTS OF A QUALITY ASSURANCE PROGRAM

Individuality, creativity, and innovation are encouraged in the implementation of the program, which may include two approaches: The newer approach involves a retrospective patient care evaluation which assesses the occurrence of clinically important postoperative problems such as the following:

Respiratory symptoms
Excessive bleeding
Persisting nausea or vomiting
Circulatory or neurologic impairment
Excessive pain
Signs of infection

This patient care evaluation can be accomplished with a form that the patient receives once home or by use of a phone call within a few days of the surgery. The older approach is the formal quality assurance audit that for many years JCAH has encouraged hospitals to undertake periodically in relation to specific perceived problems. Operationally, however, the two approaches are often undertaken in series; the retrospective patient care evaluation may suggest a problem that can be examined in detail through the quality assurance audit.

Regardless of the approach, however, the program should stress objective outcome measures, such as

Deaths
Unplanned hospital admissions or hospital transfers
Complications
Cancellations and delays
Blood transfusions
Infection rates

Even patient and surgeon satisfaction can be assessed by using objective, criteria-based rating scales rather than diffuse, freeform, subjective comments.

Once a problem is identified, its causes are sought. Depending upon the nature of the problem, staff meetings, interviews, or perhaps some other approach is used. Often, however, with a little detective work, a cause seems obvious. For example, a disproportionate number of unplanned admissions occurring among patients with asthma might prompt a more stringent preoperative assessment of such patients (e.g., electing not to treat those requiring steroids *and* bronchodilators in the ambulatory setting). Following implementation of the revised preoperative assessment, an audit is performed to monitor the effectiveness of the new policy; if the new policy is found ineffective, other changes in the selection decisions might be tried and the audit repeated until effectiveness is documented. In this way, a cycle is completed, and care is improved. A quality assurance program, thus, becomes a mechanism by which selection decisions can be modified to improve patient care. (Quality assurance is discussed further in Chap. 10.)

References

1. Abdu RA: Ambulatory herniorrhaphy under local anesthesia in a community hospital. Am J Surg 145:353, 1983
2. Abramowitz MD, Oh TH, Epstein BE et al: The antiemetic effect of droperidol following strabismus surgery in children. Anesthesiology 59:579, 1983
3. Abramson DJ: 857 Breast biopsies as an outpatient procedure. Ann Surg 163:478, 1966
4. Ackart RS, Foreman DR, Klayton RJ et al: Fiberoptic bronchoscopy in outpatient facilities, 1982. Arch Intern Med 143:30, 1983
5. Adler AG, McElwain GE, Merli GJ et al: Systemic effects of eye drops. Arch Intern Med 142:2293, 1982
6. American Heart Association: Standards and guidelines for cardiopulmonary resuscitation (CPR) and emergency cardiac care (ECC). JAMA 244:453, 1980
7. American Hospital Association: 1980 Survey of Hospital Involvement with Ambulatory Surgery. Chicago, American Hospital Association, 1980
8. American National Standard for Anesthetic Equipment—Scavenging Systems for Excess Anesthetic Gases. ANSI Z79.11-1982. New York, American National Standards Institute, January 1982
9. American Society of Anesthesiologists' Ad Hoc Committee on Effects of Trace Anesthetic Agents on Health of Operating Room Personnel: Waste Anesthetic Gases in Operating Room Air: A Suggested Program to Reduce Personnel Exposure. American Society of Anesthesiologists, Park Ridge, IL, undated.
10. Ashcraft KE, Guinee WS, Golladay ES: Clinical assessment of hematocrit and hemoglobin. Anesthesiol Rev 9(2):37, 1982
11. Bailey HAT Jr, Pappas JJ, Gay EC Jr: O.P.S.C.: Improving delivery of otolaryngological surgical care. Laryngoscope 88:1612, 1978
12. Brindle GF, Soliman MG: Anaesthetic complications in surgical outpatients. Can Anaesth Soc J 22:613, 1975
13. Brown EM: Quality assurance in anesthesiology—the problem-oriented audit. Anesth Analg 63:611, 1984
14. Bruno LA, Smith DS, Bloom MJ et al: Sudden hypotension with a test dose of chymopapain. Anesth Analg 63:533, 1984
15. Buske SM: A quality assurance program for ambulatory surgical services. In Burns LA (ed): Ambulatory Surgery: Developing and Managing Successful Programs, pp 63–81. Rockville, MD, Aspen Systems Corporation, 1984
16. Cainan J: One-day surgery for rheumatoid arthritis. Nursing Mirror, p 51, July 29, 1976
17. Cardiac catheterization plan cuts hospitalization. Hosp Prac 17(3):51, 1982
18. Carson JL, Eisenberg JM: The preoperative screening examination. In Goldmann DR, Brown FH, Levy WK et al (eds): Medical Care of the Surgical Patient: A Problem-Oriented Approach to Management, pp 16–30. Philadelphia, JB Lippincott, 1982

19. Cass E, Kadar D, Stein HA: Hazards of phenylephrine topical medications in persons taking propranolol. Can Med Assoc J 120:1261, 1979
20. Centers for Disease Control: Annual Summary 1981: Reported Morbidity and Mortality in the United States. MMWR 30(54):126, 1982
21. Centers for Disease Control: Annual Summary 1982: Reported Morbidity and Mortality in the United States. MMWR 31(54):134 and 135, 1983
22. Chiang TM, Sukis AE, Ross DE: Tonsillectomy performed on an outpatient basis: Report of a series of 40,000 cases performed without a death. Arch Otolaryngol 88:105, 1968
23. Chymopapain for herniated lumbar discs. Med Lett Drugs Ther 25:41, 1983
24. Cohen DD, Dillon JB: Anesthesia for outpatient surgery. JAMA 196:1114, 1966
25. Cohen D, Keneally J, Black A et al: Experience with day stay surgery. J Pediatr Surg 15:21, 1980
26. Cooper, JB, Newbower RS, Kitz RJ: An analysis of major errors and equipment failures in anesthesia management: Consideration for prevention and detection. Anesthesiology 60:34, 1984
27. Cork RC, Vaughan RW, Humphrey LS: Precision and accuracy of intraoperative temperature monitoring. Anesth Analg 62:211, 1983
28. Crampton RS: Ventricular defibrillation. In Jacobson S (ed): Resuscitation, pp 55–68. New York, Churchill Livingstone, 1983
29. Cullen BF, Margolis AJ, Eger EI II: The effects of anesthesia and pulmonary ventilation on blood loss during elective therapeutic abortion. Anesthesiology 32:108, 1970
30. Cullen DJ, Stevens WC, Smith NT et al: Clinical signs of anesthesia. Anesthesiology 36:21, 1972
31. Davis JE: The need to redefine levels of surgical care. JAMA 251:2527, 1984
32. Davis JE, Detmer DE: The ambulatory surgical unit. Ann Surg 175:856, 1972
33. Denlinger JK: Pneumothorax. In Orkin FK, Cooperman LH (eds): Complications in Anesthesiology, pp 173–182. Philadelphia, JB Lippincott, 1983
34. Detmer DE: Ambulatory surgery. N Engl J Med 305:1406, 1981
35. Detmer DE, Buchanan-Davidson DJ: Ambulatory surgery. Surg Clin North Am 62:685, 1982
36. Don H: Hypoxemia and hypercapnia during and after anesthesia. In Orkin FK, Cooperman LH (eds): Complications in Anesthesiology, pp 183–207. Philadelphia, JB Lippincott, 1983
37. Dornette WHL: The stethoscope—the anesthesiologist's best friend. Anesth Analg 42:711, 1963
38. Egdahl RH: Should we shrink the health care system? Harvard Business Review 61(1):125, 1984
39. Eisenberg JM, Clark JR, Sussman SA: prothrombin and partial thromboplastin times as preoperative screening tests. Arch Surg 117:48, 1982
40. Elliot DL, Linz DH, Kane JA: Electroconvulsive therapy: pretreatment medical evaluation. Arch Intern Med 142:979, 1982
41. Evans DIK, Morris Jones P, Morris P, Shaw EA: Outpatient anaesthesia for a children's leukaemia clinic. Lancet 1:751, 1971
42. Faculty expert explains steps to low hospital admission rates. Same Day Surg 6(11):136, 1982
43. Falstie-Jensen S, Jensen UH, Sondergaard-Petersen PE, Lauritzen J, Vibild HO, Kampmann J: Arthroscopy: Should it be done as an outpatient procedure or during hospitalization? Acta Orthop Scand 54:131, 1983
44. First study of freestanding outpatient surgery centers now available. Same Day Surg 8(7):80, 1984
45. Flanagan L Jr, Bascom JU: Herniorrhaphies performed upon outpatients under local anesthesia. Surg Gynecol Obstet 153:557, 1981
46. Flanagan L Jr, Bascom JU: Repair of the groin hernia: Outpatient approach with local anesthesia. Surg Clin North Am 64:257, 1984
47. Forbes AR, Gamsu G: Mucociliary clearance in the canine lung during and after general anesthesia. Anesthesiology 50:26, 1979
48. Garrioch DB, Gilbert JR, Plantevin OM: Choice of ecbolic and the morbidity of day-case terminations of pregnancy. Br J Obstet Gynaecol 88:1029, 1981

49. Gavin WA, Stewart DK, Murray JA: Outpatient coronary arteriography. Cathet Cardiovasc Diagn 7:347, 1981

50. Glassow F: Short stay surgery (Shouldice technique) for repair of inguinal hernia. Ann R Coll Surg Engl 59:123, 1976

51. Goldman L, Caldera DL, Nussbaum SR et al: Multifactorial index of cardiac risk in noncardiac surgical procedures. N Engl J Med 297:845, 1977

52. Goldmann DR, Brown FH, Levy WK et al (eds): Medical Care of the Surgical Patient: A Problem-Oriented Approach to Management. Philadelphia, JB Lippincott, 1982

53. Gravenstein JS, Paulus DA: Monitoring Practice in Clinical Anesthesia. Philadelphia, JB Lippincott, 1982

54. Greene NM: Physiology of Spinal Anesthesia, 3rd ed, p 27. Baltimore, Williams & Wilkins, 1981

55. Gronert GA: Malignant hyperthermia. Semin Anesthesiol 2:197, 1983

56. Hackett GH, Harris MNE, Plantevin OM et al: Anaesthesia for outpatient termination of pregnancy: A comparison of two anaesthetic techniques. Br J Anaesth 54:865, 1982

57. Heneghan C, McAuliffe R, Thomas D et al: Morbidity after outpatient anaesthesia: A comparison of two techniques of endotracheal anaesthesia for dental surgery. Anaesthesia 36:4, 1981

58. Herzfeld G: Hernia in infancy. Am J Surg 39:422, 1938

59. Hirsch RP, Schwartz B: Increased mortality among elderly patients undergoing cataract extraction. Arch Ophthalmol 101:1034, 1983

60. Humphreys CF, Kay H: The control of postoperative wound pain with the use of bupivacaine injections. J Urol 116:618, 1976

61. Jacobson S (ed): Resuscitation. New York, Churchill Livingstone, 1983

62. Jackson DP, Pitts HA: Biopsy with delayed radical mastectomy for carcinoma of the breast. Am J Surg 98:184, 1959

63. Jensen S, Wetchler BV: The obese patient: An acceptable candidate for outpatient anesthesia. JAANA 50:369, 1982

64. Joint Commission on Accreditation of Hospitals: Accreditation Manual for Ambulatory Health Care, pp 30–33, Chicago, Joint Commission on Accreditation of Hospitals, 1983

65. Joint Commission on Accreditation of Hospitals: Accreditation Manual for Hospitals, 1984. pp 61–68. Chicago, Joint Commission on Accreditation of Hospitals, 1983

66. Joint Commission on Accreditation of Hospitals: Accreditation Manual for Hospitals, 1984, pp 193–194. Chicago, Joint Commission on Accreditation of Hospitals, 1983

67. Jones CW: Anesthesia for outpatient surgery. JNMA 66:411, 1974

68. Kammerer WS, Gross RJ (eds): Medical Consultation: Role of the Internist on Surgical, Obstetric, and Psychiatric Services. Baltimore, Williams & Wilkins, 1983

69. Kaplan JA: The electrocardiogram and anesthesia. In Miller RD (ed): Anesthesia, pp 203–232. New York, Churchill Livingstone, 1981

70. Kaplan JA, King SB: The precordial electrocardiographic lead (V_5) in patients who have coronary artery disease. Anesthesiology 45:570, 1976

71. Katz J, Benumof J, Kadis LB (eds): Anesthesia and Uncommon Diseases: Pathophysiologic and Clinical Correlations. 2nd ed. Philadelphia, WB Saunders, 1981

72. Kay M: General anaesthesia in the private dental office. Can Anaesth Soc J 30:406, 1983

73. Keys TE: The History of Surgical Anesthesia. pp 3–31. Huntington, NY, Robert E Krieger, 1978

74. Klein W, Schulitz KP: Outpatient arthroscopy under local anesthesia. Arch Orthop Trauma Surg 96:131, 1980

75. Kingsnorth AN, Britton BJ, Morris PJ: Recurrent inguinal hernia after local anaesthetic repair. Br J Surg 68:273, 1981

76. Knight PR, Bedows E, Nahrwold ML et al: Alterations in influenza virus pulmonary pathology induced by diethyl ether, halothane, enflurane, and pentobarbital anesthesia in mice. Anesthesiology 58:209, 1983

77. Lee RH, Marzoni FA, Cannon WB et al: Outpatient adult inguinal-hernia repair. West J Med 140:905, 1984

78. Lees DE, Schuette W, Bull JM et al: An evaluation of liquid-crystal thermometry as a screening device for intraoperative hyperthermia. Anesth Analg 57:669, 1978
79. Levy ML, Coakley CS: Survey of in and out surgery—the first year. South Med J 61:995, 1968
80. Levy WK: Alcohol and drug abuse in the surgical patient. In Goldmann DR, Brown FH, Levy WK et al: Medical Care of the Surgical Patient: A Problem-Oriented Approach to Management, pp 568–577. Philadelphia, JB Lippincott, 1982
81. Lewin I, Lerner AG, Green SH et al: Physical class and physiologic status in the prediction of operative mortality in the aged sick. Ann Surg 174:2, 1971
82. Lewit EM, Marshall CL, Salzer JE: An evaluation of a plastic strip thermometer. JAMA 247:321, 1982
83. Liu LMP, Cote CJ, Goudsouzian NG et al: Life-threatening apnea in infants recovering from anesthesia. Anesthesiology 59:506, 1983
84. Marx GF, Mateo CV, Orkin LR: Computer analysis of postanesthetic deaths. Anesthesiology 39:54, 1973
85. McIntyre KM, Lewis AJ (eds): Textbook of Advanced Cardiac Life Support. American Heart Association, 1981
86. Mercier C, Page A, Verdant A et al: Outpatient management of intercostal tube drainage in spontaneous pneumothorax. Ann Thorac Surg 22:163, 1976
87. Meridy HW: Criteria for selection of ambulatory surgical patients and guidelines for anesthetic management: A retrospective study of 1553 cases. Anesth Analg 61:921, 1982
88. Miller LB: Orthopedic patients in an ambulatory surgery facility. Nurse Clin North Am 16:749, 1981
89. Miller RD: Monitoring of neuromuscular blockade. In Saidman LJ, Smith NT (eds): Monitoring in Anesthesia, 2nd ed, pp 193–225. Boston, Butterworth & Co, 1984
90. Mitchell GW, Homer MJ: Outpatient breast biopsies on a gynecologic service. Am J Obstet Gynecol 144:127, 1982
91. Modell JH: Septicemia as a cause of immediate postoperative hyperthermia. Anesthesiology 27:329, 1966
92. Molitch ME (ed): Management of Medical Problems in Surgical Patients. Philadelphia, FA Davis, 1982
93. Moss J, McDermott DJ, Thisted RA et al: Anaphylactic/anaphylactoid reactions in response to chymodiactin (chymopapain). Anesthesiology 63:S253, 1984
94. Murphy SB: Difficulties in sickle cell state. In Orkin FK, Cooperman LH (eds): Complications in Anesthesiology. pp 476–485. Philadelphia, JP Lippincott, 1983
95. National Center for Health Statistics: Utilization of Short-Stay Hospitals: Annual Summaries and Surgical Operations in Short-Stay Hospitals, US, 1981. Washington, DC, U.S. Government Printing Office
96. National Fire Protection Association: Standard for the Use of Inhalation Anesthetics. NFPA 56A. Boston, National Fire Protection Association, 1978
97. National Fire Protection Association: Safe Use of Electricity in Patient Care Areas of Hospitals. Boston National Fire Protection Association, 1980
98. National Fire Protection Association: National Electrical Code. NFPA 70. Boston, National Fire Protection Association, 1981
99. Natof HE: Complications associated with ambulatory surgery. JAMA 244:1116, 1980
100. Neufeld GR: Burns and electrocution. In Orkin FK, Cooperman LH (eds): Complications in Anesthesiology. p 677. Philadelphia, JB Lippincott, 1983
101. Nicoll JH: The surgery of infancy. Br Med J 2:753, 1909
102. Newbower RS, Cooper JB, Long CD: Failure analysis—the human element. In Gravenstein JS, Newbower RS, Ream AK et al (eds): Essential Non-Invasive Monitoring in the Operating Room. pp 269–281. New York, Grune & Stratton, 1980
103. Ogg TW, Jennings RA, Morrison CG: Day-case anaesthesia for termination of pregnancy: Evaluation of a total intravenous anaesthetic technique. Anaesthesia 38:1042, 1983
104. Orkin FK, Cooperman LH (eds): Complications in Anesthesiology. Philadelphia, JB Lippincott, 1983

105. Othersen HB, Clatworthy HW Jr: Outpatient herniorrhaphy for infants. Am J Dis Child 116:78, 1968
106. Palmer RH: Ambulatory Health Care Evaluation: Principles and Practice. Chicago, American Hospital Association, 1983
107. Physicians debate merits of mandatory intubation for elective laparoscopy. Same Day Surg 8(7):82, 1984
108. Pierce EH, Clagett OT, McDonald JF et al: Biopsy of the breast followed by delayed radical mastectomy. Surg Gynecol Obstet 103:559, 1956
109. Ponka JL, Sapala JA: Bupivacaine as a local anesthetic for hernia repair. Henry Ford Hosp Med J 24(1):31, 1976
110. Poretz DM, Eron LJ, Goldenberg RI et al: Intravenous antibiotic therapy in an outpatient setting. JAMA 248:336, 1982
111. Porterfield HW, Franklin LT: The use of general anesthesia in the office surgery facility. Clin Plast Surg 10(2):289, 1983
111a. Presurgical Chest X-ray Referral Criteria Panel Draft Report. Docket #84N-0217. Washington, DC, U.S. Food and Drug Administration, Bureau of Radiological Health and Devices, July 10, 1984
112. Rasch D, Holt J, Wilson M et al: Bronchospasm following injection of acetylcholine in a patient taking metoprolol. Anesthesiology 59:583, 1983
113. Reynolds RC, Pauca AL: Gastric perforation, an anesthetic-induced hazard in laparoscopy. Anesthesiology 38:84, 1973
114. Rosenberg TD, Wong HC: Arthroscopic knee surgery in a freestanding outpatient surgery center. Orthoped Clin North Am 13:277, 1982
115. Rutkow IM, Zuidema GD: Surgical rates in the United States. Surgery 89:151, 1981
116. Ryan JF: Unintentional hypothermia. In Orkin FK, Cooperman LH (eds): Complications in Anesthesiology, pp 284–290. Philadelphia, JB Lippincott, 1983
117. Saidman LJ, Smith NT (eds): Monitoring in Anesthesia, 2nd ed. Boston, Butterworth & Co, 1984
118. Schneider AJL: Assessment of risk factors and surgical outcome. Surg Clin North Am 63:1113, 1983
119. Shah CP: Anaesthesia for day-care surgery. I. Day-care surgery in Canada. Can Anaesth Soc J 27:399, 1980
120. Sieverts S: Ambulatory surgery and health insurance. In Burns LA (ed): Ambulatory Surgery: Developing and Managing Successful Programs. pp 177–194. Rockville, MD, Aspen Systems Corporation, 1984
121. Sidhu MS, Cullen BF: Low-dose enflurane does not increase blood loss during therapeutic abortion. Anesthesiology 57:127, 1982
122. Smith WS, McDermott DJ, Agre K et al: Chymopapain injection. JAMA 251:2515, 1984
123. Solosko D, Smith RB: Hypertension following 10% phenylephrine ophthalmic. Anesthesiology 36:187, 1972
124. Statement on cost containment. Bull Amer Coll Surg 64(7):3, 1979
125. Stein HD: Ambulatory breast biopsies: The patient's choice. Am Surg 48:221, 1982
126. Stoelting RK, Dierdorf SF (eds): Anesthesia and Co-Existing Disease. New York, Churchill Livingstone, 1983
127. Stump D: An outpatient/same-day surgery program based on peer review. QRB 9(4):112, 1983
128. Transcutaneous O_2 and CO_2 monitoring of the adult and neonate (Symposium). Crit Care Med 9:689, 1981
129. Vacanti CJ, Van Houten RJ, Hill RC: A statistical analysis of the relationship of physical status to postoperative mortality in 68,388 cases. Anesth Analg 49:564, 1970
130. Vandam LD (ed): To Make the Patient Ready for Anesthesia: Medical Care of the Surgical Patient, 2nd ed. Menlo Park, CA, Addison-Wesley, 1984
131. Vaughan RW: Definitions and risks of obesity. In Brown BR Jr (ed): Anesthesia and the Obese Patient. pp 1–7. Philadelphia, FA Davis, 1982

132. Vaughan RW, Bauer S, Wise L: Volume and *p*H of gastric juice in obese patients. Anesthesiology 43:686, 1975
133. Vickers MD (ed): Medicine for Anaesthetists, 2nd ed. Oxford, Blackwell Scientific, 1982
134. Waters RM: The down-town anesthesia clinic. Am J Surg (Anesth Suppl) 33:71, 1919
135. Wetchler BV: Anesthesia for outpatients. In Mauldin BC (ed): Ambulatory Surgery: A Guide to Perioperative Nursing Care, pp 111–158. New York, Grune & Stratton, 1983
136. Wetchler BV: Anesthesiologists serve as watchdogs in ambulatory surgical settings. Same Day Surg 8(7):83, 1984
137. Wetchler BV, Collins IS, Jacob L: Antiemetic effects of droperidol on the ambulatory surgery patient. Anesthesiol Rev 9(5):23, 1982
138. White PF: Ketamine—its use an intravenous anesthetic. Clin Anesthesiol 2(1):43, 1984
139. White PF, Coe V, Dworsky WA et al: Disseminated intravascular coagulation following midtrimester abortions. Anesthesiology 58:99, 1983
140. Willatts DG, Harrison AR, Groom JF et al: Cardiac arrhythmias during outpatient dental anaesthesia: Comparison of halothane with enflurane. Br J Anaesth 55:399, 1983
141. Wilson ME, Williams NB, Baskett PJF et al: Assessment of fitness for surgical procedures and the variability of anaesthetists' judgments. Br Med J 1:509, 1980
142. Wood GJ, Lloyd JW, Bullingham RES et al: Postoperative analgesia for day-case herniorrhaphy patients: A comparison of cryoanalgesia, paravertebral blockade and oral analgesia. Anaesthesia 36:603, 1981
143. Wright G, Goldberg M, Mark H, Petrillo MK, Wiesel B: Utilization review to increase ambulatory-based surgery: Application for surgical tooth extraction. QRB 9(4):100, 1983
144. Yag laser may bring new cases to offices, SDS offices, Same Day Surg 7:20, 1983

4

The Pediatric Patient

Burton S. Epstein, M.D.

Raafat S. Hannallah, M.D.

The concept of ambulatory or same-day surgery in infants and children is not new. Outpatient pediatric anesthesia has been reported as early as 1909 by Nicoll[56] and by Herzfeld in 1938.[40] The more recent "discovery" and growing popularity of ambulatory surgery, particularly for pediatric patients, have been dictated by our current social and fiscal needs and have created new challenges and rewarding opportunities for the pediatric anesthesiologist. This chapter reviews the fundamentals of the safe practice of pediatric anesthesia in the ambulatory surgical setting. It is based on a review of the literature, discussions with professionals who have had extensive experience with the subject, and our own personal experience.

Some authors believe that up to 50% of all surgical procedures in children can be performed safely on an outpatient basis. A recent survey by the American Academy of Pediatrics confirmed that a substantial amount of surgery is indeed being done that way.[92] Of the pediatric anesthesiologists responding to the survey, 97% reported that they perform outpatient anesthesia at their institutions. Forty percent of the respondents noted that outpatients represented 20% or less of their practice; 50% stated that such patients constituted 20% to 40% of their practice; and 6% said that outpatients accounted for some 40% of their cases.

Advantages

Some of the reasons for performing surgery on an outpatient basis are the same in both children and adults. These include

Reducing the cost of medical care

Increasing the availability of hospital beds for those who need them

Offering a level of care comparable to that received by the inpatient without its inconveniences and potential hazards

At the same time, however, ambulatory surgery has several distinct advantages that are unique to the pediatric patient:

Children rarely have systemic disease and are good anesthetic risks.

Many common surgical procedures such as herniotomy and myringotomy are simpler to perform in children than in adults and are associated with a shorter, less complicated convalescent period.

Separation from the parent is minimized.[85]

Hospital-acquired infections are reduced.[60]

The feeding schedule is less severely disrupted.

For children, the two greatest advantages of ambulatory surgery are the reductions in separation anxiety and in nosocomial infections. Steward has noted that in a well-organized program it should not be necessary to separate parent and child for much longer than the duration of anesthesia.[87] Minimizing separation from family, home, and friends is particularly beneficial for the preschooler who still depends on his or her mother as the ultimate security object during times of stress.[89] Most parents are usually enthusiastic about participating in the preparation and postoperative care of the child and prefer this to having the child admitted to the hospital. The experience may be of benefit to the whole family unit.[83]

The reduction in nosocomial infections is particularly important in infants. Othersen cites two of the few available studies concerning this issue.[60] The first, reported by Izant in 1957 involved a group of infants admitted for "clean" elective operations, of whom 17% developed signs and symptoms of enteric or respiratory infection while hospitalized or within 3 days of discharge. Izant also noted that during a 2-day hospitalization for elective herniorrhaphy, an average of 25 different potentially contaminated hospital personnel touched each infant or his or her bed. Twenty-three additional individuals were intimately involved with the care of the infant during a single visit to the operating and recovery rooms. In the second study cited by Othersen, Mintor compared 68 infants admitted for inpatient herniorrhaphy with 26 similar infants undergoing the same procedure as outpatients. He found that the incidence of postoperative cross infection was 50% to 75% lower in the outpatient group. Although the evidence seems convincing, there are no recent studies on large groups of patients that verify a reduction in cross infection among ambulatory surgical patients.

Potential Disadvantages

Although the advantages are striking, pediatric ambulatory surgery can also have its problems. Unfortunately, there is a tendency to associate outpatient surgery with "minor procedures" and "healthy patients" and to assume that all children about to undergo minor operations as outpatients have no concurrent medical problems and are psychologically well adjusted. That assumption does a disservice to those who require special consideration. When the emphasis is on increasing speed, reducing turnaround time between procedures, and minimizing the length of hospitalization, children have less time to adjust to the hospital environment. As a matter of fact, there is evidence that, from the psychological point of view, for some children hospitalization may actually be an experience that is not at all detrimental to mental health, particularly if the stay is less than 2 days.[24] Some of the reasons for this are discussed under the heading Psychological Preparation.

Assuming that all short-stay patients are a healthy and uniform group medically is a common misconception that leads to problems. Patients who have undiagnosed acute diseases such as upper respiratory infections (URI) or diarrhea, or asymptomatic patients with a previously diagnosed or even undiagnosed chronic problem, such as heart disease, may be scheduled at ambulatory surgery facilities. Unfortunately, the record of a previous consultation report, if performed, including diagnosis and recommendations for therapy, may not always be available for these patients. This usually leads to delays and hard feelings between physicians and parents.

Another potential problem results from the stipulation by many ambulatory surgical facilities that one or both parents remain with the child throughout the hospital stay. This may require that one or both parents take leave from work and that siblings at home be cared for by others. In some cases the inconvenience and out-of-pocket expense to the parents caused by this practice may be greater than the cost of hospitalization to them. In addition, some parents are apprehensive about caring for their child at home after discharge.[85] This is particularly true if the child is very young or if any problems have arisen during the recovery stay. The lack of privacy of outpatient accommodations and the potential necessity for extra visits to the hospital to obtain preoperative screening and consultations are also annoying for pediatric ambulatory surgical patients.

The question of reducing the cost of medical care to a given patient vs. the overall cost to an institution or community whose inpatient census declines because of the advent of ambulatory surgery is yet another complex issue that has generated great debate.[57]

Factors in Selection of Patients

The criteria for selecting patients and procedures for pediatric ambulatory surgery vary greatly among institutions. They are usually influenced by the condition of the patient, the attitude of the parents, the type of surgical procedure, and any special considerations for anesthetic management and recovery.[19] Since the surgeon initiates the entire process, he or she must cooperate with and understand the overall process completely. Some of the most important considerations are as follows:

The Patient

The child should be in good health or any systemic disease he or she has must be under good control. Some anesthesiologists still restrict ambulatory surgery to patients classified as ASA 1 and 2, while others[23,63,83] may accept ASA class 3 patients under special circumstances. This usually requires prior consultation with a member of the anesthesia staff and a current written statement from the attending physician about the nature of the illness and recommended therapy. Patients with a controlled convulsive disorder or well-regulated diabetes, for example, may be acceptable, while those with a bleeding tendency, liver insufficiency, incipient heart failure, uncontrolled diabetes, or infectious diseases are not. Many children with chronic diseases benefit substantially from outpatient treatment.[83] Hospital-acquired infections are a specific risk to these children, as is the emotional trauma of repeated hospitalization. A child with leukemia or one who is receiving immunosuppressant medication is particularly suitable for outpatient care. Physically handicapped, psychologically disturbed, or mentally retarded children benefit tremendously from the lack of separation and continued support of a parent or guardian that is usually fostered in outpatient facilities.

SPECIAL PROBLEMS

THE CHILD WITH A RUNNY NOSE

One of the most perplexing issues that commonly faces the anesthesiologist is the child who presents with a runny nose. Since probably 20% to 30% of all children have a runny nose a significant part of the year, the practice of *automatically* cancelling all children with a runny nose would result in inordinate hardships on the parents, the child, and the medical system. Every child with a runny nose must be evaluated on an individual basis. The subject has been recently reviewed by Berry,[9] and is summarized here.

The points to consider before making a decision are that a child who presents with a runny nose may have either a completely benign, noninfectious condition, in which case elective surgery may safely be performed, or the runny nose may be a prodrome to, or actually be, an infectious process, in which case elective surgery should be cancelled. Examples of these conditions are shown below.[9]

☐   *Differential Diagnosis of Runny Nose*

Noninfectious runny nose
  Allergic rhinitis
    Seasonal
    Perennial
  Vasomotor rhinitis
    Emotional (crying)
    Temperature
Infectious runny nose
  Viral infections—e.g., nasopharyngitis (common cold), contagious diseases (chicken
    pox/measles)
  Acute bacterial infections (e.g., streptococcal tonsillitis, meningitis)

(Berry FA: Seminars in Anesthesia 3:24–31, 1984. With permission.)

The preanesthetic assessment of these patients consists of obtaining a complete history, performing a physical examination, and examining certain laboratory data. Early in the clinical course, the history will be the most important single factor in the differential diagnosis. Specifically, allergic problems such as hay fever, sinusitis, asthma, and recurrent bronchitis should be actively sought. A history of an infectious illness in other members of the family or in the community is important. Parents are usually well aware and can tell whether their child's runny nose is "the usual runny nose" or something different. The following questions need to be answered by the parents: Is this the usual runny nose, or is it something different? Does the child have his or her normal appetite? Is the child playing and sleeping normally? If the parents say that this condition is not the usual runny nose and that it is something different, then this, by itself, is sufficient cause to cancel elective surgery. The physical examination is not always conclusive. Normal findings may be present during the early part of an infectious process. Chronic allergic rhinitis, on the other hand, may be associated with local infections within the nasopharynx resulting in purulent nasal discharge. Again, the parents can be helpful in establishing whether this is the usual discharge or not. If the remainder of the physical examination and history are normal, elective surgery may be performed. However, if there are obvious findings on physical examination such as a temperature of 38°C, viral ulcers in the oropharynx, tonsillitis, or rales, the child is considered to have an infectious process, and elective surgery is cancelled.

Useful laboratory data include a complete blood cell count and, if indicated, a chest radiograph. A white blood cell count ≥12,000 to 15,000 with a shift to the left suggests an infectious process. If a child has a runny nose and a cough and there is still a question of infectious process, he or she certainly deserves a chest radiograph before proceeding with elective surgery.

The risk associated with anesthetizing a child who has had an upper respiratory infection (URI) may be present for up to 4 to 6 weeks after an apparent recovery. Although well-controlled studies are still lacking, this appears particularly true after a flu-like syndrome that involves both the upper and lower respiratory tract. In such a case there are symptoms of the common cold plus the constitutional signs and symptoms of chills, fever, myalgias, and often a severe cough. In children who have these syndromes, perioperative respiratory complications such as laryngospasm and bronchospasm were reported during anesthesia by Tait et al.[93] McGill et al[54] noted atelectasis, which was probably related to inspissation of secretions because of residual reduction in ciliary activity caused by the previous URI.

Because of these studies it is recommended that a careful history of a URI (flu-like syndrome) in the past 4 to 6 weeks be elicited. If doubt exists as to its resolution the surgery should be postponed for at least a month following recovery. If symptoms persist, a preoperative chest radiograph should be obtained. If radiography is positive, surgery should be cancelled; if it is negative, the anesthesiologist should still be alert for signs of an irritable airway or atelectasis during or following surgery.

A common situation that poses a difficult decision is that of a child with a runny nose presenting for relatively brief or low-risk procedures such as the insertion of ventilation tubes for chronic serous otitis media. Many such children make multiple trips to the hospital for ventilation tubes, but are cancelled because of a runny nose. Many anesthesiologists are willing to proceed with this group of patients,[9,93,94] and some have reported no increase in perioperative complications associated with uncomplicated URIs.[93,94] Although one must be prepared to face the consequences of anesthetizing a child with an irritable airway such as cough, breath holding, and laryngeal spasm, one study recently suggested that the majority of complications were associated with endotracheal intubation.[93] In our experience, a gentle induction with an intravenous or inhalational agent is most appropriate. Procedures of brief duration, or those in which the airway is not very reactive, can usually be managed without intubation. If endotracheal intubation is otherwise indicated or is needed because of difficulty with airway management, then the endotracheal tube should be inserted early. The use of muscle relaxants is usually needed in this situation to facilitate early endotracheal intubation. At the termination of surgery, the airway should be cleared of secretions, and the endotracheal tube removed only after the child is fully awake.

THE PREMATURE INFANT

The age of the child is usually not important when scheduling surgery on an outpatient basis at our institution or most others.[3,44,83,85,87] One major pediatric center, however, is reluctant to discharge even a previously healthy full-term infant less than 3 to 6 months of age on the day of surgery.* This is due to the possible association of postoperative respiratory problems with sudden infant death syndrome (SIDS) in this group. The premature infant, however, is unsuitable for ambulatory surgery because of potential immaturity of temperature control, respiratory center, and gag reflexes. Hypothermia, irregular breathing, apnea, laryngeal spasm, and aspiration of liquid or food are common and may occur in the immediate postoperative period. Infants who are anemic or who have a history of apnea or aspiration with feeding, as well as survivors of respiratory distress syndrome, are considered to be especially at risk. Those who have required endotracheal intubation, with or without mechanical ventilation, for treatment of respiratory insufficiency following birth may have abnormal blood gases and pulmonary function tests for 6 months to a year following termination of therapy.[13] Two recent studies have reported perioperative complications such as apnea even in the absence of a history of respiratory distress syndrome. Liu, Coté et al noted that premature infants born before 37 weeks gestational age had a higher incidence of life-threatening apneic spells requiring postoperative ventilation than full term infants.[53] All premature infants who required ventilation were under 4 months' postnatal age. Steward also reported complications such as apnea in premature infants who had no cardiac, neurologic, endocrine, or metabolic disease.[88] Those infants who experienced apnea were all under 10 weeks' postnatal age and under 3000 g. body weight at the time of operation. The apnea occurred during the operation or up to 12 hours postoperatively. The age at which the premature infant attains physiologic maturity and no longer presents an

*Downes J: Personal communication

increased risk must be considered individually, with attention given to growth, persistent problems during feeding, time to recover from upper respiratory infections, and so forth. It would appear, however, that a premature infant without complications should not have surgery performed as an outpatient for at least 3 to 4 months after birth; however, it is much more appropriate to individualize this decision and err on the side of conservatism. If the infant has bronchopulmonary dysplasia (BPD), this period should be extended for as long as the infant is symptomatic.[9] Should any questions arise, inpatient care is recommended. (See additional discussion, Chap. 9, Case No. 6.)

By far the most common elective surgical procedure performed on infants 3 to 6 months of age is repair of an inguinal hernia—a procedure perfectly suited for ambulatory surgery. Since preterm infants have a substantially higher incidence of inguinal hernia than term infants, the former represent a significant number of those who appear on the surgical schedule for operative repair. Because of the risk of incarceration, the patients usually require "urgent" surgery. The responsibility of the medical team is to screen these patients who are considered high risk. Ideally, this is done by the surgeon's office or the screening clinic before the day of surgery. Cases that slip through that initial screening must be identified on the day of surgery. Parents of any infant under 6 months of age must be specifically asked about history of prematurity. If the child was born prematurely, then the immediate postnatal history must be carefully reviewed. Did the child have any respiratory difficulty? Did he or she need supplemental oxygen, endotracheal intubation, mechanical ventilation, and so forth? Is there a history of apnea? Was an apnea monitor needed in the hospital or at home? Is there a history of feeding difficulty, aspiration, repeated lung infections, or wheezing? This information is vital before a decision can be made to proceed with ambulatory surgery in an infant who was premature and sometimes is not spontaneously volunteered by the parents unless they are specifically questioned.

THE CHILD WITH A HEART MURMUR

A common problem in pediatric outpatient anesthesia is the child in whom a previously undiagnosed cardiac murmur is first heard during the preanesthetic examination. Even if the child is active and shows no associated signs of cyanosis, clubbing of the fingers, or congestive heart failure, it is imperative that the cause of the murmur be correctly diagnosed prior to anesthesia and surgery. A recent study has shown that a pediatric cardiologist may be the only person who can confirm that a murmur is innocent by physical examination alone.[55] A child with a confirmed cardiac lesion may not require specific preoperative cardiac therapy, or even a modification in the selection of anesthetic agents and technique, but usually needs antibiotic prophylaxis to prevent subacute bacterial endocarditis. To prevent delays and cancellations, surgeons and pediatricians must be told to have a child with a murmur fully evaluated *prior* to the day of surgery. The specific diagnosis, and recommendations for therapy, if any, should be known by the anesthesiologist in advance. For quick reference, every Department of Anesthesiology should have available the American Heart Association's guidelines for prevention of bacterial endocarditis.[5] The instruction card used at Children's Hospital National Medical Center (CHNMC) gives the following protocol:

□ *Bacterial Endocarditis Prevention in Pediatric Patients*

FOR DENTAL PROCEDURES AND SURGERY OF THE UPPER RESPIRATORY TRACT*

1. Parenteral: Aqueous crystalline penicillin G, 50,000 units/kg IV or IM, 30–60 min before procedure and then 25,000 units/kg 6 hr later.
2. Oral: Penicillin V, 2 g orally 1 hr before procedure, then 1 g 6 hr later. For children less than 60 lb use 1 g orally 1 hr before procedure, then 500 mg 6 hr later.

For children allergic to penicillin: Erythromycin, 20 mg/kg orally, 1 hr prior to procedure, then 10 mg/kg 6 hr later.

FOR GASTROINTESTINAL AND GENITOURINARY TRACT SURGERY AND INSTRUMENTATION

Ampicillin, 50 mg/kg, IV or IM

Plus

Gentamicin, 2 mg/kg IM or IV

Give initial dose 30 min prior to procedure, then 1 g oral penicillin V 6 hr later. The parenteral regimen may be repeated once 8 hr later.

For children allergic to penicillin: Vancomycin, 20 mg/kg, given IV slowly over 1 hr, starting 1 hr **before** procedure. No repeat dose is necessary.

*Note: Another regimen is used for children with prosthetic heart valves.

The Parent

Parents of pediatric outpatients should be capable of understanding and willing to follow specific instructions related to ambulatory surgery; however, in most cases it is up to the physician to educate them and make them feel secure and comfortable. In the past, the choice of outpatient care has been largely influenced by parents' wishes and the experiences of friends and family. Third-party payers are now increasingly reluctant to comply with parents' demands for hospitalization of a healthy child who is having a relatively minor superficial operation.

The Procedure

The planned surgical procedure should be brief and should be associated with only minimal bleeding and minor physiologic derangements. Reed and Ford stated that almost any operation that does not require a major intervention into the cranial vault, abdomen, or thorax can be considered.[91] Superficial procedures are selected most often. Septic cases are rarely considered because of the need for separate facilities in the recovery room.

☐ **Procedures That Must Be Done on an Outpatient Basis According to DC Medicaid Regulations**

Myringotomy (with or without tubes)
Excision of superficial lesions
Removal of ganglion
Otoplasty (older children)
Small skin graft
Circumcision
Meatotomy
Urethral dilatation
Cystoscopy and sigmoidoscopy
Examination under anesthesia
Tear duct probing

Private insurance and Medicaid guidelines in some states mandate that certain surgical procedures be performed on an ambulatory basis unless factors exist that prohibit this form of care.[61] In the District of Columbia's medicaid guidelines, the procedures listed above represent approximately 40% of the operations performed at our institution on an outpatient basis. If these procedures are performed as inpatient surgery, reimbursement to the hospital for room and board is not provided. Special, individual consideration is given, however, under the following conditions:

Patients with medical conditions, such as severe diabetes or heart disease that make prolonged postoperative observation by a nurse or skilled medical personnel a necessity

Patients who will simultaneously undergo an unrelated procedure that itself requires hospitalization

Patients who lack proper home postoperative care

Patients in whom there is a possibility that more major surgery could follow the initial procedure

Technical difficulties, as documented by admission or operative notes

A representative list of procedures that are performed commonly at CHNMC is given on next page. Of those, the five most frequently performed operations during the past 2 years were herniorrhaphy, myringotomy, adenoidectomy with or without myringotomy, circumcision, and eye-muscle surgery.

At the Surgicenter in Phoenix, Arizona, a mixed pediatric-adult surgical setting where children less than 12 years of age comprise 30% of the population, two of the five most commonly performed operations are myringotomy with or without adenoidectomy and herniotomy. Since the customary dividing line between pediatric and adult patients is defined as 17 to 18 years of age, it is no wonder that many children's hospitals and mixed facilities report that over 40% of the pediatric surgery is being performed on an ambulatory basis.

Because of the increased risk of hemorrhage, there is a continuing debate as to the advisability of performing tonsillectomy with or without adenoidectomy

☐ *Procedures Suitable for Ambulatory Surgery*

General surgery
  Hernia repair
  Excision of cyst, ganglion, skin lesion, breast mass
  Suture of lacerations; removal of sutures
  Dressing change
  Muscle biopsy
  Sigmoidoscopy, bronchoscopy, esophagoscopy and
    dilatation
  Incision and drainage of abscess
  Proctologic and vaginal procedures

Otolaryngology
  Adenoidectomy
  Myringotomy and insertion of tubes
  Removal of foreign body from ear
  Frenulectomy
  Laryngoscopy
  Closed reduction of nasal fracture

Ophthalmology
  Examination under anesthesia
  Eye-muscle surgery
  Lacrimal duct probing
  Excision of chalazion
  Insertion of lens or prosthesis

Dental
  Extraction
  Restoration

Orthopedic
  Cast change
  Arthroscopy
  Closed reduction
    of fracture
  Manipulation

Urology
  Cystoscopy
  Meatotomy
  Orchiopexy
  Circumcision
  Hydrocelectomy
  Testicular biopsy

Plastic
  Otoplasty
  Scar revision

(Gregory GA (ed): Pediatric Anesthesia. New York, Churchill-Livingstone, 1983)

as an outpatient procedure. This procedure is not currently performed on an ambulatory basis at CHNMC. In 1968, however, Chiang and his associates reported 40,000 outpatient tonsillectomies and adenoidectomies (T&As) without death.[16] In order to decrease the risk of hemorrhage, they emphasized careful selection of cases and preoperative evaluation to eliminate patients with bleeding tendencies and cardiopulmonary disease. Also, no "allergic" patient was operated on during the pollen season, and no operation was performed until 4 to 5 weeks after an acute attack of tonsillitis.

A particularly informative discussion of the T&A question was provided by Ahlgren et al.[3] Of the 977 cases they reported in 1969, 184 were T&As. Average recovery-room time for these patients was more than twice that for patients undergoing other procedures (233 vs. 102 min). The most common complication was vomiting, usually of old blood. Of the 33 patients who developed laryngeal stridor, 7 were in the T&A group. The authors noted, however, that 15% of the patients undergoing eye-muscle procedures had stridor, compared with 4% in the T&A group. Three of the ophthalmologic patients and one T&A patient who developed this complication required hospitalization. The authors concluded that, since only 2% of the T&A group required admission for bleeding (4 of the 184 patients), the incidence was not high enough to eliminate the procedure from an outpatient setting. It must be noted, however, that of the 17 patients in their series requiring hospitalization, 5 were in the T&A group.

Preoperative Preparation and Screening

From the anesthesiologist's point of view, the essential preoperative requirements for safe conduct of anesthesia in pediatric outpatients are the same as those of inpatients. A complete history and physical examination (H&P) performed by a member of the medical staff, appropriate laboratory tests, consultations when indicated, an appropriate fasting period, and a chance to personally evaluate and establish rapport with the child and the parents are the standard preanesthetic requirements. *The special challenge in ambulatory surgery, however, is to accomplish as many of these steps as possible before the child arrives in the facility for surgery and therefore to minimize delays and last-minute cancellations.* That requires proper planning and organization.

Since the surgeon is the first member of the team the parents will meet when ambulatory surgery is scheduled, the smoothness and success of the whole experience will depend on the conduct of that first visit. Because of the very brief encounter on the day of surgery, the parents (and the child, when appropriate) must have the procedure explained and have as many of their questions as possible answered in the surgeon's office. Assured, relaxed parents will be more supportive and reassuring to the child. Arrangements for preoperative laboratory testing can be made at this time, and detailed written instructions given about fasting; where and when to report the day of surgery; and whom to call for further instructions if the child develops a cold, fever, or any unexpected illness while waiting for surgery.

Since the appropriate period of preoperative fasting varies with age, it is often useful to prepare a few sets of instructions for different age groups and hand (or mail) them to the parents as appropriate. A child should not be made to fast for a prolonged period of time (beyond what is safe for his or her age). Besides the possible risk of dehydration, or hypoglycemia in young infants, children are usually more irritable and upset when hungry or thirsty. On the other hand, one should allow for some flexibility in scheduling the child for surgery earlier in the day should an unexpected cancellation occur. Jensen et al recently measured blood glucose concentrations in a group of children 6 mo to 9 yr of age undergoing inpatient and outpatient anesthesia. They reported only one case (1%) of hypoglycemia in an inpatient who fasted overnight. They concluded that, in order to minimize the risk of hypoglycemia and inhalation of vomitus on the induction of anesthesia, children older than 6 months should fast overnight and be operated on in the morning.[43] NPO requirements at CHNMC, and an example of the instruction sheet handed to parents of children 1 to 6 years of age are shown in Table 4-1 and Appendix 4-1. At the Hospital for Sick Children (HSC) in Toronto, Canada, the preoperative fasting period is shorter, and most children undergoing minor surgery as outpatients do not receive infused fluids. For comparison, the preoperative fasting orders for outpatients at the HSC are as follows.[90]

Infants under 2 years of age should be given clear fluids until 4 hours before surgery. Other feedings must be discontinued at least 6 hours before the induction of anesthesia.

Children over 2 years of age must have no food on the day of operation but may be offered clear fluids up to 4 hours preoperatively.

☐ Table 4-1. NPO Orders at CHNMC

Age	Interval between Solid Food*	Interval between Clear Liquids†
<1 yr	6 hr	4 hr
1–6 yr	MN	6 hr
>6 yr	MN	8 hr

*Includes milk or milk products
†Includes breast milk

The actual laboratory data required in children, as well as the length of time specimens can be analyzed prior to surgery, vary between hospitals. Complete blood count (CBC) and urinalysis are the usual requirements; however, a few pediatric institutions either do not demand a urinalysis or request it only when there is a history of genitourinary disease. "Routine" preoperative chest radiograph is rarely a requirement in pediatric anesthesia.[71,72]

The minimum acceptable hematocrit value for an otherwise healthy child varies with age. If the hematocrit is not in the normal range for a given age group (Table 4-2), an appropriate medical workup should be performed, and elective surgery postponed. Children with underlying medical conditions such as renal disease or leukemia may consequently have long-standing anemia and are usually accepted if otherwise suitable for a brief ambulatory procedure.

Busy day-surgery units cannot rely on the surgeon alone to present them consistently with a fully evaluated and prepared child. This is especially true when a large number of surgeons with varying interests and attitudes have privileges to practice in the unit. In order to expedite the evaluation process and ensure some degree of uniformity in the preoperative preparation of the child, personnel other than surgeons in some facilities have found it useful to participate in the preoperative screening process. The degree of involvement varies from a simple phone call to the parents by the unit clerk a day or two

☐ Table 4-2. Normal Hematocrit Values[8]

Age	Mean	Range
Birth	54	45–65
3 mo	36	30–41
5 mo–6 yr	37	33–42
6–12 yr	38	35–42

prior to surgery to the establishment of a formal screening clinic to clear all patients before admission into the operating suite.

We feel that the process proceeds most expeditiously when there is a screening clinic primarily staffed by a pediatric nurse practitioner or a physician's assistant who is responsible to, and remains in close contact with, the department of anesthesiology. One of the functions of the clinic is to telephone the parents. The parents of each child are contacted initially by telephone shortly after the operation has been posted and a second time within 48 hours of the scheduled surgery. On the initial phone call, an effort is made to identify any past or present "risk factors" (see list below). This is one method by which the anesthesiologist may determine that additional preoperative evaluation is required in advance of surgery and/or question the suitability of performing the procedure on an ambulatory basis. During the subsequent phone call, NPO orders should be reinforced, a reassessment of the patient's present health made, and any social questions answered about parking, what to bring to the hospital, the rules of the short-stay recovery unit, and so forth.

The clinic also functions as an area in which families are seen and services arranged.

☐ *Telephone Interview to Identify Risk Factors*

Breath-holding spells (apnea)
Cardiac, respiratory, and other problems
History of prematurity
   Was oxygen required?
   Was child intubated?
   Lasting effects?
Muscular problems
Developmental delays

On the day before surgery, or earlier if needed: Clinic services are available for families whose children do not have their own pediatrician to perform the H&P or for those who prefer to have the child come to the hospital in advance of the day of surgery for any other reason. Personnel in the clinic obtain all necessary information to preregister the child, perform a definitive H&P, and arrange for any needed consultations and laboratory tests.

This earlier visit, which is optional for a healthy child, is mandatory for any child who has a history of a chronic disease process that requires consultation or special management.

On the day of surgery: Children who have not been seen before the day of surgery are fully evaluated (H&P, laboratory, etc.). *All* patients are screened for acute illness (e.g., URI) and NPO status. Consultation reports are evaluated, and the need for any special preoperative psychological or pharmacologic treatment is considered before the child is routed to the operating room. The patient therefore always arrives in the operating room with a complete evaluation, including a valid permit for anesthesia and surgery. This avoids delays and unnecessary frustrations.

Preparation of the Child for Ambulatory Surgery

PSYCHOLOGICAL PREPARATION

From a psychological point of view, anesthesia and surgery on an outpatient basis can be a mixed blessing. The short stay in the hospital or surgical facility has the definite advantage of minimizing or even eliminating the trauma of separating child and parent; however, it may present other emotional problems.

Many of these problems result from the child's lack of familiarity with the hospital environment and the very brief exposure that precedes the induction of anesthesia. In many centers, the child may be taken to the operating room within 30 or 45 minutes of admission—hardly enough time for the child to become familiar with the new surroundings or to establish a rapport with the staff. In this respect, the inpatient who spends the night before surgery in the hospital has an advantage. This is especially true in institutions that offer "rooming-in" accommodations for a parent who wishes to remain with the hospitalized child overnight. Once in the ward, the inpatient gets to know the hospital routine, meets the nurses and doctors, and sees children who are recovering from surgery and who are wearing hospital gowns, bandages, and the like. The child and parents have a good chance to ask questions and get reassuring answers. This experience, which takes away some of the fears of the unknown, may make the induction of anesthesia much smoother and also makes the postoperative period less frightening.

The outpatient deserves the same opportunity. That is why preparation should start a few days before surgery, with a visit to the hospital, a tour of the facility, and a movie or a puppet show that illustrates the entire procedure in language the child understands.

At CHNMC, and in many other pediatric institutions, the children and parents are invited for a preoperative visit to the hospital. A puppet show or a movie is followed by a short tour of the hospital, conducted by a caring staff who are trained to answer all questions *honestly*, and to familiarize the child and his or her parents with what will happen on the day of surgery. The tour is oriented to the child and is conducted in a friendly, playful fashion with special attention paid to the following areas:

1. Preoperative encounters: the tour guide must carefully ascertain that the child actually knows he or she will be coming to the hospital for surgery. This is a bad time to first inform an unsuspecting child that he or she is not really here to "have a picture taken." The admission procedure is explained, and the need for laboratory tests, wearing and the use of identification bands and hospital gowns is stressed. Finally, the actual waiting area, or playroom, where child (and parents if appropriate) will eventually go on the day of surgery is visited. The children are encouraged to bring along a favorite toy or comforter. Some of them might want to try on a hospital gown at this time and get the other children to become familiar with its appearance. (For many young children, having to undress and wear that strange gown is one of the worst events they remember about the day of surgery.)
2. The operating room: the children are shown either a special operating or

induction room, or an anesthesia machine that has been set aside for this purpose. They are allowed to handle the machine, breathing circuits, masks, syringes, and so forth. Although it is often difficult to spot an unusually fearful child at this time, any such patient should be brought to the attention of the department of anesthesiology for "extra-special handling."

3. The recovery area: both the recovery room and the location where the child will stay until fit for discharge should be shown. The fact that the child may be hurting after surgery should be mentioned, with the reassurance that measures will be taken to minimize their discomfort. Any special equipment such as an intravenous line, oxygen tubing, and thermometer should be demonstrated. The child should be told where and when he or she will meet the parents, and it should be emphasized that the stay will last only one day.

Included in the tour is either a live or videotaped puppet show depicting "Clipper" undergoing the hospital experience, including anesthesia, surgery, and recovery (Fig. 4-1). The children seem to like puppet shows and can participate when the group is asked to sing along. This is followed by punch and cookies in the hospital cafeteria, where children and their parents have plenty of time to ask questions.

It would be very desirable to have different preoperative programs for adolescents and handicapped children. At the Children's Hospital of Denver, for example, a separate program for adolescents was instituted in response to

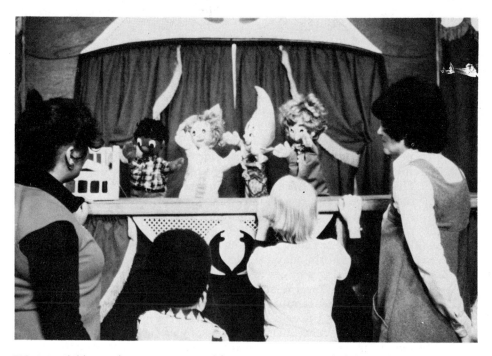

FIG. 4-1   Children and parents get many of their questions answered while watching a puppet show during the preoperative tour at CHNMC.

complaints that some of the teenagers were insulted by terms like "magic gas," which are often used to explain anesthesia induction to preschool children.

Although these recommendations represent an ideal comprehensive approach to the psychological preparation of the child for ambulatory surgery, some institutions are unable or unwilling to provide this service. In these cases, the surgeon's office usually undertakes this function. Books, pamphlets, and handouts are available that can help the parents understand their child's forthcoming surgery. The surgeon and other members of the health care team should be aware of these publications and their availability.[82] Ideally, a description of the process at the particular hospital in which the operation is scheduled should be distributed to the parent by the surgeon in the office at the time the surgery is scheduled. At that time some of the important features of the forthcoming procedure can be discussed, and the pamphlet reviewed later at home by the parents and child. An example of the introductory remarks from the coloring book used at CHNMC outlines its purpose (Fig. 4-2, next page).

Pharmacologic Premedication

The value of and need for pharmacologic premedication in pediatric day-surgery patients is a difficult question to answer in a general way. With modern agents and techniques, it is now possible to anesthetize an unpremedicated, struggling, screaming child in a few minutes with no apparent physical or physiologic harm.[76,79] As a result, premedication has now assumed more value for the emotional protection of the child rather than an adjunct to anesthesia. Although most authors usually state that if the child has been properly prepared, premedication is not necessary[25,87] or even undesirable if it prolongs recovery and delays discharge home, others feel that some form of sedation is advantageous[14,64,66,77] to facilitate anesthesia induction.

A close look at some recent studies illustrates the nature of this controversy. In one study,[14] children who were given an oral preparation of meperidine, diazepam and atropine, exhibited a significantly lower incidence of crying and secretions upon arrival in the operating room—conditions that are favorable for smooth mask induction—than those who did not receive premedication (19% vs. 34%). There was no difference in the total recovery time from anesthesia to discharge home between the medicated and the control groups (147 ±80 min vs. 156 ±78 min, respectively). Another study, however,[25] found that the oral administration of hydroxyzine, promethazine or diazepam was no better than placebo in easing the induction of anesthesia or protecting against psychological reactions in the early postoperative period. Of the inductions in these cases, however, 73% were with intravenous thiopental sodium. In no case did any of the oral preparations used for premedication cause a significant delay in recovery from anesthesia or discharge home.

In another study where intravenous thiopental was used for induction, Booker and Chapman[11] found no difference in the incidence of unacceptable behavior during induction between one group of children medicated with intramuscular morphine/atropine and another who received an oral preparation of dichloralphenazone and paracetamol. Morphine, however, had a pronounced emetic effect that lasted into the period following surgery, and many children remarked that the intramuscular injection before the operation

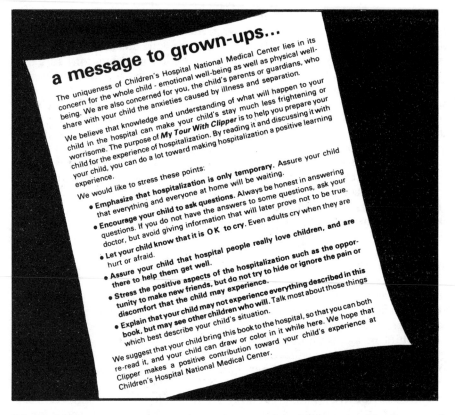

FIG. 4-2 A message to grown-ups. The inside cover of the "coloring book" information booklet mailed to children before surgery.

was the worst thing that happened to them in the hospital. Children premedicated with morphine were significantly more drowsy at home, especially following pain-free procedures, than those who received no narcotics or even those who received intravenous fentanyl (3 μg/kg) intraoperatively for more painful operations. Of particular interest in this study was the observation that 25% to 38% of the children who had exhibited an unacceptable demeanor during induction had received their premedicant drug too late to allow for full sedating effect—a common problem, especially in outpatient practice. Still another study[70] found intramuscular ketamine (3 mg/kg) an effective premedicant in children under 2 years of age who were given thiopental, nitrous oxide, oxygen, succinylcholine anesthesia for elective outpatient adenoidectomy. It was more than three times as effective as narcotic (meperidine, 1 mg/kg) in calming or sedating a child, with no prolongation in recovery time, and no difference in the emotional state following recovery.

The major problem, however, in applying the results of such studies to clinical practice is that they merely compare the effects of different premedication regimens or a placebo on a mixed group of children. The results cannot be used to predict a similar effect when dealing with the individual child who is unusually apprehensive or disturbed.

Our own feeling is that, with proper psychological preparation and establishment of a rapport with the anesthesiologists, and with limited separation of child from parents (up to the induction or including parents during the induction), the majority of children do not need preoperative sedation. But some—up to 20% of all children—do.

If a patient is to undergo repeated painful procedures, is known to be very apprehensive, or is too young to benefit from verbal reassurance, a mild tranquilizer can be ordered in advance, and given at home before the child comes to the hospital. When indicated, oral premedication with triclofos (80 mg/kg mixed in a flavored solution to conceal its bad taste),[8] or diazepam suspension (0.2–0.4 mg/kg) has been found useful.[87] An adequate time interval (1–2 hr) must be allowed for the full effect of the drugs. If drying agents are specifically indicated, oral atropine or glycopyrrolate (0.02 mg/kg) can be used. Intramuscular injections should be avoided whenever possible as a route for premedication in children. Walters et al[98] have shown in a prospective double-blind study that oral and intramuscular premedication can be equally effective in producing a cooperative and drowsy patient at anesthetic induction. If premedication is not used routinely, the anesthesiologist must be prepared to handle the occasional difficult or extremely frightened child by using a combination premedicant-induction agent such as rectal or intramuscular methohexital, or ketamine IM.[64,70] This is especially important if a mask induction has been planned. The possibility of a slightly prolonged recovery is a small price to pay for avoiding the potential psychological trauma of a stormy induction.[17] The use of cimetidine, an H_2 receptor blocker, has been suggested to decrease the gastric volume and increase the pH of gastric contents in pediatric patients.* This drug, however, is not routinely used in our ambulatory surgery unit at the present time.

Preoperative Playroom

In order to reduce the anxiety of the child without the aid of pharmacologic adjuncts, other techniques have been employed. One is the use of the preoperative holding area as a playroom. This area is usually adjacent to the operating rooms and is decorated in a style that makes the child feel at ease (Fig. 4-3). It is important that children be kept occupied while waiting for surgery. Bright colors on the walls; pictures of cartoon characters; toys, doll houses, coloring books, puzzles, and childrens' furniture all are incorporated so that the children identify the surroundings more with a friendly home or school atmosphere than with the often strange, threatening, sterile environment of a hospital or operating room. In a mixed facility, the play area can be incorporated into the general waiting room and is designed to accommodate healthy, unmedicated children and their parents up to the time of induction of anesthesia. The playroom is always supervised by a member of the hospital staff as well as volunteers who may answer questions from the child or parents or, in the absence of the latter, may act as a surrogate. Children are brought from the playroom to the operating room or induction room in a variety of ways, such as in the anesthesiologist's arms, in a red wagon, on a stretcher, or walking

*Kallar SK: Personal communication, 1984

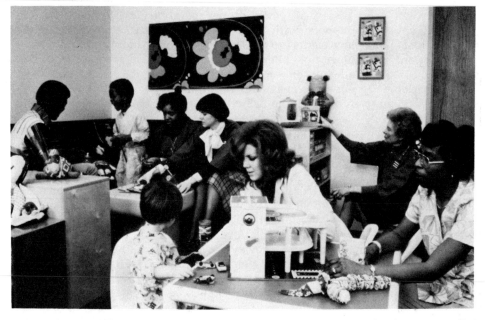

FIG. 4-3 Unmedicated children must be kept busy while waiting for surgery. The play room is staffed by volunteers.

alongside the anesthesiologist. In some institutions such as CHNMC, the parent frequently accompanies the child to an induction room.

Parental Presence during Induction

For a preschool child (ages 2-6), it is very difficult to understand why the parents, who have accompanied him through all the preoperative preparation and orientation, should have to abandon him when the "big moment" arrives. Most of us are aware of the screaming and resistance that often occurs when a young child is taken away from his or her parents for surgery. Traditionally, this unpleasant situation has been avoided by using heavy doses of premedication preoperatively. With that, the anesthetic state is in effect initiated in the parent's presence, and the anxiety of separation is minimized.

In outpatients, although it is desirable to avoid routine heavy premedication regimens, it is still essential that the goal of premedication (to make the child sedated or cause sleep before separation from the parents) not be sacrificed. One way of achieving that goal is to allow one or both parents to stay with the child during induction of anesthesia.[39]

Although for many anesthesiologists this may sound untraditional, it is becoming more accepted by others.[39,74,79] Indeed, some anesthesiologists feel that the presence of an intelligent, supportive parent during induction of anesthesia may be the best available substitute for premedication. It is largely because we encourage parents to be with their children during induction at CHNMC that our use of pharmacologic sedation is minimal, especially for outpatients.

The majority of children scheduled for elective surgery at CHNMC are unmedicated. They have anesthesia for elective surgery induced in one of the four induction rooms after coming to a preinduction play area. Both the play area and the induction rooms are located within the general operating room area, but outside the area limited to those operating room personnel who are properly attired. As a result, parents, volunteers, and staff may walk between playroom and induction rooms without changing into operating room apparel.

The parents are welcome to stay with their child during the induction of anesthesia and usually do. Other participants are at least one anesthesiologist and some other individual who can assist the anesthesiologist and/or escort the parents to the proper location following induction. This individual can be another anesthesiologist, an anesthesia aid, a surgeon, a volunteer, or an operating room nurse. We have had few problems with this concept, except that preschool children are usually more apprehensive and less cooperative than children of school age. Since induction of anesthesia is performed outside the operating room, only healthy children presenting for elective surgical procedures should be considered. Infants under 1 to 1½ years of age are rarely suitable candidates.

The method of induction can vary according to the preference of the anesthesiologist and the needs of the child. Intravenous thiopental sodium (4–6 mg/kg), intramuscular ketamine (2–3 mg/kg) or rectal methohexital (25 mg/kg) have all been used satisfactorily. Unless there are specially equipped induction rooms, or portable anesthesia machines, the use of an inhalational induction technique may not be possible. In all cases, however, equipment for airway management and resuscitation drugs must be immediately available.

There are nonetheless many possible reasons why the anesthesiologist may prefer not to have the parents present during anesthesia induction. The anesthesiologist may feel uncomfortable being "watched" by the parents. What if something goes wrong? Can the parents be critical? Furthermore there is always the question of dividing one's attention between the child and parents. An anxious parent may make the child more upset. However, experience shows that these are not common problems.[37] Parent selection and education is very important. Those who are invited to watch their child's induction must be told precisely what to expect and should have an escort to take them back to the waiting area as soon as the child is asleep. Parents must agree to leave the induction area at any moment if so asked by the anesthesiologist. Unduly anxious or hysterical parents should not be encouraged in the induction area, since they can contribute to similar anxiety in their children. Anesthesia induction occurs in the operating room when

Children are less than 1 to $1\frac{1}{2}$ years of age
There is a serious preexisting illness
Emergency surgery is scheduled
An adolescent child does not choose to have his or her parents present
Parents are unduly anxious about their participation in the experience
Premedication is considered desirable

Although there are no tightly controlled research studies, most physicians and parents are enthusiastic and find this approach very satisfactory in reducing the anxiety due to separation.

One of the major factors limiting more frequent participation of parents during anesthesia induction in many institutions is the necessity to have specially equipped areas outside the operating room where anesthesia induction can be safely performed with the parents present. That possibility should be very carefully studied by anyone involved in planning or redesigning an operating room suite.

Anesthetic Agents and Techniques

In spite of the current popularity of ambulatory surgery, there is still no agreement among major pediatric centers as to what is the best way to prepare the child or ensure a smooth induction and rapid and comfortable recovery without compromising safety. This remains a continuing challenge for the individual anesthesiologist. Smooth induction of anesthesia in the awake, unmedicated child is probably the most difficult aspect of pediatric short-stay surgery. Realizing that no single approach can be effective for all children in all situations, the anesthesiologist must be familiar with, and have confidence in, many methods of induction. The choice of an agent or technique can then be tailored to fit the needs of the individual child, and not made merely because it is the routine choice in a particular institution or is the only method with which the anesthesiologist is comfortable.

Inhalational Induction

The greatest advantage of using inhalational induction in pediatric anesthesia is its apparent simplicity. If the same agents are also used to maintain surgical anesthesia, recovery is usually prompt following most brief outpatient procedures. Successful inhalational induction, however, mandates the child's cooperation and acceptance, especially in unpremedicated outpatients. Beyond perhaps the first year of life, this can very rarely be expected until the child is at least 3 or 4 years old, when verbal communication becomes easier. Even at that age, induction by mask is not always acceptable to the fully awake child. Pediatric anesthesiologists have over the years devised many ingenious techniques to reduce the anxiety associated with gas induction and have met with variable degrees of success. These include

1. Elimination of the mask: an N_2O/O_2 mixture is blown over the child's face, while he or she is distracted with a story or a song, then halothane is gradually added to the mixture (the anesthesiologist can make believe the new smell is that of candy, perfume, jet fuel, paint, etc.).
2. Use of transparent masks: since we no longer use explosive agents, there is absolutely no need to use the traditional black conductive rubber masks. A variety of clear face masks is now available in pediatric sizes, and these should be used.
3. Use of "food flavors": as an additional method for getting the child to accept the mask near his or her face, some anesthesiologists paint the inside of the mask with a flavor or a smell of the child's choice. The child may find the smell interesting, and by allowing him or her to choose a pleasant flavor, the child becomes an active participant in the induction technique.

4. Letting the child sit up during the induction (Fig. 4-4): this is less frightening and often more acceptable to the child than being forced to lie down. The child can be given the choice to sit on the operating table or the anesthesiologist's lap. It is often less frightening to the child if the back instrument table is covered, and the anesthesiologist and assistant do not wear a mask during induction. Children are used to looking at people's faces, not just their eyes.

Inhalational Anesthetics

NITROUS OXIDE

Nitrous oxide is the most commonly used inhalational agent. It has the great advantage of being practically odorless, which makes it most suitable for starting a gas induction in the unpremedicated pediatric patient. If nitrous oxide is administered in a high inspired concentration (75%–80%) *initially*, induction is rapid and pleasant, and the child is encouraged to continue with the mask induction. Unfortunately, nitrous oxide has a limited potency (MAC >100%), and for that reason it is usually supplemented with either potent inhalational agents or intravenous anesthetics.

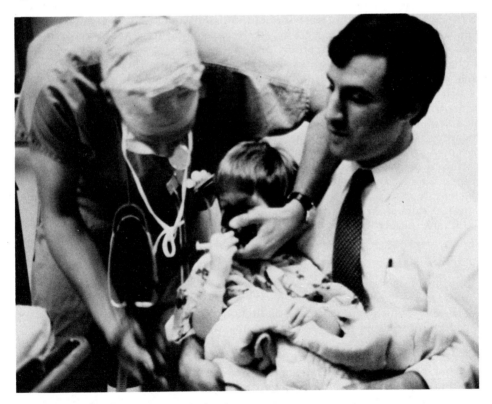

FIG. 4-4 Parent's presence, security blanket, sitting position, and allowing the child to hold his or her own mask; all contribute to a smooth inhalational induction in the unmedicated pediatric patient.

HALOTHANE

Halothane is the most commonly used potent inhalational agent in pediatric anesthesia. For the ambulatory surgery patient it offers the advantage of a rapid, smooth induction, either by direct inhalation (with nitrous oxide) or following a sleep dose of an intravenous agent.[73] Use of high inspired concentrations initially (up to 3%) will speed induction; however, this should be reduced quickly to the usual maintenance range of 0.5% to 2%. Hypotension and circulatory depression observed with halothane are dose dependent and are especially profound in the young, fasting infant.[26]

Recovery after brief halothane anesthesia is usually rapid and uneventful. Nausea and vomiting are not common. With prolonged administration of halothane, however, recovery time is longer. Although there is a tendency to avoid repeated use of halothane in adult outpatient anesthesia for fear of sensitizing the liver and possibly inducing hepatic necrosis with future exposure, it is generally believed that this is rarely a problem in the preadolescent child.[79]

ENFLURANE

Enflurane is still not as widely used as halothane in pediatric outpatient anesthesia, despite physical characteristics (low blood/gas solubility coefficient) that suggest a slightly more rapid induction and recovery. Studies that compared enflurane to halothane as the sole anesthetic agent showed that induction times were comparable, but that enflurane was associated with a higher incidence of hiccough and breath holding.[41] Following brief anesthetics, the rate of recovery of patients from enflurane anesthesia, as measured by return of eyelash reflex and swallowing, was significantly faster than that of patients who received halothane. However, full recovery times were comparable, and children anesthetized with either agent were ready to leave the recovery room at the same time. In other studies of children who received a narcotic premedication or barbiturate induction, the induction times with enflurane were found to be either longer,[84] or shorter but associated with more complications[11] than that of halothane. There was no significant difference in the length of stay in the recovery room or return to normal activities at home. These results identify enflurane as an acceptable but expensive alternative to halothane in outpatient pediatric anesthesia.[41]

ISOFLURANE

Isoflurane possesses many characteristics that make it an interesting possibility for use in pediatric outpatient anesthesia.[97] It has a low blood/gas solubility coefficient, which should make induction of anesthesia and postoperative recovery more rapid than with other inhalational agents. Isoflurane is a very stable compound, with less than 0.2% of the drug metabolized in the body, and the remainder excreted through the lungs. Thus, in the absence of significant metabolites, rapid recovery should be expected with minimal sequelae. Clinically, the rate of early postoperative recovery compares favorably with either halothane or enflurane. The return to normal status at home may be slightly more rapid than that of either of the other agents.[86] Initial studies, however, indicate that isoflurane may not yet be the ideal anesthetic in pediatric patients. Isoflurane has a more pungent smell than halothane and tends to provoke more excitement, breath holding, coughing, and laryngospasm than halothane during induction. This can be somewhat modified by starting the induction with a 60%–70% concentration of N_2O for 2 minutes, then gradually introducing the isoflurane vapor in small (0.25%) increments. In an older child, a sleep dose of intravenous thiopental can improve the acceptance of the agent. Isoflurane is less likely to sensitize the myocardium to the effects of catecholamines than halothane, which makes it more compatible with topical vasoconstrictor drugs (Table 4-3).

LIMITATIONS OF MASK INDUCTIONS

In the unpremedicated child, induction with a mask mandates the patient's acceptance and cooperation (whether spontaneous or induced). Failure to achieve such cooperation and to get the mask close to the child's face without a struggle is not uncommon (Fig. 4-5). Some anesthesiologists, realizing the unpleasantness of such a situation, decide to get the whole thing over with as quickly as possible by holding the child down and forcing the mask over his or her face with a high concentration of halothane, while promptly "smothering" the child to sleep. The struggling child will usually fall asleep quickly, while the anesthesiologist puts the blame on the stubborn child who refused to cooperate. If this type of induction is done repeatedly (and it is), the surgical team tends to become insensitive and regards it as the normal induction technique. By the end of the surgical procedure, everyone has probably forgotten how distasteful the experience was. Everyone, that is, except the child.

Although there are not many well-controlled long-term studies of the consequences of forced mask inductions, careful questioning of children or adults who still remember those horrible moments will reveal many unpleasant or even nightmarish memories that are often passed from generation to generation, consciously or unconsciously, adding a very significant element to the apprehension of anesthesia.

☐ **Table 4-3. Dose (ED$_{50}$) of Epinephrine That Produced Three or More PVCs[45]**

Agent	Dose (μg/kg)
Halothane*	2.11 ($\pm$ 0.15)
Halothane/lidocaine†	3.69 ($\pm$ 0.42)
Enflurane	10.9 ($\pm$ 8.9)
Isoflurane	6.72 ($\pm$ 0.66)

*Karl et al[46] showed that children tolerate higher doses of subcutaneous epinephrine during halothane anesthesia. At least 10 μg/kg of epinephrine infiltration may be used safely in normocarbic and hypocarbic pediatric patients without congenital heart disease.
†It is our practice to limit the volume of subcutaneous lidocaine 1% with epinephrine 1:200,000 to a maximum of 0.5 ml/kg. That volume contains the equivalent of 5 mg lidocaine +2.5 μg epinephrine/kg body weight.

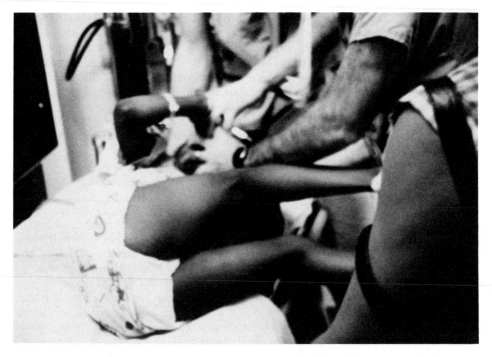

FIG. 4-5 In up to 20% of cases, mask induction may not be acceptable to unpremedicated children. An alternate induction method must be employed.

Noninhalational Induction Agents and Techniques

The major disadvantage of using any noninhalational induction agent in pediatric day-surgery patients is the possibility of prolonging the recovery period. However, with careful selection of agents, and using the minimal single dose necessary to simply induce sleep, some authors have found that the total recovery time is not significantly prolonged.[32,87] The following section is a brief review of the current indications and use of these agents in pediatric outpatient anesthesia.

INTRAVENOUS INDUCTION

Intravenous induction is the method of choice in most older children for the same reasons it has become the standard in adults. It ensures a rapid, pleasant induction with minimal struggling and no unpleasant memories of a suffocating mask or a smelly gas. The approach for young children is different than that for adults (Fig. 4-6). The drug should be injected directly in a vein on the dorsum of the hand, usually through a 25-gauge butterfly needle. An intravenous infusion need not be started prior to the drug injection. The real limitation to the more frequent use of intravenous induction in children is the anesthesiologist. No one enjoys injections, but (except in the case of a child who has a definite severe phobia about needles, which can quickly be assessed by his or her reaction to the blood test), most older children will accept intravenous induction if the proposal is made to them in a confident, supportive way. The idea of going to sleep quickly with a "scratch" or a "pinch" in the hand rather than having to breathe the "smelly" gas is more likely to generate acceptance than if the same alternatives are presented as "blowing a balloon" vs. "getting a shot." With a little practice on the part of the anesthesiologist, a small injection with a tiny concealed needle is barely felt and is much less painful than deep intramuscular injections (shots).

The age at which intravenous induction is considered practical in children varies considerably among anesthesiologists. For an experienced and skilled anesthesiologist, any child over 6 months of age with visible veins is an appropriate candidate (especially if mask induction is not accepted). Infants under 6 months of age, however, are rarely appropriate candidates for noninhalational techniques because of the higher risk of postoperative respiratory depression and the possibility of more prolonged recovery.

THIOPENTAL SODIUM

Thiopental sodium (2.5% solution) is the most commonly used induction agent for adult outpatient anesthesia. In a dose of 4 to 5 mg/kg body weight, it is equally suitable for the pediatric outpatient. There is a wide variation, however, in the pediatric patient's response to intravenous thiopental, and the response of each child during induction must be carefully monitored and used to determine the individual dose requirement. Healthy, unpremedicated children may require relatively large doses of thiopental (5 to 6 mg/kg) in order to ensure smooth and rapid transition to general inhalational anesthesia.[20] When Steward[87] compared

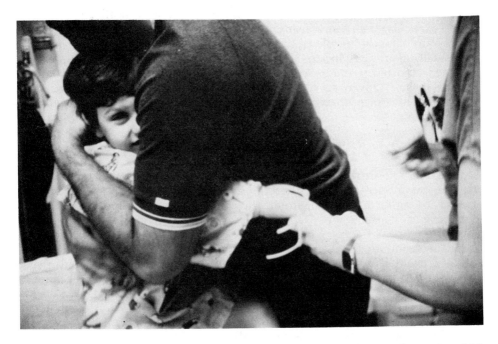

FIG. 4-6 Concealed IV induction in a child.

the recovery times in children following intravenous thiopental induction to those of children who had inhalational induction, he found that after 30 minutes there was no difference in the recovery score between the two groups. Children who had barbiturate induction, however, tended to be sleepier and required more airway support for the first 15 minutes of the recovery period. He also found that there was no difference in the eventual return to a "bright and alert" status and normal appetite at home following discharge. Repeated doses of thiopental should be avoided, as they can prolong recovery. Diazepam and opiate narcotics can also have an exaggerated depressant effect if taken in the early postoperative period following the use of intravenous thiopental for induction.[27]

METHOHEXITAL

For the outpatient, methohexital (1.5 to 2 mg/kg) offers the distinct advantage of a significantly shorter recovery than an equivalent dose of thiopental.[51] The duration of unconsciousness is similar after a single small dose of either agent. However, since metabolic breakdown products of methohexital are eliminated three times faster than those of thiopental,[42] the time required for complete psychomotor recovery is shorter. This is particularly true after large or repeated doses. When used in a 1% solution, methohexital has a lower tissue toxicity than thiopental following inadvertent subcutaneous infiltration or intra-arterial injection. Induction with methohexital is followed by an appreciable incidence of involuntary muscle movements and episodes of hiccough and coughing, which can at times be very troublesome. This can be minimized somewhat by injecting the drug slowly and using a small total dose. A severe burning sensation often develops along the course of the injected vein. This is particularly undesirable in children, because it promotes hand movement and can dislodge the needle from the vein. Pain can be minimized by mixing a very small amount of lidocaine with the methohexital (1 mg/ml).[90] Methohexital has been reported to induce epileptiform convulsions in susceptible patients.[67] Despite these disadvantages, many still consider methohexital the intravenous barbiturate of choice when rapid recovery and early ambulation are required in the outpatient.[27,42]

ETOMIDATE

Etomidate, a nonbarbiturate hypnotic agent, has been used extensively for intravenous induction of anesthesia in Europe. When used in an intravenous dose of 0.2 mg/kg in children, etomidate produces sleep rapidly and safely, with negligible side-effects on the cardiovascular system and little respiratory depression.[47]

   Pain is common following injection with etomidate, and unlike methohexital is not prevented by adding lidocaine to the solution. Myoclonia is also seen following the use of this drug. Using an analgesic agent (e.g., fentanyl as premedication or with induction of anesthesia) can reduce these problems. Some authors, however, find that the etomidate and fentanyl technique is associated with a greater frequency of nausea and vomiting, which would make early discharge from the hospital difficult.[21]

INTRAMUSCULAR INDUCTION

Intramuscular injections do not require the high degree of skill needed for intravenous induction in a struggling child. However, deep intramuscular injections are definitely more painful, and they are one of the main reasons children dislike needles and shots. Routine use of intramuscular injections for induction of anesthesia or for premedication is therefore undesirable. However, in certain situations when a struggling child cannot be managed by intravenous induction owing to lack of accessible veins (or experience on the part of the anesthesiologist), a small sedating intramuscular dose of ketamine or methohexital may be the most humane way to induce anesthesia.

The potential for prolonged recovery and emergence delirium makes ketamine undesirable for routine use in ambulatory surgical patients. There is virtually no rational indication for its intravenous use in these children. If it must be used intramuscularly, a small sedating dose (2 to 3 mg/kg) is injected into the deltoid muscle. This should provide satisfactory conditions for a mask induction within 4 to 7 minutes. Atropine (0.02 mg/kg) may be simultaneously injected to reduce the excessive secretions that can lead to airway irritation. This technique is most applicable for the 1- to 5-year-old group. When ketamine is used in this manner and followed by a thiopental, nitrous oxide, oxygen relaxant technique the recovery time is prolonged only slightly.[70] When patients are administered a low dose of ketamine *as an induction agent*, hallucinations and nightmares do not appear to be a problem. Krantz reported no instances of unpleasant dreams or emergence phenomena following administration of 2 to 2.5 mg/kg of ketamine IM used for very brief (<5 min) outpatient procedures in children. Recovery time averaged 13 ±7.6 minutes, which is satisfactory for outpatient anesthesia.[52]

Another choice for an intramuscular induction agent is methohexital, usually as a 5% solution. A dose of 6 mg/kg injected deep in the muscle has been reported to induce sleep in less than 5 minutes in patients from 1 to 3 years of age.[49] When only a single injection was used, recovery was rapid and complete. At the Children's Hospital of Michigan, methohexital sodium, 3.5% in distilled water, has been used in a dose of 7.7 mg/kg, given deep IM in the anterolateral thigh in more than 25,000 cases. Parents are allowed to hold the child on their lap during the injection and until the eyelids close. The incidence of hiccoughs was less than 8%, and clonic movements for 10 seconds' duration were seen in one patient. Although the injection is painful, no local reactions or subsequent soreness at the injection site was reported.*

RECTAL INDUCTION

Rectally administered anesthetics fell out of favor in the early 1970s because of the long duration of action and the unpredictable absorption of the agents that were given by that route (e.g., thiopental). This method is now being "rediscovered" as an easy, minimally invasive technique for last-minute premedication or anesthesia induction in very young children.

The use of methohexital is the main reason why rectal induction is again in vogue. Used as a 10% solution, in a dose of 25 mg/kg, most children fall asleep in

---

*Jewell MR: Personal communication, 1984

6 to 11 minutes, and even in outpatients, this dose did not significantly delay immediate and late recovery after short surgical procedures when compared to intravenous thiopental.[32] Occasionally, the onset of sleep may be delayed for up to 20 minutes, and very rarely the child may not fall asleep at all. If the child is at least drowsy, inhalational induction would be readily acceptable. Otherwise, one may have to either repeat the rectal injection (with the risk of prolonged recovery), or use a different induction technique. Rectal methohexital is most suitable for children 1 to 3 years of age, who would not cooperate with mask induction and have no visible veins for easy intravenous access. The older child would probably be more upset and psychologically traumatized by introducing the drug in his or her rectum than by an intravenous injection.

Kallar studied the effect of 1%, 5%, and 10% concentrations of rectal methohexital (15 mg/kg) on induction time in ambulatory surgery pediatric patients ages 1 to 5 years. The shortest induction time was observed with the 1% solution (mean 6.3 min). Failures (cases in which the patient was not asleep after administration of rectal methohexital) were observed with the 5% solution (five patients) and with the 10% solution (four patients). No failures were seen with 1% methohexital. Expulsion or defecation was observed in just under 5% of patients who received the 5% or 10% rectal solutions, but none was observed when the 1% solution was used.*

Because the administration of methohexital rectally is an easy and minimally invasive procedure, it is particularly suitable for inducing sleep in a struggling child before removing him from his parents. Airway resuscitative equipment must be immediately available to treat any airway obstruction or respiratory depression. Needless to say, the anesthesiologist must remain in attendance after the drug is administered. Other side-effects include hiccough (9%), involuntary movements, and soiling (9%). The parents must be forewarned about the latter and appropriately protected, if they are holding the child during induction.

Use of Muscle Relaxants

The intelligent use of muscle relaxants is not only safe in outpatient anesthesia, but, if used as a part of a "balanced technique," can actually reduce the need for higher concentrations of potent anesthetics and help promote promptness of recovery and early discharge.

SUCCINYLCHOLINE

Succinylcholine is most often used to facilitate endotracheal intubation without the need for an excessive depth of inhalational anesthesia. This is particularly advantageous in outpatients and in young infants who do not tolerate deep halothane anesthesia. Succinylcholine can be used intravenously in a dose of 1 mg/kg (2 mg/kg for infants under 2 years of age) or intramuscularly (4 mg/kg).

*Kallar SK: Personal communication, 1984

Succinylcholine should be combined with, or preceded by, atropine (0.02 mg/kg) when used for pediatric patients to avoid excessive bradycardia, which might otherwise follow even a single injection. Succinylcholine can also be used in repeated doses (preceded by atropine) or as an infusion for prolonged relaxation; however, this is not generally recommended in young children, because the larger doses required and the extremely variable response of small infants to succinylcholine can lead to the development of phase II block.[33]

Muscle pains, with or without excessive fasciculation, can follow rapid intravenous injection of succinylcholine in older children. This is particularly evident with the early ambulation typical of ambulatory surgery. Muscle pain can be avoided by injecting a small dose of *d*-tubocurarine (0.05 mg/kg) 2 to 3 minutes before succinylcholine. Because of curare's antagonistic effect, the dose of succinylcholine must be increased by 70% to ensure adequate relaxation. Muscle pains are seldom a problem in younger children,[15] and pretreatment is not generally recommended before the age of 6 to 8 years.

Another potential problem in using succinylcholine in outpatients is the rare possibility of prolonged apnea in children with abnormal pseudocholinesterase.[62] The prolonged paralysis (up to 6 hours with the homozygous variety) can disrupt a busy schedule, but is very simple to treat once the diagnosis is confirmed (with a nerve stimulator). Adequate ventilation (and sedation) must be continued until full muscle power returns. Hospital admission is usually recommended. Blood samples from the child and family should be drawn for analysis and confirmation of the type of the disorder at a later date.

NONDEPOLARIZING RELAXANTS

The use of *d*-tubocurarine (0.5 mg/kg) or pancuronium (0.1 mg/kg) in outpatient anesthesia is a subject of some debate. Although profound muscle relaxation is seldom, if ever, needed in the type of cases commonly performed on an outpatient basis, relaxants can be used as a part of a balanced technique.[96] They can be especially useful in children in whom anesthesia was induced with a long-acting agent like a rectal barbiturate or intramuscular ketamine, or in young infants who manifest profound cardiovascular depression after a potent inhalational agent. Provided anesthesia time is over 30 to 45 minutes, a nondepolarizing relaxant/nitrous oxide anesthesia technique, supplemented with a minimal dose of inhalational agent as necessary, can be used. With the newly introduced shorter-acting nondepolarizing relaxants such as vecuronium (0.1 mg/kg)[31] or atracurium (0.4 mg/kg),[34] even shorter procedures may be considered. It is therefore absolutely essential to ensure complete reversal at the end of surgery.[10] With careful attention to dosage, and the use of a nerve stimulator to ensure an adequate reversal dose of neostigmine (0.07 mg/kg) or edrophonium (1 mg/kg) with atropine (0.02 mg/kg) or glycopyrrolate (0.01 mg/kg), that should not be a problem. The remote possibility of "recurarization" that can result from hypothermia, acidosis, and so forth, is not likely in the healthy outpatient undergoing uncomplicated surgery. It should be understood the above statements and dosages apply to the healthy child. Special consideration must be given to the variable response of premature and mature infants to the nondepolarizing muscle relaxants, especially vecuronium.

☐ **Table 4-4.   Recommended Tracheal Tube Sizes by Age**

Age	Internal Diameter (mm)	
Premature (2.5 kg)	2.5	Noncuffed
Term newborn	3.0	
6 mo	3.5	
12 mo	4.0	
18–24 mo	4.5	
4 yr	5.0–5.5	
6 yr	5.5–6.0	
8 yr	6.0–6.5	
10 yr	6.5	Cuffed
12 yr	7.0	
14 yr	7.5	
Adult	8.0–9.5	

Children of the same age vary in size: occasionally a size 0.5 mm ID smaller or larger may be required. Cuffs are generally not used with tube size smaller than 5.5 mm. When using cuffed tube, select size 0.5 mm ID smaller. General formula for children over 2 years:

$$\text{Tube size mm ID} = \frac{\text{Age (yr)}}{4} + 4.5$$

Endotracheal Intubation

Outpatient anesthesia, per se, is not a contraindication for using an endotracheal tube. At many centers, large numbers of pediatric ambulatory surgery patients have been intubated without serious complications. The endotracheal tube size selected should enable full expansion of both lungs and normal inflation, while allowing a definite leak with pressure of 20 to 25 cm H_2O (Table 4-4). The indications and techniques of endotracheal intubation are the same as for inpatients. There is a tendency, however, to avoid "routine" intubations in outpatients for the following reasons:

1. Many outpatient procedures are of short duration and do not involve body cavities, so intubation may not be indicated.
2. Intubation of the trachea for convenience may unnecessarily complicate the anesthetic. In seeking to achieve good intubating conditions, one may come dangerously close to overdosage if halothane alone is used,[80] or a muscle relaxant may be administered that would otherwise not be needed.
3. There is a definite incidence of trauma to the larynx secondary to intubation that varies according to the skills of the anesthesiologist and size of the endotracheal tube.
4. There is a tendency to delay oral fluid intake for at least 1 hour in patients who are intubated because of the possibility of laryngeal incompetence following extubation[95] or the presence of a sore throat.

5. The most feared risk associated with the use of an endotracheal tube in ambulatory surgery patients is the possibility that the child may develop postintubation croup during recovery and especially after discharge from the hospital. However, with careful technique, and use of small implant-tested tubes with a leak, the incidence should be very small (<1%).[50] Of special importance is the time at which "significant" croup develops. Most patients develop symptoms within 1 hour of extubation; thus, many centers allow pediatric patients whose tracheas have been intubated to be discharged after 1 hour has passed.[87] In our unit, children who are intubated do not meet routine discharge criteria until 3 hours have elapsed from the time of extubation. This is an arbitrary duration, based on what we believe to be an adequate period of observation to detect possible airway problems. These children can be discharged earlier if the anesthesiologist reexamines the child, detects no signs of airway obstruction, and personally discharges the child. In any case, parents must be advised to observe and report to a previously designated physician or service any respiratory difficulty that may develop after discharge.

Pediatric Anesthesia Breathing Systems

The choice of a special breathing system for use in pediatric patients varies among individual practitioners. Currently the usual decision is between a modification of the T-piece or a circle absorption system. Each has its advantages and limitations, and, provided one understands the performance characteristics of the system, either can be used safely for the pediatric outpatient.

THE T-PIECE

The Jackson Rees modification of the original T-piece and all of the Bain-type coaxial systems have the same performance characteristics. The greatest advantages of the T-piece is its light weight, simplicity, and the convenience of a long fresh gas flow (FGF) tubing. In the absence of an absorber, changes in the inspired concentration of agents can be readily achieved by changing the dialed concentration on the machine. There are two ways to use the T-piece:

1. As a nonrebreathing system, with high FGF ($2\frac{1}{2} \times$ minute volume). This formula is generally recommended with spontaneous respiration.
2. As a partial rebreathing system, with low FGF. This method (also referred to as controlled rebreathing) requires a large minute volume to allow adequate CO_2 elimination. This can be predictably achieved only by controlling ventilation. The recommended FGF and minute ventilation[68] are
   a. FGF:
      <30 kg: 1000 ml + 100 ml/kg
      >30 kg: 2000 ml + 50 mg/kg
   b. Minute ventilation $\geq 2 \times$ FGF

Because of the need for a higher FGF (especially with spontaneous respiration) the T-piece is not usually used for older children (over 5 years or 20 kg body weight).

THE CIRCLE ABSORPTION SYSTEM

The advantages of the circle system include fresh gas economy, heat and moisture retention, and ease of scavenging. Its potential for use in all age groups eliminates the need for special pediatric systems. This can be extremely convenient in an outpatient facility that has a mixture of adult and pediatric patients.

The two major disadvantages of the circle system in pediatric anesthesia are its high resistance and large dead space. In young children that can be easily overcome by controlling ventilation and using circle tubing that has minimal dead space at the Y-connection.

Monitoring of Pediatric Patients

Safe conduct of anesthesia requires the anesthesiologist to maintain continuous vigilance. In the management of the anesthetized child, this can be greatly assisted by using a variety of monitoring devices. Some of them are common to all age groups, while others are of special value in the pediatric patient.

The minimum of monitoring aids for any pediatric patient undergoing general anesthesia include

1. A precordial (or esophageal) stethoscope. As correctly stated by Smith, the stethoscope is the most important of all monitoring devices in pediatric anesthesia, and should be used throughout all procedures in which general anesthesia is used. It allows continuous monitoring of heart rate and rhythm, volume of heart sounds, and rate and depth of respiration.[79]
2. Blood pressure measurement. In the pediatric patient the Doppler ultrasonic flowmeter or an automatic oscillometric device is a valuable adjunct to traditional blood pressure monitoring. Use of the correct size cuff is important in children. The width of the cuff should be approximately two-thirds of the length of the upper arm. If the cuff is too narrow, one will get a falsely high reading, whereas too wide a cuff will result in a falsely low reading.
3. Temperature monitoring. Special attention must be paid to temperature changes in pediatric anesthesia. Hypothermia is a constant threat to infants and can lead to delayed recovery and metabolic acidosis. Protective measures such as warm operating rooms, insulation of the extremities, heating blankets, and infrared lights should be used in small infants. Malignant hyperthermia, on the other hand, is a rare but potentially fatal complication if certain triggering agents are used in susceptible patients. For these reasons, body temperature must be continuously monitored under anesthesia. For most outpatient procedures, an external axillary thermister probe properly positioned near the axillary artery is most convenient and can be reused with no

elaborate sterilization. Alternatively, liquid crystal dots can be used to display changes in skin temperature.

4. Electrocardiogram (ECG). Although regarded as a vital monitoring device in adult anesthesia, the ECG is really the least valuable monitoring device in healthy pediatric patients.[79,90] In the absence of ischemic cardiac disease, its main value is to differentiate arrhythmias already detected by a precordial stethoscope. It is worthwhile to emphasize that a normal tracing may persist for minutes in spite of severe hypotension caused by high concentrations of potent inhalational agents, and it is important to avoid the potential false confidence conveyed by observing a normal tracing.

The inspired oxygen concentration monitor is becoming a standard safety feature on most anesthesia machines. Other monitors should be employed as needed. The amount of blood loss (expressed as a percentage of blood volume) should be measured in such procedures as adenoidectomy. A nerve stimulator can be used to avoid overdosage of muscle relaxants and to determine the degree of neuromuscular recovery at the termination of surgery. Arterial blood gas measurements are usually not needed in outpatient practice. However, if there is a serious reason to question the adequacy of oxygenation, ventilation, or acid-base status of a patient, arterial sampling is indicated.

Perioperative Fluid Management

The need for routine administration of intravenous fluids during outpatient anesthesia for children is controversial. By definition, outpatient anesthesia is administered to healthy children undergoing uncomplicated surgical procedures that do not involve major blood loss or translocations of body fluid compartments. Many believe that, if the procedure is of short duration and the anesthetic technique is one that ensures rapid recovery and return of normal appetite with minimal nausea and vomiting, these children do not really require infusion of fluids.[18,90] However, especially if fluids are not administered intravenously, the period of preoperative starvation should be minimized to avoid possible dehydration and hypoglycemia.[35] Although in many centers children over 1 year of age are usually not allowed solid food on the day of surgery, they are offered clear liquids up to 4 hours prior to surgery.

Intravenous fluid therapy during and after surgery, usually 5% dextrose in 0.3 normal saline (Table 4-5), is specifically indicated in the following circumstances:

1. Longer operations (over 30–60 min), which are more likely to result in delayed return of normal appetite
2. Procedures known to be associated with a high incidence of postoperative nausea and vomiting, such as strabismus surgery,[2] orchidopexy, and otoplasty. Not only should children undergoing these procedures have their preoperative fluid deficit replaced during surgery, but the anticipated continuing postoperative deficit should be considered when an hourly intravenous fluid rate is calculated. In this way there is less risk of dehydration if nausea and vomiting occur following discharge. By

ensuring adequate parenteral hydration, less emphasis need be placed in requiring the child to retain oral fluids postoperatively before the stomach can tolerate them. Forcing oral fluids prematurely often results in more persistent nausea and vomiting. In the absence of cardiovascular, respiratory, or renal pathology, the maximum tolerance level for fluids is high, and the risk of overloading the child is minimal.[7] In the event that persistent vomiting occurs, the intravenous fluid should be changed to normal saline or Ringer's lactate. Continued use of solutions that contain .25%, or .30% saline may result in severe hyponatremia if they are used to replace losses secondary to protracted vomiting.

3. Procedures that are associated with intraoperative blood loss, or that have the potential for postoperative bleeding, e.g., adenoidectomy or tonsillectomy

4. Young children who have been fasting for a prolonged period of time because they did not receive fluids as ordered or because a delay in the operative schedule extended the NPO period

5. Children who develop excessive cardiovascular depression and hypotension when potent inhalational agents are administered and who need rapid injection of fluids to restore normal cardiovascular function

6. Situations in which it is deemed desirable to have a readily available route for administration of intraoperative or postoperative narcotics for pain relief, or for administration of antibiotics as prophylaxis against subacute bacterial endocarditis for children with heart disease

Many anesthesiologists, on the other hand, prefer to have an infusion started in every child having surgery to guarantee a ready route for emergency administration of drugs. Apart from the extra expense, the time involved, and often the need for an extra pair of hands to begin the infusion, there is no real objection to this practice unless it is carried too far, for example, repeated attempts at venipuncture in a healthly, well-hydrated, chubby child who has been admitted for a brief, uncomplicated procedure.[79] It is reassuring to remember that the only two emergency drugs that are likely to be needed in the healthy day-surgery child are succinylcholine and atropine. In the absence of an infusion or visible veins, these two drugs are rapidly effective when administered intramuscularly (in a dose twice that used for intravenous administration).

□ **Table 4-5. Maintenance Fluid Therapy**[58]

Child's Weight (kg)	Basic Hourly Rate (ml)
<10	wt × 4
10–20	(wt × 2) + 20
>20	wt + 40

During the first hour of surgery, up to four times the basic hourly rate may be administered as a hydrating solution.

Postoperative Analgesia

Successful management of outpatient anesthesia requires that the anesthesiologist carefully evaluate and manage the child's need for postoperative pain relief. The need for analgesics depends on the nature of surgery and the pain threshold of the patient. It does not depend on whether or not the child is an outpatient or an inpatient.[8] Although many young children do extremely well postoperatively with minimal amounts of oral analgesics, or none whatsoever, many others experience pain and require an appropriate dose of a more potent analgesic. Every child deserves individual consideration! It is unfortunate that we still observe many anesthesiologists and surgeons who believe that "children don't experience pain" and deny an appropriate dose of a narcotic to a child who is in pain because "in their own experience," this procedure "usually" does not warrant it or for fear of slightly delaying discharge home.

By definition, procedures that require multiple or frequent use of potent parenteral narcotics are not appropriate for outpatient surgery. For the more typical pediatric outpatient procedures, postoperative pain or discomfort can be managed by one or a combination of the following:

MILD ANALGESICS

For infants under 6 months of age, a combination of care and nursing (or a bottle) is all that is usually needed following a procedure that is not associated with severe pain. Child-parent reunion should be allowed as soon as the child is awake.

For older infants and young children aspirin and acetaminophen (Tylenol) are the drugs most commonly used for relief of mild pain in the postoperative period. They are usually adequate for treating pain from integumental structures such as bones, joints, muscles, and teeth but inadequate for treating visceral pain. Aspirin, which is known to interfere with platelet aggregation, is best avoided following procedures that can be associated with bleeding, such as adenoidectomy, tonsillectomy, and circumcision. Acetaminophen can be used either orally or rectally in a dose of 60 mg (1 grain) per year of age. At CHNMC, Tylenol Children's Elixir is the drug most frequently used at home following discharge.

For more persistent, moderately severe pain, codeine can be used in combination with acetaminophen. Tylenol with Codeine Elixir contains 120 mg acetaminophen and 12 mg codeine/5 ml. The recommended dose is 5 ml for children 3 to 6 years, and 10 ml for the 7 to 12 age group. The analgesic action of codeine is much weaker than that of morphine, and it is less likely to produce nausea and vomiting. These factors, and the absence of respiratory depression in the normal dose range, make it a very useful oral analgesic for the outpatient.

POTENT NARCOTIC ANALGESICS

The use of potent narcotics in the pediatric ambulatory surgery patient deserves special consideration. It is well known that all narcotics given in the perioperative period may contribute significantly to postoperative drowsiness, nausea and vomiting, and delay in discharge home. However, it is also desirable that the postoperative period be as free of pain and discomfort for the child as possible. Many popular surgical procedures performed on an outpatient basis such as orchidopexy, circumcision, adenoidectomy, and herniotomy[78] are frequently associated with postoperative pain. Such pain, if untreated, may in itself delay full recovery, discourage ambulation, and increase morbidity by producing nausea and vomiting.[6,78]

The choice of the individual drug is usually a matter of individual judgment. Drugs such as morphine and meperidine are generally thought to have too long an action for outpatient use. Although their action can be reversed by antagonists like naloxone, reversal results in the immediate onset of pain and discomfort. Thus, a better approach is the use of a short-acting narcotic analgesic such as fentanyl.[73] In some units codeine is used intramuscularly in doses of as large as 1.5 mg/kg body weight, with a maximum of 60 mg.[87]

Narcotics can be used in outpatients to maintain anesthesia (with oxygen, nitrous oxide, relaxant) as a part of a balanced technique, or to supplement a "light" inhalational technique. By reducing the amount of potent inhalational or intravenous agents needed (and absorbed in fat for later release), they may actually contribute to more rapid awakening.[30,100] The residual analgesia may eliminate or reduce the need for further potent pain medication during the recovery period.

When compared to a pure inhalational technique, the intraoperative use of narcotics has been reported to cause no delay in discharge home.[14] Using psychomotor testing, however, patients who received inhalation anesthetics were found to perform significantly better at 30 to 59 minutes postoperatively than did patients who received narcotics.[28] After 1 hour, scores were essentially the same for both groups. This suggests that patients should not be discharged home if a narcotic has been administered within 1 hour.

If narcotics are indicated in the recovery period, a short-acting drug should be chosen. Intravenous use allows more accurate titration of the dose to the individual child and avoids the use of "standard" dosages based on weight which may lead to a relative overdose. Fentanyl up to a dose of 2 μg/kg is our drug of choice for intravenous use. Meperidine (0.5 mg/kg) and codeine (1–1.5 mg/kg) can be used intramuscularly if an intravenous route is not established.

Alfentanil is a new fentanyl analog with a distinctly shorter duration of action than fentanyl. Its use has not been approved by the U.S. Food and Drug Administration (FDA); however, it has been tested as an analgesic adjunct for induction, maintenance, and recovery.[100] It is still unclear whether or not an intermittent bolus injection or continuous infusion technique will be recommended for future use; however, it is obvious that a small single intravenous dose is associated with rapid analgesic effect and more rapid return of spontaneous ventilation and recovery than a comparable amount of fentanyl.[100] Youngberg et al[100] have shown that a group of children who received an initial intravenous bolus of alfentanil (35 μg/kg) at induction, followed by intermittent doses (10 μg/kg) at intervals of 12 to 15 minutes had a significantly shorter recovery time than a similar group who received halothane for surgical procedures of short duration. Pediatric ambulatory patients who received alfentanil had a significantly lower incidence and severity of pain in the recovery room. Oh et al[59] also demonstrated that 5 μg/kg alfentanil given intravenously to children in the recovery room following adenoidectomy was associated with rapid alleviation of apparent pain without complications. The length of time until discharge was comparable to that of a matched placebo group. Although studies such as this are only investigational and limited in scope, it would appear that a quick-acting, potent analgesic associated with rapid recovery such as alfentanil may be an important adjunct in the prevention or treatment of pain in the ambulatory pediatric patient.

REGIONAL ANALGESIA FOR POSTOPERATIVE PAIN

Though regional anesthesia alone is usually not popular in pediatric outpatients, many simple blocks can be combined with light general anesthesia to provide excellent postoperative pain relief and early ambulation, with minimal or no need for narcotics.

For the purpose of pain relief, a block can be performed at the end of surgery to obtain the maximum duration of analgesia in the postoperative period. For shorter procedures (<30 min), however, and with the availability of longer-acting local anesthetics (e.g., bupivacaine), there may be yet another advantage in placing the block before surgery starts, but after the child is asleep. This would help reduce the requirement for general anesthetic agents during surgery, which may result in a more rapid recovery, early discharge, return of normal appetite and less nausea and vomiting.[78]

The types of blocks that can be safely used in the pediatric ambulatory surgery patient are limited only by the skill and interest of the individual anesthesiologist. Generally, the techniques chosen should be simple and expedient to perform, have minimal or no side-effects, and not interfere with the motor function and early ambulation of the child. Although manufacturers of bupivacaine do not recommend using it in children younger than 12 years, the drug has been used extensively in pediatric anesthesia, and offers the distinct advantage of a long duration of action. Certain types of nerve blocks can be used in conjunction with general anesthesia in children. The ones more widely used in pediatric outpatients are discussed in the following sections.

ILIOINGUINAL AND ILIOHYPOGASTRIC NERVE BLOCK

The surgeon can perform this nerve block simply by infiltrating 0.5% bupivacaine solution (in doses up to 2 mg/kg) in the region medial to the anterior superior iliac spine. This block has been used successfully to provide excellent postoperative analgesia for pediatric outpatients following elective inguinal herniotomy[78] and orchidopexy.[38] In the study by Shandling and Steward,[78] the requirements for potent analgesics in the postanesthesia care unit (PACU) were significantly reduced following inguinal herniotomy. In the control group, 74 of 75 patients were given codeine in the PACU, compared with only 3 of 81 in the nerve block group. At home, analgesics were given by parents to 32 of 75 of the children in the control group and 24 of 81 of the children who had a nerve block. The only reported complication was a 4% incidence of a transient motor block of the femoral nerve resulting in a short-lived difficulty with walking. In the outpatient, this can possibly be avoided by using a more dilute solution of bupivacaine (0.25%), although the onset of the block might be less rapid.

NERVE BLOCKS OF THE PENIS

Circumcision is probably the most common outpatient procedure performed on the penis. Postoperative pain causes restlessness and agitation, and may lead the child to manipulate his penis, possibly causing infection and bleeding. To avoid the need for heavy doses of narcotics in the immediate postoperative period, dorsal nerve block of the penis has been found to provide good analgesia in 96% of cases.[81] The simple injection of 1 to 4 ml of 0.25% bupivacaine without epinephrine deep to Buck's fascia 1 cm from the midline provides over 6 hours of analgesia with no complications. Alternate approaches to penile block are either a midline injection or subcutaneous infiltration,[12] which presumably blocks the nerve after it has ramified into the subcutaneous tissue.

CAUDAL BLOCK FOR POSTOPERATIVE ANALGESIA

Caudal block is extremely easy to perform in children. It provides excellent and reproducible postoperative analgesia following a wide variety of surgical procedures such as circumcision, hypospadias repair, orchidopexy, and herniotomy. We use the technique described by Davenport with the block performed with the child on his side.[22] The block is usually completed in less than a minute, so that there is little or no delay in the rapid turnover of a busy ambulatory surgical unit.

Using bupivacaine 0.25% solution in a dose of 0.1 ml/segment/yr[75] (minimal volume 3 ml), there is virtually no risk of overdosage and no motor paralysis. Caudal block has been extensively used in ambulatory surgery by one of us* (mainly for circumcision in children 1-16 years of age), and by many others,[38,48] with most children discharged home pain-free 1 to 2 hours postoperatively. Postural hypotension resulting from sympathetic blockade is not a problem; however, blood pressure must be normal with the patient in the upright position, and ambulation must not be associated with dizziness prior to discharge. Analgesia (as measured by subsequent need of a mild oral analgesic) lasted 4 to 6 hours with this technique. Caudal block is particularly effective following orchidopexies on an outpatient basis,[38] where the pain and discomfort involved may otherwise require home use of narcotics.[18]

Recovery and Discharge Criteria

The key to understanding the reasoning behind the selection or avoidance of certain anesthetic agents and techniques in ambulatory surgery is related to recovery.

Rapid recovery and early ambulation are major objectives in pediatric ambulatory surgery. When dealing with pediatric outpatients, we must guarantee safe discharge not only from the recovery room but also from the hospital.[29] In our institution all children recover from anesthesia in the same recovery area. Ambulatory patients are then transferred to a special short-stay recovery unit (SSRU).

In order to provide uniform care and to ensure a complete legal record, some institutions have developed discharge criteria. Unlike a scoring system, all criteria should be met. At CHNMC criteria for discharge from the hospital are

Appropriateness and stability of vital signs
Ability to swallow oral fluids and cough or demonstrate a gag reflex

---

*R. Hannallah and J.K. Rosales; over 1000 cases at the Montreal Children's Hospital, Montreal, Canada

Ability to ambulate consistent with developmental age level

Absence of nausea, vomiting, and dizziness, preferably including ability to retain oral fluids

Absence of respiratory distress

A state of consciousness appropriate to developmental level

Endotracheal extubation performed within 3 hours of the time of discharge and depressant medication received within 2 hours are other factors that need to be considered. Although the intervals noted above are arbitrary, they direct our attention to two potential areas of concern within a time frame when complications might occur.

Role of the Parent in the Recovery Period

RECOVERY ROOM

Many parents want to be with their child as soon as the operation is terminated. In addition to confirming that the child has indeed survived the procedure, the parent believes that the child will relate to them better than other unfamiliar faces at a time when anxiety could result from separation. Unfortunately, most recovery rooms are not large enough or planned properly to allow parents to participate in this aspect of care. In addition, many recovery room nurses believe that early parent participation at this level may be detrimental to the care of their child and perhaps that of other children as well. Parent participation in recovery of handicapped children has proved useful in our institution in selected cases. These especially include deaf, blind, and retarded children whose ability to communicate with anyone other than the parent is compromised. In any case, parents should not have access to the recovery room until the child's vital signs have stabilized, airway obstruction is no longer a threat, and the child is awakening. They should be told in advance that their role is to provide support for their child. They should stay at the child's bedside, should not walk around the room, and should not inquire about other children in the room. The parent must understand that should the child's condition deteriorate or for any reason it seems prudent to request them to leave the unit at any time they will do so promptly and without argument. It is important that they know they are not required to stay and should feel at liberty to leave the room if they feel uncomfortable.

SHORT-STAY RECOVERY UNIT

Parents are encouraged to or may even be required to participate in the child's care in the SSRU (Fig. 4-7). Parents can care for and hold, cuddle, and feed the child, and their involvement may reduce the need for a very high nurse/patient ratio. The rules and regulations of parent participation in the SSRU should be provided in advance. An example of the issues which should be addressed is seen in Appendix 4-2.

DISCHARGE HOME

As noted by Steward[87] "every child whatever his age, must have an escort home. The journey preferably should be by private car or taxicab, and the escort

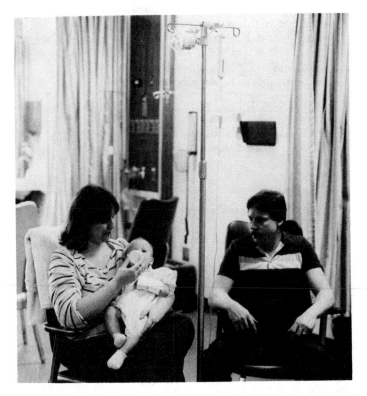

FIG. 4-7 Parents participate in the child's care in the Short Stay Unit at CHNMC.

should be provided with written instructions as to the home care of the child, and be provided with a telephone number to call for further advice or to report complications. Such service is essential in the outpatient unit." In addition to counseling the parent of each child about postoperative care, most units have designed handouts that specify the care to be provided and the signs that might herald a complication. For convenience, the handout is usually limited to postoperative instructions for one specific operative procedure. An example of such a pamphlet for patients who undergo inguinal herniorrhaphy is included in Appendix 4-3.

Complications and Admissions

COMPLICATIONS

Aside from pain, the most difficult common complication to prevent or treat is protracted vomiting, which is most commonly associated with tonsillectomy and adenoidectomy[30] and with strabismus surgery.[1,2,36,99] Vomiting is twice as common following operations that last over 20 minutes as in shorter procedures.[85] In one study of postoperative vomiting in children[69] it was noted that vomiting occurred less frequently in children less than 3 years of age but above this age varied between 42% and 51% until puberty. Although factors other than age also influenced the frequency with which postoperative vomiting occurred, a major factor was related to the operative procedure[69] (Table 4-6).

In our institution frequency of vomiting in intubated, unmedicated children receiving nitrous oxide–halothane anesthesia for strabismus surgery was reported to be as high as 85%.[1,2] Although treatment with an antiemetic agent is fraught with other potential dangers such as sedation and hypotension, the prophylactic or therapeutic use of droperidol (75 μg/kg IV 30 min before the end of surgery) was found to be highly effective in reducing the frequency and severity of vomiting in children following strabismus surgery.[2] On the average, patients who vomited and received droperidol, as well as those who did not, were unable to meet discharge criteria for 6 hours after discontinuation of the anesthetic agent and admission to the recovery room. Although this is a long recovery for an ambulatory surgery procedure, untreated patients cannot be discharged any earlier because of persistent vomiting; furthermore, they are also more uncomfortable. In our institution, severe vomiting has also been observed following orchidopexy performed on an outpatient basis. Interestingly enough, this is the one procedure noted by Cloud et al to require the use of oral narcotic agents for pain relief in the posthospitalization period.[18] Strabismus surgery and orchidopexy are examples of severe vomiting. Vomiting may be a major problem even after relatively short, uncomplicated procedures. Some patients may vomit repeatedly after oral fluids are offered. As a result, it is frequently judicious to maintain an intravenous infusion until oral fluids are tolerated. The rate of infusion should be increased to account for fluid losses. Replacement for vomiting should be done with normal saline or Ringer's lactate. Droperidol has been used successfully in doses as low as 5 μg/kg in patients with persistent vomiting following procedures other than strabismus surgery or orchidopexy.[65]

☐ **Table 4-6. Vomiting Related to Procedures or Surgical Specialty**

Procedure	No. of Patients	No. and Percentage of Patients Who Vomited		Average Number of Vomiting Episodes per Patient
Squint	33	25	(76%)	1.82
Hernia	92	50	(54%)	1.71
T&A	89	52	(58%)	1.57
Orchidopexy	64	37	(58%)	1.44
Plastic	145	71	(49%)	1.22
Hypospadias	24	11	(46%)	1.21
Circumcision	49	20	(41%)	1.20

(Based on Rowley MP, Brown TCK: Postoperative vomiting in children. Anaesth Intensive Care 10:309–313, 1982)

ADMISSIONS

Complications that result in *admission* of the patient to a hospital are usually the same types of problems discussed previously but with either greater frequency or severity.

Less than 1% of the patients operated on in our unit require admission. The most common reasons are vomiting (50%), pain (10%) and bleeding (8%). Other complications include croup, fever, and factors related to parent's apprehension about caring for the child at home.

Follow-Up

Telephone or mail questionnaires are necessary to determine the frequency of posthospitalization problems. A large percentage of parents report that their child continues to have an upset stomach, dizziness, and so forth after returning home (Table 4-7). Fortunately, most of the complications reported are mild[4,23,85] and require no treatment. A questionnaire should be designed not only to detect problems in the child but also to determine whether the parents were satisfied with the care received, and if not, to request suggestions for improvement (Fig. 4-8). A small percentage of parents respond that they would prefer to have the child hospitalized if they had it to do over again.[4,85] Some of the reasons for this have been noted previously in the section on disadvantages. In a study by Davenport,[23] this percentage was 9.2%, and in Ahlgren's, 8.0%.[3] This relatively high percentage of dissatisfaction or apprehension rarely occurs in adult ambulatory settings and seems to relate to the parent's desire to have a longer period of observation and care for their child in the hospital and a fear of potential complications at home.

Any short-stay unit should collect and analyze data for trends that might lead to correction of deficiencies and eventually to improvement in patient care. Design and modification of policy is better done by prospective review of audits than by reacting to mishaps. This leads to more uniform, safe care and minimizes medicolegal actions.

☐ **Table 4-7. Replies to Questionnaire Inquiry, "Did Your Child Have Any of the Following after Going Home?" (300 Responses)**

Symptom	None	Some	Considerable
Upset stomach	238 (79%)	50 (17%)	12 (4%)
Loss of appetite	186 (62%)	101 (34%)	13 (4%)
Dizziness	265 (88%)	33 (11%)	2 (1%)
Headache	262 (87%)	35 (12%)	3 (1%)
Sore throat	259 (86%)	30 (10%)	11 (4%)
Hoarseness	264 (88%)	29 (10%)	7 (2%)
Bad dreams	273 (91%)	20 (7%)	7 (2%)

(Ahlgren EN, Bennett EJ, and Stephen CR: Outpatient pediatric anesthesiology: A case series. Anesth Analg 50:402–408, 1971, with permission)

Dear Parents,

Your opinions and comments about the Short Stay Recovery Unit help us to meet the needs of our patients. We would appreciate your cooperation in filling out this questionnaire. Feel free to comment as well as answer the questions. Your name is not required on the questionnaire, but you may write it if you wish.

Thank you for your cooperation.

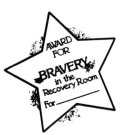

1. What was your overall impression of the Short Stay Recovery Unit (SSRU)?

   ☐ Favorable
   ☐ Unfavorable
   ☐ Indifferent

   Comments: _____
   _____
   _____

2. Did the unit meet you and your child's needs?

   ☐ Yes
   ☐ No

   Comments: _____
   _____
   _____

3. Did you receive a call the night before surgery from a nurse from the SSRU?

   ☐ Yes
   ☐ No

4. If yes, did you find the information helpful?

   ☐ Yes
   ☐ No

   Comments: _____
   _____
   _____

5. Were you informed that —

   - no siblings allowed?   ☐ Yes ☐ No
   - only two (2) adults allowed?   ☐ Yes ☐ No
   - no food or drinks allowed?   ☐ Yes ☐ No
   - one (1) adult must stay with child at all times? ☐ Yes ☐ No

6. Were you satisfied with the discharge instructions given by the nurse?

   ☐ Yes
   ☐ No

   Comments: _____
   _____
   _____

7. Did you feel comfortable taking your child home at the time of discharge?

   ☐ Yes
   ☐ No

   Comments: _____
   _____
   _____

CHNMC FORM (Rev 1/84) Disk 1601

FIG. 4-8 Short Stay Recovery Unit (CHNMC) follow up questionnaire.

References

1. Abramowitz MD, Elder PT, Friendly DS et al: Antiemetic effectiveness of intraoperatively administered droperidol in pediatric strabismus outpatient surgery. J Pediatr Ophthalmol Strabismus 18:22, 1981

2. Abramowitz MD, Oh TH, Epstein BS et al: The antiemetic effect of droperidol following outpatient strabismus surgery in children. Anesthesiology 59:579–583, 1983
3. Ahlgren EN, Bennett EJ, Stephen CR: Outpatient pediatric anesthesiology: A case series. Anesth Analg (Cleve) 50:402, 1971
4. Ahlgren EW: Pediatric outpatient anesthesia. Am J Dis Child 126:36, 1973
5. American Heart Association (AHA) Committee report: Prevention of bacterial endocarditis. Circulation 70:1123A–1127A, 1984
6. Anderson R: Pain as a major cause of postoperative nausea. Can Anaesth Soc J 23:366, 1976
7. Berry FA: Pediatric anesthesia for the practitioner-fluid balance. ASA Refresher Course Lectures Outline #221, 1976
8. Berry FA: Pediatric outpatient anesthesia. In Hershey SG (ed): ASA Refresher Courses in Anesthesiology 10:17–26, 1982
9. Berry FA: Pre-existing medical conditions of pediatric patients. Semin Anesth 3:24–31, March 1984
10. Blitt C: Nitrous-narcotic-relaxant anesthesia vs. volatile anesthesia in the adult surgical outpatient. In Brown BR (ed): Outpatient Anesthesia: Contemporary Anesthesia Practice. Philadelphia, FA Davis, 1978
11. Booker PD, Chapman DH: Premedication in children undergoing day-care surgery. Br J Anaesth 51:1083, 1979
12. Broadman LM, Belman AB, Elder PT et al: Postcircumcision pain—a prospective evaluation of subcutaneous ring block of the penis. Regional Anesth 9:48–49, 1984
13. Bryan MH, Hardie MJ, Reilly BJ et al: Pulmonary function studies during the first year of life in infants recovering from the respiratory distress syndrome. Pediatrics 52:169, 1973
14. Brzustowicz RM, Nelson DA, Betts EK et al: Efficacy of oral premedication for pediatric outpatient surgery. Anesthesiology 60:475–477, 1984
15. Bush GH, Roth F: Muscle pains after suxamethonium chloride in children. Br J Anaesth 33:151, 1961
16. Chiang TM, Sukis AE, Ross DE: Tonsillectomy performed on an outpatient basis. Report of a series of 40,000 cases performed without a death. Arch Otolaryngol 88:307, 1968
17. Clark AJM, Hurting AB: Premedication with meperidine and atropine does not prolong recovery to street fitness after outpatient surgery. Can Anaesth Soc J 28:390, 1981
18. Cloud DT, Reed WA, Ford JL et al: The surgicenter: A fresh concept in outpatient pediatric surgery. J Pediatr Surg 7:206, 1972
19. Cohen DD, Dillon JB: Anesthesia for outpatient surgery. Springfield, IL, Charles C Thomas, 1970
20. Coté CJ, Goudsouzian NG, Liu LMP et al: The dose response of intravenous thiopental for the induction of general anesthesia in unpremedicated children. Anesthesiology 55:703–705, 1981
21. Craig J, Cooper GM, Sear JW: Recovery from day-case anesthesia. Comparison between methohexitone, Althesin and etomidate. Br J Anaesth 54:447–450, 1982
22. Davenport HT: Pediatric Anaesthesia, 2nd ed. Chicago, Year Book Medical Publishers, 1973
23. Davenport HT, Shaw CP, Robinson GC: Day surgery for children. Can Med Assoc J 105:498, 1971
24. Davenport HT, Werry JS: The effect of general anesthesia, surgery and hospitalization upon the behavior of children. Am J Orthopsychiatry 5:806, 1970
25. Desjardins R, Ansara S, Charest J: Preanesthetic medication in paediatric day-care surgery. Can Anaesth Soc J 28:141, 1981
26. Diaz JH, Lockhart CH: Is halothane really safe in infancy? (abstr). Anesthesiology 51:S313, 1979
27. Dundee JW: Intravenous Anesthetic Agents. Chicago, Year Book Medical Publishers, 1979
28. Enright AC, Pace-Florida A: Recovery from anesthesia in outpatients: A comparison of narcotic and inhalational techniques. Can Anaesth Soc J 24:618, 1977
29. Epstein BS: Recovery from anesthesia. Anesthesiology 43:285, 1975
30. Epstein BS, Levy ML, Thein MH et al: Evaluation of fentanyl as an adjunct to thiopental-nitrous oxide-oxygen anesthesia for short surgical procedures. Anesthesiol Rev 2:24, 1975

31. Ferres CJ, Crean PM, Mirakhur RK: An evaluation of Org NC 45 (vecuronium) in paediatric anaesthesia. Anaesthesia 38:943–947, 1983
32. Goresky GV, Steward DJ: Rectal methohexitone for induction of anaesthesia in children. Can Anaesth Soc J 26:213, 1979
33. Goudsouzian NG, Liu LMP: The neuromuscular response of infants to a continuous infusion of succinylcholine. Anesthesiology 60:97–101, 1984
34. Goudsouzian NG, Liu LMP, Coté CJ et al: Safety and efficacy of atracurium in adolescents and children anesthetized with halothane. Anesthesiology 59:459–462, 1983
35. Graham IFM: Preoperative starvation and plasma glucose concentrations in children undergoing outpatient anaesthesia. Br J Anaesth 51:161, 1979
36. Hadaway BG, Ingram AM, Traynor MJ: Day care surgery in strabismus in children. Trans Ophthalmol Soc UK 97:23, 1977
37. Hannallah RS, Abramowitz MD, Oh TH et al: Residents' attitude towards parents' presence during anesthesia induction in children: Does experience make a difference? Anesthesiology 60:598–601, 1984
38. Hannallah RS, Broadman LM, Belman AB et al: Control of post-orchiopexy pain in pediatric patients: Comparison of two regional techniques. Anesthesiology 61:A429, 1984
39. Hannallah RS, Rosales JK: Experience with parents' presence during anaesthesia induction in children. Can Anaesth Soc J 30:286–289, 1983
40. Herzfeld G: Hernia in infancy. Am J Surg 39:422, 1938
41. Hoyal RHA, Prys-Roberts C, Simpson PJ: Enflurane in outpatient dental anaesthesia. Br J Anaesth 52:219, 1980
42. Hudson RJ, Stanski DR, Burch PG. Pharmacokinetics of methohexital and thiopental in surgical patients. Anesthesiology 59:215–219, 1983
43. Jensen BH, Wernberg M, Adersen M: Preoperative starvation and blood glucose concentrations in children undergoing inpatient and outpatient anesthesia. Br J Anaesth 54:1071–1074, 1982
44. Johnson GG: Day care surgery for infants and children. Can Anaesth Soc J 30:553–557, 1983
45. Johnston RR, Eger EI II, Wilson C: A comparative interaction of epinephrine with enflurane, isoflurane, and halothane in man. Anesth Analg 55:709–712, 1976
46. Karl HW, Swedlow DB, Lee KW et al: Epinephrine-halothane interaction in children. Anesthesiology 58:142–145, 1983
47. Kay B: A clinical assessment of the use of etomidate in children. Br J Anaesth 48:207–211, 1976
48. Kay B: Caudal block for postoperative pain relief in children. Anaesthesia 29:610, 1974
49. Khazzam A, Karkas A: Intramuscular methohexital as a sole pediatric anesthetic-analgesic agent. Anesth Analg (Cleve) 51:895, 1972
50. Koka BV, Jeon IS, Andre JM et al: Postintubation croup in children. Anesth Analg (Cleve) 56:501, 1977
51. Kortilla K, Linnoila M, Ertama P et al: Recovery and simulated driving after intravenous anesthesia with thiopental, methohexital, propanidid, or alphadione. Anesthesiology 43:291, 1975
52. Krantz EM: Low-dose intramuscular ketamine and hyaluronidase for induction of anesthesia in non-premedicated children. S Afr Med J 58:161–162, 1980
53. Liu LMP, Cóte CJ, Goudsouzian NG et al: Life-threatening apnea in infants recovering from anesthesia. Anesthesiology 59:506–510, 1983
54. McGill WA, Coveler LA, Epstein BS: Subacute upper respiratory infection in small children. Anesth Analg 58:331–333, 1979
55. Newburger JW, Rosenthal A, Williams RG, et al: Noninvasive tests in the initial evaluation of heart murmurs in children. N Engl J Med 308:61–64, 1983
56. Nicoll JH: The surgery of infancy: Br Med J 2:753–754, 1909
57. O'Donovan TR: Ambulatory Surgical Centers-Development and Management. Germantown, MD, Aspen Systems Corp, 1976
58. Oh TH: Letter: Formula for calculating fluid maintenance requirements. Anesthesiology 53:351, 1980
59. Oh TH, Abramowitz MD, Epstein BS: Analgesic effects of alfentanil in postoperative pain

control in children. Abstract presented at the American Academy of Pediatrics Section on Anesthesiology program, March 1982

60. Othersen HB, Clatworthy HW: Outpatient herniorrhaphy for infants. Am J Dis Child 116:78, 1968

61. Position statement on ambulatory surgery, October 23, 1978. Medical Society of the District of Columbia and National Capital Medical Foundation, Inc., November 10, 1980

62. Putnam LP: Pseudocholinesterase deficiency: An additional preoperative consideration in outpatient diagnostic procedures. South Med J 70:831, 1977

63. Rigg JRA, Dunn GL, Cameron GS: Paediatric outpatient surgery under general anaesthesia. Anaesth Intensive Care 8:451, 1980

64. Rita L, Cox JM, Seleny FL et al: Ketamine hydrochloride for pediatric premedication 1. Comparison with pentazocine. Anesth Analg (Cleve) 53:375, 1974

65. Rita L, Goodarzi M, Seleny F: Effect of low dose droperidol on postoperative vomiting in children. Can Anaesth Soc J 28:259–262, 1981

66. Rita L, Seleny FL: Pediatric outpatient anesthesia: Premedication versus no premedication and the choice of anesthetic agents. Anesthesiol Rev 1:9, 1974

67. Rockoff MA, Goudsouzian NG: Seizures induced by methohexital. Anesthesiology 54:333–335, 1981

68. Rose DK, Byrick RJ, Froese AB: Carbon dioxide elimination during spontaneous ventilation with a modified Mapleson D system: Studies in a lung model. Can Anaesth Soc J 25:353–365, 1978

69. Rowley MP, Brown TCK: Postoperative vomiting in children. Anaesth Intensive Care 10:309–313, 1982

70. Ryhanen P, Kangas T, Rantakyla S: Premedication for outpatient adenoidectomy: Comparison between ketamine and pethidine. Laryngoscope 90:494, 1980

71. Sagel SS, Evens RG, Forrest JV, et al: Efficacy of routine screening and lateral chest radiographs in a hospital-based population. N Engl J Med 291:1001–1004, 1974

72. Sane SM, Worsing RA, Wiens CW et al: Value of preoperative chest x-ray examinations in children. Pediatrics 60:669, 1977

73. Schmidt KF, Garfield JM, Korten K: The pharmacology of agents used in outpatient anesthesia. Int Anesthesiol Clin 14:15, 1976

74. Schulman J, Foley JM, Vernon TA et al: A study of the effect of the mother's presence during anesthesia induction. Pediatrics 39:111, 1967

75. Schulte-Steinberg O, Rahlfs VW: Spread of extradural analgesia following caudal injection in children: A statistical study. Br J Anaesth 49:1027, 1977

76. Sewall K: Preoperative medication for children. Surg Clin North Am 50:775, 1970

77. Shah CP, Robinson GC, Kinnis C et al: Day care surgery for children: A controlled study of medical complications and parental attitudes. Med Care 10:437, 1972

78. Shandling B, Steward DJ: Regional analgesia for postoperative pain in pediatric outpatient surgery. J Pediatr Surg 15:477, 1980

79. Smith RM: Anesthesia for infants and children, 4th ed. St Louis, CV Mosby, 1980

80. Smith RM: Endotracheal intubation. *In* Anesthesia for Infants and Children. 4th ed. St. Louis, CV Mosby, 1980

81. Soliman MG, Tremblay NA: Nerve block of the penis for postoperative pain relief in children. Anesth Analg (Cleve) 57:495, 1978

82. Stein, SB: A hospital story. New York, Walker, 1983

83. Steward DJ: Anaesthesia for day-care surgery: A symposium (IV) Anaesthesia for paediatric outpatients. Can Anaesth Soc J 27:412, 1980

84. Steward DJ: A trial of enflurane for pediatric outpatient anaesthesia. Can Anaeth Soc J 24:603, 1977

85. Steward DJ: Experience with an outpatient anesthesia service for children. Anesth Analg (Cleve) 52:877, 1973

86. Steward DJ: Isoflurane for pediatric outpatients (abstr). Can Anaesth Soc J 28:500, 1981

87. Steward DJ: Outpatient pediatric anesthesia. Anesthesiology 43:268, 1975

88. Steward DJ: Pre-term infants are more prone to complications following minor surgery than are term infants. Anesthesiology 56:304–306, 1982
89. Steward DJ: Psychological considerations in the pediatric patient. In Guerra F, Aldrete JA (ed): Emotional and Psychological Responses to Anesthesia and Surgery. New York, Grune & Stratton, 1980
90. Steward DJ, Creighton RE: General anesthesia for minor surgery in healthy children. In Advances in Anesthesia. Chicago, Year Book Medical Publishers, 1984
91. Surgicenter—a new idea for one day surgery. Resident Staff Phys 15:65, 1973
92. Striker TW: Results of Anesthesia Survey, American Academy of Pediatrics, Section on Anesthesia, presented at meetings of American Academy of Pediatrics, 1979
93. Tait AR, Ketcham TR, Klein MJ, et al: Perioperative respiratory complications in patients with upper respiratory tract infections. Anesthesiology 59:A433, 1983
94. Tait AR, Nahrwold ML, LaBond VA et al: Anesthesia and upper respiratory viral infections. Anesthesiology 57:A450, 1982
95. Tomlin PJ, Howarth FH, Robinson JS: Postoperative atelectasis and laryngeal incompetence. Lancet 1:1402, 1968
96. Urbach GM, Edelist G: An evaluation of the anaesthetic techniques used in an outpatient unit. Can Anaesth Soc J 24:401, 1977
97. Wade JG, Stevens WC: Isoflurane: An anesthetic for the eighties? Anesth Analg (Cleve) 60:666, 1981
98. Walters J, Christianson L, Betts EK et al: Oral vs. intramuscular premedication for pediatric inpatients (abstr). Anesthesiology 59:A454, 1983
99. Weinstock SM, Flynn JJ: Brief hospital admissions for pediatric strabismus surgery. 80:525, 1975
100. Youngberg JA, Subaiya C, Graybar GB et al: Alfentanil for day-stay surgery in children: An evaluation (abstr). Anesth Analg 63:284, 1984

Appendix 4-1. NPO Instructions for Parents

CHILDREN'S HOSPITAL NATIONAL MEDICAL CENTER DEPARTMENT OF ANESTHESIOLOGY

Instructions For Not Eating or Feeding Before Surgery (Nothing By Mouth—NPO)

In order to shorten the length of your child's stay in the hospital, your child has been scheduled for surgery as an outpatient. It is most important that your child have an empty stomach when given an anesthetic. This will reduce the danger of vomiting and inhaling stomach contents into the lungs while asleep. *You must follow* these instructions *or* your child's *surgery may be cancelled.*

If your child is 1 to 6 years old:
  A. A day before surgery call your surgeon or Children's Hospital after 5:00 P.M. at 745-3317 to find out the time surgery is scheduled (not the time you are asked to arrive at the hospital).
  B. *If surgery is* scheduled *between 7:30 A.M. and 12 noon* your child *must not eat or drink anything after midnight* the evening before the day surgery is scheduled.
  C. *If surgery is scheduled at 12 noon or later,* your child must not have any solid food, milk, or milk products after midnight the evening before surgery is scheduled. Before 6:00 A.M. the morning of surgery your

child may have up to 8 ounces of clear liquid only (Kool-Aid, apple juice, ginger ale, *but not* milk or food). *After 6:00 A.M.* your child *must have nothing* else to eat or drink before surgery.

D. If your child must take medicine by mouth for a medical condition during the period when no food or drink is allowed before surgery, please give the medicine at its scheduled time with a sip of water (no more than 2 teaspoons).

E. If you have any questions about these directions or about what your child should eat or drink before surgery; please call 745-3317 after 5:00 P.M. weekdays. We will be happy to answer your questions and discuss any special problems your child may have. You may also discuss any questions you have about feeding your child with the nurse who will telephone you a day or two before your child is scheduled for admission.

Separate forms are available for infants under 1 year, and children over 6 years old.

Appendix 4-2. Parent's Instructions for SSRU

Short Stay Recovery Unit
Children's Hospital National Medical Center
111 Michigan Avenue, N.W.
Washington, DC 20010

SHORT STAY WELCOMES YOU

Our unit is designed to care for children who have undergone surgery requiring a minimum of 1 hour of short-stay recovery time. Your child's stay in our unit will vary usually from 1 to 4 hours or longer, depending on the type of surgical procedure done and your child's individual recovery rate.

We realize that the surgical experience is stressful for both you and your child. We hope this introduction to our unit will help minimize anxiety by providing you with some important and helpful information. Feel free to let us know your specific needs, concerns, or questions so that we may work together to make your child's stay here a pleasant one.

RULES AND REGULATIONS

In order for your child to receive safe, comprehensive care, let us review a few regulations designed to promote recovery.

Visiting: For safety reasons, we require one parent or visitor to stay with your child at all times. No siblings under 12 years old, and no more than two visitors per patient are allowed on this unit.

Smoking, Eating or Drinking: These activities are not permitted on any hospital unit. You are welcome to use the cafeteria or snack bar located on the 2nd floor.

Breakfast _____ 6:30 A.M.–9:30 A.M.
Lunch _____11:00 A.M.–2:00 P.M.
Dinner _____ 4:30 P.M.–7:00 P.M.
Fast Foods _____10:00 A.M.–4:00 P.M.

WHILE YOU'RE HERE

We encourage your participation in your child's care to the point at which you feel comfortable. You and your child may watch the television located in the play room, or use the telephones provided in each room.

AFTER SURGERY

When your child returns from surgery, you may notice that an IV (intravenous fluid) bottle will be regulating fluids through an attachment to the child's arm or foot. This IV will be removed when your child can tolerate fluids without vomiting.

GOING HOME

Before being discharged from the unit to go home, your child must meet certain criteria by the medical team for the type of procedure that was performed. Your nurse will discuss these criteria with you.

Before leaving, you will receive discharge instructions and will be requested to sign your child's chart. In addition, we ask that you please answer the questionnaire to help us evaluate and improve our unit.

Thank you.

Short Stay Staff

Appendix 4-3. Home Care Instructions: Inguinal Herniorrhaphy and Hydrocelectomy

ACTIVITY

May begin normal activities but no strenuous activities such as running, skating, jumping or playing hard for two weeks. May return to *school* in 2–4 days, when child is comfortable, but no playground or gym activities for two weeks. Infants can lie on their tummies.

CARE OF INCISION

Some children have a "clear coating" over the incision; this type of dressing peels off by itself in 4 to 7 days. It does not require any special care other than keeping the area clean and dry. Other children may have a gauze-pad dressing that should not get wet and should be kept clean and dry. If the tapes become loose they can be trimmed or replaced.

It may be difficult, but try to keep your child from scratching the incision. Please do not use baby powder or creams for diaper rash for two weeks.

BATHING

May_____ May not take a bath for_____ days.

DIET

May eat regular diet at home

PAIN

Give acetaminophen_____ or aspirin _____ every 4 hours if needed for discomfort. After the second or third day there usually is no need for medicine for pain.

Generally, children should not be given aspirin or Tylenol more than four times in one day.

WHEN TO CALL DOCTOR

Any obvious bleeding. Some dried blood may be over the incision, this is normal

Redness or swelling around the incision

Fever over 101.4°F or 38°C

Drainage (pus) from the wound

Persistent pain in the incision that is not relieved by aspirin or Tylenol

ADDITIONAL INSTRUCTIONS

_____

_____

_____

_____

RETURN APPOINTMENT

_____

FOR EMERGENCIES

Doctor or clinic_____

Nursing unit _____

5

The Adult
and Geriatric
Patient

Monte Lichtiger, M.D.

Bernard V. Wetchler, M.D.

Beverly K. Philip, M.D.

Adult patients who elect to have surgery in an ambulatory setting should be in good general health, should be scheduled for procedures that are not unduly long, and should not require extensive nursing care in the postoperative period. Most patients scheduled for ambulatory surgery will be ASA class 1 or class 2 patients. Class 3 patients may also be candidates for ambulatory surgery if their systemic illnesses are well controlled.

The anesthesiologist will be integrally involved in the patient's care and therefore should be brought into the case prior to the day of surgery. In fact, the anesthesiologist is the physician most involved with the patient's care in the ambulatory setting. With the possible exception of pain centers, there is no other area in anesthetic practice in which the anesthesiologist functions so much as a primary care physician.

Preanesthesia Visit

In some ambulatory centers, the patient is either contacted by telephone or sent a history questionnaire. Figure 5-1 is the history form used at Mt. Sinai Medical Center in Miami, Florida. In this ambulatory center, we prefer to see patients for a separate preanesthesia visit 2 to 5 days prior to their scheduled surgery. When a patient makes a special trip to see an anesthesiologist, his or her attitude toward this specialist is much the same as it would be toward any other specialist. In short, a physician-patient relationship begins to develop. The

Mount Sinai MEDICAL CENTER OF GREATER MIAMI

NAME:_____ **MEDICAL RECORD NO.**_____

INSTRUCTIONS: PLEASE INDICATE YOUR ANSWER TO THE QUESTIONS BELOW BY PLACING A **CHECK,** √ IN THE APPROPRIATE BOX. **DO NOT WRITE ANYTHING ELSE ON THE SHEET.** THANK YOU.

WHAT IS YOUR AGE? [ ]

Questions For Patient

	This Space Is For Physicians Only
1.	Allergies
2.	URI
3.	Medication
	Drugs
4.	Dentition
5.	Alcohol
6.	Cigarettes
7.	Family H
8.	Surgical H
9.	Medical H Current Problems

1. Are you allergic to anything? ☐ YES ☐ NO

2. Have you recently had a cough, cold or sore throat? ☐ YES ☐ NO

3. Do you take aspirin (or a similar drug)? ☐ YES ☐ NO
   Do you take any other medicines or drugs? ☐ YES ☐ NO
   Do you use eye drops or nose drops? ☐ YES ☐ NO
   Do you wear contact lenses? ☐ YES ☐ NO

4. Do you have dentures or bridges? ☐ YES ☐ NO
   Are your front teeth capped? ☐ YES ☐ NO
   Are any teeth loose, chipped or bad? ☐ YES ☐ NO

5. Do you have an alcoholic drink more than once a day? ☐ YES ☐ NO

6. Do you smoke or did you give up smoking? ☐ YES ☐ NO

7. Have you, your family or relatives had an unexplained or serious complication during surgery or anesthesia? ☐ YES ☐ NO

8. Have you had an operation before? ☐ YES ☐ NO
   Have you ever had a blood transfusion? ☐ YES ☐ NO

9. Is it possible you may be pregnant? ☐ YES ☐ NO

10. Have you had (or still have) any of these problems? ☐ YES ☐ NO

☐ Ulcer, Hiatus Hernia	☐ Heart Murmur	☐ Back Problems
☐ Blood clots	☐ Palpitations	☐ Arthritis
☐ Swollen, Sore Legs	☐ Pacemaker	☐ Weakness
☐ Bronchitis	☐ Chest Pain, Angina	☐ Walking Problems
☐ Emphysema	☐ Kidney Problems	☐ Blackouts
☐ Phlegm	☐ Hepatitis, Liver Problem	☐ Stroke, Dizziness
☐ Pneumonia, Lung Problem	☐ Bruise or Bleed Easily	☐ Blindness/Deafness
☐ Asthma, Wheezing	☐ Anemia	☐ Epilepsy
☐ Shortness of Breath	☐ Sickle Cell Anemia	☐ Meningitis/Polio
☐ Heart Condition	☐ Thyroid Disease	☐ Headaches
☐ High Blood Pressure	☐ Diabetes	☐ Glaucoma
☐ Low Blood Pressure	☐ Cortisone Treatment	☐ Nervous Disorder
☐ Heart Attack	☐ Prednisone Treatment	☐ Any Other Problem
☐ Rheumatic Fever	☐ Persistent Indigestion	

Are there any other questions you wish to ask? ☐ YES ☐ NO

Do you have any major fears regarding your surgery or anesthesia? ☐ YES ☐ NO

I have read and understood the above questionnaire and certify that the answers given by me (or a representative for me) are correct to the best of my knowledge.

SIGNED:_____

FIG. 5-1 History form used at the ambulatory facility at Mt. Sinai Medical Center.

anesthesiologist is no longer "the one who is going to put me to sleep." He or she is a physician who takes a history, does a physical examination, orders and interprets laboratory studies, and explains to the patient what he or she is likely to experience. Patients begin to think of the anesthesiologist as a "real doctor."

During this preanesthetic visit, the patient may also be given a tour of the facility by a member of the nursing staff. This allays some of the patient's anxiety, for much of the unknown becomes visible. This tour may prompt questions from the patient that help the anesthesiologist put many fears to rest.[42,93] It should also help develop a rapport between anesthesiologist and patient. When the patient returns on the day of surgery, the people he or she encounters will already be familiar, as will the facility itself. Furthermore, if family or friends are allowed to accompany our patient into this area, we can expect less anxiety.

There are, of course, some facilities where the patients are seen just before surgery. Preoperative screening of these patients must be performed to avoid last-minute cancellations. In some institutions, a chart review including history and physical examination and laboratory reports is done 24 to 48 hours before scheduled surgery. The surgeon is contacted if any results are abnormal, and there is time to identify and possibly to correct problems. Inclusion of a health questionnaire completed by the patient can be of great value for those "forgotten" medical problems. Preoperative teaching is done partially in advance with the aid of brochures and completed by the anesthesiologist on the day of surgery. Alternatively, some anesthesiologists call their patients 2 days before the procedure, ask all of the preanesthesia questions, and discuss issues thoroughly over the telephone. They meet their patients in the waiting or holding area and answer any last-minute questions. Anesthesiologists using a same-day system feel that safety is maintained while their patients are spared the inconvenience and time away from work for an extra trip to the surgery center. If patients are not seen, tested, or called prior to the day of surgery by the ambulatory anesthesia staff, be prepared for some unusual problems on the day of scheduled surgery.

Many patients presenting for surgery will be taking medications. With the exception of the monoamine oxidase inhibitors, patients should be allowed to continue their drugs until the operation. Nonessential medications may be omitted on the morning of surgery. Patients may be instructed to take other medications with a sip of water. At Mt. Sinai Medical Center, rather than allowing patients to take their drugs at home, they are instructed to bring these medications to the surgery center. In this way, the nursing staff can supervise the administration of these drugs with minimal water intake.

Last-minute cancellations should be avoided. They cause inconvenience for the patient, surgeon, anesthesiologist, and the facility as a whole. Late cancellations are most commonly due to newly discovered abnormal physical or laboratory findings, consumption of food or fluid on the morning of surgery, or the patient's failure to arrange for a responsible escort home. Again, the preoperative interview and evaluation by a consultant anesthesiologist can identify problems in advance, determine their cause, and, after discussion with the surgeon, initiate treatment. The problem may be corrected in time for scheduled surgery. If this is not possible, a less-upsetting, earlier cancellation can permit time for correction of the problem and rescheduling at a later date. Although every effort should be made to avoid last-minute cancellations, in no way should the standard of anesthetic care be lowered for an elective ambulatory surgery procedure.

Within the framework of these issues, one can readily see how the anesthesiologist, through the preoperative evaluation, has been placed at the center of the patient's care. The anesthesiologist is the one who has evaluated the patient, ordered the tests, and uncovered any problems. It is this specialist who must then notify the surgeon and request appropriate consultations. Even if the patient is processed smoothly and no problems are found, he or she will see the anesthesiologist when admitted to the holding unit on the day of surgery, and it is the anesthesiologist who will be seeing the patient in the postanesthesia care unit and eventually determining discharge. Patients will have no doubt as to the anesthesiologist's role in their care, for he or she has been highly visible.

Premedication

Since the goal of the ambulatory surgery facility is to discharge patients promptly and awake,[116] there are many who believe that premedicant drugs should not be given. Not all patients are nervous. Egbert et al[42] found that 35% of patients without verbal or medicinal premedication did not feel nervous before their operation. If premedication is desired, the preanesthesia visit may do more to allay anxiety than any drugs that may be given to achieve this goal. In Egbert's study, of those patients who received an informative preoperative visit without additional drug, 65% were calm. Providing the patient with a pleasant waiting area equipped with magazines and television and permitting continued support from an accompanying friend or relative until the time of surgery helps the nonmedicated patient remain calm.[152,153] The routine use of little or no premedicant is advisable.[34,49]

Others believe the patients' time in the holding unit can be made more pleasant with the use of premedicant drugs.[21,145] These drugs also have some effects that may provide a smoother anesthetic and postanesthetic course (e.g., an antiemetic effect). In a study involving more than 1500 cases, Meridy showed that the use of premedicants other than long-acting narcotics did not prolong recovery (Table 5-1).[166] Narcotic premedication can cause nausea and vomiting, side-effects that can delay the patient's discharge following anesthesia.[122] Premedicant drugs may be used if needed by the patient and if drug and dosage are chosen carefully.

With these considerations in mind, we discuss a number of commonly used premedicant drugs in this chapter. They are classified as anticholinergic drugs, antacids and cimetidine, narcotics, barbiturates, and nonbarbiturate sedatives.[130]

ANTICHOLINERGIC DRUGS

Anticholinergic drugs are so named because they compete with acetylcholine at various effector organ sites. Two alkaloids, nicotine and muscarine, characteristically produce certain distinct cholinergic effects, suggesting that acetylcholine activates two types of receptors. Generally speaking, nicotinic receptors are found in autonomic ganglia, the neuromuscular junction, and the spinal cord (Table 5-2).[95] In the usual premedicant doses, anticholinergics block only the

□ **Table 5-1. Relationship Between Premedication Received by 1553 Patients and Recovery Time**

Type	No. of Patients	Recovery Time* (min)
No premedication	1015	179 ± 113
Diazepam	98	168 ± 104
Pentobarbital	25	231 ± 88
Narcotics (meperidine and morphine)	388	208 ± 101†
Hydroxyzine	92	192 ± 120

*Values are means ± SD.
†Differs significantly from patients not receiving any premedication (p < 0.001)
(Meridy HW: Criteria for selection of ambulatory surgical patients and guidelines for anesthetic management: A retrospective study of 1,553 cases. Anesth Analg 61:921, 1982)

muscarinic receptors, in the exocrine glands and the eye. With increasing dosage other muscarinic receptors are also inhibited.

When very irritant anesthetics were in vogue (e.g., diethyl ether), it was customary to treat patients with anticholinergics to minimize the secretions evoked by these anesthetic agents. Secretions can accumulate near the glottis and provoke coughing or even laryngospasm. However, the newer anesthetic agents are considerably less irritating. Furthermore, drying of mucous membranes by anticholinergics is believed to contribute to postoperative sore throat and complaints of dry mouth.[21] The lung's cleaning mechanisms may be inhibited as tracheobronchial secretions decrease and thicken, and mucociliary flow is slowed. The use of atropine premedication has also been shown to augment the tachycardia and increase the frequency of cardiac arrhythmias seen during endotracheal intubation.[54] Anticholinergics are probably not indicated for routine premedication of the ambulatory patient. Anticholinergics may, of course, be administered as indicated to control secretions from oronasal airway insertion during light anesthesia or to inhibit further secretions if a difficult intubation develops.

□ **Table 5-2. Sites of Muscarinic and Nicotinic Receptors**

Receptors	Activation
MUSCARINIC	
Exocrine glands (salivary, bronchial, sweat)	Secretion
Eye (sphincter pupillae, ciliary muscle)	Miosis, accommodation
Heart	Bradycardia, delayed A-V conduction
Smooth muscle (urinary, intestinal, respiratory)	Spasm
Central nervous system	Stimulation or inhibition
NICOTINIC	
Autonomic ganglia	Stimulation (followed by inhibition if
Neuromuscular junction	dose is large)
Spinal cord	

Some anesthesiologists administer glycopyrrolate, a quaternary ammonium compound, to provide prolonged antisecretory effect with less tachycardia and central nervous system excitement. Glycopyrrolate may also be used to decrease the volume and acidity of gastric juices.[6,128,160] Despite these potential advantages, the more prolonged and intense drying effect limits its use for short procedures.[159,160]

ANTACIDS AND CIMETIDINE

Glycopyrrolate and other anticholinergics do not adequately protect against acid aspiration.[142] In fact, they may predispose to regurgitation by decreasing lower esophageal sphincter tone.[28] Ong has demonstrated that ambulatory surgery patients may be at greater risk of aspiration than inpatients because they come to surgery with larger volumes of acidic gastric contents.[111] In another series, 60% of ambulatory anesthesia patients had gastric volumes $\geq$ 25 ml and pH $\leq$ 2.5.[99] This has prompted anesthesiologists to consider administering antacids to their patients.

Antacid therapy is directed toward increasing the pH of gastric juice. This practice has its origins in Mendelson's work, which showed that the damage to the lungs secondary to aspiration is much more severe if the pH of the aspirate is less than 2.5.[105] However, many of the antacids available are suspensions of particulate material, which has itself been shown to cause significant problems if aspirated.[91] Consequently, soluble antacids such as sodium citrate are now preferred. Antacids do reduce gastric acidity, but do not decrease the volume of the gastric contents.

Cimetidine is an H_2-receptor histamine antagonist, which may be used to decrease the risk of aspiration in ambulatory surgery patients.[82,98,141] Manchikanti and Roush studied the effects of glycopyrrolate and cimetidine on gastric volume and pH.[100] Cimetidine, 300 mg, was given orally 1 to 4 hours prior to anesthesia induction. Gastric pH was greater than 2.5 in 84% of cimetidine-treated patients, and gastric volume was less than 20 ml in 88% of patients. In contrast, the authors could not demonstrate such a decrease in gastric volume and acidity with glycopyrrolate alone and found no added protective effect of glycopyrrolate when given with cimetidine. Consequently, they recommend the addition of 300 mg of cimetidine to the preanesthetic preparation of ambulatory surgery patients. Despite convincing evidence that cimetidine increases gastric fluid pH, there are no data that demonstrate that pulmonary damage will be absent if gastric contents are inhaled by patients pretreated with cimetidine,[141] or that the use of cimetidine reduces anesthetic mortality from aspiration.[99]

Metoclopramide is a gastroprokinetic drug that has no effect on gastric acidity but increases lower esophageal sphincter tone and facilitates gastric emptying. Although it has been used to prevent emesis, Cohen did not find any significant antiemetic effect when given to ambulatory surgery patients.[24a] In one study comparing the effects on gastric fluid volume and pH in ambulatory surgery patients who received cimetidine (300 mg), metoclopramide (10 mg) or a combination of both, there were no obvious advantages with either of the metoclopramide groups over cimetidine alone.[99] However, Rao et al[119a], when studying the effects of cimetidine and metoclopramide in 80 female patients undergoing ambulatory surgery laparoscopy, found that those that received the combination of a 300-mg cimetidine tablet and a 10-mg metoclopramide tablet taken with 20 ml of water 2 hours preinduction had both a significantly lower gastric volume and a significantly higher pH than cimetidine alone, metoclopramide alone, or the control group.

At The Methodist Medical Center of Illinois, inhalation agents were administered to over 25,000 ambulatory surgery patients during a 7-year period. Postanesthesia aspiration was suspected in four patients, all of whom were admitted. Three patients remained clinically and radiologically asymptomatic during hospitalization and were discharged the next morning. A confirmed diagnosis of aspiration pneumonitis was made in a 69-year-old woman (see Case Report 19 in Chapter 8).

Until we have conclusive data that all patients should receive preanesthetic antacids or cimetidine, individual ambulatory surgery centers should make their own determinations based on past experience, the standards of care provided for their inpatients, and cost effectiveness.

NARCOTICS

The primary indication for narcotics is the relief of pain. A short-acting narcotic such as fentanyl may, therefore, be used to premedicate a patient who is scheduled for regional anesthesia. The analgesic effect of a narcotic makes the performance of the block more pleasant for such a patient. If a nitrous oxide, narcotic anesthetic is to be given, a narcotic premedicant may be given to begin the narcotic component of the anesthetic. Overall anesthetic requirement may be decreased. The use of narcotics for premedication, however, is associated with the potential for significant side-effects[64] including respiratory depression, rigidity, nausea, and postural hypotension. Effects and side-effects of narcotics are discussed in detail below, along with the use of these agents for maintenance of general anesthesia.

The use of fentanyl alone for intravenous premedication has been evaluated by Conner and colleagues.[25] After receiving 100 μg 1 hour before operation, patients reported a small decrease in anxiety and an increase in sedation. Subjective assessment of the effect of fentanyl as pleasant, however, was only 54% at 4 minutes after injection; at 24 hours, only 40% of patients reported the premedication as good to excellent. Fentanyl alone is not an effective sedative. Reasons for low patient acceptance included the short duration of drug effect. If fentanyl is to be used as a component of premedication, it should be given closer to the time of operation, within 15 to 30 minutes. Long-acting narcotics such as meperidine and morphine are not indicated for the premedication of ambulatory anesthesia patients.[106]

BARBITURATES

The so-called short-acting barbiturates such as pentobarbital and secobarbital are used widely as premedicants for inpatients. They have a good hypnotic effect and lack many side-effects such as nausea and vomiting. However, for outpatient anesthesia, the long duration of action of these drugs with their slow elimination from the body makes them poor choices as premedicants. Postanesthetic incoordination and sleepiness may persist. The ultra-short-acting barbiturates such as thiopental and methohexital may be used for the induction of anesthesia. These drugs are discussed below.

NONBARBITURATE SEDATIVES

Nonbarbiturate sedatives and tranquilizers include the phenothiazines, benzodiazepines, butyrophenones, and antihistamines. Some of these drugs have become quite popular in recent years. Table 5-3 summarizes the effects of these drugs.

PHENOTHIAZINES
The phenothiazines (e.g., prochlorperazine) are potent antiemetic drugs. This effect is secondary to inhibition of the chemoreceptor trigger zone, as well as to their anticholinergic activity, which inhibits labyrinthine impulses. However, phenothiazines tend to cause hypotension. This is due to central depression of vasomotor reflexes, peripheral adrenergic blockade, and direct vasodilation. The phenothiazines can also produce troublesome extrapyramidal effects and have been known to cause cholestatic jaundice. Duration of action is long. Because of these side-effects, phenothiazines have found little use in ambulatory anesthesia.

BENZODIAZEPINES
Benzodiazepines allay anxiety by depression of the limbic system and amygdalae, where fear, anxiety, and aggression are generated; there is little effect on the cerebral cortex. They therefore relieve anxiety and apprehension, with little soporific effect if given orally. The most commonly used drug in this class is diazepam. Peak drug levels after oral administration of 5 mg or 10 mg diazepam occurred at 60 to 90 minutes, with drowsiness persisting up to 120 minutes.[3,70] Larger doses (20 mg) resulted in more rapid peaking of drug levels and clinical effects at 30 to 60 minutes, and prolonged residual drowsiness, up to 240 minutes. Oral absorption of diazepam is slowed by the concurrent parenteral administration of atropine or narcotics and is more rapid when given with metoclopramide or oral aluminum hydroxide antacid.

Intramuscular administration of diazepam resulted in less predictable absorption and lower drug levels,[36,70] probably related to the insolubility of diazepam in water and to the lack of a true intramuscular injection. Injections into the buttock are not only painful, but they also produced the lowest drug levels.

When injected intravenously, diazepam can cause depression of the

☐ Table 5-3. Nonbarbiturate Sedatives

Indications	Effects	Contraindications

Tranquilize with little sleepiness
May reduce amount of anesthesia
  needed; potentiate narcotics
Anticonvulsant (benzodiazepines)
Amnesia (benzodiazepines)
Antiemetic (droperidol)
	Extrapyramidal signs; vasodilation;
	  antisialogic and antihistaminic;
	  long duration
		Hypovolemia

respiratory and cardiovascular systems. Although these effects are not marked, they can add to the depressant effect of other drugs such as narcotics. The recommended dose of intravenous diazepam for ambulatory surgery patients is 0.05 to 0.15 mg/kg. The intravenous administration of 10 mg diazepam to volunteers resulted in ataxia and a positive Romberg sign (8% of patients) and dizziness (16%) persisting after 60 minutes.[3] Measured by the Trieger dot test, acute recovery following intravenous diazepam, 12.5 mg to 30 mg, appeared essentially complete 90 minutes after administration (Fig. 5-2).[37] It must be remembered, though, that patients vary in their clinical response to the drug. Diazepam should be administered in small increments, particularly to the geriatric patient.

The redistribution half-life of diazepam is relatively short, about 2.5 hours. However, a recurrence of drowsiness and increase in plasma concentration occurs at 6 to 8 hours, probably owing to enterohepatic recirculation. Serum concentration has been shown to increase further when fatty solid foods were consumed 3 hours after diazepam administration.[88] This may also be related to enteric recirculation. Food at 7 hours had a similar but lesser effect, but water ingestion had none. Fatty food intake should be limited in the 7 hours after diazepam administration to avoid resedation, particularly at higher drug doses.

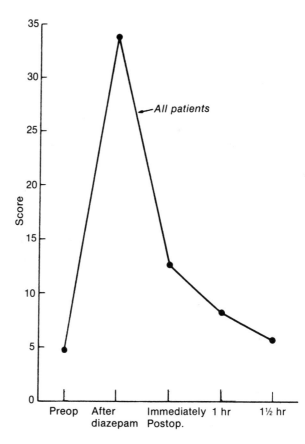

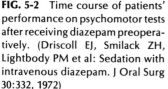

FIG. 5-2 Time course of patients' performance on psychomotor tests after receiving diazepam preoperatively. (Driscoll EJ, Smilack ZH, Lightbody PM et al: Sedation with intravenous diazepam. J Oral Surg 30:332, 1972)

The elimination half-life of diazepam is 1.5 days after primarily hepatic metabolism. Twenty-five percent of patients who received diazepam, 10 mg, intravenously felt tired for 24 hours.[3] Diazepam metabolites, notably desmethyl-diazepam, are also pharmacologically active. Plasma levels of desmethyldiazepam have been shown to rise steadily over the 48 hours after intravenous diazepam administration. The total effect of diazepam should not be considered short, and patients should be cautioned that they may feel tired for a day or more after diazepam administration.

Because diazepam is insoluble in water, it is formulated in organic solvents including propylene glycol and ethyl alcohol. Three days after 0.3 mg/kg diazepam was injected intravenously into the dorsum of the hand, all of the eight patients developed phlebitis.[57] When 5 mg diazepam was injected into the larger cephalic vein at the wrist, the incidence of sequelae at 3 days was smaller: tenderness was 19% and thrombophlebitis 17% in 47 patients.[107] One month after the injection, pain or tenderness was reported by 15.6%. In another study, the incidence of venous sequelae after diazepam increased with time: 23% after 2 to 3 days and 39% after 7 to 10 days.[67] Diazepam is available in an oil emulsion in Europe, as Diazemuls (Kabi-Vitrum, Sweden). This preparation has a lower reported incidence of pain, 1%, and thrombophlebitis, 4%.[131] After 2 weeks, the incidence of thrombophlebitis was 6%.[79] This formulation, although equally effective, is more expensive.

In the unpremedicated ambulatory surgery patient, the incidence of recall under general anesthesia has been reported to be as high as 9%.[145] Epstein[48] has stated that when diazepam, 0.15 mg/kg (up to a total dose of 5 mg), is given intravenously 2 to 3 minutes prior to anesthesia induction, the incidence of awareness experienced with a balanced anesthetic technique for laparoscopy is significantly reduced. Without diazepam, 4.9% of patients had recall for conversation, 2.1% for extubation, and 0.7% for pain.

Other benzodiazepines have been tried as oral premedications. Temazepam is rapidly absorbed and eliminated, with peak plasma levels at 20 to 40 minutes and an elimination half-life of approximately 10 hours.[9] Use of temazepam, 20 mg, 1 hour before surgery resulted in satisfactory sedation and anxiolysis in ambulatory patients.[64] Recovery was more rapid than that found after diazepam, 10 mg.[22] Oral lorazepam is an effective sedative and amnesic.[89] A 2-mg dose generated lack of recall in 30% of patients, and 4 mg caused amnesia in 70%. The delay to onset was only slightly longer than diazepam, but duration of amnesia was significantly longer, more than 240 minutes. Because of the drug's prolonged sedative and amnesic effect, the use of lorazepam by any route to premedicate ambulatory anesthesia patients is not recommended. Fluni-trazepam provides satisfactory sedation, but the duration of action is also too long for use in ambulatory anesthesia.[87]

Midazolam is a water-soluble benzodiazepine used as both a premedicant and an induction agent.[12,41] The latter effect is discussed later in this chapter under General Anesthesia. Midazolam is twice as potent as diazepam for premedication.[40] After the intravenous administration of 5 mg midazolam, sedation and anxiolysis began within 1 to 2 minutes.[41] Drug effect was reported as pleasant by 92% of patients and was acceptable to all. Marked sedation persisted for the half-hour of observation. Anterograde amnesia was present in 96% of patients at 2 minutes postinjection and declined over the ensuing 20 to 40 minutes.[26] Retrograde amnesia was not demonstrated. Recovery times were recorded after a large premedication dose of 5 mg midazolam. Motor performance recovered in 34 minutes, and subjects were fully awake, walking unaided, at 73 minutes. There was considerable variation in individual response.

Midazolam plasma levels demonstrate a half-life of 60 to 90 minutes, without evidence of enterohepatic recirculation and recurrence of drowsiness. Venous irritation is minimal with midazolam. Dundee et al reported no pain on injection and no thrombophlebitis by 2 weeks after 5 mg or 10 mg midazolam.[40]

BUTYROPHENONES

Droperidol is the most commonly used butyrophenone. Patients given this agent exhibit marked tranquilization with easy arousability. Early droperidol pharmacokinetics are acceptably rapid. After intravenous administration of 5 mg droperidol, the distribution half-life was 10 minutes,[30] and the elimination half-life was 134 minutes. Absorption after intramuscular administration was excellent. However, approximately 86% of the dose was converted to a droperidol metabolite; significant levels of the metabolite were present in plasma for 8 to 12 hours after drug administration. This correlates with the observed duration of clinical effect. Korttila and Linnoila evaluated recovery and driving-related skills after intravenous injection of 5 mg droperidol.[87] Clinical recovery as determined by a negative Romberg sign was present after 25 minutes, but tiredness or drowsiness was still reported at 10 hours by 50% of the volunteers. Tests of coordination and attention remained significantly abnormal at the final 10-hour testing. The concurrent administration of fentanyl, 0.2 mg, did not affect the results of objective tests.

A fixed-ratio combination of fentanyl, 0.05 mg/ml, and a large dose (2.5 mg/ml) of droperidol is sold as Innovar (Janssen Pharmaceutica, New Brunswick, New Jersey). The use of this product is not recommended for ambulatory premedication, since sedation may be prolonged.

Despite its long duration of action, droperidol is used in ambulatory anesthesia in small doses. Droperidol is an excellent antiemetic. This effect can be obtained with as little as 0.1 ml to 0.5 ml (2.5 mg/ml) given intravenously.[133,155] The drug, however, may potentiate the sedative effects of narcotics.

Some patients who receive droperidol may experience restlessness, anxiety, and agitation, usually at dosages ≥2.5 mg. Patients with these symptoms frequently express a feeling of "impending doom." Because of this, many anesthesiologists are reluctant to administer droperidol alone as premedication. In the authors' experience, when low doses (≤ 1.25 mg) are given with fentanyl, these symptoms appear to be minimal. Extrapyramidal symptoms and hypotension have also been reported. Droperidol does not produce clinically important respiratory depression.

ANTIHISTAMINES

Antihistamines, such as diphenhydramine and hydroxyzine, are occasionally used for their sedative and ataractic properties. Of the commonly used antihistamines, hydroxyzine seems to have the fewest troublesome side-effects. It causes little circulatory and respiratory depression and does not prolong recovery from anesthesia. In addition, it has antiemetic, antisialogogic, and analgesic effects. McKenzie compared the antiemetic effectiveness of intramuscular hydroxyzine (100 mg) with intramuscular droperidol (2.5 mg) when given immediately after induction for ambulatory surgery patients undergoing first-trimester termination of pregnancy.[102] The incidence of nausea and vomiting was significantly less in the hydroxyzine patients. All patients equaled their preoperative hand-eye coordination testings at 3 hours and were discharged at 4 hours postsurgery.

Unfortunately, antihistamines produce excessive drying of the respiratory tract; this may result in more viscous secretions that can be difficult to expectorate. Hence, their use in patients with chronic bronchitis or asthma is of questionable value. Also, hydroxyzine irritates venous endothelium and should not be given intravenously.

Anesthesia

Local, regional, and general anesthesia may be used for ambulatory surgery patients. The choice of anesthetic technique will be determined by surgical requirements, anesthetic considerations, and the patient's physical status and preferences. For example, a healthy young woman who presents for excisional biopsy of a breast mass might well be managed with general anesthesia. If the same patient were to present for arthroscopy of her knee, regional anesthesia could be an excellent choice.[125] Moreover, the octogenarian who requires eye surgery may do quite well under local block anesthesia with supplemental sedation. Whichever technique is used, the anesthesiologist's approach to the patient is most important. Conversation should be reassuring and upbeat as preparation is made to induce anesthesia. Local and regional anesthesia is discussed in Chapter 6.

Preparation also includes adequate equipment. The ambulatory surgery center must have the same type and quality of equipment that is in common use in the hospital inpatient operating suite. Each operating room must have an electrocardiograph (ECG) monitor and means for measuring blood pressure, temperature, and oxygen concentration. A defibrillator and an emergency cart must be immediately available. Furthermore, all ambulatory surgery personnel must be trained in cardiopulmonary resuscitation and be able to operate the defibrillator.

GENERAL ANESTHESIA

General anesthesia for the ambulatory patient presents special challenges. Induction must be especially rapid. Depth of anesthesia must be adequate to provide amnesia and absence of physiologic upset. However, the level of general anesthetic permissible for the inpatient is often inappropriately deep for the ambulatory surgery patient. Awakening from ambulatory general anesthesia must be carefully timed to match the end of surgery, and recovery must not be prolonged. Also, the minor morbidities of general anesthesia are more bothersome to the ambulatory patient and must be minimized. These postanesthetic sequelae can include dizziness, nausea, headache, sore throat, and muscle pains.[148] The choice of both appropriate anesthetic agents and appropriate techniques to administer these agents are critical to success.

In the evaluation of anesthetic agents and adjuvants, certain criteria should be met before any agent or drug can be considered acceptable for use in ambulatory surgery. In addition to being nonflammable, anesthetic agents must be capable of providing

Rapid, smooth, pleasant induction
Minimal or no excitement period
Readily controllable depth
No increase in secretions
Rapid, smooth, pleasant emergence
Minimal nausea/vomiting
Rapid return to rational behavior
Early return to appropriate status of ambulation

The common practice of intravenous induction followed by an inhalational or nitrous oxide, narcotic technique is well suited to the practice of outpatient anesthesia. Many rapidly acting intravenous agents that have a short duration of action may be used. These induction agents include the ultra-short-acting barbiturates and nonbarbiturate intravenous agents.

INDUCTION OF ANESTHESIA

ULTRA-SHORT-ACTING BARBITURATES

Sodium thiopental, a sulphurated barbiturate, is a yellow powder made up to a 2.5% solution in water. The solution is highly alkaline (pH 10.6). Its clinical characteristics match the list of desired characteristics well. In fact, thiopental induction reduces the incidence of nausea associated with halothane or nitrous oxide inhalation.[63]

Thiopental is discussed below as a representative intravenous anesthetic agent. Following intravenous injection, this drug is distributed to the various tissue compartments. Factors influencing the transfer of molecules across membranes and into compartments include molecular weight, fat solubility, and the degree of ionization. Anesthetic molecules are of relatively low molecular weight. The pK of a drug is the pH at which 50% of the drug is ionized and 50% is un-ionized; the pK of thiopental is 7.4. Therefore, at body pH, half of the thiopental administered is in the un-ionized form, which crosses membranes more rapidly.

When the thiopental is administered, the tissues with a high blood flow per unit volume (the vessel-rich group—heart, brain, viscera, etc.) initially take up most of the blood-borne drug. Thiopental is also very lipid soluble and readily crosses the blood-brain barrier. The drug's lipid solubility, pK, and molecular weight, when combined with high blood flow to the brain, produce a rapid induction of anesthesia.

As blood concentration of the drug falls below that of the vessel-rich group, redistribution of the drug occurs—initially to muscle and later to fat (Fig. 5-3).[117] The patient recovers consciousness from thiopental anesthesia during the initial redistribution to the muscles. Fat tissue continues to absorb thiopental for hours, but those depots play little or no part in the initial recovery of consciousness.

The extent of thiopental's dissociation depends upon the pH of the blood and tissues. If the pH increases (alkalosis) there is a greater amount of the ionized form of the drug, whereas a low pH (acidosis) causes less ionization. The un-ionized form crosses membranes more rapidly and is the active form.

% of dose

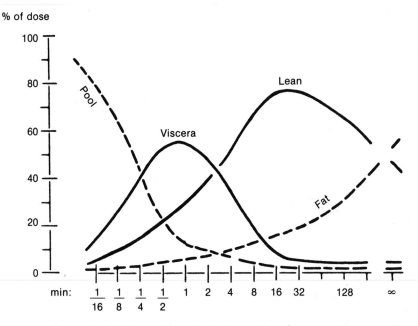

FIG. 5-3 The uptake of thiopental from body tissues. Note the geometric progression of the time scale. (Price HL, Kovnat BS, Safer JN et al: The uptake of thiopental by body tissues and its relation to the duration of narcosis. Clin Pharmacol Ther 1:16, 1960)

Thiopental is also bound to plasma proteins in an inactive form. About 70% of the drug exists in the bound form, the amount varying inversely with the plasma concentration of the drug. Thiopental is metabolized in the liver at the rate of about 10% of the amount of the drug in the body per hour.

Thiopental has a depressant effect on the heart that is dose dependent. While cardiac output decreases, systemic vascular resistance increases. Consequently, arterial blood pressure is well maintained. Barbiturates do not sensitize the myocardium to the effect of catecholamines. The ultra-short-acting barbiturates do cause respiratory depression. The sensitivity of the respiratory center to carbon dioxide is depressed at all levels of anesthesia. Responsiveness of the peripheral chemoreceptors is better maintained; however, this is also obliterated at profound depths of anesthesia. In the usual induction dose (3–4 mg/kg), tidal volume decreases while the respiratory rate increases.

Extravenous injection of thiopental may cause tissue necrosis because of the solution's alkalinity. The injection of thiopental into an artery can cause serious complications. Following intra-arterial injection, small crystals of thiopental form and cause capillary obstruction. There is a local release of norepinephrine, causing transient arteriolar spasm. Thrombosis and ischemia may occur, depending on the concentration and volume of the solution injected. Therapy is aimed at dilution of the injected drug, relief of the arterial spasm, and prevention of thrombosis. The needle or cannula should be left in the artery and 15 ml 0.5% procaine and 15 ml saline containing 50 mg papaverine should be injected. Further infiltration of local anesthetic drug around the artery may relieve pain and promote further vasodilation. Prevention of thrombosis is achieved by the administration of intravenous heparin. Oral anticoagulant therapy may be continued up to 2 weeks following the injection. A stellate ganglion block or a brachial plexus block may be performed to remove sympathetic vasoconstrictor tone. However, these blocks should not be performed in a heparinized patient. The incidence of complications secondary to intra-arterial injections has been substantially reduced with the general use of a 2.5% solution rather than a 5% or 10% solution.

Methohexital is an oxybarbiturate used clinically as a 1% solution (pH 10.6). Methohexital is 2.5 times as potent as thiopental and is less lipid soluble. Elliott et al[46] used a driving simulator to assess recovery of patients following intravenous methohexital or thiopental. At 35 minutes after injection, 78% of the methohexital (0.88 mg/kg) subjects had recovered completely, compared to only 34% of the thiopental (2.5 mg/kg) patients. Coordination tests as measured by Vickers[150] required 30 to 60 minutes to recover after methohexital 1 mg/kg and 45 to 90 minutes after 2 mg/kg. This compared to 30 to 75 minutes after 2.5 mg/kg of thiopental and 105 to 210 minutes after 5 mg/kg. Subjects reported being less sedated and mentally more clear after methohexital.

Hudson and Stanski[73] studied the pharmacokinetics of methohexital and thiopental in patients undergoing minor surgery. The study had three major objectives: (1) the disposition of a single intravenous bolus of methohexital followed by maintenance of anesthesia with other agents; (2) comparison of pharmacokinetics of methohexital and thiopental in surgical patients; and (3) determination of the relative importance of metabolism versus redistribution in the termination of anesthesia following both intravenous induction agents.

Following a single intravenous bolus induction of methohexital (m = 2.4 ±0.4 mg/kg) and thiopental (t = 6.7 ±0.7 mg/kg), similarities were found in both the rapid (m = 5.6 ±2.7 min; t = 8.5 ±6.1 min) and slow (m = 58.3 ±24.6 min; t = 62.7 ±30.4 min) distribution half-lives. Additional similarities were found in the volume of the central compartment and the volumes of distribution at steady state. The two drugs differed markedly in their clearance (m = 10.9 ±3.0 ml/kg/min; t = 3.4 ±0.5 ml/kg/min) and elimination half-life (m = 3.9 ±2.1 hr; t = 11.6 ±6 hr). Methohexital's shorter elimination half-life results solely from its greater hepatic clearance.

Although the distribution phase kinetics of the two drugs are similar, redistribution is a major factor determining the duration of sedation after a single dose of either drug. A more rapid recovery of complete psychomotor function often seen following methohexital when compared to thiopental is probably due to the more rapid metabolism of methohexital. Hudson and Stanski conclude that, based on its pharmacologic properties, methohexital would be preferable to thiopental whenever more rapid recovery from anesthesia is desired, particularly after large or repeated doses.

Significant side-effects do occur with methohexital. Respiratory upset including cough and hiccough have been reported in 26% of patients.[38] Tremors and involuntary muscle movements have been reported in 38% of patients. These muscle twitches are not associated with electroencephalographic (EEG) abnormalities in normal patients. The incidence of movement after methohexital can be reduced to 7%, the same as after thiopental, by using narcotic premedication. Judicious narcotic premedication, such as 1 μg/kg fentanyl, does not prolong recovery from methohexital. Minimizing the dose of methohexital given and injecting the drug slowly also decrease the incidence of unwanted side-effects.

Use of the ultra-short-acting barbiturates is absolutely contraindicated when equipment for ventilation and resuscitation is unavailable. They should not be used when difficulties with ventilation are likely to follow loss of consciousness. They are also contraindicated in patients with porphyria, since exacerbations of abdominal pain and paralysis may occur.

ALPHATHESIN, PROPANIDID, DIPRIVAN

Three short-acting intravenous induction agents have been used extensively in the United Kingdom for ambulatory surgery procedures. These drugs are not acceptable for clinical use in the United States because anaphylactoid reactions manifested by bronchospasm and circulatory collapse have been associated with all three agents. The reactions are due to the solvent Cremophor EL. Newer solvents are being investigated.

ALPHATHESIN

Alphathesin is a mixture of two steroids—alphaxalone and alphadolone; each milliliter contains 9 mg of the former and 3 mg of the latter. Alphaxalone has poor aqueous solubility and is dissolved in an oil base. Alphadolone increases solubility, making intravenous administration possible. Alphathesin is a rapidly acting drug of short duration.[35,109,131] It causes a drop in blood pressure, venous pressure, and stroke volume. Cardiac output remains unchanged because of a compensatory tachycardia. Tidal volume may decrease, but respiratory rate increases. Muscle tremors are occasionally seen with alphathesin. The drug does not cause ischemic sequelae if injected intra-arterially. Although recovery is more prolonged than after methohexital,[65] it is sufficiently rapid for use in ambulatory surgery patients. Dechene feels it is not a substitute for presently available intravenous anesthetics.[35]

PROPANIDID

Propanidid is a poorly soluble intravenous agent supplied as a 5% solution with Cremophor EL. When given in the usual dose (5–10 mg/kg), loss of consciousness is achieved in one circulation time.

Following injection, there is a transient fall in blood pressure and an increase in the heart rate. Respiration is increased. However, the hyperventilation is often followed by a period of hypoventilation or apnea. Recovery is quite rapid. Although initial recovery following methohexital or propanidid takes about the same time, alertness and full recovery of mental faculties occur much sooner after propanidid, allowing patients to leave the facility sooner. The rapid emergence is related to the cleavage of the ester bond by both hepatic and serum cholinesterase. Propanidid is almost completely metabolized in 20 to 30 minutes.[39] If succinylcholine is injected after propanidid, the duration of succinylcholine apnea is increased. This is probably due to competition for the same metabolic enzyme.

DIPRIVAN

Diprivan (2,6 di-isopropylphenol) is an intravenous anesthetic that, when given in a recommended dose of 2 mg/kg, causes unconsciousness in one arm-brain circulation time.[80,118] Recovery from this dose occurs in about 5 minutes. Its distribution half-life is 2.2 minutes and elimination half-life is 70 minutes; it is 96% protein bound. The rapid termination of action is due to redistribution and hepatic metabolism; no active metabolites are known.

Diprivan allows more rapid and complete recovery with fewer side-effects than does halothane anesthesia. In fact, most patients receiving this drug remarked on their alertness following anesthesia. There was also very little nausea and vomiting associated with its use. The most common side-effect of diprivan was pain on injection, which occurs in about 35% of patients. No damage to peripheral veins occurred, and most patients considered this only a minor inconvenience.

Like alphathesin and propanidid, diprivan is formulated in Cremophor EL, which is associated with hypersensitivity reactions. Another solvent, duck-egg lecithin, has been found and this new formulation of diprivan is undergoing clinical trials in the United Kingdom and the United States.[58]

ETOMIDATE

Etomidate is a short-acting intravenous anesthetic whose action is terminated by hydrolysis.[59,66,71,92,109] It is a pure hypnotic. When given in an induction dose of 0.2 to 0.4 mg/kg, it causes no significant cardiovascular effects, respiratory depression, or histamine release. Both induction time (1 min) and awakening time (4–10 min) are very rapid. There appear to be no differences in time or quality of recovery when etomidate or thiopental is used. Pain on injection (50%) and involuntary myoclonic movements (70%) occur frequently and are two of the major side-effects of this drug.[59] Myoclonic movements do not cause postoperative myalgia. Injection pain, on the other hand, has been severe enough for patients to refuse to be reanesthetized with etomidate.[92] Pain can be ameliorated by injecting into large veins and using a faster rate of injection. The incidence of pain on injection was significantly reduced from 37% to 10% by the addition of lidocaine 1% (diluted to 1 mg/ml);[17] however, a pediatric outpatient study demonstrated no reduction in pain.[84] A recent study by Giese has demonstrated that pretreatment with fentanyl, 100 μg, 3 minutes prior to induction reduced the incidence of these side-effects without compromising hemodynamic stability.[62] Fentanyl is therefore the recommended pretreatment. Another side-effect of etomidate is nausea or vomiting, which frequently occurs after emergence. Fragen compared etomidate with thiopental as induction agents and noted a 55% incidence of nausea or vomiting with etomidate and 15% with thiopental.[59] Similar results were noted when etomidate was compared to alphathesin[109] or propanidid inductions.[92] At the present time, the role of this drug for ambulatory surgery is uncertain.

MIDAZOLAM

For sleep induction, midazolam is $1\frac{1}{2}$ times as potent as diazepam[120] and 15 times as potent as thiopental.[121] However, midazolam provides a relatively slow onset of unconsciousness compared to thiopental.[10] This is typical of benzodiazepines. When volunteers were given an intravenous injection of 0.15 mg/kg midazolam, loss of lash reflex occurred at 164 seconds.[56] Giving the same dose to patients who had been premedicated with narcotic reduced induction time: loss of lash reflex occurred at 88.6 seconds. However, loss of lash reflex with midazolam did not consistently indicate loss of consciousness; some patients were still able to open their eyes on command. Both tests should be used to confirm loss of consciousness with this drug.

The injection of 0.20 to 0.25 mg/kg midazolam may be used to induce sleep. A wide variability in induction dose requirement has been noted. After 5 mg for premedication, the additional midazolam required to induce sleep was 5 mg to

2.5 mg.[26] Even this largest dose was unsuccessful in one patient. Dose requirement was not related to patients' weight, although larger doses were more often successful. Variability of response can be decreased by the preadministration of fentanyl, 1 μg/kg. Dose requirement and variability are not as great in elderly patients.

KETAMINE

Ketamine is a rapidly acting phencyclidine derivative that may be used for induction and maintenance of anesthesia. It is effective by the intravenous or intramuscular route. Ketamine produces a state of dissociative anesthesia, which is characterized by catalepsy, catatonia, amnesia, and analgesia. Adequate airway and respiration are usually maintained. Blood pressure rises transiently after intravenous administration, as does intracranial pressure. Consequently, ketamine should be used cautiously in patients who may be sensitive to these effects.

Since ketamine has a rapid onset, maintains an adequate blood pressure, and allows satisfactory ventilation, it would seem to be a good drug for ambulatory anesthesia.[78] However, this is not the case. Ketamine has been associated with postanesthetic confusion, disorientation, bad dreams, hallucinations and restlessness. Thompson compared thiopental and ketamine as induction agents for outpatient anesthesia.[145] The results of this comparison are summarized in Table 5-4. Two-thirds of the ketamine patients in this study reported that their unpleasant dreams were frightening. Although the incidence of these unpleasant dreams can be decreased with the administration of diazepam or droperidol, the addition of these drugs may further delay the patient's recovery. Patients who have received ketamine should be allowed to recover quietly; if they are disturbed frequently, there is a greater potential for excitement, restlessness, and hallucinations. This contraindicates the usual "stir up" regimen that most ambulatory surgery facilities use to promote early ambulation. Emergence from ketamine can be quite prolonged. Consequently, ketamine falls far short of the requirements of an ideal ambulatory anesthetic drug and has found little use in the management of adult patients in an ambulatory setting.[154]

☐ Table 5-4. Thiopental vs. Ketamine

	Thiopental (%)	Ketamine (%)
Alert on discharge	97	51
Dreams	6	50
Unpleasant dreams	0	50
Nausea	22	42
Vomiting	10	30
Headache	25	39
Dizziness	38	73
Recall	4	9

INHALATIONAL INDUCTION

Some anesthesiologists prefer inhalational induction, using inhalational agents alone or after only a minimal dose of intravenous agent (e.g., 50–100 mg thiopental). Induction can be quite rapid if high flows and concentrations of nitrous oxide and a potent inhalational agent are used. However, most patients have planned to go to sleep with intravenous induction; some patients may have unpleasant memories of the smell or struggle of an inhalational induction with "ether" as a child. If an inhalational induction is to be used, its characteristics should be discussed with the patient in advance.

There are techniques that can rapidly establish surgical depth of anesthesia with potent inhalational agents; these methods can also be used after an intravenous sleep induction. Appropriate techniques for ambulatory surgery patients will be discussed in association with the potent inhalational agents, in the next section.

MAINTENANCE OF ANESTHESIA

NITROUS OXIDE

Nitrous oxide is the mainstay of general anesthesia in the ambulatory setting. Its use decreases the requirement for the longer-acting agents, intravenous or inhalational, which are added to achieve surgical planes of anesthesia. A discussion of the uptake and distribution of nitrous oxide can serve as the prototype for all inhalational agents.

The blood/gas partition coefficient is a measure of the drug's relative solubility in these two phases. Agents with a low blood/gas partition coefficient, such as nitrous oxide (0.47), are relatively insoluble in blood, and induction is rapid. Emergence is similarly quick. The time needed to reach a given degree of brain saturation (anesthetic depth) with an inhaled agent depends on blood solubility as well as pulmonary ventilation, pulmonary blood flow, the distribution of arterial blood to the tissues, anesthetic solubility in different tissues, and the different tissue masses.

The uptake of nitrous oxide is further augmented by the concentration effect. Administration of high concentrations of an anesthetic agent, such as can be done with nitrous oxide, results in increased uptake of that agent by a concentrating action in the alveoli and augmentation of inspired volume. Nitrous oxide also increases the rate of uptake of other inhalational agents administered at the same time; this is the second gas effect. The use of multiples of MAC to speed induction—a technique known as overpressure—cannot be used with nitrous oxide because of its low potency. The rate of induction with nitrous oxide is limited by its lack of potency and the potential for hypoxia.

It should be remembered that the depth of anesthesia generated with a fixed percentage of nitrous oxide will decrease with increasing altitude.[76] This is directly related to the reduced partial pressure of nitrous oxide at a lower total atmospheric pressure.

NARCOTICS

Narcotics may be chosen to supplement nitrous oxide for ambulatory general anesthesia. Use of a nitrous oxide, narcotic technique may permit a lighter level of anesthetic maintenance and a more rapid emergence will result. Narcotics can also provide a smooth, pain-free awakening and recovery.[50] Hunt et al compared the use of fentanyl (approximately 1.7 μg/kg) with halothane (1%) as adjuvants to 60% nitrous oxide/oxygen anesthesia for ambulatory dilatation and curettage.[75] Patients who received fentanyl reported less abdominal pain both in hospital and after returning home. Interestingly, there was no increase in the frequency of nausea and vomiting in the fentanyl group. Other complications such as headache, dizziness, drowsiness, and muscle ache were also comparable.

Pollard[115a] compared the clinical differences between an intravenous technique employing fentanyl/droperidol and an inhalational technique employing isoflurane in ambulatory surgery patients undergoing procedures of 30 minutes or less estimated duration. The advantages of the fentanyl/droperidol group included more rapid onset of action, more rapid recovery to consciousness and orientation, and less need for postoperative analgesics.

For surgical procedures of short duration in ambulatory patients, the ideal narcotic adjuvant is one that has a rapid onset and short duration of action, potent analgesic affect, minimal effect on vital signs, and least post-anesthetic hangover. Fentanyl has proven to be an excellent narcotic for ambulatory surgery anesthesia. Onset of analgesia after intravenous administration is rapid, within 2 minutes, and duration of analgesia is equally short,[101] approximately 45 minutes. Doses of 1 to 2 μg/kg are recommended for the ambulatory patient.

The use of fentanyl is not without problems, however. Fentanyl causes respiratory depression. A dose of 1.3 μg/kg resulted in depression of CO_2 response slope comparable in magnitude and duration to that seen after 0.12 mg/kg morphine,[123] with both responses remaining below 80% of control at 4 hours. There is also evidence of a recurrence of respiratory depression, accompanied by decreases in PaO_2 and pH and increase in $PaCO_2$. Respiratory depression occurred first at 30 to 60 minutes and again thereafter, with wide individual variation. These delayed effects may be due to secretion of fentanyl into gastric juice and reabsorption from the small intestine, or to the return of unchanged active fentanyl from peripheral compartments such as muscle, when increased patient activity caused increased muscle blood flow. The clinician should be aware that somnolence, respiratory depression requiring ventilatory support, and respiratory arrest have occurred $\frac{1}{2}$ to 4 hours after apparent recovery from fentanyl administration.[1] The addition of droperidol (given as Innovar) did not alter the respiratory depression caused by fentanyl.[8]

Truncal and extremity rigidity may occur after fentanyl administration and may be of sufficient severity to interfere with ventilation by bag and mask. Glottic rigidity and partial to complete glottic closure have contributed to the inability to ventilate.[129] This problem has also been seen with morphine and meperidine. Rigidity after fentanyl may recur in the postoperative period, associated with the secondary increase in plasma fentanyl level. Rigidity is common with high-dose fentanyl inductions, but rare in ambulatory surgery patients given appropriately low drug doses. Moderate-dose fentanyl, 3.9 μg/kg, caused rigidity in 4% of patients undergoing minor gynecologic surgery.[157] For ambulatory surgery patients who will be intubated, increments of fentanyl may be given after the pretreatment dose of a nondepolarizing muscle relaxant (e.g., 3 mg d-tubocurarine), to minimize the possibility of rigidity. Rigidity may also be treated by small doses of a nondepolarizing muscle relaxant such as pancuronium, 0.5 mg to 1 mg, or by succinylcholine, 10 mg to 20 mg. Naloxone is also effective but is not recommended, since it can reverse analgesia as well.

Naloxone has been used to reverse other narcotic side effects, primarily respiratory depression. Naloxone, however, has sequelae of its own. Analgesia may be terminated. Hypertension, pulmonary edema, ventricular arrhythmias, and cardiac arrest in healthy patients have been reported after 0.1 mg to 0.4 mg naloxone.[144] The routine "prophylactic" use of naloxone after fentanyl administration cannot be recommended. Other nonspecific analeptics such as aminopyridine, almitrine, and doxapram have also been tried for reversal of fentanyl-induced respiratory depression, with some success but with side-effects of their own.

Other side-effects, such as bronchoconstriction and bradycardia, that have been reported with high-dose fentanyl are rarely seen in the ambulatory patient given 1 to 2 μg/kg. The narcotic should be administered by slow intravenous injection in small, 25-μg to 50-μg increments.

The limitations and side-effects of traditional opioid and synthetic narcotics have stimulated the search for improved analgesics with fewer undesirable effects.[74] From this search has come mixed agonist/antagonist agents, three of which have found clinical application: pentazocine, butorphanol, and nalbuphine. A common characteristic of these drugs is a ceiling on the analgesia, sedation, and respiratory depression produced at increasing dosage, which limits their value as anesthetic *agents* but affords them greater safety as *adjuvants* in the ambulatory setting. They also tend to produce less nausea and vomiting, particularly in patients with a history of emesis after administration of other narcotics.

Pentazocine, in doses of 20 mg to 30 mg, is equipotent to morphine, 10 mg. At higher doses, dysphoria and psychotomimetic effects are intolerable to most patients and have been responsible for illicit use. It antagonizes the analgesia of opioid narcotics that might be administered later. Of particular concern in patients with coronary artery disease is its tendency to raise heart rate, systemic, pulmonary artery, and left ventricular end-diastolic pressures, cardiac work, and presumably cardiac oxygen utilization. Although this drug produces a smaller increase in biliary tract pressure than conventional narcotic agents, this advantage is insufficient to outweigh its many disadvantages.

Butorphanol is more potent but less psychotomimetic and cardiodepressive than pentazocine. In doses of 2 mg to 3 mg, it is equipotent to morphine, 10 mg, and generally more useful in the ambulatory setting. A poorer narcotic antagonist, butorphanol does not impair the effectiveness of subsequent narcotics. Recently, butorphanol, in a dose of 14 to 28 μg/kg administered intravenously, has been found to be a satisfactory substitute for fentanyl (e.g., 0.75–1.5 μg/kg) prior to a balanced general anesthetic consisting of thiopental induction, nitrous oxide and light isoflurane, for short gynecologic procedures (e.g., pelvic laparoscopy, D&C).* It has also proved more satisfactory than diazepam when used during facial plastic surgery: butorphanol, 8 mg to 10 mg, is infused slowly intravenously until the patient responds only to his or her name, local anesthesia is administered, then the infusion is slowed to a rate of about 2 mg/15 min. At these higher dosages, mild hypertension occurred but was not associated with increased bleeding or other problems and ceased with termination of the infusion.[27] We do not recommend this technique for routine ambulatory anesthesia. Fine and Finestone used large doses of these drugs for cystoscopy (butorphanol 60 μg/kg and nalbuphine 300 μg/kg) and found the incidence of side-effects and duration of recovery greater than with fentanyl (3 μg/kg).[55] Wetchler et al, in evaluating butorphanol and fentanyl as supplementation to inhalational anesthesia (nitrous oxide, isoflurane, 0.5%–1%) for

*Orkin FK: Personal communication, 1984

laparoscopy, found no statistically significant differences in PACU problems or length of stay between butorphanol, 20 μg/kg, and fentanyl, 2 μg/kg.[161] The use of butorphanol, 40 μg/kg, resulted in a significantly longer PACU length of stay (mean 199 min, range 111–303 min) compared to fentanyl, 2 μg/kg (mean 154 min, range 105–280 min).

Least psychotomimetic and cardiodepressive of these drugs, nalbuphine is as potent as morphine. As a result, it may prove the most valuable; however, its potency as a morphine antagonist limits the effectiveness of subsequent narcotics. It has been recommended as part of a technique for sedation in cases performed under local anesthesia: nalbuphine, 0.4 mg/kg, slowly intravenously, is followed 5 minutes later by droperidol, 35 μg/kg; 1 hour later, another 0.14 mg/kg and 35 μg/kg, respectively, may be added.[86] Onset of action for either butorphanol or nalbuphine occurs within 2 minutes after intravenous administration. Unfortunately, their duration of effective action is long, similar to morphine. The place for reduced doses of these agonist-antagonist narcotics has not been fully evaluated.

The needs of outpatient anesthesia have also prompted the search for new short-acting narcotic analgesics. Alfentanil is a fentanyl analog with approximately one-quarter the potency and one-third the duration of action of the older drug.[24,112,127] Pharmacokinetic investigation by Bovill and colleagues revealed a rapid redistribution half-life, 11.6 minutes.[14] The elimination half-life of 94 minutes is considerably shorter than that of fentanyl (219 min). This difference is the result of the higher protein binding and lower lipid solubility of alfentanil. Also, the volume of distribution of alfentanil is smaller, with less potential for drug accumulation in tissues. Since alfentanil is available for metabolic clearance, prolongation of drug effect after large or repeated doses is less likely.[72] No secondary increases in alfentanil plasma concentration have been reported.

Coe et al see alfentanil as a clinically superior intravenous adjuvant for ambulatory general anesthesia.[24] Comparing fentanyl and alfentanil in patients who underwent termination of pregnancy, they found a higher incidence of chest wall rigidity and ventilatory depression in the fentanyl group, a higher incidence of mild bradycardia and moderate hypotension in the alfentanil group, and no significant difference in the incidence of nausea, vomiting, dizziness, or excessive drowsiness. The fentanyl:alfentanil potency ratio was 6:1 based on total dose administered. Kay compared recovery in ambulatory cystoscopy patients following fentanyl and alfentanil and found no significant difference in time to early recovery of consciousness.[85] However, in Maddox-Wing and digit substitution tests to assess later recovery, at 1 hour postanesthesia, the patients who received alfentanil scored consistently better.

Kallar and Keenan evaluated and compared recovery time following alfentanil and fentanyl in 43 patients scheduled for termination of pregnancy. In the operating room, all patients received droperidol, 0.625 mg, intravenously followed by a small loading dose of either alfentanil (6–8 μg/kg) or fentanyl (2 μg/kg). Anesthesia was induced with methohexital (1 mg/kg) and maintained with 70% nitrous oxide and oxygen. Supplemental doses of alfentanil (2–5 μg/kg), fentanyl (0.5–1.5 μg/kg), or methohexital (20 mg) were administered as needed. The median time to establish alertness was significantly shorter for the alfentanil group (16 min), than for the fentanyl group (25 min). Although the percentage of completely recovered alfentanil patients was significantly greater than fentanyl patients at 20 and 30 minutes postoperatively, at 60 minutes postanesthesia recovery room scores indicating alertness were the same in both groups.*

POTENT INHALATIONAL AGENTS

Halothane, enflurane, and isoflurane are the potent anesthetic vapors now in common use.[44] These agents are often used in conjunction with nitrous oxide to maintain general anesthesia by a primarily inhalational technique. Advantages of the inhalational technique for maintenance include the potential for more rapid recovery.[47] These agents are eliminated primarily by excretion through the lungs; renal or hepatic metabolism are minimal. Enright and Pace-Floridia reported that in the 30 to 59 minutes after operation, patients who received inhalational agents for ambulatory procedures were more alert than those who received narcotics, despite longer anesthetic time.[47] Nausea and vomiting may also be less with the inhalational agents. In practice, many anesthesiologists combine the advantages of inhalational and narcotic techniques by supplementing nitrous oxide and low-dose narcotic with potent vapors when needed. This approach results in the administration of lower amounts of each agent.

Pharmacokinetic principles as discussed under nitrous oxide apply, of course, to the potent vapors as well. The concentration effect plays no role, however, because high concentrations cannot be administered. Instead, appropriate anesthetic depth can be rapidly achieved with overpressure, a technique that is effective with these more potent agents. Torri et al showed that, with enflurane from a nonrebreathing circuit, the time needed to reach surgical anesthesia could be reduced from approximately 4 minutes with the patient breathing 3.5% enflurane (approximately 2 MAC) to 2 minutes with the patient breathing 5% enflurane (3 MAC).[146]

The inspired concentration needed to reach 1 MAC in the alveoli within several breaths can be calculated for each agent.[43] Theoretically, these concentrations should be 3.9 MAC (3.0%) for halothane, 3.4 MAC (5.7%) for enflurane, and 2.8 MAC (3.1%) for isoflurane, using a nonrebreathing circuit.[115] It is the interaction of alveolar ventilation and cardiac output at these inspired concentrations that rapidly produces 1 MAC in the alveoli and blood. Inspired anesthetic concentration must then be decreased for maintenance of anesthesia to compensate for anesthetic returning to the alveoli from venous blood. With this approach, the speed of induction can be made equivalent for all three agents. The common conception that solubility limits speed of induction is not valid if comparable overpressure is used.

If 1 MAC of a vapor such as enflurane is inspired as the sole agent, particularly with spontaneous ventilation, anesthesia will not be achieved in time for surgery (Fig. 5-4).[115] Rapid and safe establishment of adequate anesthetic depth can be achieved in practice, with a potent vapor as the primary agent. At the Brigham and Women's Hospital, sufficient intravenous barbiturate is given to obtund consciousness. Delivered anesthetic concentration is rapidly increased to several multiples of MAC in order to maximize the concentration gradient between the inspired gas and the alveoli. High fresh gas flows and high minute ventilation, usually with controlled respiration, are also necessary. Problems with respiratory tract irritation are minimal. The course of

*Kallar SK: Personal communication, 1984

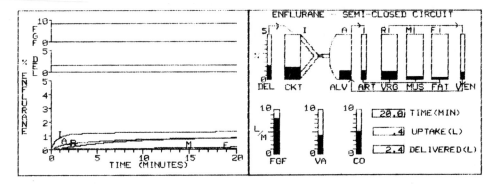

FIG. 5-4 Simulated anesthetic administration of 1 MAC enflurane with a semiclosed circuit.[115] In the graphic display (*left*), the time course of partial pressure of enflurane (expressed in percentage of one atmosphere) is shown for inspired gas (I), alveolar gas (A), vessel-rich tissue group (R; brain and heart), muscle (M) and fat (F). Note that 1 MAC enflurane is not reached in the alveolar gas. The pictorial display (*right*) also indicates the partial pressure delivered from the anesthesia machine (DEL) and breathing circuit (CKT), as well as the selected fresh gas flow (FGF) of 8 Liters/min, alveolar ventilation (VA) of 4 Liters/min, and cardiac output (CO) of 5 Liters/min.

such an anesthetic, as for dilatation and curettage, is shown in Fig. 5-5.[115] Anesthetic administration is discontinued early enough to permit awakening at the end of the operation. Rate of anesthetic elimination is inversely related to each agent's blood/gas partition coefficient; awakening is rapid if the surgery has been brief. When nitrous oxide is added, less of the potent vapor is needed.

Of the potent agents, halothane is the least irritating to the airways. However, its blood/gas solubility is relatively high (2.4), and emergence is therefore relatively slow. Recovery is further delayed by high tissue/blood solubility and considerable uptake into fat. Metabolic degradation of halothane may play a role in the development of halothane hepatotoxicity; the incidence of this complication is in the range of 1 in 35,000 administrations. The use of

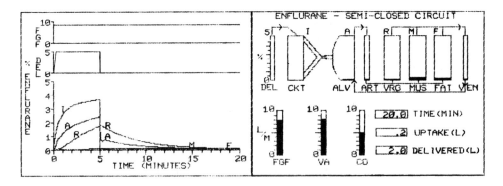

FIG. 5-5 Graphic (*left*) and pictorial (*right*) displays after a brief simulated anesthetic administration of 3 MAC enflurane (5%) through a semiclosed circuit.[115] At 5 min, the breathing circuit is "emptied" of anesthetic (I to zero), and the "patient" breathes 100% oxygen. Anesthetic elimination is rapid. See Fig. 5-4 for explanation of symbols.

halothane in ambulatory anesthesia should be reserved for those patients with specific indications, including asthmatics, heavy smokers, and bronchitics, particularly when mask anesthesia without supplemental paralysis is planned.

Enflurane has lower blood/gas (1.8) and blood/tissue solubility. Emergence is therefore more rapid. After 7 minutes of 2-MAC enflurane or halothane for dilatation and curettage (D&C), patients were able to respond to their name after 5.7 minutes with enflurane as compared with 7.6 minutes with halothane.[138] However, postoperative physical complaints[90,147] and intellectual or perceptual-motor function[143] were comparable between the two anesthetic agents. Enflurane is metabolized to a lesser degree (2%–3% vs. 15%–25% for halothane), and enflurane-associated hepatitis occurs very rarely.[94] In all, enflurane has excellent induction, maintenance, and recovery characteristics for ambulatory anesthesia, with minimal potential for delayed side-effects.

Isoflurane has the lowest blood/gas partition coefficient (1.3) and the fastest elimination. Of the three volatile agents in common use, isoflurane also undergoes the least metabolism.[44,151] This reduces patient exposure to metabolites with the potential for delayed toxicity. In the postanesthesia care unit, patients who received isoflurane required analgesics significantly more frequently than those who received enflurane or halothane.[147] On the first postoperative day, isoflurane recipients experienced more dizziness, nausea, coughing, pungent smell, and headache. Although at present isoflurane's cost is considerably more than the other volatile agents, its rapidity of action and minimal metabolism make it a good choice for ambulatory general anesthesia.

Early ambulation and discharge does not depend solely on the general anesthetic technique. Many ambulatory surgery facilities add local anesthetic infiltration to the management of their patients. Use of 0.25% bupivacaine infiltration during surgery allows the anesthesiologist to maintain his patient at lighter levels of anesthesia. This will, of course, hasten emergence. Infiltration may also be performed at the end of the procedure to provide postoperative analgesia. Less narcotic will be required in the recovery area, and the patient can be mobilized more rapidly.

CONTINUOUS INTRAVENOUS ANESTHESIA

Many intravenous anesthetics, narcotics, and muscle relaxants can be combined to provide anesthesia without additional inhaled drug.[81] True intravenous anesthetic agents are those that can induce and maintain a state of anesthesia alone in a spontaneously breathing patient. Narcotics alone are not categorized as intravenous anesthetics because, although they can produce anesthesia, they can only do so in doses that suppress spontaneous ventilation. True intravenous anesthetics are metabolized in the blood or by the liver and have short elimination half-lives. Consequently, most of these drugs do not show cumulative effects within the first several hours of continuous intravenous infusion. Emergence from anesthesia is, of course, determined by the rates of elimination of these agents. Potentially usable drugs, alone or in combination, include methohexital, fentanyl, alfentanil, ketamine, and the intravenous induction agents available in the United Kingdom.[78] Recovery after thiopental infusion has been excessively long.[158]

Dose requirements for intravenous anesthetics are given as minimum infusion rates (MIR), equivalent to MAC for inhalational agents. The MIR is the infusion rate (measured in μg/kg/min) that prevents movement in half of the patients during surgical incision. Like MAC, MIR is affected by the patient's age, by the addition of other analgesics and anesthetics, and by premedication. Prys-Roberts maintains that ensuring the proper depth of anesthesia with intravenous agents is no more difficult than doing so with inhalational anesthetics.[119] The common practice of intermittently injecting intravenous drugs causes rapid increases and decreases in blood and brain concentrations of these drugs.[157] Intravenous anesthetics can be more controllable if given by continuous infusion. An infusion technique minimizes the "peaks and valleys" of drug concentrations, decreasing the total amount of drug required and shortening recovery time. Another advantage of this technique over that of intermittent injections is the possible reduction in side-effects of these drugs.

Continuous infusions of fentanyl, alfentanil, and ketamine have been studied in ambulatory surgery patients. After a 100-μg loading dose, fentanyl was administered as 0.1 μg/kg/min of a 2-μg/ml infusion solution, rather than in intermittent 50-μg-bolus increments,[157] resulting in a 45% decrease in the total dose for a 23-minute procedure. With the lower dose, intraoperative motor and cardiovascular side-effects were less frequent and time to awakening decreased by 62%. Excessive postoperative sedation decreased from 48% to 4%, and discharge times were decreased by 29%. Coe et al showed that use of alfentanil by infusion rather than intermittent bolus resulted in a 33% decrease in total dose and a 15% decrease in time to ambulation, but no difference in the incidence of respiratory depression or muscular rigidity.[24] In their study, a loading dose of 250-μg to 500-μg alfentanil was followed by 0.6 to 1.1 μg/kg/min of a 10-μg/ml solution.

Ketamine has been given as a continuous infusion of 50 μg/kg/min after a 50-mg loading dose.[157] A 1-mg/ml concentration was used. The total dose required to supplement outpatient thiopental, nitrous oxide anesthesia, using the infusion, was decreased by 43%—101 mg for a 22-minute procedure. The time to awakening was decreased by 60% and the time to discharge by 13%. However, the reduction in ketamine dose was not accompanied by a reduction in emergence symptoms.

There are, of course, disadvantages and problems associated with the continuous infusion technique. These include the preparation of the solutions in the appropriate concentrations, the need for infusion pumps, and the maintenance of the proper infusion rate. Furthermore, patients differ in the way they handle drugs; the metabolic degradation of a given drug varies from patient to patient. Consequently, the anesthesiologist must be concerned with the possible accumulation of an intravenous agent in a given patient and the toxic effects of excessive drug levels. In short, as with any anesthetic agent or technique, its advantages must be weighed against its disadvantages.

MUSCLE RELAXANTS

The clinical use of muscle relaxant drugs has changed the practice of general anesthesia over the past 35 years. Deep anesthesia can be avoided with their use without compromising the intra-anesthetic course; this translates into more rapid emergence and earlier patient discharge from the facility.[69] There are, however, potential problems related to the use of muscle relaxants. They may cause lingering weakness, which may prolong the patient's discharge, or they may be responsible for postoperative myalgia.

Booij and Crul feel the ideal neuromuscular blocking drug should meet the following requirements:[13]

Nondepolarizing mechanism of action
Rapid onset of action
Short duration of action
Rapid recovery
Noncumulative action
No cardiovascular side-effects
No histamine release
Reversibility by cholinesterase inhibitors
High potency
Pharmacologically inactive metabolites

Until 1984, anesthesiologists' choices were limited when managing the ambulatory surgery patient. Short procedures call for short-acting muscle relaxants, and the only appropriate muscle relaxant available was succinylcholine. Succinylcholine is a depolarizing muscle relaxant that has a rapid onset and a short duration of action. It may be used as a bolus to facilitate endotracheal intubation or as an infusion to provide relaxation during the surgical procedure. Churchill-Davidson in 1954 first drew attention to the muscle pain experienced by patients following the administration of succinylcholine.[20] Pain is most frequently reported in the neck and shoulder muscles and may be mild to severe. Churchill-Davidson found the incidence and severity of myalgia significantly greater in outpatients (66%) than inpatients (13.9%); outpatients are more awake and active sooner. Postoperative muscle pain has been associated with the fasciculations seen after succinylcholine administration.[19,20,68] These fasciculations are contractions of the muscle fibers of a motor unit and can be explained by prejunctional activation of the motor nerve by the succinylcholine. However, there is no correlation between the development of postoperative pain and the intensity of the fasciculations. In fact, postoperative myalgia can occur in patients receiving succinylcholine who did not have clinical evidence of fasciculation. Myalgia often develops or worsens after discharge from the ambulatory surgery unit, during the first postoperative day.[19] Succinylcholine usage is also associated with a transient rise in serum potassium level and occasionally with signs of muscle injury such as a rise in serum creatine phosphokinase and myoglobinemia. In addition, succinylcholine is associated with postoperative sore throat and hoarseness, even in the absence of endotracheal intubation.[19]

Pretreatment with a variety of drugs has been reported to lessen and even eliminate myalgia following succinylcholine (ScH) usage. Perry and Wetchler evaluated the effects of varying pretreatment regimens on outpatients having oral surgery procedures.[114] Tables 5-5 and 5-6 compare the effects of pretreatment on the incidence and severity of fasciculation and postoperative myalgia. Regardless of which method of pretreatment was used, moderate to severe complaints of myalgia were never less than 8% (*d*-tubocurarine pretreatment) in any group. It was additionally noted that the optimum time for succinylcholine administration following *d*-tubocurarine pretreatment was 2 minutes. Gallamine (20 mg) or metocurine (1 mg) is also useful; pancuronium may decrease fasciculation but not prevent myalgia.[11,16] The use of nondepolarizing muscle relaxants (particularly 3 mg *d*-tubocurarine) given prior to

☐ **Table 5-5. The Incidence and Severity of Fasciculation**

Group (N = 25)	0*	+1	+2	+3
Diazepam, 0.05 mg/kg, followed in 5 min by ScH	3	7	9	6
dTc, 0.05 mg/kg, followed in 5 min by ScH	22	3	0	0
dTc, 0.05 mg/kg, followed by ScH when "eyelids heavy"	13	5	2	5
ScH, 1.5 mg/kg	1	5	9	10
"Self-Taming" ScH	1	9	8	7
Ca Gluconate, 1000 mg, followed in 1 min by ScH	4	4	6	11

*0, no fasciculation; +1, fine movement of face and fingers; +2, medium movement of face, fingers, and chest muscles; +3, coarse movement of face, fingers, toes, chest, and abdominal muscles.

succinylcholine to decrease the incidence of fasciculation and postoperative myalgia has become routine in many centers.[33]

Other pretreatment techniques have been evaluated. Fahmy[53] reported that pretreatment with 0.05 mg/kg of diazepam was superior to pretreatment with *d*-tubocurarine in preventing postsuccinylcholine myalgia. Other investigators have not found diazepam useful.[51,144] Baraka reported on pretreatment

☐ **Table 5-6. The Incidence and Severity of Postanesthesia Myalgia**

Group (N = 25)	None	Slight	Moderate or Severe Cases	Percentage Moderate or Severe Cases
Diazepam, 0.05 mg/kg, followed in 5 min by ScH	15	1	9	36%
dTc, 0.05 mg/kg, followed in 5 min by ScH	21	2	2	8%
dTc, 0.05 mg/kg, followed by ScH when "eyelids heavy"	21	2	2	8%
ScH, 1.5 mg/kg	17	2	6	24%
"Self-Taming" ScH	13	5	7	28%
Ca Gluconate, 1000 mg, followed in 1 min by ScH	9	7	9	36%

with a small dose (10 mg) of succinylcholine itself; he found this "self-taming" dose reduced the incidence of muscle pains.[5] However, Brodsky and Brock-Utne and Siler found that although the incidence and severity of fasciculations was decreased by a pretreatment dose of succinylcholine, it had no effect on postoperative myalgia.[15,135] Shrivastava pretreated succinylcholine with 10 ml 10% calcium gluconate and reported a significant decrease in the incidence of postoperative muscle pains.[134] Giving succinylcholine by infusion (0.1%) rather than as a 1-mg/kg bolus reduced the incidence of myalgia from 68% to 30%.[19] When these aches and pains related to anesthesia outlast the pain of surgery, they are a source of great consternation to both anesthesiologist and patient.[45,134]

Succinylcholine's short duration of action is related to its rapid breakdown by plasma cholinesterase. Some patients may be receiving anticholinesterase drugs (i.e., for the treatment of glaucoma), which can decrease the activity of pseudocholinesterase and thereby prolong the action of succinylcholine. Organophosphate insecticides have the same effect. There is also a genetic variant that produces an atypical form of the cholinesterase enzyme. This atypical enzyme hydrolyzes succinylcholine and other esters (e.g., local anesthetics) at markedly reduced rates. Patients with decreased pseudocholinesterase activity may have prolonged paralysis following the use of succinylcholine. Consequently, the anesthesiologist must exercise extreme caution when administering this drug to any patient who gives a personal or family history of suspicious respiratory problems during anesthesia or in the recovery room.[2] Should prolonged succinylcholine apnea occur, ventilatory support must be provided until the effects of the drug have dissipated. However, unless sedation is also provided, the paralyzed patient will be awake and aware of the problem. At this point, he or she should be informed of the problem and reassured about its outcome. Despite the potential problems, succinylcholine remains the muscle relaxant most frequently used for the ambulatory surgery patient.

Nondepolarizing muscle relaxants have also been available. These include d-tubocurarine, metocurine, pancuronium, and gallamine. The autonomic side-effects of each drug usually determine its appropriateness in a given clinical situation. However, use of any of these nondepolarizing relaxants for the ambulatory surgery patient is limited because of their relatively long duration of action.

Two intermediate-acting nondepolarizing relaxants were approved in 1984 that are useful in outpatient anesthesia: atracurium and vecuronium. Both drugs are relatively devoid of cardiovascular side-effects in their clinical dose range;[7] vecuronium causes no histamine release, but the two agents differ as to their mode of catabolism. Whereas vecuronium undergoes hepatic excretion, atracurium breaks down spontaneously at body pH and temperature. The latter drug would therefore seem preferable in a patient with renal or hepatic disease.

Atracurium is an interesting example of molecular engineering.[139] It was designed to block the neuromuscular junction, be water soluble, and undergo Hofmann elimination (the spontaneous breakdown of a molecule at body pH and temperature). Its metabolites are devoid of neuromuscular blocking activity and hemodynamic effects in the clinical dose range. These properties produce a drug that does not have a cumulative effect in the patient. This, coupled with its intermediate duration of action, may make atracurium a good muscle relaxant for the ambulatory surgery patient.[4,113]

Stirt et al consider atracurium an acceptable alternative to succinylcholine when speed of intubation is not critical.[140] Intubating conditions were compared at 2.5 minutes following administration of atracurium (0.4 or 0.5 mg/kg) and 1 minute after succinylcholine (1 mg/kg). Excellent or good intubating conditions were noted in 67% of patients with 0.4 mg/kg and 90% of patients with 0.5 mg/kg atracurium, compared to 100% with succinylcholine. Patients who received 0.5 mg/kg of atracurium therefore compared favorably to the succinylcholine group as to the level of neuromuscular block, but speed of onset was four times faster following succinylcholine. Increasing the intubating dose of atracurium above 0.5 mg/kg increases histamine-related side-effects. When using 0.4 to 0.5 mg/kg, particularly in combination with a major inhalation agent, length of action may be longer than desired for a short ambulatory surgery procedure. Sokoll et al found 0.3 mg/kg of atracurium produced a block lasting 44 minutes with a narcotic anesthetic compared to 67 minutes with isoflurane.[137]

Pearce and Wetchler have both studied the use of atracurium in ambulatory surgery patients.[113,156] Pearce feels 0.25 mg/kg is the lowest dose compatible with adequate intubating conditions. In 18 oral surgery patients, intubating conditions were excellent (10), good (7), or inadequate (1). The time to onset of block can be shortened and good intubating conditions provided if split dosages of nondepolarizing agents are given.[61] Wetchler studied 25 patients and found excellent (22) to good (3) intubating conditions when using a pretreatment atracurium dose of 0.075 mg/kg followed by 0.3 mg/kg in $2\frac{1}{2}$ minutes. Intubation was performed 2 minutes after the 0.3 mg/kg dose.[156]

Vecuronium is another safe and predictable relaxant. Foldes,* in attempting to decrease the time before a nondepolarizing agent could provide suitable intubation conditions, uses a technique called the *priming principle.* When vecuronium is the muscle relaxant, it is administered in the following manner:

1. "Priming dose," which is 15% (0.015 mg/kg) of the usual intubation dose
2. Patient preparation and induction takes place during a 5 to 7 minute interval.
3. A "primed intubation dose," which is 50% (0.05 mg/kg) of the usual intubating dose

Clarke compared vecuronium (0.1 mg/kg) with succinylcholine (1 mg/kg) and found the overall incidence of satisfactory intubating conditions to be the same.[23] Fragen and Shanks used vecuronium (0.045 mg/kg) for outpatient gynecologic laparoscopy.[60] Time to maximum block (condition suitable for intubation) was approximately 5 minutes. Duration of action was longer when vecuronium was used with inhalational agents than when it was used with narcotics (as with atracurium). With narcotic anesthesia, recovery to 50% depression of twitch height was seen at 15 minutes, and with isoflurane anesthesia at 20 minutes. In Fragen and Shanks' study, pharmacologic reversal of the muscle relaxant with edrophonium (0.5–0.6 mg/kg) and atropine (7–10 μg/kg) was given at the conclusion of surgery if less than 80% recovery of train-of-four was present. (Operative time was 40.0 min ±13.4 min). Reversal was necessary in 11 in 20 of the fentanyl group and 9 in 20 of the isoflurane group. Of those requiring reversal, 3 in 9 and 2 in 11, respectively, needed a second

*Foldes FF: Personal communication, 1984

dose of edrophonium. In view of a reported shorter duration of action, vecuronium may have an advantage over atracurium.[13,124]

It is imperative that the reversal of these nondepolarizing relaxants be complete at the end of the procedure. Such reversal can be accomplished by the appropriate use of facilitatory drugs—quaternary ammonium compounds that facilitate cholinergic transmission (Fig. 5-6). Their actions are secondary to both anticholinesterase and direct cholinomimetic effects. An anticholinergic drug (e.g., atropine) is administered with the facilitatory drug to minimize its muscarinic effects. Such reversal agents have different dynamics.[32,83,110] For example, the antagonism produced by neostigmine usually lasts for 90 minutes. If the proper amount of muscle relaxant has been administered, the residual muscle relaxant should be eliminated in this time. If an excessive dose of relaxant has been given, however, weakness may develop after the neostigmine effect is terminated. It is therefore imperative that a patient be observed in the recovery area until the effects of facilitatory drugs are gone.

These facilitory drugs differ in their time of onset and duration of action. Edrophonium has the fastest onset time but has weaker muscarinic activity than neostigmine. Pyridostigmine, which also has less muscarinic activity than neostigmine, has the slowest onset of these drugs, requiring 10 to 15 minutes to achieve significant reversal. Controlled studies in anesthetized patients have shown that the duration of edrophonium does not differ from that of neostigmine.[31] Furthermore, Morris et al have shown that all three drugs are cleared from the plasma at the same rate (Table 5-7). In a dose of 0.5 mg/kg, edrophonium antagonism appears to be equal to neostigmine, 0.04 mg/kg, or pyridostigmine, 0.2 mg/kg. In an early study, Katz failed to fully restore twitch height in half of the patients studied with 10-mg to 20-mg doses of edrophonium. However, more recent studies with larger doses of edrophonium have shown that it can fully reverse a curariform block.

In an ambulatory surgery setting, as anesthesiologists balance the various drugs used to achieve a goal of early home readiness for the patient, they must be aware of the effects certain anesthetic agents (such as isoflurane) have on the degree of muscle relaxation and length of action of nondepolarizing muscle relaxants. Isoflurane will produce the same degree of muscle relaxation

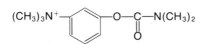

Neostigmine

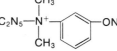

Edrophonium

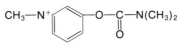

Pyridostigmine

FIG. 5-6 Molecular structure of facilitatory drugs. (Lichtiger M, Moya F: Introduction to the Practice of Anesthesia, 2nd ed. Hagerstown, Harper & Row, 1978)

☐ **Table 5-7. Duration of Action of Anticholinesterase Drugs During Halothane Anesthesia**

Drug	Dose (mg/kg)	Elimination Half-Life (min)
Neostigmine	0.04	80
Edrophonium	0.5	110
Pyridostigmine	0.35	112

with lower doses of muscle relaxants.[44] Decreasing the amount of relaxant required for surgery should result in fewer problems related to these drugs.

ENDOTRACHEAL INTUBATION

When outpatient anesthesia was in its infancy, there was some hesitation about endotracheal intubation in patients who were to be discharged so soon after surgery. The initial concern was with the patient who might develop calamitous airway problems at home, such as laryngospasm or airway swelling and closure. Thus, how long should a patient be kept in the recovery room after extubation? As the subspecialty has matured, it has become apparent that, if such problems are going to develop, they will manifest within 1 to 2 hours following extubation. There have been very few adult ambulatory surgery patients who have required hospital admission because of problems related to intubation.

Endotracheal intubation is associated with significant minor morbidity, however. Minor anesthetic complications can assume distressingly large proportion if associated with only minor surgery when the patient is up and about soon. Two of the potential complications of endotracheal intubation that concern the ambulatory patient and ambulatory anesthesiologist are postanesthesia myalgia and sore throat. The first is discussed above, with succinylcholine, under Muscle Relaxants.

The incidence of sore throat in outpatients undergoing mask anesthesia is 15% to 22%.[19] In this circumstance, sore throat may be due to the inhalation of dry gases, the use of anticholinergics, or the use of oral or nasal airways. After an endotracheal tube has been employed, the incidence of sore throat in ambulatory surgery patients rises to 46%.[97] The risk of producing a sore throat can be reduced to 25%, by the use of a low-*volume* cuffed tube. Limiting cuff volume (cuff area touching the trachea) is more important than avoiding high intracuff pressure for very short intubations. Postintubation sore throat may also be reduced by avoiding lidocaine jelly to lubricate the tube; this practice has been associated with a 90% incidence of sore throat.[97] Lubrication with lidocaine solution, water-soluble lubricant or saline does not affect the incidence of this complication. It should also be mentioned that the use of succinylcholine without intubation, even after curare pretreatment, results in sore throat in 45% of patients.[19] This may be related to minor injury of the striated muscles of the pharynx during fasciculation.

The Geriatric Patient

At the present time, about 10% of all Americans are 65 years of age or older. Current projections are that this will increase to 16% by the year 2000. With improvements in medical care, more of these patients are coming to surgery. In 1961, the perioperative mortality rate in the geriatric population approached 20%. However, a steady improvement has reduced that figure to less than 5% by 1980. Although much of this reduction may be accounted for by advancements in medical knowledge and care, the anesthesiologist's application of this new technology and knowledge in the operating theater has been one of the most important factors contributing to this decreased mortality. All of these facts, coupled with the growing emphasis on cost containment in the delivery of medical care, will bring greater numbers of elderly patients into the ambulatory setting.

There are two factors that must be considered in the elderly patient: the patient's preexisting disease and the physiologic changes associated with aging. In this discussion, it is most important to realize that *patients with multiple medical problems must be carefully evaluated before being accepted as candidates for ambulatory surgery.*

When dealing with the elderly patient, a primary concern should be to keep hospitalization as brief as possible. The older patient is less able to cope with a new environment and frequently has fewer psychologic and physiologic defenses to cope with stress. Elderly patients tend to ask fewer questions of physicians and do not like to bother them with questions they feel may not be important. The anesthesiologist should be aware of this attitude, attempt to find out the concerns the patient has, and provide appropriate information about anesthetic techniques. Over one-half of hospitalized geriatric patients experience some transient confusional state postoperatively. This high incidence can be decreased in the ambulatory surgery geriatric patient because of a quicker return to natural surroundings as well as a significant decrease in the number of medications the patient will be subjected to during their procedure.[149]

PREEXISTING DISEASE

Many physicians feel the geriatric patient's postoperative mortality rate is directly proportional to the number and severity of any preexisting diseases.[52,77] Some of the more common disease states of the elderly are outlined on next page. Many of these diseases, although not curable, are amenable to medical therapy and can be controlled. It is important they be controlled prior to anesthesia and surgery.

CARDIOVASCULAR PROBLEMS

Patients with coronary artery disease are frequently treated with beta-blocking drugs and calcium channel blockers. If congestive heart failure is part of the clinical picture, these patients may be receiving digitalis and diuretics. During the preoperative visit, the anesthesiologist's attention must be directed toward estimating how well-compensated the patient is. Should the patient require any alteration in therapeutic regimen, it should be done preoperatively.

☐   *Common Diseases of the Elderly*

Cardiovascular problems
  Coronary artery disease
  Hypertension
Respiratory diseases
  Chronic obstructive pulmonary disease
  Restrictive disease (often related to arthritis)
Central nervous system problems
  Cerebrovascular accidents
  Parkinsonism
  Emotional problems
Endocrine disease
  Diabetes mellitus
Urinary tract problems
  Prostatism
  Nephrosclerosis

Patients with hypertension should continue their antihypertensive therapy up to the time of surgery and should resume taking applicable medication as soon as possible in the postoperative period. If their hypertension is poorly controlled, they should be reevaluated by their internists and brought into good control prior to anesthesia and surgery. Inadequately treated hypertensive patients tend to have a decreased blood volume with a smaller intravascular space. With the induction of anesthesia, and its attendant expansion of the intravascular space, precipitous decreases in blood pressure may result. Furthermore, patients who are receiving diuretics as part of their antihypertensive therapy may have a severe total body deficiency of potassium. All too frequently, serum potassium determinations underestimate this potassium loss.

RESPIRATORY DISEASES
Geriatric patients with respiratory diseases should be carefully evaluated in the preoperative period. The importance of a good history and physical examination cannot be overemphasized. Pulmonary function tests should be obtained if they are indicated. A reasonable assessment of respiratory function can be gained with an arterial blood gas study.

Chest physiotherapy and control of chronic pulmonary infection may be required prior to surgery for the patient to be in optimal condition. The patient who has problems with copious secretions will benefit from physical therapy, whereas the patient whose sputum is yellow (or darker) must be considered to have infection. A preoperative course of pulmonary therapy with bronchodilators, coupled with the administration of a broad-spectrum antibiotic, can reduce the incidence of postoperative pulmonary complications.

It is also important to have the patient experience the kinds of therapy that will be used in the postoperative period. Thus, if incentive spirometry will be used, the patient should be instructed in it preoperatively because there may be significant impairment in his or her ability to function postoperatively. Elderly patients may be somewhat confused after surgery. They will also be less responsive to instruction while they are experiencing pain and the effects of analgesic drugs and residual anesthesia. Therefore, it is vital that, preoperatively, they fully understand the importance and use of the devices that will be employed postoperatively. Obviously, if a patient has lung disease that will require this type of postoperative care, he or she cannot be considered a candidate for ambulatory surgery.

CENTRAL NERVOUS SYSTEM PROBLEMS

Unfortunately, there is very little that can be done to control central nervous system disorders. The anesthesiologist must be aware of the patient's diseases to conduct a safe anesthetic. The patient with cerebrovascular disease, for example, should be maintained near his or her normal blood pressure and relatively normocarbic. The head should be kept in a neutral position, for excessive turning could seriously compromise the vertebral circulation.[96]

The patient with parkinsonism should be allowed to continue taking L-dopa until the time of surgery. The significant therapeutic effect of this drug should not be lost just because the patient is scheduled for surgery. Furthermore, certain drugs (e.g., phenothiazines and butyrophenones) that have an antidopaminergic effect should be avoided.

Emotional problems are, at best, difficult for the anesthesiologist to treat. We can only hope that these elderly patients have adjusted to some of their problems. We should do whatever we can to keep them comfortable and in contact with what has become familiar to them. For example, if their hearing is impaired, we can allow them to come to the ambulatory center with their hearing aids. Friends and relatives should be allowed to be with them in the holding area and should rejoin them postoperatively as soon as possible. In fact, ambulatory surgery itself serves to keep patients in environments familiar to them and should not be denied them.

ENDOCRINE DISEASE

Maturity-onset diabetes is another controllable disease common in the geriatric patient. Surgery represents a particularly stressful situation to the diabetic patient. Even well-controlled diabetics may have problems related to the stress of surgery, fluid and nutritional changes, and altered physical activity. The method required to control the patient's blood sugar is indicative of the extent of the diabetic's problems.

Patients who are controlled by diet alone rarely present problems. These patients have (1) a prolonged response from their own insulin secretion, (2) lower fasting blood sugars than normal patients, and (3) frequent hypoglycemic episodes. It is this tendency toward hypoglycemia with which the anesthesiologist must be most concerned. (See list below.) Hypoglycemia is also a major concern in patients taking oral hypoglycemic agents (e.g., chlorpropamide).

☐ *Signs of Hypoglycemia During General Anesthesia*

Sweating
Dilatation of pupils
Tachycardia
Hypertension

There are many regimens for managing the insulin-dependent diabetic during and after surgery. Most often, the decision of which mode of therapy will be used is made in the preoperative period, before the anesthesiologist is involved. It may range from withdrawal of the patient from the usual insulin with coverage on a "sliding scale" to keeping the patient on the usual insulin preparation with a preoperative reduction in dosage. However, in the ambulatory surgery setting, the anesthesiologist may be the one who determines the management of the diabetic patient. At Mt. Sinai Medical Center, patients taking oral hypoglycemic drugs are instructed not to take their medication on the morning of surgery. Furthermore, if they are taking an oral hypoglycemic with a reasonably long duration of action (e.g., chlorpropamide), they are told to omit an evening dose if they are on such a regimen. We try to schedule these patients early in the day and they are given dextrose-containing infusions. We also strive to restore their usual dietary and medical therapy as soon as possible in the postoperative period.

Insulin-dependent diabetics can be candidates for ambulatory surgery if their diabetes is stable and well controlled and the planned procedure allows them to reestablish their dietary habits soon after surgery. For short procedures in insulin-dependent diabetics, some simply withhold their insulin until after the procedure. It is the fear of intraoperative hypoglycemia that has prompted this course of action. Of course, blood sugar is monitored in these patients, and insulin administration is based on any undue rise in blood sugar.

The more prevalent approach to those patients involves the administration of one-third to one-half of their customary dose of intermediate-acting insulin. An intravenous infusion with dextrose is simultaneously started to counteract any untoward reactions. This concept is supported by studies that show that when ketosis develops in insulin-dependent diabetics, there is no reactive insulin secretion. Furthermore, the stress of surgery stimulates catecholamine release, which increases blood sugar. Thus, the diabetic with some insulin "on board" is expected to do better with a little extra sugar than one with less sugar and no insulin in his system. Additional information on the management of the insulin-dependent diabetic can be found in Chapter 8 and Chapter 9, Case No. 16.

If the patient has a urinary catheter in place, urine sugar and acetone can be followed intraoperatively. A catheter should not be inserted solely for this purpose, since diabetic patients have a high incidence of serious urinary tract infections (e.g., necrotizing papillitis). Instead, the blood sugar level can be followed in the operating room by using Dextrostix (Ames Division, Miles Laboratories, Elkhart, Indiana).

URINARY TRACT PROBLEMS

There is little that can be done to control urinary tract problems in the preoperative period. Nephrosclerosis is a complication of hypertension. Its presence, as manifested by an elevated blood urea nitrogen, serum creatinine, and urinary protein, implies poor control of a hypertensive state. Consequently, our attention is directed back to the control of the patient's arterial blood pressure.

Prostatism is another common problem of the elderly. If a patient gives a history consistent with benign prostatic hypertrophy, the anesthesiologist must be concerned about postoperative urinary retention. This is a frequent occurrence in patients with prostatism who receive large intraoperative fluid volumes. It may result from bladder distention in the intraoperative period, which causes a loss of detrusor tone. The bladder musculature probably needs reasonably good function to propel the urine through its partially obstructed urethra. A rational approach to fluid therapy in these patients, coupled with other modes of therapy (e.g., urinary catheterization) to prevent bladder distention, will help to prevent this complication. Patients with prostatism, however, should demonstrate their ability to void prior to their discharge from an ambulatory surgery facility.

THE PHYSIOLOGY OF AGING

The aging process involves many physiologic and pathologic changes which may alter the patient's response to anesthesia and surgery (Fig. 5-7).[96,108] There is, for example, a general reduction in physiologic reserve; this decreases the patient's ability to respond to stress with an increase in organ activity. However, it is difficult to separate this general deterioration in function from the effects of disease on these same organ systems. Some of the more common diseases in the geriatric patient have been discussed. Our focus must now shift to physiologic changes that are not usually categorized as disease entities.

PHARMACOKINETICS

When a drug is administered parenterally, its uptake and redistribution to rapidly equilibrating tissues is relatively unaffected by age. However, gastrointestinal absorption is affected. There are changes in gastric acidity, intestinal motility, and intestinal perfusion which decrease the uptake of drugs given by this route. This must be considered when a predictable response to premedicant drugs is wanted.

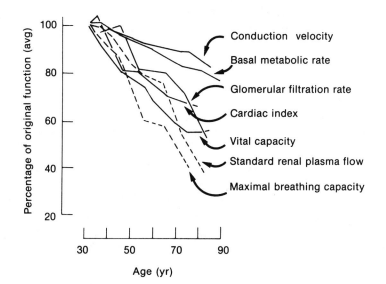

FIG. 5-7 Changes in physiologic function with age in humans expressed as percentage of mean value at age 30 years. (Miller RD: Anesthesia for the elderly. In Miller RD (ed) Anesthesia. New York, Churchill Livingstone, 1981)

Once the drug has gained access to the circulation, it rapidly equilibrates with the vessel-rich group of tissues. However, the elderly patient has increased body fat, decreased body mass, and a decreased muscle mass. These changes, coupled with decreases in perfusion, tend to delay redistribution to the more slowly equilibrating tissues, particularly for drugs that are highly lipid soluble. Thus, the half-life of such lipid-soluble drugs is markedly prolonged. Furthermore, drug metabolism may be delayed by a reduction in both hepatic perfusion and liver microsomal enzyme activity. The metabolites of these drugs will also be excreted more slowly because of changes in renal function. Obviously, drugs that depend on renal excretion for their elimination will also have more prolonged effects. Consequently, an increase in a drug's half-life is common in the geriatric patient. This can result in the accumulation of a drug following repeated doses.[77,96]

Other factors have also been cited as contributing to the elderly patient's response to drugs. Decreased muscle mass, mentioned above, will permit the anesthesiologist to achieve good muscle relaxation with a lower dose of neuromuscular blocking agent. In this example, it is the decreased muscle tone and the decreased number of receptor sites that cause the increased drug effect. Another factor is the decreased plasma protein binding of drugs. It is not only a decrease in the amount of plasma protein that causes this, but also a change in the quality of this protein such that its drug-binding potential is decreased. The net result of this decrease in protein binding is a marked increase in the free drug available in the blood. Since it is this free drug that has access to the receptor sites, a smaller quantity of drug may produce the desired effect.

MEDICATIONS

Most geriatric patients are receiving a multitude of drugs for their varied ailments. They are usually not aware of the names of these drugs, although they know why they are taking them. Patients should be asked to bring their medications to the ambulatory unit to identify them. Many of these drugs can cause problems during anesthesia, and the anesthesiologist must be aware of the patient's medications. The more commonly used drugs are listed in Table 5-8 along with some of the problems associated with their use.[77] This list is

☐ Table 5-8. Problems Associated with Commonly Used Drugs

Drug	Problem
Diuretics	Hypokalemia (dysrhythmogenicity)
Digitalis	Cardiac irritability (accentuated by hypokalemia)
Tranquilizers	Dependency
Barbiturates	Dependency, enzyme induction
Alcohol	Dependency, liver disease
Echothiophate drops	Plasma cholinesterase inhibition
Antibiotics	Muscle-relaxant interaction
Beta-blockers	Decreased myocardial contractility
Methyldopa, reserpine	Decrease MAC, sympathetic denervation hypersensitivity
Guanethidine	Denervation hypersensitivity

obviously incomplete. However, when we consider the number of drugs that are administered during an anesthetic, even this partial list points out the potential for drug interactions.

AIRWAY PROBLEMS

Elderly patients may be edentulous or have loose teeth associated with periodontal disease. They also tend to have alterations in the structure of their mandibles. These changes complicate intubation and create difficulties with mask fit. Cervical arthritis and temporomandibular problems will accentuate these difficulties. A further consideration is the potential for aspiration, since protective airway reflexes are diminished and hiatal hernia is common.

RENAL FUNCTION

Most notable of the physiologic changes of aging is a decrease in tissue elasticity. Elastic changes in the vascular system cause irregular changes in blood flow throughout the body; renal blood flow, for example, is severely affected. By 75 years of age, renal blood flow is decreased by more than 50%. Therefore, glomerular filtration decreases, and the distribution of renal blood flow is altered such that a greater proportion of the blood goes to the renal medulla. The geriatric patient is therefore more susceptible than others to renal failure. This change in physiology should not influence one's decision as to whether or not a geriatric patient is a candidate for ambulatory surgery; it is just a part of the aging process.

PULMONARY FUNCTION

Geriatric patients who do not have specific lung diseases still have significant changes in their pulmonary function. Not only is the elastic recoil of the lung affected by the general changes in tissue elasticity, but the chest wall also becomes stiffer, probably because of arthritic changes in the chest. Pulmonary blood flow also decreases, leading to changes in the ventilation:perfusion ratio. This ratio is also affected by the closing volume and the dead space, both of which increase with age. These changes result in an increase in the alveolar-arterial oxygen tension difference so that arterial oxygen tension decreases. Residual volume and functional residual capacity increase as lung elasticity decreases. Vital capacity and forced expiratory volume are likewise reduced.

CIRCULATORY FUNCTION

The decreased elasticity already referred to leads to decreases in vessel compliance and the development of hypertension. These decreases in vessel compliance can also affect autoregulation in various organ systems. Such changes in the ability of the vasculature to alter its pattern of flow decrease the ability of the organism to respond to stress. The decreasing cardiac index adds to this inability to respond well to stress. Changes in the coronary vasculature also occur with age.

PATIENT SELECTION

When considering the diseases and physiologic changes seen in the geriatric patient, it may at first seem odd to consider them as candidates for ambulatory surgery. However, there are certain factors that must be considered. Not all elderly patients have all of the problems enumerated above, nor do they all have them to the same degree. Physiologic age is more important than chronologic age. Is the patient in question a young 80 or an old 65? A physiologic profile consisting of past medical history, current level of physical activity, and present physical condition will serve as a better indicator of the patient's ability to tolerate the planned procedure than an evaluation of the patient on age alone.

Of equal importance is the capability and emotional maturity of the responsible party who will take the patient home and provide care in the perioperative period. Proper postoperative home care is one of the most important factors in geriatric ambulatory surgery. Family members who are unreliable or not physically able may not be capable of providing such care. Should this be the case, the safety of the patient's postoperative course is in question. Consequently, it is just as important to evaluate the responsible person during the preoperative visit. Is this person able to follow instructions and to do what will be required of him or her?

The type of surgery performed is also important. Ambulatory surgery should be limited to procedures that do not require extensive postoperative nursing care. Furthermore, it must be asked what would be gained if the patient were to be admitted to a hospital. If there is little to be gained and the responsible person is capable of caring for the patient, ambulatory surgery may be safely performed. Remember that the geriatric patient may benefit from having close friends and family members nearby. Ambulatory surgery should not be denied to the geriatric patient solely on the basis of age.

THE CATARACT PATIENT

The most common surgical procedure on the elderly patient is cataract removal. In 1886 it was shown that early ambulation following cataract extraction caused no unusual ill effects.[18] The trend is away from inpatient hospitalization and toward outpatient care. In the future we will not have to justify ambulatory eye surgery; instead, we may need to justify hospitalization for eye surgery. Anesthesiologists will be expected to manage these procedures in an outpatient setting—either hospital affiliated, freestanding or office based. Ophthalmologists have already established an association specifically devoted to ambulatory eye surgery—the Outpatient Ophthalmic Surgery Society. Total anesthesia involvement can include the anesthesiologist performing the retrobulbar block. Unless appropriately trained during a residency program to perform this block, anesthesiologists often over-react when first requested to perform it. However, who is better trained in administering regional block and more aware of the effects of local anesthetic drugs than an anesthesiologist?

Except for the anesthesia risk, hospitalization for the average cataract patient is unnecessary. Given a simple choice of "do you want to be asleep or awake during your surgery," most patients want to be asleep. Being awake carries with it certain fears. If carefully questioned, cataract patients usually admit they are afraid of seeing the surgeon operate on the eye; some believe the eye is removed, surgery is performed, and the eye is then replaced. When dealing with a cataract patient, it is important to dispel these fears, discuss the safety of regional block anesthesia, and stress the importance of an early return to a familiar home environment. If presented with the facts in a concerned, nonthreatening manner, the majority of elderly patients willingly enter into cataract extraction under "local anesthesia."

Intense patient education is very important in ambulatory surgery. McMahan provides patients and families with preoperative teaching by way of a video recording that fully explains the procedure from start to finish.[103,104] Patients are also given written material and detailed instructions about what to expect before, during, and after surgery. The informed geriatric patient feels less threatened.

A retrobulbar block in a nonsedated patient can be stressful as the needle approaches the eye and painful as the injection is made. To make the procedure more acceptable, small doses of intravenous sedation can be provided, or a 50% mixture of nitrous oxide, oxygen can be inhaled for approximately 5 minutes.[104]

At the Methodist Medical Center Ambulatory Surgery Center, in Peoria, Illinois, anesthesiologists perform the retrobulbar block. Preblock analgesia is provided by a Nitronox unit (Ohmeda, Orchard Park, New York) equipped with a scavenging device (Fig. 5-8) that delivers a 50% nitrous oxide, oxygen mixture by means of a hand-held demand valve (inspiratory effort 1 cm H_2O). After trying various methods of mask administration (oronasal, nasal) in the often edentulous elderly patient population, a pliable lip seal mask (from the days of intermittent positive-pressure breathing) has proven to be the most satisfactory (Fig. 5-9). The effects of nitrous oxide are seen within 3 to 5 minutes, and once inhalation is discontinued, the effects are reversible in approximately the same length of time. A discussion of inhalation analgesia can be found in Chapter 6; additional information on retrobulbar technique, drug dosages, and complications can be found in *Anesthesia for Otolaryngology and Ophthalmology,* by John C. Snow.

Respiratory arrest has been reported following retrobulbar injection of bupivacaine (0.75%). Kirk reported four instances of sudden apnea that required intubation and mechanical ventilatory support for 15 to 20 minutes following the block.[136] Cardiopulmonary arrest has also occurred.[126] No fatalities were noted in either report. When performing retrobulbar block, anesthesiologists should take the following precautions:

Use the smallest volume of the local anesthetic.
Use the least effective concentration of the local anesthetic.
Provide frequent aspiration before injection.
Monitor cardiac status during and after the block.
Closely observe ventilatory status during and after the block.
Make sure resuscitation equipment is readily available.

ANESTHETIC MANAGEMENT

The type of anesthesia the geriatric patient will receive depends on the following factors:

The surgical procedure
The patient's general health
The patient's emotional state

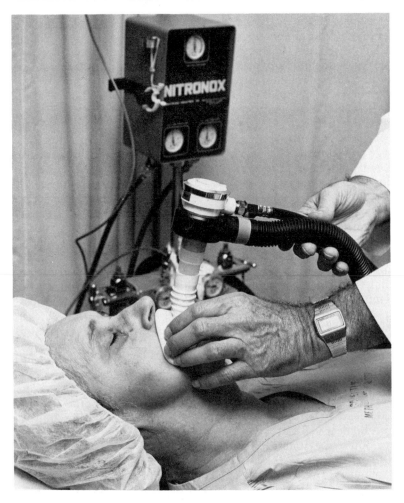

FIG. 5-8 Administration of 50% nitrous oxide–oxygen with a Nitronox analgesia unit.

The third factor refers not only to the patient's emotional stability, but also to his or her ability to accept local or regional anesthesia. Curiously, many elderly patients fear general anesthesia more than regional anesthesia. They have a fear of going to sleep and not awakening: they desire to maintain some control of the situation. Consequently, most geriatric patients receive regional anesthesia or local anesthesia with supplemental sedation. The Methodist Medical Center Ambulatory Surgery Center managed 2951 patients over the age of 60 between 1981 and 1983. Ninety percent of the patients had local or regional anesthesia. The admit rate for the patients over 60 years old was 0.8%; this is only 0.2% higher than the admit rate for all patients.

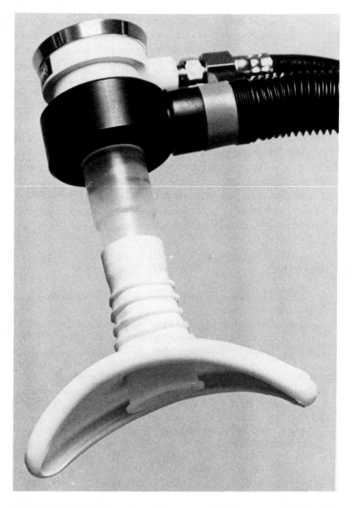

FIG. 5-9 Pliable lip seal mask for use with Nitronox analgesia unit.

SPECIAL CARE AND HANDLING

Surgery for the aged presents a special challenge for all members of the ambulatory surgery team. The geriatric patient presents with more numerous, and totally different, problems than those seen in younger patients. Crawford recommends ambulatory surgery facilities provide a lot of "high touch" for their geriatric population.[29] "High touch" is a term used by John Naisbitt in *Megatrends* to offset all the "high tech" in today's society. Quiet kindness should replace excessive urgency, a slower time scale will allow unrushed opportunities for patient care and contact, and a friendly family spirit helps replace what is missing in the lives of many elderly patients.[108]

You may want to bring your geriatric patients in earlier than usual on the morning of surgery. Geriatric patients take longer to get from the parking area to the facility, longer to register, longer to answer questionnaires, and longer to change their clothes. Don't rush them. Don't make them feel like they're keeping you waiting. Give them a little extra time and consideration; take a little extra time with explanations. Explain what you are going to do each step of the way. Do not expose these patients unnecessarily; reassure them as much as possible.

Whereas confusion and agitation frequently occur following surgery and anesthesia in the geriatric inpatient, this is rarely the case for the geriatric ambulatory surgery patient because there is less frequent disruption in routine, diet, medication, and sleep.

Goethe said, "no skill or art is needed to grow old, the trick is to endure it." And the trick of caring for elderly patients surgically is how to help them endure what must eventually affect all of us.[108]

References

1. Adams AP, Pybus DA: Delayed respiratory depression after use of fentanyl during anaesthesia. Br Med J 1:278, 1978
2. Ali HH, Savarese JJ: Monitoring of neuromuscular function. Anesthesiology 45:216, 1976
3. Baird ES, Hailey DM: Delayed recovery from a sedative: Correlation of the plasma levels of diazepam with clinical effects after oral and intravenous administration. Br J Anaesth 44:803, 1972
4. Baird WLM, Kerr WJ: Reversal of atracurium with edrophonium. Br J Anaesth 55:63S, 1983
5. Baraka A: Self-taming of succinylcholine-induced fasciculations. Anesthesiology 46:292, 1977
6. Baraka A, Saab M, Salem MR et al: Control of gastric acidity by glycopyrrolate premedication in the parturient. Anesth Analg 56:642, 1977
7. Basta SJ, Savarese JJ, Ali HH et al: Histamine-releasing potencies of atracurium, dimethyltubocurarine, and tubocurare. Br J Anaesth 55:105S, 1983
8. Becker LD, Paulson BA, Miller RD et al: Biphasic respiratory depression after fentanyl-droperidol or fentanyl alone used to supplement nitrous oxide anesthesia. Anesthesiology 44:291, 1976
9. Beechey APG, Eltringham RJ, Studd C: Temazepam as premedication in day surgery. Anaesthesia 36:10, 1981
10. Berggren L, Eriksson I: Midazolam for induction of anaesthesia in outpatients: A comparison with thiopentone. Acta Anaesth Scand 25:492, 1981
11. Blitt CD, Carlson GL, Rolling GD et al: A comparative evaluation of pretreatment with nondepolarizing neuromuscular blockers prior to the administration of succinylcholine. Anesthesiology 55:687, 1981
12. Boas RA, Newson AJ, Taylor KM: Comparison of midazolam with thiopentone for outpatient anesthesia. N Z Med J 96:210, 1983
13. Booij L, Crul J: A comparison of vecuronium with the hypothetical ideal neuromuscular blocking drug. Clinical Experiences with Norcuron Symposium, Geneva, 1983
14. Bovill JG, Sebel PS, Blackburn CL et al: The pharmacokinetics of alfentanil (R39209): A new opioid analgesic. Anesthesiology 57:439, 1982
15. Brodsky JB, Brock-Utne JG: Does "self-taming" with succinylcholine prevent postoperative myalgia? Anesthesiology 50:265, 1979
16. Brodsky JB, Brock-Utne JG, Samuels SI: Pancuronium pretreatment and post-succinylcholine myalgias. Anesthesiology 51:259, 1979
17. Brown PM, Moss E: Reduction of pain on injection of etomidate. Anaesthesia 36:814, 1981

18. Bruns HD: The ambulant after-treatment of cataract extraction. Trans Am Ophthalmol Soc 14:473, 1916
19. Capan LM, Bruce DL, Patel KP et al: Succinylcholine-induced postoperative sore throat. Anesthesiology 59:202, 1983
20. Churchill-Davidson HC: Suxamethonium (succinylcholine) chloride and muscle pains. Br Med J 74:209, 1954
21. Clark AJM, Hurtig JB: Premedication with meperidine and atropine does not prolong recovery to street fitness after out-patient surgery. Can Anaesth Soc J 28:390, 1981
22. Clark G, Erwin D, Yate P et al: Temazepam as premedication in elderly patients. Anaesthesia 37:421, 1982
23. Clark RS, Mirakahur RK: Intubating conditions after vecuronium: A study with three doses and a comparison with suxamethonium and pancuronium. Clinical Experiences with Norcuron Symposium, Geneva, 1983
24. Coe V, Shafer A, White PF: Techniques for administering alfentanil during outpatient anesthesia—a comparison with fentanyl. Anesthesiology 59:A347, 1983
24a. Cohen SE, Woods WA, Wyner J: Antiemetic efficacy of droperidol and metoclopramide. Anesthesiology 60:67, 1984
25. Conner JT, Herr G, Katz RL et al: Droperidol, fentanyl and morphine for i.v. surgical premedication. Br J Anaesth 50:463, 1978
26. Conner JT, Katz RL, Pagano RR et al: RO 21-3981 for intravenous surgical premedication and induction of anesthesia. Anesth Analg 57:1, 1978
27. Cook TA: Butrophanol tartrate: An intravenous analgesic for outpatient surgery. Otolaryngol Head Neck Surg 91:251, 1983
28. Cotton BR, Smith G: Comparison of the effects of atropine and glycopyrrolate on lower oesophageal sphincter pressure. Br J Anaesth 53:875, 1981
29. Crawford F: Geriatric patients merit special care and respect. Same Day Surgery 7:98, 1983
30. Cressman WA, Plostnieks J, Johnson PC: Absorption, metabolism and excretion of droperidol by human subjects following intramuscular and intravenous administration. Anesthesiology 38:363, 1973
31. Cronnelly R, Morris RB: Antagonism of neuromuscular blockade. Br J Anaesth 54:183, 1982
32. Cronnelly R, Morris RB, Miller D: Edrophonium: Duration of action and atropine requirement in man during halothane anesthesia. Anesthesiology 57:261, 1982
33. Cullen DJ: The effect of pretreatment with nondepolarizing muscle relaxants on the neuromuscular blocking action of succinylcholine. Anesthesiology 35:572, 1971
34. Dawson B, Reed WE: Anaesthesia for adult surgical outpatients. Canad Anaesth Soc J 27:409, 1980
35. Dechene JP: Alphathesin, a new steroid anaesthetic agent. Can Anaesth Soc J 23:163, 1976
36. Divoll M, Greenblatt DJ, Ochs HR et al: Absolute bioavailability of oral and intramuscular diazepam: Effects of age and sex. Anesth Analg 62:1, 1983
37. Driscoll EJ, Smilack ZH, Lightbody PM et al: Sedation with intravenous diazepam. J Oral Surg 30:332, 1972
38. Dundee JW: Clinical studies of induction agents. VII. A comparison of eight intravenous anaesthetics as main agents for a standard operation. Br J Anaesth 35:784, 1963
39. Dundee JW, Clarke RSJ: Comparison of barbiturates with propanidid. Acta Anaesth Scand 25:(Suppl):413, 1966
40. Dundee JW, Samuel IO, Toner W et al: Midazolam: A water-soluble benzodiazepine. Anaesthesia 35:454, 1980
41. Dundee JW, Wilson DB: Amnesic action of midazolam. Anaesthesia 35:459, 1980
42. Egbert LD, Battit GE, Turndorf H et al: The value of the preoperative visit by an anesthetist. JAMA 185:553, 1963
43. Eger EI: Anesthetic uptake and action. Baltimore: Williams & Wilkins, 1974
44. Eger EI: Isoflurane (forane). Madison, WI, Airco, 1982
45. Eisenberg M, Balsley S, Katz RL: Effects of diazepam on succinylcholine-induced myalgia,

potassium increase, creatine phosphokinase elevation, and relaxation. Anesth Analg 58:314, 1979

46. Elliott CJR, Green R, Howells TH et al: Recovery after intravenous barbiturate anesthesia. Lancet 1:68, 1962

47. Enright AC, Pace-Floridia A: Recovery for anaesthesia in outpatients: A comparison of narcotic and inhalational techniques. Can Anaesth Soc J 24:618, 1977

48. Epstein BS: Outpatient anesthesia. ASA Refresher Course. Las Vegas, 1982

49. Epstein BS: Outpatient anesthesia. In Hershey SG (ed): ASA Refresher Courses in Anesthesiology. Philadelphia, JB Lippincott, 1974

50. Epstein BS, Levy ML, Thein MH et al: Evaluation of fentanyl as an adjunct to thiopental-nitrous oxide-oxygen anesthesia for short surgical procedures. Anesth Rev 2(3):24, 1975

51. Erkola O, Salmenpera M, Tammisto T: Does diazepam pretreatment prevent succinylcholine-induced fasciculations? A double-blind comparison of diazepam and tubocurarine pretreatments. Anesth Analg 59:932, 1980

52. Evans TI: Problems in general anaesthesia—geriatrics. Aust Fam Physician 6:339, 1977

53. Fahmy NR, Malek NS, Lappas DG: Diazepam prevents some adverse effects of succinylcholine. Clin Pharmacol Ther 26:395, 1979

54. Fassoulaki A, Kaniaris P: Does atropine premedication affect the cardiovascular response to laryngoscopy and intubation? Br J Anaesth 54:1065, 1982

55. Fine J, Finestone SC: A comparative study of the side-effects of butorphanol, nalbuphine and fentanyl. Anesth Rev 8(9):13, 1981

56. Forster A, Gardaz JP, Suter PM et al: Midazolam as an induction agent for anaesthesia: A study in volunteers. Br J Anaesth 52:907, 1980

57. Forster A, Gardaz JP, Suter PM et al: Respiratory depression by midazolam and diazepam. Anesthesiology 53:494, 1980

58. Fragen RJ: New intravenous drugs for induction and maintenance of anesthesia. Current Reviews in Clinical Anesthesia Lesson 16;4:135, 1984

59. Fragen RJ, Caldwell N: Comparison of a new formulation of etomidate with thiopental—side effects and awakening times. Anesthesiology 50:242, 1979

60. Fragen RJ, Shanks CA: Neuromuscular recovery after laparoscopy. Anesth Analg 63:51, 1984

61. Gergis SD, Sokoll M, Mehta O et al: Intubation conditions after atarcurium and suxamethonium. Br J Anaesth 55:835, 1983

62. Giese JL, Stanley TH, Pace NL et al: Fentanyl pretreatment reduces side effects associated with etomidate anesthetic induction. Anesthesiology 59:A320, 1983

63. Gold MI: Postanesthetic vomiting in recovery room. Br J Anaesth 41:143, 1969

64. Greenwood BK, Bradshaw EG: Preoperative medication for day-case surgery. Br J Anaesth 55:933, 1983

65. Hannington-Kiff JG: Comparative recovery rates following induction of anaesthesia with althesin and methohexitone in out-patients. Postgrad Med J 116, 1972

66. Hebron BS, Edbrooke DL, Newby DM et al: Pharmacokinetics of etomidate associated with prolonged IV infusion. Br J Anaesth 55:281, 1983

67. Hegarty JE, Dundee JW: Sequelae after the intravenous injection of three benzodiazepines—diazepam, lorazepam, and flunitrazepam. Br Med J 2:1384, 1977

68. Hegarty P: Postoperative muscle pains. Br J Anaesth 28:209, 1956

69. Herbert M, Healy TEJ, Bourke JB et al: Profile of recovery after general anaesthesia. Br Med J 286:1539, 1983

70. Hillestad L, Hansen T, Melsom H et al: Diazepam metabolism in normal man. Clin Pharmacol Ther 16:479, 1974

71. Horrigan RW, Moyers JR, Johnson BH et al: Etomidate vs. thiopental with and without fentanyl—a comparative study of awakening in man. Anesthesiology 52:362, 1980

72. Hudson RJ, Stanski DR: Metabolism versus redistribution of fentanyl and alfentanil. Anesthesiology 59:A243, 1983

73. Hudson RJ, Stanski DR, Burch PG: Pharmacokinetics of methohexital and thiopental in surgical patients. Anesthesiology 59:215, 1983
74. Hug CC: New narcotic analgesics and antagonists in anesthesia. Semin Anesth 1:14, 1982
75. Hunt TM, Plantevin OM, Gilbert JR: Morbidity in gynaecological day-case surgery. Br J Anaesth 51:785, 1979
76. James MFM, Manson EDM, Dennett JE: Nitrous oxide analgesia and altitude. Anaesthesia 37, 238, 1982
77. Janis K: Anesthesia for the geriatric patient. In Hershey SG (ed): ASA Refresher Courses in Anesthesiology. Philadelphia, JB Lippincott, 1979
78. Jastak JT, Goretta C: Ketamine HCl as a continuous-drip anesthetic for outpatients. Anesth Analg 52:341, 1973
79. Jensen S, Huttel MS, Schou Oleson A: Venous complications after i.v. administration of diazemuls (diazepam) and dormicum (midazolam). Br J Anaesth 53:1083, 1981
80. Jones DF: Recovery from day-case anaesthesia: comparison of a further four techniques including use of the new induction agent diprivan. Br J Anaesth 54:629, 1982
81. Jones D, Lawrence AS, Thornton JA: Total intravenous anaesthesia with etomidate-fentanyl. Anaesthesia 38:29, 1983
82. Joyce TH, Turner P, Benson D et al: Aspiration of gastric contents post cimetidine. Anesthesiology 55:A312, 1981
83. Katz RL: D-tubocurarine, edrophonium and neostigmine. Anesthesiology 28:327, 1967
84. Kay B: A clinical assessment of the use of etomidate in children. Br J Anaesth 48:207, 1976
85. Kay B, Venkataraman P: Recovery after fentanyl and alfentanil for minor surgery. Br J Anaesth 55:169S, 1983
86. Klein DS: Nalbuphine and droperidol combination for local standby sedation. Anesthesiology 58:397, 1983
87. Korttila K, Linnoila M: Skills related to driving after intravenous diazepam, flunitrazepam or droperidol. Br J Anaesth 46:961, 1974
88. Korttila K, Mattila MJ, Linnoila M: Prolonged recovery after diazepam sedation: The influence of food, charcoal ingestion and injection rate on the effects of intravenous diazepam. Br J Anaesth 48:333,1976
89. Kothary SP, Brown ACD, Pandit UA et al: Time course of antirecall effect of diazepam and lorazepam following oral administration. Anesthesiology 55:641, 1981
90. Kreienbuhl G: Subjektive beschwerden nach halothan-lund nach enfluraneanaesthesie bei ambulanten (tagesklinik-) patienten. Anaesthetist 27:533, 1978
91. Kumar N, Pandit SK, Detmer MD: Pulmonary lesions after antacid and cimetidine aspiration. Anesth Analg 59:547, 1980
92. Less NW, Hendry JGB: Etomidate in urological outpatient anaesthesia. Anaesth 32:592, 1977
93. Leigh JM, Walker J, Janaganathan P: Effect of preoperative anaesthetic visit on anxiety. Br Med J 2:987, 1977
94. Lewis JH, Zimmerman HJ, Ishak KG et al: Enflurane hepatotoxicity. Ann Intern Med 98:984, 1983
95. Lichtiger M, Moya F: Introduction to the Practice of Anesthesia, 2nd ed. Hagerstown, Harper & Row, 1978
96. Lichtiger M, Moya F: Physiologic and pathologic considerations in the geriatric patient. Curr Rev Nurs Anesthetists 1:1, 1978
97. Loeser EA, Stanley TH, Jordan W et al: Postoperative sore throat: Influence of tracheal tube lubrication versus cuff design. Can Anaesth Soc J 27:156, 1980
98. Manchikanti L, Kraus JW, Edds SP: Cimetidine and related drugs in anesthesia. Anesth Analg 61:595, 1982
99. Manchikanti L, Marrero TC: Effect of cimetidine and metoclopramide on gastric contents in outpatients. Anesthesiol Rev 10:9, 1983
100. Manchikanti L, Roush JR: Effect of preanesthetic glycopyrrolate and cimetidine on gastric fluid pH and volume in outpatients. Anesth Analg 63:40, 1984

101. McClain DA, Hug C: Intravenous fentanyl kinetics. Clin Pharmacol Ther 28:106, 1980

102. McKenzie R, Wadhwa RK, Lim Uy NT et al: Antiemetic effectiveness of intramuscular hydroxyzine compared with intramuscular droperidol. Anesth Analg 60:783, 1981

103. McMahan LB: Ambulatory eye surgery. J Miss State Med Assoc 24(7):181, 1983

104. McMahan LB: Nitrous-analgesia for cataract surgery. Ophthalmic Surg 13:307, 1982

105. Mendelson CL: Aspiration of stomach contents into lungs during obstetric anesthesia. Am J Obstet Gynecol 53:191, 1946

106. Meridy HW: Criteria for selection of ambulatory surgical patients and guidelines for anesthetic management: A retrospective study of 1,553 cases. Anesth Analg 61:921, 1982

107. Mikkelsen H, Hoel TM, Bryne H et al: Local reactions after i.v. injections of diazepam, flunitrazepam, and isotonic saline. Br J Anaesth 52:817, 1980

108. Moore AR: Surgery and the aged. Aust Fam Physician 7:1045, 1978

109. Morison DH, Dunn GL, deGraft-Johnson A: Alphathesin and etomidate for minor out-patient anaesthesia. Can Anaesth Soc J 29:622, 1982

110. Morris R, Cronnelly R, Miller RD et al: Pharmacokinetics of edrophonium and neostigmine when antagonising d-tubocurarine neuromuscular blockade in man. Anesthesiology 54:399, 1981

111. Ong BY, Palahniuk RJ, Cumming M: Gastric volume and pH in outpatients. Can Anaesth Soc J 25:36, 1978

112. Patrick M, Eagar B, Toft DF et al: Alfentanil supplemented anesthesia for short procedures: A double blind comparison with fentanyl. Anesthesiology 59:A346, 1983

113. Pearce AC, Williams JP, Jones RM: The use of atracurium for short surgical procedures in day-case patients. Anesthesiology 59:A265, 1983

114. Perry J, Wetchler BV: Outpatient anesthesia: The effects of diazepam pretreatment of succinylcholine on fasciculation or postoperative myalgia. AANA 52(1):48, 1984

115. Philip JH: GAS MAN—Understanding Anesthesia Uptake and Distribution. Menlo Park: Addison-Wesley, 1984

115a. Pollard J: Clinical evaluation of intravenous vs inhalational anesthesia in the ambulatory surgical unit: A multicenter study. Curr Therap Res 36(4):617, 1984

116. Prescott RJ, Espley AJ, Davie IT et al: Double-blind clinical trial of anaesthetic premedication for use in major day surgery. Lancet May, 1976

117. Price HL, Kovnat BS, Safer JN et al: The uptake of thiopental by body tissues and its relation to the duration of narcosis. Clin Pharmacol Ther 1:16, 1960

118. Prys-Roberts C, Davies JR, Calverly RK et al: Haemodynamic effects of infusions of disopropyl phenol (ICI35868) during nitrous oxide anaesthesia in man. Br J Anaesth 55:105, 1983

119. Prys-Roberts C, Sear JW, Low JM et al: Hemodynamic and hepatic effects of methohexital infusion during nitrous oxide anesthesia in humans. Anesth Analg 62:317, 1983

119a. Rao TLK, Madhavareddy S, Chinthagada M et al: Metoclopramide and cimetidine to reduce gastric fluid pH and volume. Anesth Analg 63:1014, 1984

120. Reves JG, Corssen G, Holcomb C: Comparison of two benzodiazepines for anaesthesia induction: Midazolam and diazepam. Can Anaesth Soc J 25:211, 1978

121. Reves JG, Vinik R, Hirschfield AM et al: Midazolam compared with thiopentone as a hypnotic component in balanced anaesthesia: A randomized, double-blind study. Can Anaesth Soc J 26:42, 1979

122. Riding JE: Post-operative vomiting. Proc Soc Land 53:671, 1960

123. Rigg JRA, Goldsmith CH: Recovery of ventilatory response to carbon dioxide after thiopentone, morphine and fentanyl in man. Can Anaesth Soc J 23:370, 1976

124. Robertson EN, Booij L, Fragen RJ et al: A clinical comparison of atracurium and vecuronium. Br J Anaesth (Submitted for publication)

125. Rosenberg TD, Wong HC: Arthroscopic knee surgery in a freestanding outpatient surgery center. Orthop Clin North Am 13:277, 1982

126. Rosenblatt RM: Cardiopulmonary arrest after retrobulbar block. Am J Ophthalmol 90:425, 1980
127. Rosow CE, Latta WB, Keegan CR et al: Alfentanil and fentanyl in short surgical procedures. Anesthesiology 59:A345, 1983
128. Salem MR, Wong AY, Mani M et al: Premedicant drugs and gastric juice pH and volume in pediatric patients. Anesthesiology 44:216, 1976
129. Scamman FL: Fentanyl-O_2-N_2O rigidity and pulmonary compliance. Anesth Analg 62:332, 1983
130. Schmidt KF, Garfield JM, Korten K: The pharmacology of agents used in outpatient anesthesia. Int Anesth Clin 14(2), 1976
131. Schou Oleson A, Huttel MS: Local reactions to i.v. diazepam in three different formulations. Br J Anaesth 52:609, 1980
132. Sear JW, Prys-Roberts C: Plasma concentrations of alphaxalone during continuous infusion of Althesin. Br J Anaesth 51:861, 1979
133. Shelley ES, Brown HA: Antiemetic effect of ultra low dose droperidol. ASA Abstracts 633, 1978
134. Shrivastava OP, Chatterji S, Kachawa S et al: Calcium gluconate pretreatment for prevention of succinylcholine-induced myalgia. Anesth Analg 62:59, 1983
135. Siler JN, Cook FJ, Ricca J: Does "self-taming" decrease postoperative myalgia in outpatients? Anesthesiology 52:98, 1980
136. Smith LJ: Retrobulbar bupivacaine can cause respiratory arrest. Ann Ophthalmol 1005, 1982
137. Sokoll MD, Gergis SD, Mehta M et al: Safety and efficacy of atracurium (BW33A) in surgical patients receiving balanced or isoflurane anesthesia. Anesthesiology 58:450, 1983
138. Stanford BJ, Plantevin OM, Gilbert JR: Morbidity after day-case gynaecological surgery. Br J Anaesth 51:1143, 1979
139. Stenlake JB, Waigh RD, Urwin J et al: Atracurium: Conception and inception. Br J Anaesth 55:3S, 1983
140. Stirt JA, Katz RL, Murray AL et al: Intubation with atracurium in man. Anesthesiology 59:A266, 1983
141. Stoelting RK: Gastric fluid pH in patients receiving cimetidine. Anesth Analg 57:675, 1978
142. Stoelting RK: Responses to atropine, glycopyrrolate, and riopan of gastric pH and volume in adult patients. Anesthesiology 48:367, 1978
143. Storms LH, Stark AH, Calverley RK et al: Psychological functioning after halothane or enflurane anesthesia. Anesth Analg 59:245, 1980
144. Taff RH: Pulmonary edema following naloxone administration in a patient without heart disease. Anesthesiology 59:576, 1983
145. Thompson GE, Remington JM, Millman BS et al: Experiences with outpatient anesthesia. Anesth Analg 52:881, 1973
146. Torri G, Damia G, Fabiani ML et al: Uptake and elimination of enflurane in man. Br J Anaesth 44:789, 1972
147. Tracey JA, Holland AJC, Unger L: Morbidity in minor gynaecological surgery: A comparison of halothane, enflurane and isoflurane. Br J Anaesth 54:1213, 1982
148. Urbach GM, Edelist G: An evaluation of anaesthetic techniques used in an outpatient unit. Can Anaesth Soc J 24:401, 1979
149. Vandam LD: To make the patient ready for anesthesia: Medical care of the surgical patient. Reading, MA, Addison-Wesley, 1980
150. Vickers MD: The measurement of recovery from anaesthesia. Br J Anaesth 37:296, 1965
151. Wade JG, Stevens WC: Isoflurane: An anesthetic for the eighties? Anesth Analg 60:666, 1981
152. Wetchler BV: Anesthesia for outpatients. In Mauldin BC (ed): Ambulatory Surgery: A guide to perioperative nursing care. New York, Grune & Stratton, 1983
153. Wetchler BV, Anesthesia for outpatient surgery. AORNJ 34:283, 1981
154. Wetchler BV: For ambulatory surgery patients, use ketamine with caution. Same-Day Surgery 8(1):11, 1984

155. Wetchler BV, Collins IS, Jacob L: Antiemetic effects of droperidol in the ambulatory surgery patient. Anesth Rev 9:23, 1982
156. Wetchler BV, Perry J: Limiting post-operative myalgia in the outpatient: Succinylcholine versus atracurium. Presented at the Medical College of Virginia Symposium on Anesthesia for Ambulatory Surgery. Williamsburg, Virginia, 1984
157. White PF: Use of continuous infusion versus intermittent bolus administration of fentanyl or ketamine during outpatient anesthesia. Anesthesiology 59:294, 1983
158. White PF, Dworsky WA, Horai Y et al: Comparison of continuous infusion fentanyl or ketamine versus thiopental—determining the mean effective serum concentrations for outpatient surgery. Anesthesiology 59:564, 1983
159. Wyant GM: Glycopyrrolate methobromide. Can Anaesth Soc J 21:230, 1974
160. Wyant GM, Kao E: Glycopyrrolate methobromide: Effect on salivary secretion. Can Anaesth Soc J 21:230, 1974
161. Wetchler BV, Alexander CD, Shariff MS et al: A comparison of butorphanol and fentanyl in ambulatory surgery patients. Third Annual Symposium on Anesthesia for Ambulatory Surgery, Williamsburg, Virginia, 1985

6

Local and Regional Anesthesia

Beverly K. Philip, M.D.

Benjamin G. Covino, Ph.D., M.D.

Local anesthesia may be defined as a temporary loss of sensation due to the inhibition of nerve endings in a specific part of the body. Local anesthesia is often performed by a surgeon for relatively minor procedures. Regional anesthesia may be defined as the interruption of impulses in specific nerve fibers innervating a larger body area. Regional anesthetic techniques are usually performed by an anesthesiologist, for more complex procedures. Local and regional anesthesia have long been used for ambulatory surgery; in 1963 and 1964, 56% of ambulatory procedures at the University of California, Los Angeles were performed by these techniques.[22] Success with local and regional anesthesia for ambulatory patients begins with appropriate preparation. A team of anesthesiologist, surgeon, and nurse who enthusiastically support these techniques for the patient must be assembled. The patient must be psychologically suitable and medically free of contraindications. His or her cooperation must be gained by appropriate education. Local anesthetic drugs must be chosen that are effective in the desired time frame, and anesthetic techniques employed that will provide patient and surgeon with satisfactory operative conditions. Premedication and supplemental sedation, both verbal and medicinal, may be used to augment the block-induced analgesia, but should not delay discharge. Finally, the complications of local and regional anesthesia must be known, avoided when possible, and appropriately treated if they occur.

Preparation

Excellent conditions for ambulatory surgery that will satisfy patient, surgeon and anesthesiologist can be obtained with local and regional anesthesia. To achieve this optimal outcome, all members of the team must be carefully selected. Also, the inherent limitations of local and regional anesthesia itself must be appreciated.

The anesthesiologist must have the personality and skills to communicate well with patients and be able to gain trust rapidly. He or she must be confident, competent, and gentle. The anesthesiologist also functions as an educator. This has particular importance for regional ambulatory anesthesia, because the prepared patient is better able to cooperate. Information needed by the patient includes the minor discomforts often associated with administration of local or regional anesthesia, such as intradermal injection for skin analgesia, insertion of block needle, or paresthesias. The anesthesiologist must also teach the patient to expect sensations that will not be blocked by the anesthetic, such as pressure and movement, and about the often disquieting sensations of numbness, paralysis, and dissociation of the involved body part. The quality of sensation as it returns and postoperative discomforts need also to be discussed. The anesthesiologist must forewarn about sights, sounds, or smells the awake patient may experience during the course of the surgery. Potential complications of the planned anesthetic technique should be discussed, and the patient should be instructed to call the ambulatory surgery unit if any develop. The anesthesiologist who plans to use regional anesthesia must know and be able to discuss the relative benefits of regional anesthesia in an informative but nonthreatening manner.

This detailed preoperative explanation of expected intraoperative and postoperative sensations should be made before the patient is in the operating room. Preoperative teaching can be completed in a quiet office or waiting area in the ambulatory unit on the day of surgery. Anesthesia screening clinics have been established to which the patient comes either on the day of the preoperative surgical appointment or at some time between the scheduling of surgery and the day of operation. A separate anesthesia evaluation and discussion, before the day of surgery, does allow a more relaxed presentation of the benefits and experiences of regional anesthesia.

It is self-evident that the anesthesiologist who plans to perform local or regional anesthesia for ambulatory procedures must be technically skilled. A day surgery unit is not the place to learn regional blocks. The anesthesiologist's expertise must include choice of the appropriate technique, anesthetic drug, and, if indicated, appropriate sedation to supplement the block. In summary, satisfactory regional anesthesia for ambulatory surgery requires preoperative education, intraoperative analgesia from proper local anesthetic placement, and possibly intravenous supplementation.

For regional anesthesia to be successful for the ambulatory surgical patient, the surgeon must support it. Surgeons with experience in operating on patients under local or regional anesthesia in ambulatory surgery have enthusiastically recommended this anesthesia to other surgeons for herniorrhaphies, laparoscopies, and anorectal and urologic procedures. Support must begin preoperatively, with the surgeon suggesting and encouraging the use of regional blocks to the patient. At the time of operation, the surgeon should be tolerant of extra time that is sometimes required for performance of the regional anesthetic procedure and for analgesia to develop fully. Inserting the slower-onset epidural or brachial plexus block early, in a holding area or induction room, can be a decided advantage. Preoperative and intraoperative communication between the surgeon and anesthesiologist about duration and extent of surgery is imperative. Since not all sensations are blocked by regional anesthesia, the surgeon must be gentle with patient's tissues and use careful surgical technique. The particular challenge of operating on an awake and listening patient should also be appreciated.

The surgical procedure must also be compatible with ambulatory regional anesthesia. The body part involved must be accessible by local or regional block. A related issue is the need for the surgeon often to tailor surgical technique to accommodate the not-total loss of sensation that occurs even with good local or regional blockade. For laparoscopic tubal ligation to be well tolerated by the awake patient, surgeons have advocated the use of nitrous oxide rather than carbon dioxide as the insufflating gas, limiting intraperitoneal gas volume and pressure, using only moderate Trendelenburg position, and applying local anesthetic solution to the uterine and tubal surfaces before manipulation or fulguration.[95] Enthusiastic participation of the ambulatory surgical nurse is invaluable in teaching, encouraging, and preparing a regional anesthesia patient for the procedure.

Local and regional anesthesia has several specific advantages that recommend it to the patient. Recovery time is significantly shorter. For a variety of ambulatory surgical procedures recovery after local and regional anesthesia required 136 minutes, as compared to 207 minutes after general anesthesia.[85] For patients undergoing laparoscopic tubal sterilization, recovery time was reduced from 176 minutes under general anesthesia to 103 minutes under lumbar epidural block.[13] The likelihood of postoperative hospital admission is also less. In the same series of various ambulatory procedures,[85] 2.9% of the patients who had general anesthesia required admission, compared to 1.2% of those who had local or regional blockade. Another advantage is the postoperative analgesia that can be provided with numbness limited to the operative site. Surgical complications can be reduced; blood loss after therapeutic abortion is least in the patients receiving local anesthesia. Also, complications specific to procedures, such as pneumothorax with laparoscopy, can be detected earlier in a conscious patient. Avoidance of the discomforts of general anesthesia may be most important to the patient. Sore throat, muscle pains, airway trauma, and dizziness are minimized. In a series of patients receiving lumbar epidural rather than general anesthesia for laparoscopy, the incidence of nausea and vomiting was reduced from 38% to 4%.[13] Also, some patients would rather not "go to sleep." This stems from a curiosity about the surgical experience, a desire to be aware and retain some control over the situation, or from a strong fear of general anesthesia.

The primary requirement for successful ambulatory anesthesia remains proper patient selection. Regional anesthesia requires ongoing cooperation by the patient; patients must be chosen who are psychologically suitable. Education and preparation of the patient by surgeon and anesthesiologist can be decisive in achieving success. Of 116 appropriately chosen and educated patients, 98% were able to complete laparoscopies under local anesthesia.[26] On the other hand, patients who overreact to minor discomforts or who are severely apprehensive or anxious are better excluded. Mentally retarded patients can be handled successfully under ambulatory regional anesthesia with appropriate sedation. These patients often have medical and surgical problems that suggest the use of local or regional anesthesia, and, on the whole, the handicapped patients' needs may be better met by same-day surgery, which allows them to return to their home or institution rapidly. In a recent series of 132 handicapped patients, 53% were able to complete dental restorations without general anesthesia.[62] The young child may not be able to understand enough to cooperate with the insertion of a block and maintenance of regional anesthesia. However, caudal anesthesia applied during the surgical general anesthetic can be successfully used to provide intraoperative and postoperative analgesia even for newborn infants.[84] The elderly patient may be a particularly good candidate for regional anesthesia. Pain sensation is decreased, allowing better tolerance of minor discomforts. The incidence of postdural puncture headache after spinal anesthesia decreases with age. Protective airway reflexes are also attenuated in the elderly,[110] which may increase the possibility of aspiration under general anesthesia.

On the other hand, the older patient is less tolerant of adverse physiologic changes that may occur, such as hypotension with spinal or epidural anesthesia. Decreased sympathetic-nervous-system activity and a reduced intravascular volume, due to drugs or decreased fluid intake, combine to increase the incidence of hypotension. The dose of local anesthetic for epidural anesthesia may need to be reduced with age.[17] The duration of spinal anesthesia may be prolonged in the elderly because of decreased blood flow in the vessels surrounding the subarachnoid space and therefore decreased anesthetic removal. Blocks can be more difficult to perform because of intervertebral narrowing and calcification. Drugs for supplemental sedation may generate unexpectedly large effect owing to decreased liver and kidney function. Elderly individuals are more likely to have cardiovascular, respiratory, or other systemic disease; ASA status 3 older patients can be offered ambulatory regional anesthesia after individual anesthetic consultation if their underlying diseases are stable. However, these patients may be better cared for in a hospital (integrated, separated) unit. The elderly may also have associated problems that will interfere with the success of a regional anesthetic, such as tremors, inability to communicate due to deafness or blindness, and disorders of mentation such as confusion and disorientation.[86] Regional anesthesia is a good choice for the older patient, but should be used with knowledge and care.

Ambulatory patients receiving local or regional anesthesia must be as carefully evaluated and prepared as those who receive general anesthesia. Preoperative requirements should include a written history and physical examination for all patients. Surgery under local anesthesia alone can result in cardiorespiratory complications. Meyers reported that 5.6% of approximately 1000 cataract surgery procedures under local anesthesia generated emergency calls for an anesthesiologist.[86] Prompt and appropriate intervention requires definite knowledge of the patient's underlying physical conditions as documented in the history and physical examination report. Appropriate laboratory evaluations are needed for patients who are receiving intravenous sedation or regional block and are suggested for patients undergoing local anesthesia.

Intraoperative monitoring is essential to the safety of local and regional ambulatory anesthesia. Monitoring begins with the assessment of mental status by verbal communication. This is adequate for minor procedures under purely local anesthesia. For more complex procedures requiring intravenous sedation or more extensive anesthesia or regional blockade, additional monitoring is needed. Audible and visible devices displaying cardiac rhythm and blood pressure should be used. A stethoscope placed on the precordium or at the sternal notch monitors respiration as well. An automated blood pressure device is particularly convenient if the circulating nurse is also responsible for watching the patient. However, if intravenous sedation is necessary to complete the procedure, an anesthesiologist should be present. This individual is specifically trained in the safe dosage and duration of action of anesthetics, sedatives, and analgesics, and in the identification and treatment of complications of these agents. He or she is responsible solely for monitoring the effects of drug administration on the patient, without being distracted by the need to obtain supplies or assist surgery.

Before any local or regional anesthetic is administered, facilities must be present to support a full resuscitation. "Local anesthesia rooms," which may not have a dedicated anesthesia machine, must have immediate access to equipment able to support ventilation, including a manual resuscitation bag; masks; and oral, nasal, and endotracheal airways. Sources of 100% oxygen and suction are needed, as are intravenous fluids and the equipment to start an infusion. These supplies, plus drugs for cardiopulmonary resuscitation and treatment of convulsions, should be stored together in a well-organized and labeled container, such as a mobile crash cart. This equipment must be inspected regularly and staff familiarized with its use. All patients receiving intravenous sedation or any regional block must have an intravenous access line.[96]

The question is often raised whether ambulatory patients for regional anesthesia should be fasting. Ambulatory surgery patients are at risk for pulmonary sequelae of acid aspiration; 60% of ambulatory surgery patients in one study had gastric aspirates of low pH, ≤ 2.5, and elevated volume, ≥ 25 ml.[80] Cigarette smoking also increases outpatient gastric volume.[134] Surgeons should be aware that excessive amounts of local anesthetic can cause a systemic reaction with convulsions or loss of consciousness, which may result in aspiration. Even without a toxic reaction, the ambulatory regional anesthesia patient can be at risk because of supplemental medications given. The use of 50% nitrous oxide to supplement local anesthesia has been shown to cause laryngeal incompetence and tracheal soiling in 20% of patients.[110] Heavy neuroleptanalgesia has been shown to have the same effect in 100% of patients.[16] Supplemental medications, particularly narcotics, may nauseate the patient or cause vomiting. "Heavy sedation" may well be in fact general anesthesia. The ambulatory regional anesthesia patient is already at risk for aspiration; increasing that potential by adding a full stomach is adding unacceptable additional hazard.

Drug interaction is also an important consideration. Ambulatory surgery patients may be taking medicines that interact or interfere with the administration of regional anesthesia. Anticoagulation with coumadin or heparin is a contraindication to major regional anesthesia (spinal and epidural) because of the risk of epidural hematoma formation and paraplegia. Anticoagulation should also be evaluated cautiously for other blocks with a significant possibility of large vessel puncture, such as brachial plexus anesthesia. Large doses of aspirin may also interfere with coagulation;[31] if major regional block is considered in these patients, bleeding, clotting, and platelet studies should be performed. The safety of performing regional anesthesia for patients on "minidose" heparin anticoagulation is still in some doubt.

Antihypertensive agents with effects on the sympathetic nervous system can alter patients' response to the vasopressors that may be needed for spinal or epidural anesthesia. Rauwolfia alkaloids deplete norepinephrine stores in postganglionic sympathetic nerves, so that hypotension during major regional anesthesia may be more difficult to treat. Guanethidine and alpha-methyldopa sensitize postsynaptic effector sites to norepinephrine. The intraoperative response to direct-acting sympathomimetic drugs such as phenylephrine and methoxamine may therefore be exaggerated, and the response to indirect vasopressors such as ephedrine may be attenuated. Treatment of hypertension or coronary artery disease often includes beta-adrenergic antagonist drugs such as propranolol. The usual compensatory mechanisms for intraoperative hypotension may be lost owing to drug effect, resulting in inability to increase myocardial contractility or heart rate and inability to vasoconstrict unblocked segments. Correction of intraoperative hypotension in the presence of these drugs requires increased doses of beta-adrenergic agonist drugs acting through blocked pathways; drugs with significant alpha-adrenergic effect such as metaraminol or phenylephrine should be used if the response is inadequate. Atropine and calcium are also effective. Propranolol and cimetidine can decrease the clearance rate of lidocaine from plasma. Since lidocaine is cleared largely by the liver, this effect is due to either a reduction in cardiac output and hepatic blood flow or to competition for hepatic enzyme systems that degrade lidocaine. Systemic lidocaine effects, particularly toxicity, may be enhanced in patients taking propranolol or cimetidine.

Antidepressant drug therapy may also interact with regional anesthetic administration. Tricyclic antidepressants inhibit norepinephrine uptake at postganglionic neurons in the periphery and within the central nervous system.[31] The patient's response to epinephrine and indirect vasopressors during regional anesthesia may be exaggerated. Monamine oxidase inhibitors (MAOIs) may also precipitate an excessive response to indirect vasopressors; epinephrine and norepinephrine are tolerated because of alternate metabolic pathways.[33] The catastrophic interaction between MAOIs and drugs used for supplemental sedation, particularly meperidine, must also be remembered. Butyrophenone derivatives used for supplementation, such as haloperidol or droperidol, may antagonize L-dopa and exacerbate the symptoms of parkinsonism. Other chronic medications may also interact. In patients receiving cimetidine, diazepam clearance is delayed and sedation increased. Exposure to organophosphate insecticides or to cancer chemotherapeutic drugs such as cyclophosphamide and the nitrogen mustards decreases plasma cholinesterase levels. The patient may experience a prolonged regional block if the anesthetic agent chosen is an ester. Echothiophate eye drops are used to constrict the pupil for glaucoma therapy; decreased plasma pseudocholinesterase levels result from systemic absorption, with a similar clinical result on the duration of ester anesthetic block.

Procedure-specific complications are different under local or regional anesthesia than under general anesthesia. The overall complication rate, however, may be the same. Grimes et al found an incidence of 0.35% for complications after abortion under general anesthesia, with greater risk of uterine perforation, cervical injury, and intra-abdominal hemorrhage.[58] Under local anesthesia, the incidence was 0.30% (not statistically different), with increased risk of fever and convulsions. Local and regional blocks themselves do have morbidity. Interscalene block may cause phrenic paralysis and intercostal block may result in spinal anesthesia. Limb exsanguination, as would be performed for intravenous regional anesthesia, has caused a fatal pulmonary embolus.[100] Furthermore, the use of excessive sedation in conjunction with a local or regional block may interfere with a patient's cooperation and jeopardize the success of the procedure.

Evaluation of recovery from regional anesthesia and criteria for discharge are discussed in Chapter 7.

Use of Premedication and Supplemental Sedation

GENERAL CONSIDERATIONS

Premedication serves to reduce fear and anxiety. In addition, premedication and supplemental sedation can provide analgesia, facilitate venipuncture, prevent postoperative nausea and vomiting, and, possibly, provide amnesia. Premedicant and supplemental drugs can improve patient tolerance and acceptance of regional anesthetic techniques, particularly when the patient would rather not be fully awake. However, the use of drugs to premedicate patients for ambulatory regional anesthesia is not without problems. The recovery time from local anesthesia with sedation can be longer than from a general anesthetic, and discharge on the day of surgery may be delayed. Premedicant drugs have their own complications, particularly if an inappropriate drug or dose is given. Premedicant drugs should be carefully tailored to the needs of the patient and requirements of the procedure, to produce desired effects while minimizing undesired side-effects. When premedication is not needed for the ambulatory regional anesthesia patient, it should not be used to make the anesthesiologist more comfortable.

Oral medications are preferred by some patients to "another needle." Timing of administration is important. If a premedicant is to be given orally, it should be given early enough to be working by the time anxiety-provoking preparations begin. Oral drugs must therefore be given 1 to 2 hours in advance. Supervised administration of the pill to ensure a limited fluid intake is preferable. The anxious patient who regularly takes a sedative at home may on occasion be permitted to continue his or her chronic medication, with appropriate preoperative instruction. The oral premedication chosen should have a duration of action adequate to continue until insertion of the regional block and surgery, but sufficiently limited neither to interfere with patients' ability to comprehend postoperative instructions nor to delay resumption of usual activities. Intramuscular premedication is not recommended, since a similarly tardy onset and duration of effect is obtained only after a painful injection well before the procedure.

Premedication can also be given intravenously, shortly before the local or regional anesthetic. This is the preferred route, since it avoids the need for the patient to be in the ambulatory unit for a long time before operation. The patient is not chemically sedated before preparations begin, but medication is given promptly after venipuncture and is soon effective. The patient becomes relaxed and is more prepared for the insertion of the regional block. Intravenous sedation should be given in small, incremental doses and the effect titrated carefully. Intravenous premedication can then be continued as intraoperative sedation. Intraoperative supplementation may be given in repeated small doses or as a continuous infusion. Administration by continuous infusion may result in lower total drug dose and fewer side-effects. However, close attention is needed for frequent readjustment of dosage and infusion rate in response to changing surgical stimulation. Use of a predetermined continuous infusion rate may result in inappropriate dosing.

Is amnesia an appropriate attribute of ambulatory premedication? Brief amnesia may be useful during painful or lengthy series of local anesthetic injections. Thompson[118] noted that patients who appeared in distress during endoscopy, but who did not remember it as unpleasant because of supplemental medication, were satisfied with their experience. Drug choice and dosage remain important. It should also be emphasized that a lack of recall of perioperative events may be disturbing to some patients, particularly those who chose regional anesthesia to remain in contact with the proceedings.

Perhaps the most effective and innocuous premedication for ambulatory regional anesthesia is verbal reassurance. Egbert et al reported that the patients who were visited by an anesthesiologist and received an explanation of what was to happen were not drowsy but were subjectively and objectively calm.[46] Many patients facing surgery, particularly those facing minor surgery on the genitourinary tract, are afraid of the procedure, anesthesia, and possible complications. Patients are afraid of the unknown, of general hazards including pain, injury, and death, and of specific hazards such as nausea, vomiting, and loss of consciousness and control. Fear of local or regional anesthesia may stem from a lack of understanding of what is involved. This fear is best combated by providing knowledge and information.

Verbal reassurance does not end when the block is inserted. Reassurance and explanations must continue throughout the operation so that the regional anesthesia patient remains calm. Need for supplemental medications will thereby be decreased. The patient can be helped to remain calm by limiting surgery-related noise of instruments and loud conversation. Distraction with music through headphones is frequently used in our institution to supplement regional anesthesia. The patient is requested to bring in tapes of preferred music. Alternatively, the institution may provide a modest assortment of music of different styles. Radio or taped music played over speakers in the operating room is also useful but is less effective, becoming part of the general background clatter.

The ambulatory surgery patient receiving regional rather than general anesthesia must be more in control of anxieties and fears in order to cooperate in making surgery under block successful. The ambulatory regional patient cannot simply accede passively to preparations until consciousness is lost. There is, therefore, more of a need for premedication and supplemental sedation in the regional anesthesia patient. Certain characteristics of regional blocks and their administration and maintenance also recommend the use of supplemental medication. Regional blocks can be painful on insertion and, once in effect, may not be able to obliterate all sensation, particularly from the viscera. Supplemental medication can also help the patient to lie still for relatively long periods of time on a hard operating table. The use of sedation increases the acceptability of regional anesthesia for patients who do not desire to be completely awake in the operating room. In the absence of a general anesthetic, judiciously given premedicants are less likely to delay a patient's discharge.

Tables 6-1 and 6-2 provide summaries of approximate drug dosages.

☐ Table 6-1. Use of Selected Drugs for Premedication and Supplemental Sedation

Class	Drug	Suggested Dose
Ataractics	Diazepam	
	Oral	0.07–0.15 mg/kg
	IV	0.05–0.15 mg/kg
	Midazolam, IV	0.03–0.15 mg/kg
	Droperidol, IV	8–17 µg/kg
Analgesics	Fentanyl, IV	1–3 µg/kg
	Alfentanil, IV	5–20 µg/kg
Inhalation analgesia	Nitrous oxide	30%–50%
	Enflurane	0.5%
Temporary loss of consciousness	Thiopental, IV	1–4 mg/kg
	Methohexital, IV	0.5–2 mg/kg
	Midazolam, IV	0.2–0.25 mg/kg
	Ketamine, IV	0.5 mg/kg

ATARACTICS

DIAZEPAM

Diazepam is the benzodiazepine most widely used for premedication and supplemental sedation. Diazepam is well absorbed orally, and serum drug levels correlate with clinical effect.[40,66] Relaxation and drowsiness are seen 10 to 15 minutes after a 10-mg dose. Diazepam is suitable for oral premedication; 5 mg, or 10 mg for the large or very anxious patient, may be given an hour before the procedure and preparation. Use of larger doses will result in prolonged drowsiness.

The intravenous route is preferred for rapid preoperative effect. Diazepam, 10 mg, given intravenously resulted in clinical sedation within 2 to 3 minutes. Peak serum drug levels were three times those noted after oral administration.[7] Intravenous doses of diazepam should be decreased accordingly, to avoid excessive effect. For premedication and supplemental sedation, diazepam in 2.5 mg increments should be used. It should also be remembered to allow 3 minutes for the drug to take effect before administering more, to avoid oversedation. The total dose of intravenous diazepam should be limited to avoid prolonged

☐ Table 6-2. Use of Supplemental Drugs by Continuous Infusion

Drug	Concentration (ml^{-1})	Loading Dose (kg^{-1})	Maintenance (kg^{-1} · min^{-1})
Alfentanil	10 µg	8 µg	1 µg
Fentanyl	2 µg	1.6 µg	0.1 µg
Ketamine	1 mg	0.8 mg	50 µg
Methohexital	1–2 mg	0.5–2 mg	.15 mg
Thiopental	3–5 mg	1–4 mg	.3 mg

effects. Ataxia and dizziness sufficient to delay discharge were present in 8% and 16% of subjects, respectively, 1 hour after administration of 10 mg.[7] After 20 mg, these causes of delayed discharge were present in 40% and 30% of subjects, respectively. Tests of coordination and reaction time were abnormal until 6 hours after 0.15 mg/kg intravenous diazepam.[68] Individual dose response is widely variable, and drug requirement is less in the elderly.

The major drawback of diazepam administered intravenously for supplemental sedation is local pain and phlebitis. A faster rate of injection is associated with a higher incidence of pain. Flushing the vein vigorously with saline may reduce thrombophlebitis.[69]

Diazepam to supplement regional anesthesia is given by some until slurred speech and drooping eyelids occurs. This has resulted in doses averaging 0.31 mg/kg for dental procedures[53] and 0.45 mg/kg for outpatient endoscopies.[142] Korttila and Linnoila studied the effect of 0.30 and 0.45 mg/kg diazepam on skills related to driving.[68] Although a negative Romberg test was achieved after 36 minutes, impairment of coordination and reactive skills persisted until 10 hours. Tests of attention were minimally affected. Narcotics are often given in conjunction with diazepam to supplement sedation; this combination delays the return of normal function. Patients should be cautioned not to drive or operate dangerous machinery for 10 hours after sedation with diazepam and 24 hours after diazepam with long-acting narcotics.[67]

Clinical overdoses of diazepam may be given accidently; various antagonists have been tried. Naloxone, 0.4 mg, physostigmine, 1 mg to 2 mg, and aminophylline, 1 mg/kg, have all been used with inconsistent success and with significant side-effects including nausea, vomiting, changes in blood pressure, and cardiac dysrhythmias. The routine use of any of the above drugs to antagonize diazepam effects is not recommended. Specific benzodiazepine antagonists are being investigated.

Diazepam is particularly useful as premedication before regional anesthesia, since it has been shown to increase the seizure threshold for lidocaine.[37] This should not be construed as a reason to increase the dose of local anesthetic given. Diazepam should not be given without monitoring respiration. Doses of 0.14 mg/kg intravenously depressed the ventilatory response to CO_2, increased the dead space to tidal volume ratio, and increased arterial pCO_2. These effects were present within 1 minute and lasted 25 to 30 minutes.[59] Depression of ventilatory response correlated with drowsiness.

Benzodiazepines are noteworthy for their ability to cause amnesia. This effect is least marked after oral premedication. Intravenous diazepam is a more reliable amnesic. Lack of recall after 5 mg to 10 mg intravenous diazepam developed in 50% and 90% of patients, respectively. The percentage of volunteers who developed amnesia was increased by accelerating the rate of diazepam injection and by increasing the dose.[69] Anterograde amnesia was present at 1 minute, peaked at 2 to 3 minutes, and persisted for approximately 30 minutes. Retrograde amnesia after intravenous diazepam has been variably reported. Diazepam given intravenously may be used to produce brief amnesia in the ambulatory surgery patient receiving regional anesthesia, as for the insertion of the block. Although 10-mg intravenous bolus doses have been studied, the use of 2.5-mg increments is preferred in the ambulatory patient, to avoid oversedation. This may limit the amnesia obtained. It should also be remembered that some patients become distressed when they cannot recall perioperative events; this effect should be discussed with the patient in advance. Midazolam will be discussed later in this chapter under Temporary Obtundation of Consciousness.

DROPERIDOL

Droperidol has been used for many years as a supplement to surgical and diagnostic procedures under local or regional anesthesia. This butyrophenone derivative produces sedation and a sense of detachment. Amnesia is minimal. Droperidol does not significantly affect respiration, although wide individual variation of response occurs.[101] When droperidol is administered with a narcotic, neuroleptanalgesia results. Early enthusiastic use of droperidol alone and in neurolept combinations generated many reports of complications including prolonged and excessive sedation, hypotension, extrapyramidal symptoms, and apprehension and anxiety despite apparent drowsiness.[48,60] Studies included use of the drug for premedication and for supplementation. Doses given were 2.5 mg to 10 mg in adults; similar effects were seen at similar doses in children, 0.1 to 0.17 mg/kg.[43] Patients sometimes became anxious, agitated, and confused to the extent that they cancelled previously desired elective surgery. The incidence of refusal was 4.7% in a series of 121 military patients for plastic surgery[14] and 0.7% in a series of 1438 private patients scheduled for sterilization or plastic procedures.[72]

Droperidol, 2.5 mg/ml, is sold alone and in combination with fentanyl, 0.05 mg/ml, as Innovar (Janssen Pharmaceutica, New Brunswick, New Jersey). In general, this combination is not appropriate for premedication or sedation of ambulatory patients undergoing regional anesthesia. The dose of butyrophenone is too large and the effect too long-acting relative to the short-acting analgesic.

Droperidol is a potent antiemetic. Lower doses of 0.005 to 0.017 mg/kg (0.625–1.25 mg in adults) have been shown to be significantly effective in reducing the incidence of postoperative vomiting in adults and children.[108,128] Excessive sedation, extrapyramidal symptoms, or anxiety were not seen. The use of low-dose droperidol can therefore be recommended for the ambulatory local or regional anesthesia patient.

ANALGESICS

FENTANYL

Fentanyl is a potent narcotic analgesic cogener of meperidine. After intravenous administration, analgesia began within 2 minutes and lasted 30 to 60 minutes.[82] Termination of effect was due to redistribution into blood and peripheral tissues; the redistribution half-life of fentanyl was 13.4 minutes. Of the injected dose, 98.6% was cleared from plasma in 60 minutes. These rapid drug kinetics illustrate why fentanyl has become the narcotic of choice to supplement ambulatory surgery regional anesthesia. Fentanyl is effective both when given before the insertion of a block and when used to supplement the maintenance of local or regional anesthesia. Increments of 25 μg to 50 μg fentanyl may be given intravenously to achieve desired analgesia, with an initial dose totaling 50 μg to 200 μg (1–3 μg/kg). Additional doses may be given in 30 to 60 minutes as clinically indicated. The elderly require reduced drug doses. If an ongoing need for fentanyl supplementation of regional anesthesia is anticipated, the continuous infusion technique may be advantageous.[129]

OTHER OPIOIDS

The need for an even shorter-acting narcotic than fentanyl resulted in the synthesis of alfentanil and sufentanil. The pharmacokinetics of alfentanil suggest that it be used by continuous infusion for the supplementation of ambulatory surgery regional anesthesia.[12]

Some longer-acting opioid analgesics have been popular in specific institutions, usually as a holdover from inpatient use. Morphine and meperidine are two such drugs. The use of longer-acting opioids results in a longer duration of sedation and of other side-effects such as nausea and dizziness. Meperidine in particular is not recommended for outpatient use. Intramuscular meperidine is associated with syncope after standing up. Tests of coordination and reaction time remain abnormal 12 hours after the administration of 75 mg meperidine.[67] The use of longer-acting opioid analgesics should be avoided as premedication or supplementation for the ambulatory regional anesthesia patient.

INHALATION ANALGESIA

Anesthetic gases and vapors administered at subanesthetic concentrations provide analgesia and sedation. These effects can be used to supplement local and regional anesthesia for the ambulatory surgery patient. Advantages of inhalation over intravenous analgesia are related to the mode of drug administration—ventilation through the lung. These advantages include rapid reversibility and easier maintenance of a constant blood concentration and therefore constant anesthetic effect.[98] A disadvantage is the need to administer the gas or vapor through a tight-fitting mask or mouthpiece, to avoid contamination of operating room air. Inhalation analgesia is particularly useful for minor surgery on closed-space infections, which are difficult to block with local anesthetic.[50] Pediatric, adult, and mentally retarded patients are all satisfactory candidates.

Most inhalation anesthetic agents have been used for analgesia. Trichlorethylene and chloroform are no longer commercially available. Diethyl ether and cyclopropane are not recommended for the ambulatory surgery setting because they are flammable. Halothane is not effective for analgesia at subanesthetic concentration.[42] Agents currently in use for inhalation analgesia include nitrous oxide, enflurane, and methoxyflurane.

Methoxyflurane is effective for inhalation analgesia given intermittently at concentrations of 0.2% to 0.5% (1.2–3.1 MAC).[23] However, onset of analgesia and recovery are relatively slow because of high blood solubility. In addition, methoxyflurane is metabolized in part to inorganic fluoride, and serum fluoride levels above 50 μM/l have been associated with polyuric renal failure. This level has been reached in patients self-administering methoxyflurane for obstetric analgesia.[79] The use of methoxyflurane analgesia for ambulatory surgery regional anesthesia patients is not recommended, because of its slow effect and the possibility of renal damage.

Nitrous oxide has achieved widespread popularity particularly as an adjunct to dental regional anesthesia. Concentrations of 10% to 60% in oxygen are used. Onset of analgesia is rapid, as is termination of the effect once administration ceases.[42] Psychomotor effects have also been studied.[64] During the inhalation of 30% end-tidal nitrous oxide, impairment of word recall, the ability to do arithmetic problems, and eye-hand coordination were seen. Impairment was maximal 7 minutes after beginning inhalation and remained at that level for the half-hour of gas administration. Subjects reported a significant increase in physical and mental sedation and in relief of tension (relaxation). Recovery of normal function was complete 22 minutes after administration ceased. An appropriate period of postanesthetic supervision is necessary for any ambulatory patient after nitrous oxide inhalation.

Subanesthetic concentrations of enflurane have also been used for supplemental analgesia. Enflurane was shown to impair digit memory, audiovisual reaction time, and manual dexterity at concentrations greater than .09 MAC (0.15% alveolar).[25] Dose-related amnesia was also seen. At 0.24 MAC enflurane (0.4% alveolar and 0.53% inspired), sufficient drowsiness developed to preclude completing the tests. Abboud et al reported similar maximal levels for effective analgesia without loss of consciousness at approximately 0.5% inspired enflurane or 40% inspired nitrous oxide in obstetric patients.[1] Satisfactory analgesia was reported by 89% and 76% of the parturients for the two agents, respectively; the difference was not significant. Complete amnesia (of delivery) developed in 7% and 10% of patients, respectively. Inhalation analgesia to supplement regional anesthesia may be obtained by using 30% to 40% nitrous oxide or 0.5% enflurane; impairment of psychomotor abilities and sometimes amnesia occur at these doses.

The actual percentage of nitrous oxide reaching the patient, and therefore level of analgesia obtainable, is very dependent on the method of administration. Lichtenthal et al used the ratio of nitrous oxide concentration delivered to the system to the steady-state end-expiratory concentration as a measure of the efficiency of several delivery systems.[73] Nasal prongs at 7 to 8 Liters/min delivered only 19% of the preset concentration: administered "50%" nitrous oxide reached the patient as 9%. A see-through rebreathing mask, such as might be used during regional anesthesia, delivered 34% of preset concentration; with this device, administered "50%" yielded 17% end-expired nitrous oxide. To achieve expired concentration approaching that preset, 95% to 98%, a tight-fitting nonrebreathing mask was needed. The true yield of nitrous oxide from a dental-type nasal mask will depend as well on what fraction of respiration occurs through the nose and on how much nitrous oxide is entrained through the nose during oral respiration.

Patient-controlled self-administration of nitrous oxide or methoxyflurane has also been used to provide supplemental analgesia and sedation. Inhalers are available that will deliver 0.3% to 0.9% methoxyflurane in air,[23] or 50% nitrous oxide in oxygen, either premixed[115] or from tandem cylinders.[50] A supposed safety advantage of these devices is the need for patient cooperation in maintaining a tight mouthpiece or mask seal in order to receive anesthetic.[23,115] This is intended to limit excessive anesthesia, with resultant risks of excitement, vomiting, and aspiration. Such failsafes can, of course, be circumvented, as by propping the inhaler on a pillow. Furthermore, methoxyflurane inhalers are able to deliver concentrations of several times 1 MAC, sufficient to produce surgical anesthesia if inspired continuously. Patient-controlled devices are intended to be safe enough to use without an anesthesiologist present. However, the patient receiving self-administered inhalation analgesia still requires a trained individual in constant attendance; this attendant must terminate or decrease the anesthetic if drowsiness, confusion, or excitement develops. Devices for self-administered inhalation analgesia should not be used in "local rooms" of an ambulatory surgery suite without such precautions.

The degree of analgesia obtained is strongly influenced by the expectation of pain or its relief. Pain threshold and tolerance of electrical tooth pulp stimulation are ordinarily increased with 33% inhaled nitrous oxide.[44] Patients were given suggestions that nitrous oxide causes an enhanced sensitivity and awareness of body sensations; afterwards, pain responses were actually heightened during gas inhalation. On the other hand, establishing an expectation of the analgesic effectiveness of nitrous oxide will reduce perceived pain. More subjective relief and decreased anxiety were obtained using the same 15% to 45% inhaled nitrous oxide when the dental stimulation was performed in a pain-research laboratory rather than in a dental clinic.[45] Anxiety and expectation of pain can be reduced by eliminating stressful environments.

Side-effects of nitrous oxide inhalation analgesia have been reported. Lichtenthal et al reported that concentrations of over 30% sometimes caused excitement.[73] Stewart et al[115] evaluated 50% nitrous oxide in oxygen. They reported a 20.6% incidence of minor side-effects, including nausea or vomiting (5.7%), dizziness or lightheadedness (10.3%), excitement (3.7%), and numbness (0.3%).[115] These authors did not include as complications the 7.6% of patients who became drowsy or fell lightly asleep. Oversedation can, however, eliminate one of the advantages of inhalation analgesia—the preservation of airway reflexes. Twenty percent of patients breathing 50% nitrous oxide in oxygen through a nasal mask aspirated dye placed in the mouth during simulated dental treatment.[110]

TEMPORARY OBTUNDATION OF CONSCIOUSNESS

BARBITURATES

Regional anesthetic blocks can be painful when administered. Administration may become uncomfortable when multiple injections are needed, as with intercostal nerve blocks. A particularly sensitive operative area may be involved, as with anorectal procedures. Also, a combination of both factors may be present, as with the multiple injections required for facial cosmetic surgery. One technique for alleviating the discomfort of these situations is the administration of intravenous agents that will briefly obtund consciousness and prevent memory.

The barbiturates are well-suited for this purpose. Thiopental induces unconsciousness after 1 to 4 mg/kg injected slowly. A single bolus of 2.6 mg/kg caused sleep lasting for 120 seconds,[47] during which local or regional anesthesia may be established. Five minutes after injection of this bolus, subjects were able to walk and answer questions. Use of larger doses leads to prolongation of recovery. Thiopental may also be administered as a 0.3% to 0.5% solution, suitable to eliminate awareness during the maintenance of a regional anesthetic.[130] Recovery after a 4-mg/kg loading dose plus 428 mg of thiopental infusion, given over 21 minutes, required 10 minutes to awakening, 20 minutes to orientation, and 1.9 hours until patients were fit for discharge.

One other barbiturate has gained widespread acceptance in ambulatory anesthesia and is useful to supplement regional blockade. This barbiturate is methohexital. Methohexital is administered in a dose of 0.5 to 2 mg/kg to induce sleep. After a single bolus of 0.88 mg/kg, volunteers slept for 143 seconds. Recovery is more rapid than after thiopental,[47] and after larger or cumulative doses, the relative advantage of methohexital over thiopental became even more pronounced. Methohexital may also be used in a 0.1% to 0.2% solution for continuous infusion to maintain basal narcosis during regional anesthesia. Smaller total doses and speedier recovery would be expected with this mode of administration. With intravenous fentanyl premedication, methohexital is the barbiturate of choice to obtund consciousness and supplement regional anesthesia for ambulatory patients.

Methohexital has been widely used by dentists to supplement regional anesthesia. Narcotic and sedative premedication, usually including diazepam, are employed in conjunction with the barbiturate. A typical combination included 5-mg to 15-mg diazepam, in increments, until the patient was sedated, then methohexital in 5-mg to 10-mg increments, during which the local anesthetic was injected and the procedure performed. Perception of painful tooth stimulation was not abolished under barbiturate sedation, even with the addition of alphaprodine 30 mg;[49] local analgesia must be used. Patients remained conscious and able to obey commands, but complete amnesia of the injection and procedure were usually reported. Under this combined-drug sedation, significant decreases in cardiac output (21%), cardiac rate (30%), and minute work (28%) were found in volunteers.[49] As would be expected, recovery was prolonged. Performance of the Trieger dot test had recovered to normal by 3 hours, but tests of perceptual and cognitive ability revealed that residual impairment was still present at that time.[54]

MIDAZOLAM

Midazolam may be useful to blunt consciousness temporarily during ambulatory surgery regional anesthesia. The half-life and therapeutic effect of midazolam are shorter than those of other available benzodiazepines, 60 to 90 minutes.[24,106] Secondary increases in plasma concentration have not been seen. Another major advantage of this drug is its water solubility and therefore minimal pain or venous irritation. Successful trials of midazolam for premedication and sedation encouraged the evaluation of its use as a short-acting sleep-inducing agent. To obtund consciousness during the insertion of a regional block, an injection of 0.20 to 0.25 mg/kg midazolam may be necessary. A wide variability in induction dose requirement has been noted.

A dose of 0.1 to 0.15 mg/kg midazolam is effective in achieving basal sedation.[24,52] Drowsiness lasted for 128 minutes in volunteers who received 0.15 mg/kg midazolam. 50% of the subjects lost consciousness with this dose for an average duration of 304 seconds. Apnea occurred in 40% of patients and lasted for 30 seconds. Amnesic effect is significant. After 0.15 mg/kg, 100% of subjects developed anterograde amnesia for 40 minutes; they did not remember standing or walking at 22 minutes.

KETAMINE

Ketamine is another agent that has been used to blunt consciousness temporarily during administration of regional anesthesia. In a dose of 2 mg/kg, ketamine produced excellent sedation for the insertion of intercostal blocks.[132] However, unpleasant emergence reactions are consistently a problem with high doses of ketamine. Delirium, vivid hallucinations, and unpleasant dreams have been reported in up to 40% of patients; symptoms may recur for several weeks. In order to decrease the incidence of these reactions, lower doses of ketamine have been tried.

Bovill and Dundee reported that analgesia persisted up to 40 minutes after ketamine anesthesia had terminated.[11] It was also observed that subanesthetic doses of parenteral ketamine, approximately 0.5 mg/kg, could be used for postoperative analgesia.[111] At this lower dose, analgesia developed within 5 minutes after intramuscular injection and lasted 60 to 90 minutes. Side-effects were experienced by 35% of patients, but were of lesser severity. Dizziness, incoordination, blurred vision, and difficulty in communication were most common, but one case of severe agitation was also reported. Patients remained conscious and oriented. Ketamine analgesia is also effective by the oral route, with a longer onset of action, 30 minutes.

On the basis of this subdissociative analgesic effect, ketamine at low doses (0.4–0.5 mg/kg) has been used before administering local anesthesia. In a series of 200 plastic surgery patients, 87% had significant amnesia and no unpleasant memories. An additional 8.5% had unpleasant memories but were cooperative. One patient had unpleasant dreams for 3 days after surgery. It should be noted that this low dose was inadequate for maintenance of the procedure; injection of local or regional anesthesia was required during the period of amnesia.[126]

Various premedications have been tried in order to decrease the incidence of unpleasant emergence reactions. Combinations of droperidol, opiates, and scopolamine have all been shown to decrease emergence delirium and dreams. Benzodiazepines are the most effective, whether given as premedication or at the end of the procedure. This may be due to their ability to generate amnesia;[132] patient acceptance of ketamine is not related to an observer's report of difficult induction or emergence delirium. Diazepam, 5 mg to 10 mg is the agent of choice.[12,65] Patients who received 0.15 mg/kg diazepam with 0.5 mg/kg ketamine for supplementation after regional anesthetic blockade had a similar incidence of dreaming and similar postoperative nursing care needs compared with control patients receiving no supplementation. However, the incidence of visual disturbances remained high. Increasing the dose of diazepam to 30 mg resulted in more postoperative anxiety, confusion, and terrifying dreams, and in a need for increased postoperative nursing supervision.

Lorazepam, 4 mg, is highly effective by any route of administration in reducing ketamine sequelae and greatly improving patient acceptance. The combination of lorazepam with ketamine led to prolongation of recovery, however, and is not recommended for ambulatory surgery patients.

A chemical derivative of phencyclidine, ketamine may also have significant abuse potential as a hallucinogen. It should be avoided in patients with a history of psychiatric problems. This drug has several additional disadvantages as a supplement for ambulatory regional anesthesia. It is associated with increased postoperative vomiting. Airway reflexes are not consistently preserved, and there is a risk of aspiration.[117] Any drugs used to treat vomiting or emergence symptoms prolong the duration of anesthetic action, making ketamine less suitable for ambulatory surgery patients. Despite the administration of ketamine by low-dose infusion and the selection of appropriate premedication, emergence reactions remain a significant issue. Specific indications should be weighed before ketamine is used for supplementation of ambulatory regional anesthesia.

Local Anesthetic Drugs

Local anesthesia, like many other therapeutic modalities, originated among the natives of South America. In 1860, cocaine was isolated from the leaves of a Peruvian bush *Erythroxylon coca* but its medicinal use remained obscure until 1884, when Koller reported the use of cocaine for topical anesthesia in ophthalmology. Since that time, numerous topical and injectable anesthetic agents have been introduced, and several may be used for ambulatory anesthesia. Local anesthetic drugs are unique, since they produce a loss of sensation and muscle paralysis in a circumscribed area of the body by a localized effect on peripheral nerve endings or fibers.

MECHANISM OF LOCAL ANESTHESIA

Neural excitation depends on depolarization of the nerve membrane from a resting potential of approximately −90 mV to a threshold potential level of approximately −60 mV. Attainment of the threshold potential results in spontaneous and complete nerve depolarization followed by a phase of repolarization that leads to reestablishment of the original resting potential. This entire process occurs within 1 msec, the depolarization phase being completed in 0.3 msec and repolarization requiring 0.7 msec. Nerve conduction requires only that depolarization occur in a localized segment of nerve which, in turn, will activate the adjacent segment such that a self-perpetuating wave of depolarization will proceed along the entire length of the nerve fibers.

The changes in membrane potential during and after nerve excitation are related to changes in permeability of the cell membrane to various electrolytes, particularly sodium and potassium. During depolarization, sodium permeability increases, allowing sodium ions to flow passively from the extracellular space into the cell. Repolarization is associated with a decrease in sodium permeability, which results in a passive efflux of potassium ions from the interior to the exterior of the cell membrane. At the conclusion of the repolarization phase, the "sodium-potassium" pump actively extrudes sodium from inside the nerve cell and returns potassium to the intracellular space.

Local anesthetic drugs interfere with the initial step in the excitation-conduction process by decreasing the rate and degree of depolarization without altering the resting potential, threshold potential, or repolarization phase.[28] When the degree of depolarization is sufficiently depressed that the threshold potential is not achieved, then a propagated action potential fails to develop and nerve conduction is blocked. Since depolarization is related to an influx of sodium ion from the exterior of the cell, it was logical to assume that local anesthetics depress depolarization by inhibiting sodium conductance across the membrane. Indeed, all local anesthetics tested markedly decrease sodium permeability with minimal effects on potassium flux. Isolation of the biotoxin tetrodotoxin from puffer fish ovaries provided the most convincing evidence for the mechanism of local anesthesia. This substance, which specifically inhibits sodium conductance and nerve depolarization alone, is the most potent local anesthetic substance studied to date in animal models.

In summary, the mechanism of action of local anesthetic agents is related to the following sequence of events:

Binding of local anesthetic molecules to receptor sites in the nerve membranes

Reduction in sodium permeability
Decrease in the rate of depolarization
Failure to achieve threshold potential level
Lack of development of a propagated action potential
Conduction blockade

The receptor site for local anesthetic agents is believed to reside at the nerve membrane. However, the specific receptor location varies according to the type of local anesthetic employed. The conventional agents, such as lidocaine and procaine, are believed to bind at receptor sites located on the inner surface of the nerve membrane. Biotoxins, such as tetrodotoxin and saxitoxin, act at receptor sites located on the external surface of the membrane. Finally, agents such as benzocaine and benzyl alcohol act by penetrating the nerve membrane, causing membrane expansion and a decrease in the diameter of the sodium channel.

ACTIVE FORM OF LOCAL ANESTHETIC AGENTS

Most of the clinically useful anesthetic preparations are available in the form of solutions of a salt; lidocaine, for example, is usually prepared as an 0.5% to 2.0% solutions of lidocaine hydrochloride. In solution, the salts of these local anesthetic compounds exist as uncharged molecules (B) and as positively charged cations (BH^+). The relative proportion between the uncharged base (B) and charged cation (BH^+) depends on the pK_a of the specific chemical compound and the pH of the solution, that is, $pH = pK_a - \log (BH^+/B)$. Since pK_a is constant for any specific compound, the relative proportion of free base and charged cation depends essentially on the pH of the local anesthetic solution ($BH^+ \rightleftharpoons B + H^+$). As the pH of the solution is decreased and H^+ concentration increased, the equilibrium will shift toward the charged cationic form, more cation will be present than free base. Conversely, as the pH is increased and H^+ concentration decreased, the equilibrium will be shifted toward the free base form and more of the local anesthetic agent will exist in the free base form. Both the uncharged base form (B) and the charged cationic form (BH^+) of local anesthetic agents are involved in the process of conduction block. The uncharged base form diffuses more easily through the nerve sheath and so is required for optimal penetration, which is reflected clinically in onset of anesthesia. Following diffusion through the epineurium, equilibrium reoccurs between B and BH^+, and the charged cation actually binds to the receptor site in the nerve membrane. Therefore, the cationic form is ultimately responsible for the suppression of electrophysiologic events in peripheral nerve, which is reflected clinically in the profoundness of anesthesia.

STRUCTURE-ACTIVITY RELATIONSHIP

Chemical compounds that demonstrate local anesthetic activity usually possess the following chemical arrangement:

Aromatic portion—Intermediate chain—Amine portion

The agents of clinical importance can be categorized into two distinct chemical groups. Local anesthetics with an ester link between the aromatic portion and the intermediate chain are referred to as aminoesters and include procaine, chloroprocaine, and tetracaine. Local anesthetics with an amide link between the aromatic end and intermediate chain are referred to as amino-amides and include lidocaine, mepivacaine, prilocaine, bupivacaine, and etido-caine. The basic differences between the ester and amide compounds reside in the manner in which they are metabolized and their allergic potential. The ester agents are hydrolyzed in plasma by pseudocholinesterase, whereas the amide compounds undergo enzymatic degradation in the liver. Para-aminobenzoic acid is one of the metabolites formed from the hydrolysis of ester-like compounds. This substance is capable of inducing allergic reactions in a small percentage of the general population and so is responsible for the allergies reported in association with ester-like local anesthetic agents. The amide, lidocaine-like drugs are not metabolized to para-aminobenzoic acid, and reports of allergic phenomena with these agents are extremely rare.

Chemical alterations within a homologous group produce quantitative changes in physicochemical properties such as lipid solubility and protein-binding that can alter the anesthetic properties of the compounds (Table 6-3). For example, within the ester series, the addition of a butyl group to the aromatic end of the procaine molecule increases lipid solubility and protein-binding and results in tetracaine, a compound that has a greater intrinsic anesthetic potency and longer duration of anesthetic activity. In the amide series, the addition of a butyl group to the amine end of mepivacaine transforms this agent into bupivacaine, a compound that is more lipid soluble, is more highly protein bound, and biologically possesses a greater intrinsic potency and longer duration of action. In the case of lidocaine, substitution of a propyl for an ethyl group at the amine end and addition of an ethyl group to the alpha carbon in the intermediate chain yield etidocaine, which is more lipid soluble, more highly protein bound, and, biologically, a local anesthetic agent of greater potency and longer duration.

On the basis of differences in anesthetic potency and duration of action, it is possible to classify the clinically useful injectable local anesthetic compounds into three categories:

Group I—agents of low anesthetic potency and short duration of action (procaine and chloroprocaine)

Group II—agents of intermediate anesthetic potency and duration of action (lidocaine, mepivacaine and prilocaine)

Group III—agents of high anesthetic potency and long duration of action (tetracaine, bupivacaine, and etidocaine). These are rarely used for ambulatory surgery anesthesia.

PHYSIOLOGIC DISPOSITION OF LOCAL ANESTHETIC AGENTS

The vascular absorption, tissue distribution, metabolism, and excretion of local anesthetic agents is of particular importance in terms of their potential toxicity.[119] Absorption varies as a function of site of injection, dosage, addition of a vasoconstrictor agent, and specific agents employed. Absorption occurs most rapidly after intercostal nerve blockade, followed by injection into the caudal canal, lumbar epidural space, brachial plexus and sciatic femoral sites, and

☐ **Table 6-3. Chemical Structure and Physicochemical and Anesthetic Properties of Various Local Anesthetic Agents**

	Chemical Structure			Lipid Solubility	Protein Binding	pKa	In Vitro Potency	Anesthetic Duration	Onset Time
	Aromatic End	Intermediate Chain	Amine End						
AMINO ESTERS									
Procaine	H₂N—	—COOCH₂CH₂—N	C₂H₅ / C₂H₅	1	5	8.9	1	Short	Slow
2-Chloroprocaine	H₂N— (Cl)	—COOCH₂CH₂—N	C₂H₅ / C₂H₅	1	?	9.1	2	Short	Fast
Tetracaine	H₉C₄ N—H	—COOCH₂CH₂—N	CH₃ / CH₃	80	85	8.6	16	Long	Slow
AMINO AMIDES									
Lidocaine	CH₃ / CH₃	NHCOCH₂—N	C₂H₅ / C₂H₅	4	65	7.7	4	Moderate	Fast
Prilocaine	CH₃	NHCOCH—N	C₃H₇ / H, CH₃	1.5	55	7.7	3	Moderate	Fast
Etidocaine	CH₃ / CH₃	NHCOCH—N (C₂H₅)	C₂H₅ / C₃H₇	140	95	7.7	16	Long	Fast
Mepivacaine	CH₃ / CH₃	NHCO—N (CH₃)		1	75	7.6	2	Moderate	Fast
Bupivacaine	CH₃ / CH₃	NHCO—N (C₄H₉)		30	95	8.1	16	Long	Moderate

subcutaneous tissue. For example, the intercostal administration of 400 mg of lidocaine without epinephrine results in an average peak venous plasma level of approximately 7 μg/ml, whereas the same dose of lidocaine employed for brachial plexus block yields a mean maximum blood level of approximately 3.5 μg/ml.

The blood level of local anesthetic agents is related to the total dose of drug administered rather than the specific volume or concentration of solution employed. A linear relationship tends to exist between the amount of drug administered and the peak anesthetic blood level. For example, the maximum blood level of lidocaine increases from approximately 1.5 μg/ml to 4 μg/ml as the total dose administered into the lumbar epidural space is raised from 200 mg to 600 mg. Depending on the site of administration, a peak blood level of 0.5 to 2 μg/ml is achieved for each 100 mg of lidocaine or mepivacaine injected.

Addition of a vasoconstrictor to local anesthetic solutions decreases the rate of absorption of certain agents from various sites of administration. Epinephrine

(1:200,000), 5 μg/ml, significantly reduces the peak blood levels of lidocaine and mepivacaine, irrespective of the site of administration. Epinephrine decreases the peak blood levels of prilocaine, bupivacaine, and etidocaine achieved after peripheral nerve blocks, but has little influence on the absorption of these drugs following lumbar epidural administration. Phenylephrine and norepinephrine (1:20,000) can also reduce local anesthetic absorption, but not as effectively as epinephrine 1:200,000.

The rate and degree of vascular absorption varies among various agents. Lidocaine and mepivacaine are absorbed more rapidly than prilocaine, whereas bupivacaine is absorbed more rapidly than etidocaine. The lower blood levels of prilocaine probably reflect its tendency to produce less vasodilation than lidocaine or mepivacaine. The lower peak blood levels of etidocaine compared to bupivacaine may be related to the greater lipid solubility and uptake by peripheral fat of etidocaine.

Following absorption from injection site, local anesthetic agents distribute throughout total body water. An initial rapid disappearance from blood (alpha phase) occurs, which is related to uptake by rapidly equilibrating tissues, that is, tissues with a high vascular perfusion. A secondary slower disappearance rate (beta phase) reflects distribution to slowly perfused tissue and metabolism and excretion of the compound. The disappearance rate of prilocaine is significantly more rapid than that of lidocaine or mepivacaine. The rate of tissue redistribution for the latter two agents is similar. Although all tissues will take up local anesthetics, the highest concentrations are found in the more highly perfused organs, such as lung and kidney. The greatest percentage of an injected dose of a local anesthetic agent distributes to skeletal muscle because of the large mass of this tissue in the body.

The metabolism of local anesthetic agents varies according to their chemical classification. The ester-like or procaine-like agents undergo hydrolysis in plasma by the enzyme pseudocholinesterase. Chloroprocaine shows the most rapid rat of hydrolysis (4.7 μmol/ml/hr) compared to procaine (1.1 μmol/ml/hr) and tetracaine (0.3 μmol/ml/hr). Less than 2% of unchanged procaine is excreted, whereas approximately 90% of para-aminobenzoic acid, which is the primary metabolite of procaine, appears in urine. On the other hand, only 33% of diethylaminoethanol, the other major metabolite of procaine, is excreted unchanged.

The amide-like or lidocaine-like agents undergo enzymatic degradation primarily in the liver. Prilocaine undergoes the most rapid rate of hepatic metabolism. Lidocaine, mepivacaine, and etidocaine are intermediate in terms of rate of degradation, whereas bupivacaine is metabolized most slowly. Some degradation of the amide-like compounds may occur in non-hepatic tissue as indicated by the formation of certain metabolites following the incubation of prilocaine with kidney slices. Complete metabolism for all the amide compounds has not been elucidated. Lidocaine, which has been studied most extensively, undergoes primarily oxidative de-ethylation to monoethylglycinexylidide, followed by a subsequent hydrolysis to hydroxyxylidine. Less than 5% of unchanged amide-like drugs is excreted into the urine. The major portion of an injected dose appears in the form of various metabolites. For example, 73% of lidocaine can be accounted for in human urine by hydroxyxylidine. The renal clearance of the amide agents is inversely related to their protein-binding capacity. Prilocaine, which has a lower protein-binding capacity than lidocaine, has a substantially higher clearance value than lidocaine. Renal clearance also is inversely proportional to the pH of urine, suggesting urinary excretion by nonionic diffusion.

Anesthetic Techniques

On the basis of anatomic considerations, regional anesthesia for the ambulatory surgery patient may be divided into three categories: infiltration, peripheral nerve blockade (minor and major), and central neural blockade (epidural, caudal, and spinal). Since surgical procedures performed on an ambulatory basis are, by definition, relatively brief, the long-acting local anesthetic agents are rarely used for ambulatory surgery anesthesia. Therefore, the following discussion will be limited to the agents of short or moderate duration. The reader is encouraged to refer to any of the standard anesthesia textbooks for a detailed description of the various anesthetic techniques. Surgical indications for the various techniques are summarized in Table 6-4.

INFILTRATION ANESTHESIA

Infiltration anesthesia involves administration of a local anesthetic agent into an extravascular or intravascular site and subsequent diffusion to nerve endings where excitation is inhibited. Extravascular infiltration anesthesia includes the

☐ **Table 6-4. Surgical Indications for Ambulatory Anesthetic Technique**

Technique	Surgical Indication
INFILTRATION	
Extravascular	Any superficial surgical procedure
	Herniorrhaphy
	Laparoscopy
	Endoscopy
	Postoperative analgesia
Intravascular	Orthopedic or plastic hand procedure
	Orthopedic or plastic foot procedure
PERIPHERAL NERVE BLOCKADE	
Minor nerve block	Orthopedic or plastic hand procedure
	Orthopedic or plastic foot procedure
Major nerve block	Orthopedic procedures involving arm, hand, leg, foot
	Plastic procedures involving arm, hand, leg, foot
	Vascular procedures on arm or leg
CENTRAL NEURAL BLOCKS	
Epidural and spinal	Orthopedic procedures of lower limbs
	Vascular procedures of lower limbs
	Minor gynecologic procedures
	Herniorrhaphy
	Hemorrhoidectomy

□ **Table 6-5.** **Infiltration Anesthesia for Ambulatory Surgery**

Agent	Concen-tration (%)	Plain Solutions			Epinephrine-Containing Solutions		
		Max. Adult Dose (mg)	Max. Dose (mg/kg)	Duration (min)	Max. Adult Dose (mg)	Max. Dose (mg/kg)	Duration (min)
SHORT DURATION							
Procaine Chloroprocaine	1–2	800	11	15–30	1000	14	30–90
MODERATE DURATION							
Lidocaine	0.5–1	300	4	30–60	500	7	120–360
Mepivacaine	0.5–1	300	4	45–90	500	7	120–360
Prilocaine	0.5–1	600	7	30–90	Not available		

injection of local anesthetic into or around the operative site, as well as topical administration to mucous membranes or peritoneum. Intravascular infiltration anesthesia consists of the injection of anesthetic drug into the vasculature of a tourniquet-occluded limb such that the drug cannot enter the central circulatory compartment but instead diffuses from the peripheral vascular bed to nonvascular tissue such as nerve endings.

EXTRAVASCULAR INFILTRATION
In terms of frequency of adequate analgesia, 1% to 2% procaine, 0.5% to 1% lidocaine, 2% chloroprocaine, 0.5% to 1% mepivacaine, and 1% prilocaine are equivalent. Onset of action is almost immediate for all agents following intradermal or subcutaneous administration. Absorption from mucous membranes is almost as rapid as after intravenous injection. However, the various agents can be differentiated according to duration of infiltration anesthesia (Table 6-5). Procaine and chloroprocaine have a short duration, whereas lidocaine, mepivacaine, and prilocaine are agents of moderate duration. Epinephrine may be added to prolong infiltration anesthesia, and thereby provide intraoperative and postoperative analgesia. The effect is most pronounced when epinephrine is added to solutions of lidocaine. Epinephrine should be used in concentrations no higher than 1:200,000. Its use is contraindicated in infiltration anesthesia and minor nerve blocks of the hands, feet, and digits in the presence of coronary artery disease and when blood supply to the area is compromised by severe peripheral vascular disease.

The dosage of a local anesthetic required for adequate infiltration anesthesia depends on the extent of the area to be anesthetized and the expected duration of the surgical procedure. It is frequently necessary to anesthetize large surface areas for surgical procedures performed under infiltration techniques. In order not to exceed the maximum dosage limits of the various agents and thus avoid possible toxic reactions, large volumes of dilute anesthetic solutions should be employed. For example, 500 mg with epinephrine is considered the maximum single dose of lidocaine. Surgical procedures involving a large surface area may require the use of 75 ml to 100 ml of anesthetic solutions. In such a situation a 0.5% solution of lidocaine with epinephrine should be employed rather than the 1% solution. In most infiltration procedures 0.5% lidocaine will provide an adequate depth and duration of analgesia.

For topical administration to mucous membranes, the permissible dose of local anesthetic does not change. However, higher concentrations are needed, such as 4% lidocaine or 1% tetracaine for the oronasopharynx and proximal digestive tract. Therefore, only limited volumes may be used.

Infiltration in and around the surgical site at the end of an operation can provide postoperative analgesia. Patient comfort is greatly increased and recovery-room narcotic requirement decreased. Time to discharge may also be reduced. Extravascular infiltration is effective particularly for anorectal surgery, circumcision, and herniorrhaphy in adults and children. This is one of the indications for a long-acting anesthetic agent in ambulatory anesthesia. Bupivacaine, 0.25%, plain or with epinephrine 1:200,000, will provide 3 to 7 hours of pain relief. Maximum recommended adult doses are 175 mg and 225 mg, respectively.

INTRAVASCULAR INFILTRATION (INTRAVENOUS REGIONAL)

The essential features of intravascular infiltration are its simplicity and relatively rapid disappearance of analgesia following tourniquet release.[32] The procedure involves the intravascular administration of a local anesthetic agent into a tourniquet-occluded limb. It is imperative that the venous flow from the involved limb be completely obstructed in order to prevent the rapid entrance of local anesthetic drug into the central vascular compartment, which could result in serious toxicity. If properly performed, satisfactory analgesia and muscle relaxation are consistently obtained. Only the fingertips are sometimes not anesthetized.

Tourniquet. Both the safety and efficacy of this regional anesthetic procedure depends on the interruption of blood flow to the involved limb. Calibration of the occlusive cuff is of vital importance, since a malfunctioning cuff can lead to inadequate occlusion and potential side-effects due to the rapid introduction of local anesthetic agents into the central circulatory compartment. The tourniquet should be inflated to 100 mm Hg above systolic blood pressure. It should remain inflated for at least 15 to 30 minutes, to permit adequate tissue binding of the anesthetic drug. At the conclusion of surgery, intermittent tourniquet release has been advocated as a means of increasing the safety of this procedure. Since peak blood concentrations of local anesthetic agents occur within 30 seconds following cuff deflation, the cyclic deflation/inflation procedure should take place at 10 to 15 second intervals in order to decrease the peak concentrations of local anesthetic drug in the central circulatory compartment. Use of a double pneumatic cuff also has been advocated as an additional safety precaution and as a means of decreasing ischemic pain associated with the tourniquet. For the latter purpose, analgesia is established with the proximal cuff; the distal cuff is then inflated on the anesthetized limb.

Preinjection Exsanguination. Exsanguination of the involved limb appears to be of value from a safety and efficacy point of view, since less drug is required to achieve adequate anesthesia if the limb has been exsanguinated prior to injection. Most commonly, the extremity is elevated to ensure gravity drainage and then tightly wrapped, distal to proximal, in an Esmarch bandage. When applied prior to the reduction of fracture, compression by the Esmarch bandage may cause pain. A longer period of gravity drainage (5 min) should be used for exsanguination in these cases, instead of the bandage.

Injection Site. The majority of studies of intravenous regional anesthesia have involved surgical procedures on the upper limbs. It is considerably more difficult to obtain a satisfactory degree of surgical analgesia with this technique in the lower limbs because of the greater mass of tissue involved. However, short procedures of the foot can be successfully performed under intravenous regional anesthesia without larger amounts of local anesthetic. The tourniquet may be safely applied below the knee with the precaution of avoiding pressure over the superficial peroneal nerve as it runs around the neck of the fibula. The tourniquet then should be applied just below the fibular neck, and extra padding applied over the anterior lateral aspect of the leg. The particular blood vessel in the occluded area chosen for injection does not appear to influence the adequacy of analgesia.

Drug-Related Considerations. Lidocaine has been the agent used most frequently for intravenous regional anesthesia. Prilocaine, mepivacaine, chloroprocaine, and procaine also have been used successfully for the production of intravascular regional anaesthesia. However, thrombophlebitis has been reported in several patients in whom chloroprocaine was used. Residual analgesia following cuff deflation persists for approximately 5 to 10 minutes with agents such as prilocaine and lidocaine. The recent reports of cardiotoxicity with bupivacaine indicate that this agent should not be recommended for intravenous regional anesthesia.

The concentration and volume of local anesthetic solution influences analgesic adequacy and potential safety of intravascular regional anesthesia. In general, the use of large volumes of more dilute solutions provides the optimum conditions for satisfactory anesthesia and enhanced safety.

Most commonly, 40 ml of a 0.5% solution of lidocaine (200 mg) has been found to produce satisfactory analgesia for the upper arm, which would correspond to a dosage of approximately 3 mg/kg. Since large volumes of local anesthetic solution are required for procedures involving the lower limbs, the use of 75 ml to 100 ml of a dilute anesthetic solution has been advocated, for example, 0.25% to 0.35% lidocaine (to a 300-mg maximum). Intravascular regional anesthesia is also quite successful in children, with 3 to 5 mg/kg of 0.25% to 0.5% lidocaine.

PERIPHERAL NERVE BLOCKADE

Regional anesthetic procedures that involve the inhibition of conduction in nerve fibers of the peripheral nervous system can be classified together under the general category of peripheral nerve blockade.[87] This form of regional anesthesia has been subdivided arbitrarily into minor and major nerve blocks. Minor nerve blocks are defined as procedures involving single nerve entities, such as the ulnar or radial nerves at the wrist and the anterior or posterior tibial nerves at the ankle. Major nerve blocks comprise those procedures in which two or more distinct nerves or a nerve plexus are blocked, for example, brachial plexus blockade.

MINOR NERVE BLOCKS

A classification of the various agents according to their duration of action reveals that procaine and chloroprocaine possess a short duration of anesthetic activity, whereas lidocaine, mepivacaine, and prilocaine are agents of moderate duration (Table 6-6). The duration of both sensory analgesia and motor blockade is prolonged significantly when epinephrine is added to various local anesthetic solutions. As observed for infiltration anesthesia, lidocaine appears to benefit most by the addition of epinephrine.

MAJOR NERVE BLOCKS

Brachial plexus blockade is the most common major nerve block employed for ambulatory surgical procedures of the upper extremity. A 'flooding' technique is frequently employed to achieve satisfactory brachial plexus blockade. This involves the use of large volumes, up to 40 ml, of local anesthetic solution in order to maximize diffusion to the nerve plexus. The axillary approach to the brachial plexus is the safest and simplest to perform. Use of this technique reduces the risk of complications such as pneumothorax, which may become symptomatic after discharge. Interscalene, supraclavicular and infraclavicular approaches may also be used to achieve somewhat different areas of anesthesia. For children, doses of 0.5 ml/kg may be employed.

Onset Time. The onset of complete anesthesia usually requires 10 to 20 minutes for brachial plexus blockade, even with agents such as chloroprocaine and lidocaine, which have a relatively rapid onset of action. Considerable variation in onset time exists based on the technical skill of the anesthesiologist.

Duration of Anesthesia. The greatest duration of anesthesia usually occurs following major nerve blocks (Table 6-7). In general, the agents of moderate duration, such as lidocaine and mepivacaine, produce anesthesia of 2 to 4 hours, whereas short-acting drugs such as chloroprocaine will provide 1 to 2 hours of anesthesia. This prolonged duration of effect is due to several factors. In general, a greater dose of local anesthetic agent is used for major nerve blocks as

□ **Table 6-6. Minor Nerve Blocks for Ambulatory Surgery**

		Plain Solutions			Epinephrine Containing Solutions
Agent	Usual Concentration (%)	Usual Adult Volume (ml)	Usual Adult Dosage (mg)	Average Duration (min)	Average Duration (min)
Procaine Chloroprocaine	2%	5–20	100–400	15–30	30–60
Lidocaine Mepivacaine Prilocaine	1%	5–20	50–200	60–120	120–180

☐ **Table 6-7. Major Nerve Blocks for Ambulatory Surgery**

Agent	Usual Concentration (%)	Plain Solutions				Epinephrine Containing Solutions			
		Usual Adult Volume (ml)	Max. Adult Dose (mg)	Usual Onset (min)	Usual Duration (min)	Usual Adult Volume	Max. Adult Dose	Usual Onset	Usual Duration
Chloroprocaine	2–3	25–40	800	10–20	30–50	30–60	1000	10–20	60–120
Lidocaine	1–1.5	20–30	300	10–20	60–90	30–50	500	10–20	120–140
Mepivacaine	1–1.5	20–30	300	10–20	60–120	30–50	500	10–20	180–300
Prilocaine	1–2	30–50	600	10–20	60–120	Not available			

compared with other types of regional anesthetic procedures. In addition, the region of the brachial plexus is poorly vascularized, which results in a slow rate of vascular absorption and a greater uptake of drug by the major nerves. Epinephrine will prolong the duration of most local anesthetic agents employed for major nerve blocks and therefore should be used only when indicated.

CENTRAL NEURAL BLOCKADE

EPIDURAL ANESTHESIA

Lumbar epidural anesthesia is useful for surgical procedures involving the lower abdomen, pelvis, perineum, and lower extremities.[17] Epidural anesthesia may be used for laparoscopy, but the patient should be forewarned that shoulder pain will be felt. This referred diaphragmatic irritation can be minimized by modifying the surgical technique, as suggested under Preparation, above. (The same provisos are applicable for laparoscopy under spinal anesthesia.) Caudal anesthesia is usually reserved for pelvic and perineal surgery. In children, caudal epidural anesthesia is most often administered under basal sedation or light general anesthesia, to provide postoperative analgesia. Both lumbar and caudal epidural are particularly applicable for use after induction of general anesthesia, since their success does not depend on obtaining paresthesias. Care must be taken to avoid airway obstruction when these blocks are performed in the lateral position under inhalation anesthesia.

Volume and Concentration of Anesthetic Solutions. Lumbar epidural administration in adults usually requires the use of 10-ml to 20-ml volumes to achieve satisfactory analgesic results. Cranial spread occurs more easily than sacral spread following lumbar epidural injections, owing in part to negative intrathoracic pressure and to the resistance afforded by the narrowing of the epidural space at the lumbosacral junction. A significant delay in or an absence of analgesia at the first and second sacral segments is frequently observed following lumbar epidural injections. This has been attributed in part to the narrowing of the epidural space at the lumbosacral junction and also to the thickness of spinal roots in this region. Caudal anesthesia usually requires greater amounts of drug (20 ml to 30 ml), owing to loss of solution through the anterior sacral foramina and the rapid vascular absorption from this site. Little cranial spread beyond the lumbosacral junction occurs following caudal injections because of the peculiar anatomy of the epidural space in this region. Concentrations of 1.5% to 2.0% lidocaine or mepivacaine, 2% prilocaine, and 2% to 3% chloroprocaine are most commonly employed for lumbar epidural and caudal anesthesias. For children, the recommended dosage for lumbar or caudal epidural anesthesia can be calculated for 1% lidocaine, 1% mepivacaine, and 0.25% bupivacaine by using the formula 0.1 ml per year per segment (±0.2 ml). The formula is applicable up to the age of 12 in caudal epidural block. For a caudal block, it is often easier to use 0.5 ml/kg of one of these solutions, since this amount will consistently spread to L2–3 and sometimes to T10–11.[113]

Patient Position.   Posture has been demonstrated to influence the quality of epidural analgesia. Larger quantities of anesthetic drug are required to achieve the same dermatomal level in patients in the sitting position than in the horizontal position. Lumbar epidural anesthesia is often performed with the patient in the sitting position in obstetrics to obtain satisfactory perineal analgesia.

Age and Height.   Discrepancies exist among studies in which the influence of age and height on epidural anesthesia has been assessed by clinical means, that is, analgesic dermatomal levels, and by radiographic observations. Bromage has reported that dose-per-segment requirements of epidurally administered anesthetic agents are directly proportional to patient height; dose requirements are directly proportional to patient age until 18 years, then inversely proportional to age after age 18.[17] However, other investigators have failed to demonstrate any correlation in adults between age and height, on the one hand, and the spread of radio-opaque material in the epidural space, on the other.

Anesthetic Agent.   Lidocaine, mepivacaine, and prilocaine are commonly used for surgical procedures of 1 to 2 hours, whereas chloroprocaine is employed most often for procedures of less than 1 hour (Table 6-8). The use of epinephrine (1:200,000) may significantly prolong the duration of the effects of these agents, and it should be added only when indicated and when adequate time for recovery is available. Onset of epidural anesthesia usually occurs within 5 to 15 minutes following administration of chloroprocaine, lidocaine,

☐ **Table 6-8. Epidural Blockade for Ambulatory Surgery**

Agent	Usual Concentration (%)	Plain Solutions				Epinephrine Containing Solutions			
		Usual Adult Volume (ml)	Total Adult Dose (mg)	Usual Onset (min)	Usual Duration (min)	Usual Adult Volume	Max. Adult Dose	Usual Onset	Usual Duration
Chloroprocaine	3	15–25	150–750	5–15	30–60	15–30	150–900	5–15	30–90
Lidocaine	1–2	15–30	150–300	5–15	60–90	15–30	150–500	5–15	60–180
Mepivacaine	1–2	15–30	150–300	5–15	60–120	15–30	150–500	5–15	60–180
Prilocaine	1–3	15–30	150–600	5–15	60–120		Not available		

mepivacaine, and prilocaine. Procaine is rarely used for epidural anesthesia because of its slow onset of action.

Hemodynamic Considerations. Interruption of sympathetic impulses can lead to cardiovascular alterations following the establishment of epidural anesthesia. However, since autonomic blockade occurs slowly, cardiovascular changes may not be very marked. On the other hand, profound hypotension may be observed in some patients following the onset of epidural anesthesia. The changes in blood pressure, heart rate, and cardiac output are related to the level of blockade, the amount of drug administered, the specific local anesthetic agent employed, the inclusion of a vasoconstrictor in the anesthetic solution, and the cardiovascular status of the patient.

Level of block. The higher the block, the greater the number of sympathetic fibers that are affected, leading to a reduction in vascular tone. Thus, peripheral resistance decreases, but a fall in arterial pressure may be prevented by vasoconstriction in unblocked segments. Thus, blocks below T_5 are seldom associated with marked hypotension. Higher blocks, however, not only prevent compensatory vasoconstriction but also affect the cardiac sympathetic nerves, which arise in the T1-5 segments. At these dermatomal levels of block, a fall in heart rate and cardiac output may occur. The blockade of sympathetic fibers to the heart and the failure to block the vagus nerves can cause vasovagal attacks, which are associated with profound bradycardia and in some patients transient cardiac arrest. This may, in fact, represent the most common cause of profound hypotension following high levels of epidural anesthesia. As the veins forming the capacitance vessels will also be affected by the sympathetic block, venous pooling can occur if the venous return is obstructed by gravity or abdominal tumors including pregnancy. Thus, patients are very susceptible to the head-up posture, which causes expansion of the capacitance vessels and can lead to a marked decrease in venous return and cardiac output.

Drug dosage. Relatively large amounts of local anesthetic drug are required to achieve a satisfactory degree of epidural blockade. The local anesthetic agents are absorbed rapidly and significant blood levels may be achieved. The absorbed local anesthetic agent may produce systemic effects involving the cardiovascular system. Most local anesthetic agents produce a biphasic effect on the cardiovascular system. For example, it has been shown that blood levels of lidocaine of less than 4 μg/ml following epidural blockade resulted in a slight increase in blood pressure due mainly to an increase in cardiac output. Doses of epidural lidocaine that produce blood levels in excess of 4 μg/ml caused hypotension due in part to the negative inotropic action and the peripheral vasodilator effect of lidocaine.

Specific agents. Differences in the onset of epidural anesthesia occur as a function of the specific agent employed and the concentration used. In general, local anesthetics commonly used for epidural blockade in ambulatory surgery can be classified as agents of rapid and moderate onset. Chloroprocaine and lidocaine produce a fairly rapid onset of anesthesia, whereas mepivacaine and prilocaine are relatively slower in onset. With all agents there is a tendency for onset to be faster as the concentration is increased. The more rapidly acting agents tend to produce a more profound degree of hypotension due to the more rapid blockade of sympathetic fibers.

Addition of vasoconstrictors. Epinephrine may be added to local anesthetics intended for epidural use in order to decrease the rate of vascular absorption and prolong the duration of anesthesia. Absorbed epinephrine itself may produce transient cardiovascular alterations. A more profound degree of hypotension has been reported to occur following the use of epinephrine containing local anesthetics for epidural blockade. The absorbed epinephrine is believed to stimulate β-2-adrenergic receptors in all peripheral vascular beds, leading to an enhanced state of vasodilation and a fall in diastolic pressure. The β-1-adrenergic receptor stimulating effect of epinephrine results in an increase in heart rate and cardiac output that will counteract the peripheral vasodilator state to some extent. Although absorbed epinephrine may cause the early cardiovascular changes observed following epidural block, the prolonged hypotension seen with local anesthetics containing epinephrine is probably related to the achievement of a more profound degree of sympathetic blockade.

Blood volume status. The cardiovascular alterations described above relate primarily to changes occurring in normovolemic subjects. Cardiovascular depression is more severe and more dangerous following the production of epidural anesthesia in hypovolemic subjects. Epidural anesthesia in mildly hypovolemic volunteers was found to provoke vasovagal attacks associated with profound hypotension and bradycardia. Hypovolemia is usually accompanied by compensatory vasoconstriction that will be abolished by the block, and cardiovascular collapse may ensue.

SPINAL ANESTHESIA
The analgesic properties of subarachnoid blockade may be influenced by a number of factors that can be related to the patient, the anesthetic solution, and anesthetic technique.[56]

Patient Factors. Patient position during and immediately following subdural administration of a local anesthetic agent will influence the spread of spinal anesthesia. Since hyperbaric anesthetic solutions are commonly used for subarachnoid blocks, the spread in cerebrospinal fluid will be affected by gravity. For example, the patient in a sitting position at the time of injection will experience a lower-level block than the patient who is supine.

A decrease in the spinal fluid capacity of the subarachnoid space will markedly affect the degree of analgesia and the dose requirements for satisfactory spinal anesthesia. Inferior vena cava compression, usually due to pregnancy, is the most common cause of engorgement and distention of the vertebral system, decreasing the capacity of the subarachnoid space for spinal fluid. The dosage requirements for spinal anesthesia are significantly lower in pregnant patients, from midgestation to term, than in nongravid subjects.

Anesthetic Factors. Relatively few agents are prepared in a form specifically intended for subarachnoid administration (Table 6-9). Lidocaine, 5.0%, is the anesthetic of choice for ambulatory surgery patients. Tetracaine may also be used if surgery is scheduled sufficiently early in the day to permit recovery and discharge. Hyperbaric tetracaine may then be useful for arthroscopic surgical procedures. Hypobaric and isobaric solutions of tetracaine have also been used for specific operative situations, such as anorectal surgery, in which it may be advantageous to maintain the patient in a head-down position.

Lidocaine and mepivacaine essentially provide a short duration of spinal anesthesia, whereas tetracaine, dibucaine, and bupivacaine are considered agents of long duration. An average total analgesic duration for lidocaine and

☐ **Table 6-9. Spinal Anesthetic Agents for Ambulatory Surgery**

Agent	Usual Concentration (%)	Usual Adult Volume (ml)	Total Adult Dose (mg)	Baricity	Glucose Concentration (%)	Usual Anesthetic Duration (min)
Lidocaine	5	1–2	50–100	Hyperbaric	7.5	45–60
Tetracaine	0.25–1	1–4	5–20	Hyperbaric	5	75–150
	0.1–0.3			Hypobaric		
	0.5			Isobaric		
Dibucaine	0.25	1–2	2.5–5	Hyperbaric	5	75–180
	0.5	1–2	5–10	Isobaric		
	0.06	5–20	3–12	Hypobaric		
Bupivacaine	0.5	3–4	15–20	Isobaric		75–150
	0.75	2–3	15–22.5	Hyperbaric	8	75–150

mepivacaine of 45 to 60 minutes has been reported following the use of 5% lidocaine and 4% mepivacaine. Tetracaine in doses of 4 mg to 15 mg has been reported to provide 75 to 105 minutes of surgical anesthesia for intra-abdominal procedures and 120 to 150 minutes of surgical anesthesia for perineal and lower-extremity procedures. Dibucaine, 5 mg to 10 mg, and bupivacaine, 15 mg to 20 mg, produce a duration of spinal anesthesia similar to those reported for tetracaine. Onset of spinal anesthesia is extremely rapid, particularly with an agent such as lidocaine. To reduce the risk of postdural puncture headache, 25- or 26-gauge spinal needles should be used for ambulatory surgery patients.

As in other forms of regional anesthesia, vasoconstrictor agents may prolong the duration of spinal anesthesia. The addition of 0.2 mg to 0.3 mg epinephrine to lidocaine solutions will produce a 50% prolongation of spinal anesthesia, for procedures lasting 60 to 90 minutes. An increase in the duration of tetracaine subarachnoid block has also been reported following the addition of epinephrine or phenylephrine, 1 mg to 5 mg. However, the addition of a vasoconstrictor to spinal anesthetic solutions of tetracaine is not recommended for ambulatory surgery because of the prolonged duration of blockade.

Spinal anesthesia is frequently associated with a fall in systemic blood pressure. The degree of hypotension is related primarily to the extent of the spinal blockade. Subarachnoid blocks which extend to the T10 level are rarely associated with a significant fall in pressure. Extension of block to the T5 dermatomal level usually results in a fall in blood pressure due to a decrease in peripheral vascular resistance that is a direct result of the inhibition of sympathetic outflow below the level of block. Analgesic dermatomal levels above T5 may be associated with a more profound degree of hypotension due to a fall in cardiac output. The decrease in cardiac output may be related, in part, to a decrease in venous return and to the inhibition of sympathetic fibers innervating the heart.

The degree of spinal hypotension may be influenced by patient position. Maintenance of a slight head-up posture following spinal anesthesia usually will lead to a more pronounced fall in blood pressure due to a decrease in venous return. Placement of patients in a slight head-down position will tend to maintain normal venous return so that the degree of hypotension is lessened.

Differences also exist among different agents in terms of spinal hypotension. Lidocaine produces a more rapid onset of block than tetracaine, which usually results in a more profound degree of hypotension. A comparison of tetracaine and dibucaine or bupivacaine indicated that tetracaine caused a significantly greater fall in blood pressure, despite the fact that the level of analgesia produced by the drugs was similar.

Hypovolemia will clearly result in a profound degree of hypotension following spinal anesthesia. Patients should be well hydrated prior to the performance of a subarachnoid block. Hypotension in a normovolemic patient is easily reversed by placing the patient in a slight Trendelenburg position or administering either a crystalloid solution or a vasoconstrictor agent such as ephedrine or phenylephrine.

Doses of spinal anesthetic agents suitable for pediatric ambulatory surgery have been determined (Table 6-10). These agents are all hyperbaric and contain glucose, although other formulations could be used. The increased dose requirement for lidocaine spinal anesthesia in infants is due to a higher volume of cerebrospinal fluid relative to body weight.

Complications of Local and Regional Anesthesia

The potential complications of regional anesthesia include headache, neurologic sequelae, systemic toxicity, and allergic reaction. All may occur in ambulatory surgery patients. With a better understanding of the pathophysiology involved, these complications can often be prevented. If complications do occur, early diagnosis and appropriate treatment should result in a satisfactory outcome.

HEADACHE

Headache is a common postoperative complaint. It may be due to nonanesthetic causes such as dehydration or the psychogenic reactions of tension and depression. Anesthetic causes of headache include postdural puncture and meningeal irritation or infection.

The postdural puncture headache (PDPH) may be of variable intensity. It is described as a dull or aching pressure that begins at the occiput and extends down the neck and over the head to the frontal region. It may be unilateral or generalized. The postdural headache is postural. It occurs, or is at least

□ **Table 6-10. Spinal Anesthetic Agents for Pediatric Ambulatory Surgery**

Agent	Concentration (%)	Dose (mg/kg)
Lidocaine	5	2 (under 3 yr)
		1 (3–10 yr)
Tetracaine	1	0.2
Dibucaine	0.5	0.2

aggravated, when the patient sits or stands and is relieved upon reclining or with abdominal compression. The PDPH typically begins during the second postoperative day and lasts usually 1 to 4 days. Since headache onset is expected to occur after discharge from the ambulatory unit, it is important to instruct patients to contact the facility if PDPH develops. Symptoms associated with PDPH include nausea and vomiting, dizziness, visual disturbances such as blurred vision and rare abducens palsy, and auditory disturbances such as tinnitus and stuffiness.

The etiology of the pain of PDPH was first proposed by Bier in 1899. The hypothesis is that cerebrospinal fluid (CSF) leaks out through a hole in the dura made by the needle, resulting in a decrease in CSF pressure. With diminishing CSF pressure, the brain is displaced caudad, with traction on pain-sensitive blood vessels and supporting parts of the dura (falx and tentorium cerebelli). Pain is conducted by way of the trigeminal nerve to the anterior head and by way of the glossopharyngeal, vagus, and upper cervical nerves to the posterior head and neck.

The incidence of headache after spinal anesthesia has been evaluated in many studies. It ranges from 3.5% to 11% in large surgical series, although rates as low as 0.4% have been reported.[56,99,125] The incidence of PDPH specifically in an ambulatory surgery population is not known. An estimation may be gained by examining series of comparable procedures under spinal anesthesia. Burke reported 1.3% headache in 1063 women undergoing laparoscopy.[19] The incidence of PDPH after inguinal hernia repair in men has been reported to be 1.9% to 3.4%.[71,121] For comparison, the incidence of (nonspinal) headache after general anesthesia is 17% to 26%.[120]

Several factors have been associated with a decreased incidence of PDPH after spinal anesthesia. Factors that decrease the incidence but are not subject to control include male sex and increasing age. Female surgical patients develop fewer headaches than obstetric patients. Factors under the anesthesiologist's control, and therefore usable for prevention, include needle size and hydration. A decrease in incidence of headache from 41% with a 20-gauge needle to 0.4% with a 26-gauge needle has been demonstrated.[56] In patients who were given fluids, 2.5 Liters/day, the incidence of headache was decreased for all needle sizes. The consistently low incidence of PDPH in modern series of patients undergoing procedures suitable for ambulatory surgery[19,71,121] is probably due to increased awareness of the effectiveness of smaller needle size; 25-gauge or 26-gauge needles should be used for spinal anesthesia in ambulatory patients. Early ambulation has no significant effect on headache occurrence.[20,63,125]

Treatment of PDPH includes bed rest; hydration, intravenous if necessary; increased abdominal pressure by wearing a binder and lying prone; analgesic drugs, from aspirin to narcotics; and psychological support of reassurance and encouragement.[96] All of these therapies are symptomatic. There are, however, treatments that attempt to act on the cause of PDPH—leakage of CSF. Rice and Dabbs first reported the use of epidural placement of saline.[106] Injecting an average of 82 ml through caudal and lumbar catheters, they achieved immediate relief of headache in 99.5% patients. Subsequent studies report 69% to 87.5% success when epidural saline placement was used postpartum for headache prophylaxis, either by continuous infusion or by repeat injections.[29,30] Permanent, immediate cures are thought to be due to inversion of a flap valve preventing further CSF leak. However, epidural saline therapy is often only temporarily successful. Rice and Dabbs reported a 54% recurrence rate. Usubiaga and colleagues[123] demonstrated an increase in CSF and epidural pressures immediately after epidural saline injection. This provided relief of the PDPH, but pressures returned to baseline in 3 to 10 minutes, possibly explaining the transitory effect. Epidural placement of 50 ml to 100 ml of normal saline without preservative is somewhat successful in preventing PDPH, and can be given slowly through the epidural catheter *in situ*. However, a permanent cure for headache may not be achieved with this therapy.

Epidural blood patch (EBP) is another therapy that acts on the cause of PDPH. First described by Gormley,[55] the technique now used at Brigham and Women's Hospital consists of identification of the epidural space at the level at which dural puncture was performed, venipuncture and withdrawal of 10 ml to 20 ml blood under aseptic conditions, and injection of the blood into the epidural space.[96] Patient tolerance determines the final dose; injection should be terminated if back or radicular pain develops. The patient rests supine for 30 minutes with knees flexed over pillows to decrease the lumbar lordosis, and 1 Liter of intravenous crystalloid is given. Limited activity, and particularly avoidance of Valsalva straining, is recommended for the rest of the day to prevent dislodging the clot. EBP is easily performed on an outpatient basis. Relief often occurs immediately or within 24 hours. The success rate for EBP has been reported to be 91% to 100%.[39,55] The mode of action of EBP has been investigated by DiGiovanni et al.[39] They performed epidural injections of autologous blood in goats after dural puncture with a 18-gauge needle. At 24 hours, the goats' epidural space contained intact unorganized blood cells with no fibrous reaction. Fibroblastic activity began at 48 hours and therefore could not play a major role in the immediate relief of headache symptoms. Rather, EBP acts by formation of gelatinous tamponade, which prevents leakage of CSF, allowing the dural tear to undergo normal healing. Subarachnoid pressure studies during EBP show pressures are sustained at 71.4% peak for 15 minutes after completion of the epidural injection.[9] By 3 months after EBP, collagen has been laid down by fibroblasts, with the resulting tissue essentially undistinguishable from underlying dura.[39] Successful epidural anesthesia has been reported 7 to 380 days after EBP.[2,93] Epidural blood placement does not obliterate the epidural space and does not preclude the use of regional block for later surgical or obstetric procedures.

Criteria for use of EBP are that the headache should be identified as PDPH, not migraine or other chronic headache, it should have lasted at least 2 or 3 days, it should be severe enough to interfere with patients' ability to function at daily activities, and conservative therapy should have been ineffective. At the Boston Hospital for Women (one of the predecessors of the present Brigham and Women's Hospital), we examined our need for EBP after spinal anesthesia for obstetric delivery from January 1976 to June 1977.[96] In 1999 patients, 10% developed headache, but only 0.67% required EBP. We also examined the data for 61 patients who sustained an unintentional dural puncture with a 17-gauge needle during attempted epidural anesthesia. Of these patients, 33% developed PDPH, but only 6.7% required EBP. Based upon these data, the majority of PDPH appear to resolve with conservative therapy alone.

Palahniuk and Cumming present additional evidence against the use of prophylactic EBP.[94] They evaluated obstetric patients who sustained unintended dural puncture with a 16-gauge Tuohy needle; some were given autologous blood through a correctly placed epidural catheter at the termination of the anesthetic. The incidence of headache was unchanged: 54% for the patients who received epidural blood therapy and 59% for those patients who did not. Loeser et al studied the success rate of EBP in patients with PDPH relative to the time from dural puncture.[77] The patients given EBP within 24 hours of dural puncture had a 29% success rate, whereas those patients who were given EBP after 24 hours had a 96% success rate. The high failure rate of prophylactic EBP may be due to the following factors: (1) blood may not be placed directly over the hole produced by the dural puncture, especially if injected through an epidural catheter, and (2) the pressure and/or volume of leaking CSF may be sufficient to prevent organization of the clot over the dural hole. The use of EBP for headache prevention is not recommended because the prophylactic patch is of limited effectiveness and because the majority of headaches resolve with conservative therapy.

No permanent adverse effects of epidural blood patch have been reported. Transient backache and paresthesias or radicular pain may be experienced. Reassurance of the patient is essential. The dura may be punctured again during EBP, but the subarachnoid injection of autologous blood (in dogs) was not associated with neurologic deficits.[104] A major contraindication to the performance of EBP is the presence of infection, either generalized septicemia or local infection in the area of needle insertion. Other major contraindications are coagulopathy and active neurologic disease.

A second class of headaches complicating regional anesthesia is the headache of meningeal inflammation. Aseptic meningitis has been reported after spinal and epidural anesthesia. The headache of aseptic meningitis is severe, generalized, and nonpostural and may be accompanied by fever, photophobia, and other signs of meningeal irritation. Symptoms appear within several hours of the anesthetic and last 2 to 4 days. A diagnostic lumbar puncture will reveal clear to slightly cloudy CSF with elevated pressure, increased protein, normal sugar, and leukocytosis—usually polymorphonuclear. Peripheral leukocytosis is also seen. Cultures of the CSF are negative and no bacteria or pathogens are seen on microscopic examination. Aseptic meningitis has been sporadically reported, but its occurrence is rare; in Dripps and Vandam's series of 10,098 spinals and Lund's series of 10,000 epidurals, none occurred.[41,78] The etiology of this syndrome is uncertain but is thought to include local toxicity due to impurity or overdose of local anesthetic; the introduction of blood, skin, or antiseptic into the subarachnoid space; and the irritative effect of residual detergents used to clean equipment or soak ampules of local anesthetic. Therapy for aseptic meningitis is conservative and consists of analgesics and fluids. Recovery is usually complete.

Septic meningitis is another possible cause of headache following spinal anesthesia. Signs and symptoms of septic meningitis are the same as those of the aseptic variety, but when a diagnostic lumbar puncture is performed, a purulent exudate with decreased sugar content is found; pathogenic organisms, usually cocci or gram-negative rods, are seen on microscopic examination or culture. The incidence of septic meningitis following spinal anesthesia is rare, 0.005%. Treatment consists of analgesics, fluids, and appropriate antibiotics.

NEUROLOGIC SEQUELAE

Neurologic complications of regional anesthesia occur primarily associated with spinal and epidural anesthesia. Direct trauma from needle or catheter may injure nerve roots. Sensory rather than motor roots are more often affected, and limited damage occurs over the distribution of the nerve. Needle trauma may also be seen after techniques that elicit paresthesias, such as brachial plexus blocks. Symptoms usually resolve. Injury to the spinal cord itself is accompanied by sharp pain and occasionally loss of consciousness; damage tends to be more extensive and irreversible. Trauma to the bones and ligaments results in backache. Transient backache due to the instrumentation has been reported in 1.6% of patients after epidural and 2.7% of patients after spinal anesthesia.[78,99] Vertebral bodies and intervertebral discs have been penetrated by an anesthetic needle. Direct trauma by needle or catheter can injure blood vessels, usually veins. Significant symptoms may occur if the patient is anticoagulated or has a clotting disorder.

Ischemic injury to the spinal cord is another relatively common cause of neurologic sequelae to regional anesthesia. Ischemia may be caused by arterial hypotension, whether anesthetically induced or accidental.[122] The use of epinephrine in epidural anesthetic solutions may reduce spinal cord circulation. This vasoconstriction is not usually significant in man unless accompanied by hypotension, arteriosclerosis, or both. Vascular spasm may result in ischemic injury in the absence of actual obstruction. The severity of the ischemic neurologic injury is proportional to the distance of the vascular lesion from the spinal cord. Interruption of flow at the level of the aorta or vertebral arteries may lead to complete transverse necrosis of the cord, whereas more distal lesions cause more circumscribed damage. Occlusion of the anterior spinal artery results in a syndrome of motor paralysis with preservation of sensation. With ischemic damage to the anterior two-thirds of the cord, the prognosis for recovery is poor. Posterior spinal artery syndrome is rare and consists of anesthesia below the level of ischemic injury with segmental loss of skin and tendon reflexes.

Compression of the cord may indirectly cause ischemic injury. The resulting neurologic deficit is a function of the severity of the compression, the rapidity of onset of compression, and the function of the compressed tissue. Anesthesia-related causes of ischemic cord compression include epidural abscess and epidural hematoma. Symptoms of epidural abscess include fever and localized back pain and tenderness. Lower extremity root pain, weakness, and flaccid paralysis develop over 1 to 4 days. Peripheral blood cultures may be positive. Epidural abscesses are usually located dorsal to the spinal cord; pus may be aspirated while a diagnostic lumbar puncture is being attempted. Lumbar puncture with manometrics reveals evidence of block; CSF has elevated protein, moderate pleocytosis with lymphocytes, normal glucose, and negative smear and cultures. Epidural abscess is often associated with sepsis or infection elsewhere in the body; antecedent trauma to the back or chronic debilitation from alcoholism or diabetes are also predisposing factors. The development of an epidural abscess in relation to spinal or epidural anesthesia is rare (<.0015%). More often, epidural abscesses occur spontaneously, not associated with anesthesia. Treatment is decompression by prompt surgical drainage of the abscess. Recovery may be complete when minimal neurologic deficit has developed and treatment is instituted rapidly, but delays may result in permanent neurologic sequelae.

Epidural hematoma is the second common cause of spinal cord injury from ischemic compression. Epidural hematoma formation is often heralded by sharp pain in the distribution of the affected portion of cord, followed shortly by weakness and flaccid paralysis. Onset is usually sudden and progression to paralysis rapid. Fever does not occur. Lumbar puncture reveals clear fluid, sometimes with elevated protein; myelography shows extradural compression. Disseminated intravascular coagulation (DIC) has been reported within 2 hours after second-trimester abortions by dilatation and evacuation; the presumed stimulus is amniotic fluid or placental thromboplastin.[133] These patients should be evaluated carefully, including indicated hematologic tests, before a regional anesthetic is administered for removal of retained products of conception. Hematomas may occur after spinal or epidural anesthesia or after lumbar puncture without anesthesia. Intracranial subdural and intracerebral hematomas have also been reported after spinal anesthesia, possibly related to the decrease in CSF pressure and traction on intracranial blood vessels. Prognosis for recovery of neurologic function is best if surgical decompression with evacuation of the clot is done promptly.

Infection is now a rare cause of neurologic sequelae of regional anesthesia. Extrinsic sources of infection include contaminated equipment or drugs. Aseptic technique with good skin preparation and sterile equipment are necessary. Infection may arise from internal local sources or from elsewhere in the body, transported by the bloodstream or lymphatics. Infections may develop anywhere along the path of the anesthetic needle or catheter. Infections in the spinal cord itself cause localized edema, vascular occlusion, and neuronal destruction, as well as ascending and descending degeneration. Paralysis, sensory deficit, and loss of sphincter control may occur. Prognosis is poor despite antibiotics or decompressive laminectomy.

Exposure to chemical toxic agents is another cause of neurologic sequelae. Neurolytic agents such as alcohol, collodion, hypertonic saline, propylene glycol, and several preservatives, including benzyl alcohol and methyl hydroxybenzoate, have been injected into the epidural and subarachnoid spaces, resulting in temporary or permanent neurologic deficits. Alcohol can be found in antiseptics used for skin cleansing; care should be taken to avoid contamination of equipment with these solutions. Local anesthetic ampules should not be soaked in alcohol because minute cracks in the glass may allow entry of the toxic substance into the solution to be injected. Accidental detergent contamination has also been implicated in the development of neurologic sequelae. Equipment used for regional anesthesia should be thoroughly rinsed in water before undergoing sterilization.

Excessively high concentrations of some local anesthetics may also be neurotoxic. The hyperosmolality of these solutions is thought to be at fault. Radiopaque contrast materials are also neurotoxic with a 0.22% incidence of sequelae;[122] complications due to injection of contrast material may be incorrectly ascribed to an ongoing regional anesthesia. Clinical symptoms of chemical neurologic toxicity usually appear as a mild aseptic meningitis. Rarely, a chronic proliferative adhesive arachnoiditis may develop. The specific neurologic deficit depends on the particular location and density of the inflammatory reaction; pain, sensory and motor deficits, and loss of rectal and bladder sphincter control may be seen. Onset of the adhesive arachnoiditis syndrome may be delayed weeks or months, and symptoms are often progressive. Recovery is rare.

Exacerbation of preexisting pathology is a common cause of neurologic sequelae ascribed to regional anesthesia. Preexisting disease may be vascular or neurologic. Vascular pathology may be in the form of anatomic malformations, either congenital or acquired. Embolization of any of the vessels supplying the cord may also cause vascular insufficiency and neurologic deficit. Generalized vascular disease may also predispose to ischemic neurologic injury. Such diseases include atherosclerosis, diabetes mellitus, syphilis, thromboangiitis obliterans, and periarteritis nodosa.

Preexisting neurologic pathology may be aggravated coincident with regional anesthesia. Nerve injury may actually be due to mechanical compression from a prolapsed intervertebral disc, spondylosis, developmental laminar stenosis, or a uterine leiomyoma. Tumor, another cause of neurologic damage, may be first suspected after regional anesthesia. Metastatic epidural tumors causing compressive ischemic injury are the most common, but primary and subdural neoplasma also occur. Neurologic disease affecting the spinal cord, such as multiple sclerosis and tabes dorsalis, may worsen at the time of regional anesthesia, and the deficit may be ascribed to anesthesia. However, stable chronic neurologic disease in itself is not a contraindication to receiving regional anesthesia; the course of such disease is probably not affected by the anesthesia. Informed consent by the patient is, as always, needed.

Extrinsic nonanesthetic factors may also cause neurologic damage during regional anesthesia by means of vascular or direct traumatic mechanisms. Interference of vascular supply to the spinal cord can be a result of surgical section. Causes of direct nerve trauma include improper positioning of the patient on an operating table or in stirrups and the use of retractors. Recovery of function may require several months, but is often complete.

When neurologic injury occurs following regional anesthesia, its cause must be immediately and thoroughly investigated. Anesthesia can often be proved or disproved as the cause of the sequelae. The first step in the differential diagnosis is a complete neurologic examination, followed by diagnostic lumbar puncture unless definite contraindications exist. Myelography should be performed if there is evidence of subarachnoid block. The single most important diagnostic test is electromyography. Electromyography can differentiate between intradural and extradural neuropathies; the latter cannot be caused by spinal anesthesia, so the block may be exonerated. Electromyography can also be used to determine the precise level of spinal cord damage and the duration of injury, thereby identifying the lesion as antedating the anesthesia. Marinacci and Courville used electromyography to evaluate 542 patients with neurologic deficit ascribed to spinal anesthesia.[81] They were able to rule out an anesthesia cause in all but four of the cases.

Neurologic sequelae have been reported since the introduction of regional techniques, but are rare with modern anesthetic agents. Dripps and Vandam (1954) followed 10,098 spinal anesthesias and found no cases of postanesthetic paralysis.[41] Phillips et al (1969) also reported no cases of major neurologic deficit in their series of 10,440 spinals.[99] These authors also evaluated their patients for minor peripheral nerve symptoms. Dripps and Vandam reported an incidence of 0.7% of areas of numbness or pain in the lower extremities or perineum; most symptoms had resolved by the 6-month postanesthetic evaluation. Phillips et al reported a 0.36% incidence of any symptoms of peripheral nerve injury. Their incidence of persistent peripheral neuropathy after spinal anesthesia was 0.02%.

Epidural anesthesia has also been evaluated for its incidence of neurologic complications. Dawkins reviewed 32,718 lumbar epidural anesthesias and found 0.02% developed permanent and 0.1% transient paralysis.[34] Usubiaga reviewed a separate 780,000 epidural anesthesias.[122] He found the incidence of major paralytic complication to be 0.01%, of which 13% recovered "almost completely." In two larger subseries totaling 100,000 anesthesias, Usubiaga reported that 0.005% patients developed major neurologic injury; more experienced groups appear to have a lower rate of complication. Caudal epidural anesthesias have a similarly low rate of neurologic sequelae; Dawkins reported 0.005% patients with permanent paralysis and 0.02% with transient paralysis in his review of 22,968 caudal anesthesias.[34]

Neurologic deficits have been reported after regional anesthesia with all modern local anesthetic agents including lidocaine, mepivacaine, bupivacaine, and etidocaine.[21,102] Recently, several cases of prolonged neurologic sequelae have been reported after the unintentional subarachnoid injection of relatively large volumes of 2-chloroprocaine. Six patients developed persistent neurologic deficit with symptoms of adhesive arachnoiditis or anterior spinal artery syndrome.[90] Two additional patients made complete recovery in 72 hours and in 6 months. Covino et al evaluated the data and suggested that a cause may be the low pH of commercially prepared chloroprocaine, which is 2.167 for the 2% CE solution and 3.126 for the 3% solution.[27] However, low pH in itself is probably not the sole cause of the reported deficits. Ravindran et al showed no sequelae from the subarachnoid placement of pH 3.0 saline.[105] Chloroprocaine, 3.3%, was used by Foldes and McNall in 1952 for spinal anesthesia in 214 patients with no neurologic sequelae; they used a less stable formulation with pH of 4.8.[51] Neuropathy may be dose related. Moore et al[90] pointed out that patients who received larger doses (> 400 mg) had longer or persistent residual deficits. The question has also been raised of whether 2-chloroprocaine is a direct nerve tissue irritant.[109] Ravindran and colleagues placed chloroprocaine subarachnoid in dogs, using a drug volume approximately that of the total canine CSF volume.[105] Of the 20 animals, 35% developed hind limb paralysis, with subpial necrosis of the spinal cord seen on microscopic section. No such effect was seen in dogs given 0.75% bupivacaine or low pH (3.0) saline. Questions of species specificity and the effect of treatment on control groups arise with these studies. The contributions of spinal cord barotrauma and of the preservative bisulfite at low pH to the production of neurologic sequelae are also being investigated.* The safety of 2-chloroprocaine, particularly for epidural use, is an issue that still requires resolution. New formulations are being evaluated.

To avoid possible neurologic sequelae, care should be taken not to give chloroprocaine intrathecally. An adequate test dose should be given through the needle or catheter: 3 ml of 3% chloroprocaine should be used, and 3 to 4 minutes should be allowed to elapse to give time for development of a possible subarachnoid anesthetic. Repeated fractional doses of 3 ml to 5 ml should be used rather than a single large bolus. If a full anesthetizing dose is given intrathecally, the volume of solution given (at least 10 ml, if possible) should be withdrawn. Irrigation of the subarachnoid space with preservative-free normal

---

*Gissen A: Personal communication, 1984

saline may be considered.[27] Chloroprocaine should be avoided for epidural use if an accidental dural puncture has occurred.

SYSTEMIC TOXICITY

Another of the complications of regional anesthesia is the systemic toxic reaction. These reactions occur when local anesthetic is administered so that the rate of absorption is greater than the rate of destruction. This imbalance can be due to the injection of an excessive dose, either excessive concentration or excessive volume, or both. An increased rate of absorption may result from the presence of lacerated veins or normally rich vascularity at the site of injection, or from application to mucous membranes or abraded skin. The rate of injection also affects the development of systemic toxicity; a faster rate of injection results in a decreased tolerance to the anesthetic. Toxic reactions may be due to an unintentional intravascular injection, even of a therapeutic dose, because it is the sudden increase in systemic concentration that causes the reaction. Intravenous injection may be accomplished directly, through a needle, or indirectly, as with an epidural catheter, which may find its way into a vein either at the time of initial placement or anytime thereafter. Arterial injection is less likely to cause a toxic reaction, because the longer circuit through the peripheral vascular bed allows time for dilution and ester hydrolysis. However, reverse arterial blood flow has been proposed as another possible cause of systemic toxic reaction. Effects in the cerebral vascular system have been demonstrated after brachial, radial, and femoral intra-arterial injection. Systemic toxic reactions may also be due to a decreased rate of detoxification of the local anesthetic. The detoxification rate depends on the chemical composition of the drug, and therefore its mode of metabolism, the functional ability of the detoxifying organ, and the patient's metabolic rate. Other factors that influence the development of a toxic reaction include the effect of concurrent medications, the patient's acid-base balance (acidosis decreases the threshold), general physical status, and variable and unpredictable individual sensitivity.

The signs and symptoms of central nervous systemic toxic reactions occur along a concentration related spectrum.[124] Among the early subjective signs of local anesthetic toxicity, drowsiness is noted first. Patients may also complain of lightheadedness, dizziness, a metallic taste, nausea, tinnitus, circumoral tingling or numbness, or blurred vision. Objectively, confusion, slurred speech, nystagmus, and muscle tremors or twitches can be seen. An inverse relationship exists between the relative potency of local anesthetic agents and the blood levels required to generate toxic symptoms. For lidocaine, a level of 4 μg/ml was the threshold for beginning symptoms. With more potent bupivacaine and etidocaine, toxicity appears in the 2 to 3 μg/ml range.[114] Cortical electroencephalography (EEG) at this stage shows only drowsiness.

Further in the spectrum of toxicity are frank convulsions. Drowsiness proceeds to loss of consciousness, and muscle twitches to generalized tonic-clonic seizures. Ventilation may be impeded by seizure activity and cyanosis may develop. Pulse and blood pressure may rise as a result of the sympathetic response to hypoxia and hypercarbia, although hypotension sometimes develops due to depressant effects of the local anesthetic. This level of systemic toxicity has also been correlated with lidocaine blood levels. Wikinski et al, using lidocaine for psychiatric shock therapy, found a mean plasma level of 22 μg/ml at the time of convulsion.[133] Usubiaga et al watched the electroencephalogram in human volunteers who were given lidocaine until they convulsed.[124] Slow waves and irregular spiking were seen, which progressed to synchronous epileptiform discharges. Convulsive doses of lidocaine in cats block inhibitory pathways in the cerebral cortex; facilitatory neurons function unopposed, resulting in central nervous system excitation. Subcortical electroencephalograms in experimental animals show that local anesthetics block inhibitory relays, leading to excitation of an epileptogenic focus in the amygdala.[127]

Local anesthetic agents can produce profound effects on the cardiovascular system. The systemic administration of these agents can exert a direct action both on cardiac muscle and on peripheral vascular smooth muscle. In general, the cardiovascular system appears to be more resistant to the effects of local anesthetic agents than the central nervous system. Studies in dogs and sheep have indicated that doses of local anesthetic agents which cause significant cardiovascular effects are approximately three times higher than the dose of these agents which will have distinct effects on the central nervous system.[76,92]

The sequence of cardiovascular events that usually occurs following the systemic administration of local anesthetic agents is as follows: at relatively nontoxic blood levels of these agents, either no change in blood pressure or a slight increase in blood pressure may be observed. The slight increase in blood pressure may be related to a slight increase in cardiac output and heart rate which have been seen in some animal preparations and is believed due to an enhancement of sympathetic activity by these agents. In addition, the direct vasoconstrictor action of local anesthetics on certain peripheral vascular beds at low concentrations may be responsible in part for a slight increase in systemic blood pressure.

As the blood level of local anesthetic approaches toxic concentrations, a fall in blood pressure is usually the first cardiovascular sign. Studies with both the ester and amide agents in intact dogs have demonstrated that the initial hypotension observed is probably not related to peripheral vasodilation and a subsequent decrease in peripheral vascular resistance.[74,75] Rather, initial hypotension appears to be correlated with the negative inotropic action of these agents which results in a decrease in cardiac output and stroke volume. This depression in blood pressure is transient in nature and spontaneously reversible in most patients. However, if the amount of local anesthetic administered is excessive, an irreversible state of cardiovascular depression occurs. Profound peripheral dilation develops due to a direct relaxant effect on vascular smooth muscle. At high concentrations the depressant effect of these agents on the excitability of cardiac tissue will also become evident as a decrease in sinus rate and as AV conduction block. Ultimately, the combined peripheral vasodilation, decreased myocardial contractility and depressant effect on rate and conductivity will lead to cardiac arrest and circulatory collapse.

Most investigations have shown that a general relationship exists between the potency of various agents as local anesthetic drugs, and their depressant effect on the cardiovascular system.[74,75] In recent years there has been some suggestion that the more potent, highly lipid soluble and highly protein bound local anesthetic agents, such as bupivacaine and etidocaine, may be relatively more cardiotoxic than the less potent, less lipid soluble and protein bound local anesthetics such as lidocaine.[4] Several case reports have appeared in the literature in which bupivacaine and etidocaine were associated with rapid and profound cardiovascular depression. These cases differed from the usual cardiovascular depression seen with local anesthetics in several respects. The onset of cardiovascular depression occurred relatively early. In some cases severe cardiac arrhythmias were observed, and the cardiac depression appeared resistant to various therapeutic modalities. Studies in intact animals to evaluate the relative cardiovascular toxicity of various local anesthetics have been somewhat contradictory. The cardiovascular depression produced by local anesthetic agents appears related to the potency of the various drugs.[74,75] On the other hand, a narrower margin of safety may exist between the dose of bupivacaine or etidocaine to cause CNS toxicity and the dose to cause cardiovascular toxicity, as compared to lidocaine.[35,91] In addition, it has been reported that bupivacaine can induce cardiac arrhythmias in awake animals, whereas no such changes were observed with lidocaine.[38,70]

Changes in acid-base status will alter the potential cardiovascular toxicity of local anesthetic agents. As described previously, hypercarbia and acidosis will decrease the threshold of local anesthetic agents for convulsive activity. Similarly, hypercarbia, acidosis and hypoxia will tend to increase the cardio-depressant effect of local anesthetic agents. Studies on isolated atrial tissues have shown that hypercarbia, acidosis and hypoxia will tend to potentiate the negative chronotropic and inotropic action of lidocaine and bupivacaine.[112] It has been postulated that the cardiovascular depression observed with the more potent agents such as bupivacaine may be related in part to the severe acid-base changes that occur following the administration of toxic doses of these agents.

The clinical picture associated with massive local anesthetic overdose is collapse at times without convulsions. Ultimately, death occurs due to respiratory arrest. The incidence of any systemic toxic reaction was 0.2% in one series of 66,366 epidurals.[34] In another series of 93,102 patients receiving a variety of regional anesthetics (epidural, caudal, spinal, and peripheral blocks), the incidence of mild toxic reactions was 0.38% and of convulsions 0.12%.[87]

The best treatment for systemic toxic reactions is prevention. Therefore, aspirate carefully before injecting at any site, inject slowly, and use the optimum dose—minimum concentration and volume—for the desired effect. Ten milliliters of preservative-free normal saline or air can be injected into the epidural space prior to the insertion of a catheter;[97] this may reduce the incidence of blood vessel puncture by the catheter, and therefore prevent intravascular anesthetic injection. Large volumes (>3–5 ml) of local anesthetic should not be given as a bolus.[96]

If a patient undergoes a mild reaction, observe him closely because the reaction may progress. Administer oxygen by face mask. If a convulsion occurs, ventilation should be assisted with 100% oxygen by bag and mask. Anti-convulsive drugs should be given. Diazepam, 5 mg to 10 mg, can be given intravenously to terminate lidocaine-induced convulsions and increase the lidocaine seizure threshold.[37] Another choice is thiopental, which is readily available; 50 mg to 100 mg can be given. Convulsions usually last less than sixty seconds, but if prolonged, succinylcholine and endotracheal intubation may be needed to assure an adequate airway and oxygenation.

If cardiorespiratory collapse occurs, all of the above measures may be needed, including ventilation with 100% oxygen and anticonvulsive drug. In addition, the circulation must be supported with fluid and vasopressors. Closed-chest cardiac massage and drugs for resuscitation should be given as indicated.

Moore et al have demonstrated the development of profound hypoxia and metabolic and respiratory acidosis within one to three minutes of the onset of a convulsive toxic reaction, further predisposing the patient to cardiac arrest.[89] Because of the possibility of this full range of reactions, an intravenous line is required before commencing ambulatory regional anesthesia.

ALLERGIC REACTIONS

The anesthesiologist often must evaluate a patient needing or desiring regional anesthesia who claims to be "allergic" to local anesthetics. True allergic reactions to local anesthetic drugs are rare;[116] it is estimated that 99% of adverse reactions do not involve allergic mechanisms. In order to distinguish whether or not a reaction is allergic, a careful clinical history must be taken first.[6] The patient and attending physician or dentist must be interviewed, and the chart consulted. The exact drug given should be identified, including vasoconstrictors or preservatives, as well as the dosage and route of administration. The time of onset and duration of the reaction, and a clear description of the reaction itself and of any treatment given, are also needed. Most commonly, adverse reactions incorrectly labelled "allergy" are in fact systemic toxicity due to relative or absolute local anesthetic overdose. Reaction to epinephrine, vasovagal syncope, allergy to other drugs or dental alloys, and surgical orofacial swelling must also be ruled out.

True allergic reactions are mediated primarily by histamine released from mast cells and basophils. Release of histamine can be triggered by any one or combination of four mechanisms. IgE antibodies specific for a local anesthetic may have been produced on previous exposure to the drug; this is anaphylaxis. Activation of the complement system may occur with IgG or IgM antibody-drug interaction, or directly by local anesthetic activation of complement C_3. Histamine-releasing cells may be stimulated directly by the local anesthetic; this anaphylactoid reaction is more common in patients with multiple allergies or after repeated exposure to a drug. However, complement-mediated and anaphylactoid pathways of histamine release do not require previous exposure to the offending agent.[116]

Once histamine is released, the clinical syndrome is similar regardless of the trigger. Severity varies according to the individual's susceptibility. Symptoms in the skin are seen first. Erythema of the face, arms, and upper chest appear, due to capillary dilation. Pruritic hives or wheals form secondary to increased capillary permeability. Angioedema of the eyelids is common. Upper airway edema including the larynx can develop, and airway obstruction may occur. Rhinitis and conjunctivitis are also the result of local edema and inflammation. Blood pressure falls, reflecting increased capillary permeability and intravascular hypovolemia. Cardiac dysrhythmias may be caused by local histamine release in the heart as well as histamine-stimulated catecholamine secretion. Patients may complain of abdominal pain and vomiting, caused by hyperperistalsis. Bronchospasm is a potentially severe and life-threatening respiratory complication. Cardiorespiratory collapse can occur immediately and abruptly following drug administration.

An ongoing regional anesthetic may modify the presentation of anaphylaxis caused by another drug given at the same time.[8] Cephalosporin anaphylaxis during spinal anesthesia appeared initially as cardiovascular collapse without respiratory, laryngeal or cutaneous manifestations. Institution of external cardiac massage led to the appearance of a diffuse rash. Sympathetic blockade due to the spinal anesthetic combined with increased vascular permeability due to the anaphylactic reaction may have generated cardiac arrest by a catastrophic reduction in venous return.

If an allergic reaction occurs, stop the administration of the suspect local anesthetic drug. Epinephrine, 5 μg/kg (0.3–0.5 ml of 1:1000), should be given immediately, subcutaneously or into a muscle, or by the intravenous route if the reaction is severe. Epinephrine probably acts by inhibiting degranulation and release of chemical mediators from mast cells and basophils. The antihistamine diphenhydramine, 0.5 to 1 mg/kg, should also be given to block unoccupied receptors. Supplemental oxygen should be administered and an endotracheal tube inserted if airway edema is in question. Vascular volume should be maintained by crystalloid or colloid infusion, and vasopressors may be needed. Aminophylline, 3 to 5 mg/kg intravenously, is used to treat sustained bronchospasm. Hydrocortisone 100 mg is also often administered, although its theoretical basis is unclear.

Ester local anesthetics such as benzocaine, procaine and tetracaine are relatively more likely to cause true allergic reactions. These agents are metabolized to para-aminobenzoic acid (PABA) and related compounds, which are highly antigenic. Amide local anesthetics such as lidocaine, prilocaine, mepivacaine, and bupivacaine are rarely the cause of allergic reactions; only one case has been well documented, with bupivacaine.[18] Paraben derivatives are frequently present as preservatives in local anesthetic solutions, both in multidose vials and dental cartridges, and in numerous over-the-counter preparations. Parabens are structurally similar to para-aminobenzoic acid, and may cause allergic reactions directly or by cross-sensitization with ester local anesthetics. Cross reactivity of ester anesthetics has also been reported with para-aminobenzoic acid in sunscreens. Patients allergic to procaine may exhibit cross-sensitization with procaine penicillin.[5]

If a patient appears to be allergic to a local anesthetic drug, regional anesthesia probably can safely be given with a preservative-free anesthetic of unrelated structure.[61] If further in vivo testing is needed, the intradermal test may be used. Intradermal injection of 0.1 ml of local anesthetic is made into the skin of the medial forearm. One percent procaine, 0.5% lidocaine, mepivacaine, or prilocaine, 0.25% tetracaine or bupivacaine, and/or 0.1% methylparaben may be used. Preservative-free normal saline should also be injected intradermally, to control for false positives due to local histamine release from needle trauma or tissue distension. False-positive reactions may also occur because of isolated skin hypersensitivity to procaine and tetracaine, which is unassociated with systemic allergy.[5] If the identity of the offending local anesthetic is not certain, skin testing for drug tolerance should be performed with a preservative-free amide anesthetic. A negative reaction probably indicates safety for use. Patients should be tested at least one month after an acute allergic reaction, and should not be taking drugs that modify the immune response, such as antihistamines or steroids. A positive reaction consists of a 10 mm or larger wheal appearing within 15 minutes and lasting for at least 30 minutes. Equipment and personnel to support cardiopulmonary resuscitation must be available during intradermal testing, since a systemic reaction may occur.

Intradermal testing was able to demonstrate a lack of reactivity to the suspect local anesthetic drug in up to 92% of patients.[61] Attempts to confirm lack of reactivity by giving increasing intramuscular doses provided no additional information.[6] Testing by intravenous drug challenge carries excessive risk. *In vitro* diagnostic approaches such as IgE inhibition, leukocyte histamine release, and radioallergosorbent tests are currently in use but are expensive and not easily available.[116]

Patients with a strong history of allergies or who need to receive a suspect local anesthetic may be premedicated to attenuate a response. Both H_1- and H_2-receptor antagonists should be used; diphenhydramine, 0.5 to 1 mg/kg, and cimetidine, 4 to 6 mg/kg, can be given orally. Prednisone, 50 mg, has been helpful to attenuate reaction to radiographic contrast media. Prednisone may be given orally every 6 hours for 1 day, with the last dose 1 hour before the procedure.

Local and regional anesthesia can provide optimal conditions for ambulatory surgery. With regional block, intraoperative and postoperative analgesia can be obtained without postanesthetic central depression. With the use of appropriate agents and techniques for anesthesia and supplemental sedation, disadvantages of regional blockade can be minimized and potential complications may be avoided. Ambulatory regional anesthesia can satisfy patient, surgeon, and anesthesiologist.

References

1. Abboud TK, Shnider SM, Wright RG et al: Enflurane analgesia in obstetrics. Anesth Analg 60:133–137, 1981
2. Abouleish E, Wadhwa RK, de la Vega S et al: Regional anesthesia following epidural blood patch. Anesth Analg 54:634–636, 1976
3. Adams AP, Pybus DA: Delayed respiratory depression after use of fentanyl during anaesthesia. Br Med J 1:278–279, 1978
4. Albright GA: Cardiac arrest following regional anesthesia with etidocaine or bupivacaine. Anesthesiology 51:285–287, 1979
5. Aldrete JA, Johnson DA: Evaluation of intracutaneous testing for investigation of allergy to local anesthetic agents. Anesth Analg 49:173–183, 1970
6. Aldrete JA, O'Higgins JW: Evaluation of patients with history of allergy to local anesthetic drugs. South Med J 64:1118–1121, 1971
7. Baird ES, Hailey DM: Delayed recovery from a sedative: Correlation of the plasma levels of diazepam with clinical effects after oral and intravenous administration. Br J Anaesth 44:803–808, 1972
8. Barnett AS, Hirschman CA: Anaphylactic reaction to cephapirin during spinal anesthesia. Anesth Analg 58:337–338, 1979
9. Bart AJ, Wheeler AS: Comparison of epidural saline and epidural blood placement in the treatment of post-lumbar-puncture headache. Anesthesiology 48:221–223, 1978
10. Becker LD, Paulson BA, Miller RD et al: Biphasic respiratory depression after fentanyl-droperidol or fentanyl alone used to supplement nitrous oxide anesthesia. Anesthesiology 44:291–296, 1976
11. Bovill JG, Dundee JW: Alterations in response to somatic pain associated with anaesthesia. XX: Ketamine. Br J Anaesth 43:496–498, 1971
12. Bovill JG, Sebel PS, Blackburn CL et al: The pharmacokinetics of alfentanil (R39209): A new opioid analgesic. Anesthesiology 57:439–443, 1982
13. Bridenbaugh LD, Soderstrom RM: Lumbar epidural block anesthesia for outpatient laparoscopy. J Reprod Med 23:85–86, 1979
14. Briggs RM, Ogg MJ: Patients' refusal of surgery after Innovar premedication. Plast Reconstr Surg 1973; 51:158–161, 1973

15. Brindle GF, Soliman MG: Anaesthetic complications in surgical out-patients. Can Anaesth Soc J 22:613–619, 1975
16. Brock-Utne JG, Winning TJ, Rubin J et al: Laryngeal incompetence during neuroleptanalgesia in combination with diazepam. Br J Anaesth 48:699–701, 1976
17. Bromage PR: Epidural analgesia. Philadelphia, WB Saunders, 1978
18. Brown DT, Beamish D, Wildsmith JAW: Allergic reaction to an amide local anesthetic. Br J Anaesth 53:435–437, 1981
19. Burke RK: Spinal anesthesia for laparoscopy: A review of 1,063 cases. J Reprod Med 21:59–62, 1978
20. Carbaat P, van Crevel H: Lumbar puncture headache: Controlled study on the preventive effect of 24 hours' bed rest. Lancet 2:1131–1135, 1981
21. Chloroprocaine Labeling Revised. FDA Drug Bull 10:23–24, 1980
22. Cohen DD, Dillon JB: Anesthesia for outpatient surgery. JAMA 196:98–100, 1966
23. Cohen SE: Inhalation analgesia and anesthesia for vaginal delivery. In Shnider SM, Levinson G (eds): Anesthesia for Obstetrics, 121–138. Baltimore, Williams & Wilkins, 1979
24. Conner JT, Katz RL, Pagano RR et al: RO 21-3981 for intravenous surgical premedication and induction of anesthesia. Anesth Analg 57:1–5, 1978
25. Cook TL, Smith M, Winter PM et al: Effect of subanesthetic concentrations of enflurane and halothane on human behavior. Anesth Analg 57:434–440, 1978
26. Coupland GAE, Townend DM, Martin CJ: Peritoneoscopy-use in assessment of intra-abdominal malignancy. Surgery 89:645–649, 1981
27. Covino BG, Marx GF, Finster M, et al: Prolonged sensory/motor deficits following inadvertent spinal anesthesia. Anesth Analg 59:399–400, 1980
28. Covino BG, Vassallo HG: Local Anesthetics: Mechanisms of Action and Clinical Use. New York, Grune & Stratton, 1976
29. Craft JB, Epstein BS, Coakley CS: Prophylaxis of dural-puncture headache with epidural saline. Anesth Analg 52:228–231, 1973
30. Crawford SJ: The prevention of headache consequent upon dural puncture. Br J Anaesth 44:598–600, 1972
31. Cullen BF, Miller MG: Drug interactions and anesthesia: A review. Anesth Analg 58:413–423, 1979
32. D'Amato H, Wielding S (eds): Intravenous regional anesthesia. Acta Anaesth Scand 36(Suppl), 1969
33. Davie IT: Specific drug interactions in anesthesia. Anaesthesia 32:1000–1008, 1977
34. Dawkins CJM: An analysis of the complications of extradural and caudal block. Anaesthesia 24:554–563, 1969
35. deJong RH, Bonin JD: Deaths from local anesthetic-induced convulsions in mice. Anesth Analg 59:401–405, 1980
36. deJong RH, Heavner JE: Diazepam prevents local anesthetic seizures. Anesthesiology 34:523–531, 1971
37. deJong RH, Heavner JE: Diazepam prevents and aborts lidocaine convulsions in monkeys. Anesthesiology 41:226–230, 1974
38. deJong RH, Ronfeld RA, DeRosa RA: Cardiovascular effects of convulsant and supraconvulsant doses of amide local anesthetics. Anesth Analg 61:3–9, 1982
39. DiGiovanni AJ, Galbert MW, Wahle WM: Epidural injection of autologous blood for postlumbar-puncture headache. Anesth Analg 51:226–232, 1972
40. Divoll M, Greenblatt DJ, Ochs HR et al: Absolute bioavailability of oral and intramuscular diazepam: Effects of age and sex. Anesth Analg 62:1–8, 1983
41. Dripps RD, Vandam LD: Long-term follow-up of patients who received 10,098 spinal anesthetics: Failure to discover major neurological sequelae. JAMA 156:1486–1491, 1954
42. Dundee JW, Moore J: Alterations in response to somatic pain associated with anesthesia. IV: The effect of sub-anaesthetic concentrations of inhalation agents. Br J Anaesth 32:453–459, 1960
43. Dupre LJ, Stieglitz P: Extrapyramidal syndromes after premedication with droperidol in children. Br J Anaesth 52:831–833, 1980

44. Dworkin SF, Chen ACN, LeResche L et al: Cognitive reversal of expected nitrous oxide analgesia for acute pain. Anesth Analg 62:1073–1077, 1983

45. Dworkin SF, Schubert MM, Chen ACN et al: Analgesic effects of nitrous oxide with controlled painful stimuli. JADA 107:581–585, 1983

46. Egbert LD, Battit GE, Turndorf H et al: The value of the preoperative visit by an anesthetist. JAMA 185:553–555, 1963

47. Elliott CJR, Green R, Howells TH et al: Recovery after intravenous barbiturate anesthesia. Lancet 1:68–70, 1962

48. Ellis FR, Wilson J: An assessment of droperidol as a premedicant. Br J Anaesth 44:1288–1290, 1972

49. Everett GB, Allen GD: Simultaneous evaluation of cardiorespiratory and analgesic effects of intravenous analgesia in combination with local anesthesia. JADA 81:926–931, 1970

50. Flomenbaum N, Gallagher EJ, Eagen K et al: Self-administered nitrous oxide: An adjunct analgesic. JACEP 8:95–97, 1979

51. Foldes FF, McNall PG: 2-Chloroprocaine, a new local anesthetic agent. Anesthesiology 13:287–296, 1952

52. Forster A, Gardaz JP, Suter PM et al: I.V. midazolam as an induction agent for anaesthesia: A study in volunteers. Br J Anaesth 52:907–911, 1980

53. Gale GD: Recovery from methohexitone, halothane and diazepam. Br J Anaesth 48:691–698, 1976

54. Gelfman SS, Gracely RH, Driscoll EJ et al: Comparison of recovery tests after intravenous sedation with diazepam-methohexital and diazepam-methohexital and fentanyl. J Oral Surg 37:391–397, 1979

55. Gormley JB: Treatment of postspinal headache. Anesthesiology 21:565–566, 1960

56. Greene BA: A 26 gauge lumbar puncture needle: Its value in the prophylaxis of headache following spinal analgesia for vaginal delivery. Anesthesiology 11:464–469, 1950

57. Greene NM: Physiology of spinal anesthesia, 3rd ed. Baltimore, Williams & Wilkins, 1981

58. Grimes DA, Schulz KF, Cates W, et al: Local versus general anesthesia: Which is safer for performing suction curettage abortions? Am J Obstet Gynecol 135:1030–1035, 1979

59. Gross JB, Smith L, Smith TC: Time course of ventilatory response to carbon dioxide after intravenous diazepam. Anesthesiology 57:18–21, 1982

60. Herr GP, Conner JT, Katz RL et al: Diazepam and droperidol as i.v. premedicants. Br J Anaesth 51:537–542, 1979

61. Incaudo G, Schatz M, Patterson R et al: Administration of local anesthetics to patients with a history of prior adverse reaction. J All Clin Immunol 61:339–345, 1978

62. Indresano AT, Rooney TP: Outpatient management of mentally handicapped patients undergoing dental procedures. JADA 102:328–330, 1981

63. Jones RJ: The role of recumbency in the prevention and treatment of postspinal headache. Anesth Analg 53:788–796, 1974

64. Korttila K, Ghoneim MM, Jacobs L et al: Time course of mental and psychomotor effects of 30 per cent nitrous oxide during inhalation and recovery. Anesthesiology 54:220–226, 1981

65. Korttila K, Levanen J: Untoward effects of ketamine combined with diazepam for supplementing conduction anaesthesia in young and middle-aged adults. Acta Anaesth Scand 22:640–648, 1978

66. Korttila K, Linnoila M: Absorption and sedative effects of diazepam after oral administration and intramuscular administration into the vastus lateralis muscle and the deltoid muscle. Br J Anaesth 47:857–862, 1975

67. Korttila K, Linnoila M: Psychomotor skills related to driving after intramuscular administration of diazepam and meperidine. Anesthesiology 42:685–691, 1975

68. Korttila K, Linnoila M: Recovery and skills related to driving after intravenous sedation: Dose-response relationship with diazepam. Br J Anaesth 47:457–463, 1975

69. Korttila K, Mattila MJ, Linnoila M: Prolonged recovery after diazepam sedation: The influence of food, charcoal ingestion and injection rate on the effects of intravenous diazepam. Br J Anaesth 48:333–340, 1976

70. Kotelko DM, Shnider SM, Dailey PA et al: Bupivacaine-induced cardiac arrhythmias in sheep. Anesthesiology 60:10–18, 1984

71. Leaverton GH, Garnjobst W: Comparison of morbidity after spinal and local anesthesia in inguinal hernia repair. Am Surg 38:591–593, 1972

72. Lee CM, Yeakel AE. Patient refusal of surgery following Innovar premedication. Anesth Analg 54:224–226, 1975

73. Lichtenthal P, Philip J, Sloss LJ et al: Administration of nitrous oxide in normal subjects. Chest 72:316–322, 1977

74. Liu P, Feldman HS, Covino BM et al: Acute cardiovascular toxicity of intravenous amide local anesthetics in anesthetized ventilated dogs. Anesth Analg 61:317–322, 1982

75. Liu P, Feldman HS, Covino BM et al: Acute cardiovascular toxicity of procaine, chloroprocaine and tetracaine in anesthetized ventilated dogs. Reg Anesth 7:14–19, 1982

76. Liu PL, Feldman HS, Giasi R et al: Comparative CNS toxicity of lidocaine, etidocaine, bupivacaine and tetracaine in awake dogs following rapid IV administration. Anesth Analg 62:375–379, 1983

77. Loeser EA, Hill GE, Bennett GM et al: Time vs. success rate for epidural blood patch. Anesthesiology 49:147–148, 1978

78. Lund PC: Peridural anesthesia: A review of 10,000 administrations. Acta Anaesth Scand 6:143–159, 1962

79. Maduska LA, Tielens DR: Plasma and cerebrospinal fluid fluoride levels following the obstetrical use of methoxyflurane analgesia. Anesthesiol Rev 3:40–41, 1976

80. Manchikanti L, Marrero TC: Effect of cimetidine and metoclopramide on gastric contents in outpatients. Anesthesiol Rev 10:9–16, 1983

81. Marinacci AA, Courville CB: Electromyogram in evaluation of neurological complications of spinal anesthesia. JAMA 168:1337–1345, 1958

82. McClain DA, Hug CC: Intravenous fentanyl kinetics. Clin Pharmacol Ther 28:106–114, 1980

83. McDonnell TE, Bartkowski RR, Williams JL: ED_{50} of alfentanil for induction of anesthesia in unpremedicated young adults. Anesthesiology 60:136–140, 1984

84. McGown RG: Caudal analgesia in children. Anaesthesia 37:806–818, 1982

85. Meridy HW: Criteria for selection of ambulatory surgery patients and guidelines for anesthetic management: A retrospective study of 1553 cases. Anesth Analg 61:921–926, 1982

86. Meyers EF: Problems during eye surgery under local anesthesia. Anesthesiol Rev 6:23–25, 1979

87. Moore DC: Administer oxygen first in the treatment of local anesthetic-induced convulsions. Anesthesiology 53:346–347, 1980

88. Moore DC: Regional block, 3rd ed. Springfield, IL, Charles C Thomas, 1961

89. Moore DC, Crawford RD, Scurlock JE: Severe hypoxia and acidosis following local anesthetic-induced convulsions. Anesthesiology 53:259–260, 1980

90. Moore DC, Spierdijk J, vanKleef JD et al: Chloroprocaine neurotoxicity: Four additional cases. Anesth Analg 61:155–159, 1982

91. Morishima HO, Pederson H, Finster M et al: Etidocaine toxicity in the adult, newborn, and fetal sheep. Anesthesiology 58:342–346, 1983

92. Morishima HO, Pedersen H, Finster M et al: Toxicity of lidocaine in adult, newborn and fetal sheep. Anesthesiology 55:56–61, 1981

93. Naulty JS, Herold R: Successful epidural anesthesia following epidural blood patch. Anesth Analg 57:272–273, 1978

94. Palahniuk RJ, Cumming M: Prophylactic blood patch does not prevent post-lumbar puncture headache. Can Anaesth Soc J 26:132–133, 1979

95. Penfield AJ: Laparoscopic sterilization under local anesthesia. Obstet Gynecol 49:725–727, 1977

96. Philip BK: Complications of regional anesthesia in obstetrics. Regl Anesth 8:17–30, 1983

97. Philip BK: Effect of epidural air injection on catheter complications. Regl Anesth 10:21–23, 1985

98. Philip JH: GAS MAN: Understanding anesthesia uptake and distribution. Menlo Park, Addison-Wesley, 1984

99. Phillips OC, Ebner H, Nelson AT et al: Neurologic complications following spinal anesthesia with lidocaine. Anesthesiology 30:284–289, 1969
100. Pollard BJ, Lovelock HA, Jones RM: Fatal pulmonary embolism secondary to limb exsanguination. Anesthesiology 58:373–374, 1983
101. Prokocimer P, Delavault E, Rey F et al: Effects of droperidol on respiratory drive in humans. Anesthesiology 59:113–116, 1983
102. Ramanathan S, Chalon J, Richards N et al: Prolonged spinal nerve involvement after epidural anesthesia with etidocaine. Anesth Analg 57:361–364, 1978
103. Ravindran RS, Bond VK, Tasch MD et al: Prolonged neural blockade following regional analgesia with 2-chloroprocaine. Anesth Analg 59:447–451, 1980
104. Ravindran RS, Tasch MD, Baldwin SJ et al: Subarachnoid injection of autologous blood in dogs is unassociated with neurologic deficit. Anesth Analg 60:603–604, 1981
105. Ravindran RS, Turner M, Miller J: Neurologic effects of subarachnoid injection of 2-chloroprocaine-CE, bupivacaine, and low pH normal saline in dogs. Anesth Analg 61:279–283, 1982
106. Reves JG, Corssen G, Holcomb C: Comparison of two benzodiazepines for anaesthesia induction: Midazolam and diazepam. Can Anaesth Soc J 25:211–214, 1978
107. Rice GG, Dabbs CH: The use of peridural and subarachnoid injections of saline solution in the treatment of severe postspinal headache. Anesthesiology 11:17–23, 1950
108. Rita L, Goodarzi M, Seleny F: Effect of low dose droperidol on postoperative vomiting in children. Can Anaesth Soc J 28:359–362, 1981
109. Rosen MA, Baysinger CL, Shnider SM et al: Evaluation of neurotoxicity after subarachnoid injection of large volumes of local anesthetic solutions. Anesth Analg 62:802–808, 1983
110. Rubin J, Brock-Utne JG, Greenberg M et al: Laryngeal incompetence during experimental "relative analgesia" using 50% nitrous oxide in oxygen. Br J Anaesth 49:1005–1007, 1977
111. Sadove MS, Shulman M, Hatano S et al: Analgesic effects of ketamine administered in subdissociative doses. Anesth Analg 50:452–457, 1971
112. Sage D, Feldman H, Arthur GR et al: Differential sensitivities of mammalian nerve fibers during pregnancy. Anesth Analg 63:1–7, 1984
113. Schulte-Steinberg O: Neural blockade for pediatric surgery. In Cousins MJ, Bridenbaugh PO (eds): Neural Blockade in Clinical Anesthesia and Management of Pain. Philadelphia, JB Lippincott, 1980
114. Scott DB: Evaluation of the clinical tolerance of local anesthetic agents. Br J Anaesth 47:328–331, 1975
115. Stewart RD, Paris PM, Stoy WA et al: Patient-controlled inhalational analgesia in prehospital care: A study of side-effects and feasibility. Crit Care Med 11:851–855, 1983
116. Stoelting RK: Allergic reactions during anesthesia. Anesth Analg 62:341–356, 1983
117. Taylor PA, Towey RM: Depression of laryngeal reflexes during ketamine anaesthesia. Br Med J 2:688–689, 1971
118. Thompson DG, Evans SJ, Murray RS et al: Patients appreciate premedication for endoscopy. Lancet 2:469–470, 1980
119. Tucker GT, Mather LE: Clinical pharmacokinetics of local anaesthetics. Clin Pharmacokinet 4:241–278, 1979
120. Urbach GM, Edelist G: An evaluation of anaesthetic techniques used in an outpatient unit. Can Anaesth Soc J 24:401–407, 1977
121. Urbach KF, Lee WR, Sheely LL et al: Spinal or general anesthesia for inguinal hernia repair? JAMA 190:25–29, 1964
122. Usubiaga JE: Neurological complications following epidural anesthesia. Intern Anesth Clin 13(2):1–153, 1975
123. Usubiaga JE, Usubiaga LE, Brea LM et al: Effect of saline injection on epidural and subarachnoid space pressures and relations to post-spinal anesthesia headache. Anesth Analg 46:293–296, 1967
124. Usubiaga JE, Wikinski J, Ferrero R et al: Local anesthetic-induced convulsions in man. Anesth Analg 45:611–620, 1966

125. Vandam LD, Dripps RD: Long-term follow-up of patients who received 10,098 spinal anesthetics: Syndrome of decreased intracranial pressure. JAMA 161:586–591, 1956
126. Vinnick CA: An intravenous dissociation technique for outpatient plastic surgery: Tranquility in the office surgical facility. Plast Reconstr Surg 67:799–805, 1981
127. Warnick JE, Kee RD, Yim GKW: The effects of lidocaine on inhibition in the cerebral cortex. Anesthesiology 34:327–332, 1971
128. Wetchler BV, Collins IS, Jacob L: Antiemetic effects of droperidol on the ambulatory surgery patient. Anesthesiol Rev 9:23–26, 1982
129. White PF: Use of continuous infusion versus intermittent bolus administration of fentanyl or ketamine during outpatient anesthesia. Anesthesiology 59:294–300, 1983
130. White PF, Coe V, Dworsky WA et al: Disseminated intravascular coagulation following midtrimester abortions. Anesthesiology 58:99–101, 1983
131. White PF, Dworsky WA, Horai Y et al: Comparison of continuous infusion fentanyl or ketamine versus thiopental-determining the mean effective serum concentrations for outpatient surgery. Anesthesiology 59:564–569, 1983
132. White PF, Way WL, Trevor AJ: Ketamine—its pharmacology and therapeutic uses. Anesthesiology 56:119–136, 1982
133. Wikinski JA, Usubiaga JE, Morales RL et al: Mechanism of convulsions elicited by local anesthetics. Anesth Analg 49:504–510, 1970
134. Wright DJ, Pandya A: Smoking and gastric juice volume in outpatients. Can Anaesth Soc J 26:328–330, 1979

7

Problem Solving in the Postanesthesia Care Unit

Bernard V. Wetchler, M.D.

Surgery is finished, anesthesia has been discontinued, and the patient now enters the postanesthesia care unit (PACU). If you have not developed a philosophy of care for the ambulatory surgery patient that is different from the way you traditionally manage the hospitalized patient postoperatively, you may find yourself admitting more patients into the hospital than is necessary. In addition, methods of caring for postoperative pain, nausea and vomiting, and fluid intake are not identical. Patients are not recovering from their surgery; wounds take the same length of time to heal regardless of whether the procedure is done on an outpatient or an inpatient basis. Patients are recovering from their anesthesia. Of equal importance to the type and depth of anesthesia the patient has received is the immediate care provided in the PACU.

The patient, responsible person, postanesthesia care nurse, surgeon, and anesthesiologist all play a role in achieving a common goal of early home readiness for the patient (see next page). Major roles are played by the anesthesiologist and the PACU nurse, both of whom are present until the last patient of the day is discharged from the facility. There is no one better qualified than the anesthesiologist to determine when the patient is "home ready." In ambulatory surgery the anesthesiologist can have greater visibility as a physician (evaluation, PACU care, discharge examination) in the eyes of both patient and family.

The Facility

Levy and Coakley stressed the need to separate ambulatory patients in the PACU from inpatients because of the psychological and emotional impact that

☐ **Participants in Achieving Early Home Readiness**

PATIENT

Is motivated to go home
Is willing and able to follow instructions

SURGEON

Carries out appropriate scheduling
  Patient
  Procedure
Provides
  Written discharge instructions
  Prescription for home medications
  Follow-up appointment

PAC NURSE

Monitors vital signs
Manages common PACU problems
Encourages home readiness
Ambulates patient
Checks discharge criteria
Reviews discharge instructions
Evaluates responsible person

RESPONSIBLE PERSON

Encourages home readiness
Takes patient home
Provides assistance at home

ANESTHESIOLOGIST

Makes final preanesthesia patient evaluation
Provides appropriate ambulatory anesthesia
Treats common PACU problems
Examines and discharges patient

---

patients who have had more extensive surgical procedures may have on the reactive alert outpatient.[73] Separation should start with the presurgical waiting area and proceed into the recovery room.

Other disadvantages in mixing outpatient with inpatient are differences in the type, timing, and philosophy of nursing care in dealing with the nonsedated outpatient. It is difficult for postanesthesia care nurses trained in inpatient care to adjust their techniques several times a day to accommodate patients returning to a hospital room as well as those returning to their bed at home. If it is not practical to have separate postanesthesia care units, then screens should be used to separate an area within the PACU and designate it for the ambulatory surgery patient. Grouping ambulatory surgery patients together and having nursing staff work with these patients on a regular basis will minimize problems.

As our patient gradually goes from postanesthesia somnolence to home readiness, we look at varying phases in the patient's recovery. This process is best managed in a designated ambulatory surgery PACU divided into two phases and best accomplished with two separate areas or rooms. We have had great success in motivating our patients for early home readiness under this system.

In developing policies and procedures that will determine time spent in the ambulatory surgery PACU, it is best if patients are required to meet specific criteria for discharge rather than assigning specific time periods as a requirement for length of stay. If one uses traditional inpatient methods of assigning a minimum stay in the PACU of 1 or 2 hours, there can be a great deal of overload in the ambulatory facility because the majority of procedures take less than 1 hour. Whenever you handle short procedures with quick turnover time between cases, you have the potential to overload your PACU. You can't tell staff bringing in patients that there will be a delay before a runway is available, that they are in a holding pattern, that they will have to circle the PACU until space is available. The question in this situation is, "How much space is needed?"

For adequate recovery-room space, Brody recommends a ratio of 1.5 recovery station per operating room if a mix of cases (inpatient, outpatient) is being cared for.[18] If operating rooms are dealing only with short, simple procedures on relatively healthy patients, then four recovery stations are needed per operating room. Short procedures have comparably short recovery times. Consequently, flexibility should be the keyword in the postoperative management of the ambulatory surgery patient. Build flexibility into your guidelines, but never at the expense of patient safety. Don't etch your PACU length of stay in stone. Don't establish discharge criteria you are unable to follow. Make policies practical for your day-to-day situations, and you will find a 2:1 or at most a 3:1 ratio will provide sufficient space needs.

At The Methodist Medical Center of Illinois, our two-phase, two-room PACU with an adjacent holding and dressing area has provided us with flexibility and space (Fig. 7-1). We do not specify absolute times that have to be spent in either of our recovery phases. We rely on a postanesthesia recovery scoring system to determine when our patients can be moved from one phase of recovery to another, and this scoring system plays a part in determining when we consider our patients home ready.

Postanesthesia Scoring Systems

The majority of acceptable postanesthesia recovery scoring systems have similarities to the method of evaluation of the newborn proposed by Apgar in 1953 at the 27th Congress of the International Anesthesia Research Society.[9] For any scoring system to be useful, it must be a practical and simple method of evaluating the patient. It must also be easy to remember and be applicable to all postanesthesia situations. In a busy PACU, the assessment of the patient's condition only by the commonly observed physical signs will avoid any added burden on postanesthesia care personnel. If a scoring system is used, it should not create busy work for the nursing staff and take away from patient care.

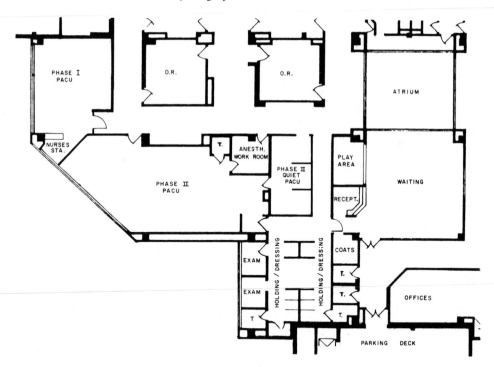

FIG. 7-1 Partial floor plan of Methodist Ambulatory Surgery Center, The Methodist Medical Center of Illinois, Peoria, Illinois.

By assigning numeric values to parameters indicating patient recovery, progress becomes more obvious than it would if vital signs were merely charted with accompanying nurses notes, such as, "Patient reacting—appears able to go home." In a discussion of a patient's postoperative condition, a numbered system is more easily understood, and it allows physicians and nurses to communicate with a common language. A scoring system is a simple way of providing uniform assessment for all patients and may have added medicolegal value when used in addition to the usual subjective means of assessing a patient's home readiness.

An early scoring system proposed by Carignan et al[22] in 1964 lacked common acceptance because of its complexity. Aldrete and Kroulik devised a postanesthesia recovery scoring system analogous to the Apgar method (Table 7-1). Activity, respiration, circulation, consciousness, and color were assigned numeric scores of 0, 1, or 2, a score of 10 indicating that the patient was in the best possible condition for discharge from the PACU.[5]

Steward feels a serious limitation of scoring systems is the inclusion of factors such as color, which lacks consistency in interpretation, and blood pressure, which may have little constant relationship to recovery from anesthesia.[5,22,45,105] In Steward's modification only three areas are evaluated (Table 7-2). These were chosen because they were easily classified into well-recognized stages and demonstrated a series of progressive changes relating to

☐ Table 7-1 Aldrete Scoring System

Postanesthesia Recovery Score	In	15	30	45	Hrs	Out
ACTIVITY						
Able to move voluntarily or on command						
4 extremities	2	2	2	2	2	2
2 extremities	1	1	1	1	1	1
0 extremities	0	0	0	0	0	0
RESPIRATION						
Able to deep breathe and cough freely	2	2	2	2	2	2
Dyspnea, shallow or limited breathing	1	1	1	1	1	1
Apneic	0	0	0	0	0	0
CIRCULATION						
Preoperative blood pressure ___ mm						
BP ± 20 mm of preanesthesia level	2	2	2	2	2	2
BP ± 20 to 50 mm of preanesthesia level	1	1	1	1	1	1
BP ± 50 mm of preanesthesia level	0	0	0	0	0	0
CONSCIOUSNESS						
Fully awake	2	2	2	2	2	2
Arousable on calling	1	1	1	1	1	1
Not responding	0	0	0	0	0	0
COLOR						
Normal	2	2	2	2	2	2
Pale, dusky, blotchy, jaundiced, other	1	1	1	1	1	1
Cyanotic	0	0	0	0	0	0

DISMISSAL CRITERIA: Total score of 10, plus stable vital signs   Total ___
A physician's order is required for discharge with lower score.

the recovery process and indicating a significant return of protective functions. A total score of 6 indicates a fully recovered patient.

The scoring system of Robertson et al, used to measure arousal from general anesthesia in ambulatory surgery patients, incorporated certain features of the scoring system suggested by Steward (Table 7-3).[91] It is more cumbersome to use than other systems because a variety of numeric scores is given for the varying parameters. A score of 9 indicates complete recovery to the aware state.

Two-Phase Postanesthesia Care Unit

Regardless of which scoring system is used, the majority of nonpremedicated patients having short surgical procedures will reach a score indicating early recovery from anesthesia in approximately 30 minutes. We use the Aldrete scoring system, and upon scoring 10, the patient is moved from phase one postanesthesia care into phase two. Our phase one PACU has all the usual

☐ Table 7-2   Steward Scoring System

Criterion	Score
CONSCIOUSNESS	
Awake	2
Responding to stimuli	1
Not responding	0
AIRWAY	
Coughing on command or crying	2
Maintaining good airway	1
Airway requires maintenance	0
MOVEMENT	
Moving limbs purposefully	2
Nonpurposeful movements	1
Not moving	0
Total	___

(Steward DJ: A simplified scoring system for the post operative recovery room. Can Anaesth Soc J 22(1):111, 1975)

☐ Table 7-3   Robertson Scoring System

Criterion	Score
CONSCIOUSNESS	
Fully awake; eyes open; conversing	4
Lightly asleep; eyes open intermittently	3
Eyes open on command or in response to name	2
Responding to ear-pinching	1
Not responding	0
AIRWAY	
Opening mouth or coughing or both, on command	3
No voluntary cough, but airway clear without support	2
Airway obstructed on neck flexion but clear without support on extension	1
Airway obstructed without support	0
ACTIVITY	
Raising one arm on command	2
Nonpurposeful movement	1
Not moving	0
Total	___

(Robertson GS, MacGregor DM, Jones CJ: Evaluation of doxapram for arousal from general anesthesia in outpatients. Br J Anaesth 49:133, 1977) equipment one expects to find in any recovery area. The majority of our patients ambulate into the operating room, and only at the conclusion of their surgical procedures are they placed on a stretcher for phase one PACU care.

In our phase two PACU, reclining lounge chairs are used (Fig. 7-2). Here, family members are actively engaged in attending the patient and encouraging activity in preparation for discharge home. We initially position the reclining chair in an almost flat stage, and gradually, over a period of approximately 30 minutes, the patient is moved into a sitting position. A patient can progress from a cart to a recliner much earlier than to a regular chair. The recliner is more comfortable and can be positioned appropriately if nausea or orthostatic hypotension occur. Patients are usually discharged sooner if their activity is increased to the recliner stage after surgery than if they recover completely on a cart or are transferred to a bed.[101]

In the two-phase postanesthesia care room at the North Carolina Memorial Hospital the first phase is called the *recovery room* and the second phase is called *day op room*. The time spent by patients in the day op room exceeds the time spent in the first-phase recovery room. By having a second room, they have relieved a single recovery room of a tremendous number of patient hours and potential overcrowding.[84]

In our own busy ambulatory surgery service, in which over 7000 patients are seen per year, we would have been unable to manage recovery care of our

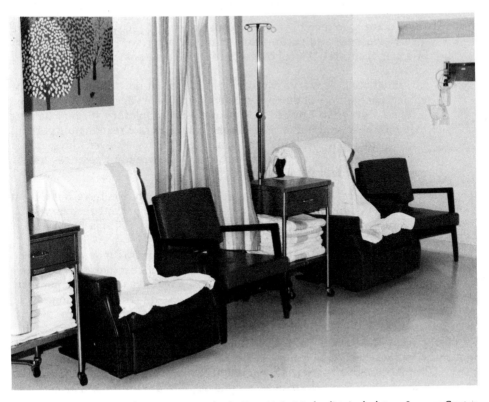

FIG. 7-2 Phase II Postanesthesia Care Unit, Methodist Ambulatory Surgery Center.

patients in a single room having a 1.5:1 or 2:1 ratio of recovery spaces to operating rooms. On busy days, we also use our holding area for patient observation prior to discharge. This gives us the flexibility of a three-phase recovery area. If a surgeon doing a procedure under local anesthesia (no sedation, no anesthesia standby) wishes the patient to be observed in the recovery area, the patient can go directly to the holding area for observation before going home.

An ambulatory surgery PACU must be equipped to handle all emergencies. Ambulatory surgery procedures are not as invasive as procedures performed on hospitalized patients, and the level of sophisticated monitoring to which patients in the PACU are subjected usually reflects this. Procedures are shorter, patient population is healthier, and with patients responding quickly following their anesthetic, not every patient need be monitored by machines. This does not mean the facility can cut corners. The ambulatory surgery PACU must have electrocardiographic (ECG) monitoring capabilities, appropriate ventilatory support apparatus, plus a fully stocked crash cart capable of managing emergencies (e.g., cardiopulmonary, respiratory, hyperthermic).

Measuring Recovery from Anesthesia

Steward divided recovery from general anesthesia into three stages:[107]

I. Immediate recovery: Return of consciousness, recovery of protective airway reflexes and resumption of motor activity. This stage is short and can accurately be followed by the use of a postanesthesia scoring system.
II. Intermediate recovery: Return of coordination; disappearance of subjective feelings of dizziness. Following a short anesthetic, this stage lasts no more than 1 hour. At this time, the ambulatory surgery patient may be considered home ready in the company of a responsible person.
III. Long-term recovery: This stage may last hours or even days and is dependent on the length of anesthesia. Measurement requires use of precise psychomotor testing.

A variety of clinical, pencil-and-paper, and psychomotor tests have been used, singly or in combination, as a means of measuring patient recovery from anesthesia. The majority are too involved and impractical for a busy clinical setting.

Korttila measured patient recovery following intravenous sedation.[69] Psychomotor tests revealed considerable impairment of reactive and coordinative skills at $2\frac{1}{2}$ hours, whereas neither the clinical nor the pencil-and-paper tests (used in Finland as sensitive indicators in assessing the performance of suspected drunken drivers) demonstrated significant impairment of performance 1 half-hour after injection (see next page).

Cohen and MacKenzie gave patients a series of five tests of mental function just prior to anesthesia and during the second and third hour after entry into the PACU.[25] Although all patients appeared to have normal cognitive functioning at the time of discharge, there was a considerable degree of impairment of psychomotor ability.

☐ *Combination of Tests Used by Korttila*

CLINICAL

Walking on a straight line
Romberg test with open eyes
Picking up matches
Numerical countdown test
Horizontal nystagmus
Postrotary nystagmus

PENCIL-AND-PAPER

Bender motor gestalt
Burdon-Wiersma

PSYCHOMOTOR

Reactive skills
Coordinative skills
Attention
Critical flicker fusion

(Korttila K: Recovery after intravenous sedation: A comparison of clinical and paper and pencil tests used in assessing later effects of diazepam. Anaesthesia 31:724, 1976)

Doenicke et al studied the effectiveness of psychological testings and feel they do not adequately reflect the variations in cerebral function during the hours and days following anesthesia; fatigue plays a major role in the inaccuracies following repetitive testing.[36] To rule out the effect of fatigue on results, electroencephalography was used to assess depth and recovery from anesthesia following administration of different intravenous anesthetics.[37]

Boas et al compared a group of ambulatory surgery patients recovering from anesthesia induction with midazolam with a group recovering from thiopental.[17] Patients had to recognize previously shown pictures, repeat a series of numbers, and place dots in small squares. The dose of midazolam was 0.125 to 0.2 mg/kg and that of thiopental was 5 mg/kg. Induction time took longer with midazolam, although subsequent transition to halothane inhalation anesthesia was smooth and uneventful. Recovery was more prolonged with midazolam, tests of memory and aided mobility showing greater impairment 1 hour after anesthesia.

The majority of these tests are too involved for practical clinical use. The development of a simple objective test to measure patient recovery from anesthesia is definitely of clinical value and in some respects might be considered more objective from a medicolegal standpoint. One such test used at several ambulatory surgery centers has been found an effective means of assessing patient recovery. The Trieger dot test[80] (Fig. 7-3) is an adaption of the Bender motor gestalt test. Patients are asked to connect a series of dots (usually done in the waiting room) prior to the start of anesthesia and surgery. The patient should be observed and timed. Adding the number of dots not touched by the connecting pencil line to the time it takes to complete the drawing is the simplest method of determining the patient's score. This test can be repeated following entry into the PACU and prior to discharge. To be considered ready for discharge, a patient's score should be equal to, or better than, the initial score. On occasion, a patient may have achieved a score in the preanesthesia period that cannot be matched in the postanesthesia period, and therefore it is well to include modifiers that will allow the postanesthesia score to be acceptable for discharge. The Trieger test is a simple, direct, self-administered objective test that measures sensorimotor performance, a critical determinant of recovery.

Denis et al, in comparing reliability and validity of psychomotor tests as measures of recovery in ambulatory surgery patients, found the Bender gestalt track tracer a reliable and valid measure of recovery from anesthesia.[33] The track tracer consists of a square and a circle. The patient is instructed to trace or follow the track of the square and circle without touching the sides. The test, which can be completed in approximately 60 seconds, is reliable, valid, objective, noninvasive, inexpensive, and easily understood by patients. Any staff member can administer it, there is a permanent record on paper, and, like the Trieger

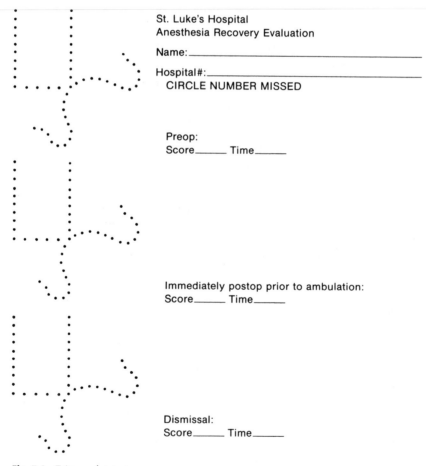

St. Luke's Hospital
Anesthesia Recovery Evaluation

Name:_____

Hospital#:_____
CIRCLE NUMBER MISSED

Preop:
Score_____ Time_____

Immediately postop prior to ambulation:
Score_____ Time_____

Dismissal:
Score_____ Time_____

Fig. 7-3 Trieger dot test.

test, it can be considered an objective means of assessing patient recovery from anesthesia.

Once discharge criteria have been met, the clinical judgment of the physician examining the patient becomes the single most important factor in determining the patient's home readiness. Psychological tests whose results do not coincide with clinical judgment in no way indicate that the patient should not be sent home. The patient should be allowed home once clinical discharge criteria have been met, but should be transported home and watched over by a responsible person.

Perhaps in no other area must anesthesiologists be more acutely aware of the variations that occur in the PACU following anesthetic intervention than when dealing with the ambulatory surgery patient. The literature can be helpful in decision making; however, only by personal evaluation of the effects that the varying agents have on individual patients such as nausea, vomiting, headache, dizziness, drowsiness, and length of stay in the PACU can anesthesiologists decide which agents are more desirable than others for their ambulatory surgery patients.

Complications: Reasons for Admission

The time interval between admission into the PACU and patient departure with a responsible person will vary depending on the use of premedication, the length and complexity of the surgery, anesthetic agents administered, and the degree of severity of common postoperative problems such as drowsiness, dizziness, pain, nausea, and vomiting. Perioperative problems can be of such a nature and severity that they may result in admission or transfer into the hospital.

During a 4-year period at George Washington University Hospital, PACU complications were reviewed in a group of 5516 outpatients.[73] Of these patients, 185 (3.4%) had complications requiring treatment. In order of frequency, these were nausea and vomiting, pain, emergence delirium, bleeding, syncope, hypoventilation, and arrhythmias. During 1983, out of a total of 4065 cases, 44 patients (1%) were admitted. Of those admissions, only 21% were considered anesthesia related, compared to 64% related to surgery. The remaining admissions (15%) occurred for medical or social reasons.*

At the Phoenix Surgicenter, the hospital transfer rate is approximately 0.2% for all patients, increasing to 0.59% for patients over 65 years of age and to 1.41% for patients who are ASA physical status 3.[31] The most common causes for transfer are bleeding, inadequate pain control, and the need for further elective operation. Meridy reports a transfer into the hospital of 2.44% of patients.[78] Of that number, 0.64% were judged to have complications secondary to anesthesia and 1.8% to have complications secondary to surgery. Of the patients transferred to the hospital, 87% received some form of general anesthesia, whereas 13% received only local anesthesia. Of patients admitted to the hospital because of anesthetic complications, all received a general anesthesia (Table 7-4). No single general anesthetic appeared superior to any other in reducing postoperative morbidity.

*Levy M-L: Personal communication, 1984

☐ **Table 7-4   Complications Resulting in Hospital Transfer**

Complication	No. of Patients
ANESTHESIA RELATED	
Nausea and vomiting	8
Epistaxis	1
Atrial flutter	1
SURGERY RELATED	
Pain	9
Bleeding	4
Temperature	3
Observation	2
Surgical misadventure	3
Errors in diagnosis	7

(Meridy HW: Criteria for selection of ambulatory surgical patients and guidelines for anesthetic management: A retrospective study of 1,553 cases. Anesth Analg 61(1): 921, 1982)

Laparoscopy is one of the most frequently performed ambulatory surgery procedures. Following laparoscopy, patients have reported weakness (66%), drowsiness (58%), dizziness (42%), vomiting (31%), visual disturbances (15%), and headache (13%) when leaving the PACU.[34] None of the symptoms were severe enough to require admission into the hospital. Ninety-three percent of the patients felt they required an escort home. There were no significant differences in immediate postoperative morbidity among patients who received halothane, enflurane, or fentanyl.

Complications caused by creation of a pneumoperitoneum, although rare, may present as subcutaneous emphysema, pneumothorax, and pneumo-mediastinum.[35,97] In the PACU, patients may present with palpable subcutaneous crepitus over the upper chest, shoulders, and neck or, in the case of pneumothorax, signs of respiratory embarrassment. Chest radiograph and blood gases should be checked in the PACU. These patients are usually hospitalized for observation and on rare occasion may require insertion of a chest tube. Batra et al reported one case of moderately severe respiratory distress from pneumothorax that disappeared quickly and spontaneously, permitting patient discharge the same day without prolonged thoracentesis and with no adverse outcome.[13] The patient remained overnight in a hotel-like facility next door to the hospital and was monitored as an outpatient for 2 days. It was felt the pneumothorax resulted from gas diffusing from the distended peritoneal space to the pleural space.

At our own ambulatory surgery facility, we have taken care of 45,326 patients from September 15, 1977 through September 14, 1984. Of that number, 27,372 received services of the anesthesia department, while 17,954 had local anesthesia (but no sedation) administered by the surgeon. We have admitted 310 patients (0.68%) for perioperative problems. Of the patients admitted, 303 (97.7%) were managed by the anesthesia department, while 7 (2.3%) had only local anesthesia. Reasons for admission, although not always easily delineated, can usually be divided among patient, procedure, and postanesthesia care (Table 7-5).

In the procedure-related group, 98 patients were admitted for more extensive surgery than planned. Initially, the inability to perform a laparoscopy and the need to perform a laparotomy meant automatic admission; currently, laparotomy does not require admission. Hospital admission results more frequently in our facility from bleeding as the reason for performing the initial surgery (i.e., epistaxis, incomplete abortion) than from bleeding occurring as a complication of the surgery.

Further breakdown of reasons for admission in our facility revealed that the 61 anesthesia-related problems (nausea/vomiting, syncope, arrhythmias, compromised ventilatory status) accounted for only 19.7% of all admissions

☐ **Table 7-5 Reasons for Hospital Admission from Methodist Ambulatory Surgery Center**

Reason	No. of Patients
PATIENT	
Refused to go home	13
No responsible person	9
PROCEDURE	
More extensive surgery	98
Positive biopsy	39
Misadventures	38
Bleeding	
Uterine perforation	
Bladder puncture	
Bowel burn	
Pneumothorax	
IVP dye reaction	4
Postspinal headache	1
PAC	
Bleeding	28
Syncope	21
Drowsiness	
Dizziness	
Decreased blood pressure	
Pain	18
Pulmonary	15
Asthma	
Aspiration	
Croup	
Nausea/vomiting	13
Arrhythmias	11
Hypertension	2

☐ **Table 7-6 Breakdown of Hospital Admissions from Methodist Ambulatory Surgery Center**

No. of Patients	Related to	Percentage of Patients
188	Procedure	60.6
61	Anesthesia	19.7
39	Pathology	12.6
22	Patient	7.1

(Table 7-6). One hundred eighty-eight admissions (60.6%) were related to the surgical procedure and 39 (12.6%) to pathology found on biopsy; a total of 227 admits (73.2%) were therefore related to the surgery itself. The remaining 7.1% of admits were related to patients refusing to go home or to lack of a responsible person being present to take the patient home and take care of his or her needs.

Of the 28 patients in whom bleeding was first noted in the postanesthesia recovery unit, 13 followed tonsillectomy or adenoidectomy (T&A) (Table 7-7). Our overall ambulatory surgery T&A bleed is 1.5%.

A 41-year-old woman never recovered after her procedure. Within the first 30 minutes in the PACU, she developed signs of a neurologic deficit and was admitted into the hospital. She was appropriately worked up (CT scan), and was diagnosed as having had an inoperable massive cerebral bleed from a ruptured congenital A-V malformation. She died 9 hours after tubal surgery. Postmortem examination confirmed the radiographic diagnosis.

Premedication

The anesthesiologist has little control over unexpected length and complexity of surgery, but does have control over premedicant drugs and anesthetic agents administered. The larger the dose and the more long-acting depressant premedication given, the greater is the chance of prolonging recovery with potential for drowsiness, dizziness, hypotension, or vomiting.[44] Anesthesiolo-

☐ **Table 7-7 Postanesthesia Care Bleeding at the Methodist Ambulatory Surgery Center**

Procedure	No. of Patients
T&A	13
Cervical biopsy	4
Oral surgery	4
Prostatic biopsy	3
Laparoscopy	2
Bartholin cyst	1
A-V malformation	1

gists differ in opinion as to whether premedication should be used prior to ambulatory surgery. The majority believe little or no premedication should be given because it may prolong recovery time to the point at which the patient may have to be admitted to the hospital,[31,104] whereas others feel premedication should be considered a part of good patient care.[23] At George Washington University Hospital no premedication is used.[24,74] The Phoenix Surgicenter, where over 95,000 patients have been anesthetized since 1970, attributes their patients' rapid recovery following general anesthesia to the absence of using narcotic or sedative premedication.[31]

Some facilities use only belladonna drugs.[3,79] At our facility, where 7000 patients are cared for annually and over 4000 are managed by the anesthesia department, either atropine alone or no premedication is used. Without atropine, patient complaint of dry mouth in the PACU is decreased.[72] Premedication is fully discussed in Chapter 5.

Pain

Medications given in the PACU must be closely monitored and given in small, immediately effective doses. Intramuscular narcotic analgesic injection for pain control of surgical patients in the PACU is probably more a custom than a well-thought-out process.[4] In patients recovering from anesthesia, analgesics must have a rapid onset in order to alleviate pain promptly, and this is best achieved by the intravenous route. Faster onset and more precise blood levels can be obtained when drugs are given intravenously. When the intramuscular route is used, undertreatment is possible, since drugs may be deposited into subcutaneous rather than muscular tissue.

Pain must be treated quickly and effectively. If pain is allowed to linger and become severe before instituting treatment, larger doses of narcotics will be required for relief. Untreated pain will result in nausea and vomiting. In our facility, we have found that fast and effective treatment of pain lessens the amounts of narcotics required and limits postoperative nausea and vomiting. To facilitate the smooth functioning of our ambulatory surgery facility, we have established routine orders and policies for pain control that allow our postanesthesia care nursing staff to administer small intravenous doses of narcotic analgesics without having to call a physician for every order.

Postoperative pain control should be started intraoperatively by supplementing inhalation anesthesia with short-acting narcotic analgesics or regional block. Patients wake up quickly in the PACU following anesthesia with currently used major inhalation agents and quickly complain of pain. By making appropriate use of short-acting narcotic analgesics or regional block intraoperatively, awakening will be smoother and discharge home will occur sooner.

In a group of patients undergoing voluntary interruption of pregnancy or dilatation and curettage (D&C) procedures who were given thiopental, nitrous oxide, oxygen or thiopental, nitrous oxide, oxygen with supplemental fentanyl, Epstein found a significantly higher incidence of pain and a slightly higher incidence of excitement during recovery in the patients who did not receive fentanyl.[42] Analgesics were required in only one of fourteen patients in the fentanyl group and five of 25 in the thiopental group. Although there was a higher incidence of nausea in the fentanyl group, this group of patients recovered statistically sooner than those who received no narcotic supplementation during anesthesia. In the D&C group in the immediate postoperative period, there was reduction in pain, a shorter time to walk without support and stand with negative Romberg, and less time spent in the PACU. In a 24-hour postoperative period, there was reduction in pain compared to the group that did not receive fentanyl (see below). Hunt added a single dose of fentanyl (75–125 μg) intravenously immediately before induction to a group of ambulatory surgery patients undergoing D&C.[61] The addition of fentanyl significantly reduced the frequency of abdominal pain in the PACU and during the first evening at home, but did not increase the frequency of other postoperative sequelae such as nausea and vomiting. In using fentanyl in over 20,000 ambulatory surgery procedures, we have found it to be associated with the shortest recovery time and the least amount of postanesthetic hangover when used in a supplemental dose of 1 to 2 μg/kg.[112]

☐ *Advantages of Fentanyl as an Adjunct to Thiopental, Nitrous Oxide, Oxygen*

Operative period
   Smoother course of anesthesia
   Reduction in dose of thiopental
Immediate postoperative period
   Reduction in pain
   Shorter time to walk without support, stand with negative Romberg, and to discharge
Twenty-four hour postoperative period
   Reduction in pain

(Epstein BS, Levy ML, Thein MH et al: Evaluation of fentanyl as an adjunct to thiopental-nitrous oxide-oxygen anesthesia for short surgical procedures. Anesth Rev 2(3):24, 1975).

The use of regional blocking techniques as a means of postoperative pain control is discussed in Chapter 4; however, additional comment is indicated at this time. Shandling and Steward feel that children over 6 months of age almost invariably require some postoperative analgesics following inguinal hernia repair.[94] Struggling, crying, and restlessness in the immediate postoperative period may result in bleeding into the wound, resulting in delayed healing. Postoperative vomiting (15%–20%) is more common in pediatric patients than in adults following hernia repair.[103] Fewer analgesics are required in the postanesthesia recovery period in some facilities where narcotic analgesics have been included as part of the anesthetic technique. When regional block supplementation is provided to the patient, there is both a decrease in pain and vomiting during both the recovery period and the first 48 postoperative hours.

At our facility, we have used regional blocking techniques in both our pediatric and adult patients undergoing inguinal hernia surgery with excellent results. Asking our surgeons to block the ilioinguinal and iliohypogastric nerves has resulted in a much smoother postoperative course and earlier home readiness.

The technique is not without its problems. If the local anesthetic is injected near the femoral nerve, it may take 3 to 4 hours for quadriceps functions to return. We have never had this problem occur using 0.25% bupivacaine, but it has been reported when 0.5% bupivacaine was used.[94] The pediatric patient can be carried home, but in the adult patient it is wise to wait for this function to return before considering the patient home ready.

In Chapter 4, we refer to the bupivacaine manufacturers' caution about the drug's use in children under the age of 12. I feel, as do Epstein and Hannallah, that sufficient evidence supports bupivacaine as an acceptable local anesthetic drug in the pediatric patient when appropriately administered.

We have used a transcutaneous nerve stimulator to relieve postoperative pain following inguinal hernia repair. Patients were instructed on the use of the unit prior to surgery. Immediately following surgery, with the patient still on the operating room table, electrodes were put in place. The patient used the unit in the PACU and at home for 48 hours. Among patients who had a unilateral hernia repair, mild to moderate relief of pain in the first 24 hours was felt by 78%, and marked pain relief was noted during the second 24 hours by 93%. All patients were allowed to take oral pain medications. For patients who had bilateral repairs done during separate procedures performed 1 week apart, the transcutaneous nerve stimulator was provided for only one of the procedures. Significantly less pain medication was taken by all four patients following the procedure for which the transcutaneous nerve stimulator was provided.

Postoperative morbidity following laparoscopic tubal sterilization is low and primarily related to pain. There is no incisional pain, but abdominal discomfort, shoulder pain, and nausea and vomiting frequently delay discharge. The level of discomfort will vary, depending on the type of sterilization performed; less pain and cramping follow cautery compared to Yoon fallopian ring sterilization.

We evaluated the effects of intraoperative local block of the mesosalpinx in the area of the Yoon ring placement.[6] One hundred eighty-six patients were involved in our double blind study. They were divided into four groups: control (no injection), normal saline, 1% lidocaine, and 0.5% bupivacaine. The intensity of deep pain complaint in the 0.5% bupivacaine-injected group was lower (statistically significant) during the PACU stay and when patients dressed to return home. In addition, the bupivacaine group complained of a lower level of pain intensity 24 hours after surgery.

In a study from the University of Massachusetts Medical Center comparing types of anesthesia and their effect on recovery following laparoscopic tubal ligation, the use of a longer-acting narcotic, meperidine (1–1.5 mg/kg), instead of fentanyl (2 µg/kg) intraoperatively, did not delay recovery from anesthesia or patient discharge. Techniques that provided the best postoperative pain relief, least nausea, and a most rapid tolerance of postoperative fluids were meperidine and epidural anesthesia. Based on observations of the postanesthesia care nurses, the epidural group had the best scores in every parameter. The study concluded that anesthetic techniques that provide the best pain relief in the first 2 hours following surgery have a lower incidence of overall morbidity and more rapid recovery.[99]

McGlinchey et al supplemented general anesthesia with regional block of the dorsal nerve of the penis (0.5% bupivacaine) in a group of adult outpatients undergoing circumcision.[77] None of the patients required analgesia in the 6 hours following surgery, unlike a control group in which all required strong narcotic analgesic supplementation in the recovery stages.

Surgeons may resist injecting local anesthesia during the procedure because they are concerned about

Hemorrhage into the wound
Infection
Reaction to local anesthetic drug
Numbness which may allow the patient to inflict some type of self-injury

In addition, the surgeon may see no surgical or technical advantages to injecting local anesthesia and may object on the grounds that it will prolong surgery time.

You are going to have to sell the surgeon on the advantages of regional block supplementation:

Less pain in the PACU
Less analgesics needed in the PACU
Less postoperative minor morbidity
Earlier "home readiness"

By having the anesthesiologist communicate problem-solving techniques to the surgeon, patients can be provided with a smoother course in the PACU and the immediate postoperative period at home. Whenever simple regional supplemental block can be performed, make use of it; your patients will certainly be appreciative.

In our PACU, pain in both adults and children is managed with a short-acting narcotic analgesic. Fentanyl has been our drug of choice. A policy on postoperative pain management has been approved by our medical staff. This policy allows our postanesthesia care nurses to administer small intravenous doses of fentanyl without the need for a specific physician's examination or order. Intravenous fentanyl, 12.5 μg (0.25 ml), is given at 5-minute intervals up to a total dose of 50 μg (1 ml). Pain control is instituted at the first sign of discomfort. This works satisfactorily in more than 98% of our patients (see below). If pain persists after 50 μg of fentanyl has been administered, an anesthesiologist checks the patient to see if there is a reason for the persistence before any additional analgesia is given.

☐ *Adult Patient PACU Pain Management at the Methodist Ambulatory Surgery Center*

This policy applies to patients who are at least 12 years old and weigh more than 80 lb.

1. Fentanyl, 12.5 μg, IV (0.25 ml)
2. Repeat at 5-min intervals as needed.
3. Question patients as to disappearance of pain after administering each dose.
4. Total dose not to exceed 50 μg (1.0 ml)
5. Contact a member of the anesthesiology department if pain is not relieved.

Pediatric patients also have an established fentanyl dosage based on weight (see next page). We feel more secure in allowing our nursing staff to administer intravenous fentanyl in this manner rather than having them calculate the patients' needs in micrograms per kilogram of body weight. For pediatric patients, the initial fentanyl dosage can be repeated only once before we require examination by an anesthesiologist. Our policy allows for the routine use of acetaminophen elixir in our pediatric patients, and we have enjoyed great success using a combination of intravenous and oral pain medications in this population group. At Children's Hospital National Medical Center (CHNMC) fentanyl 1 μg/kg to 2 μg/kg is given intravenously for postoperative pain management. (See Postoperative Analgesia in Chap. 4.)

☐ *Pediatric Patient PACU Pain Management at the Methodist Ambulatory Surgery Center*

This policy applies to patients who are less than 12 years old and weigh less than 80 lb. The following table shows total dosages for specific patient weights:

WEIGHT (LB)	INITIAL DOSAGE	TOTAL DOSAGE
20–40	5 μg (0.1 ml)	10 μg (0.2 ml)
41–50	7.5 μg (0.15 ml)	15 μg (0.3 ml)
51–60	10 μg (0.2 ml)	20 μg (0.4 ml)
61–80	12.5 μg (0.25 ml)	25 μg (0.5 ml)

1. Fentanyl intravenously according to the dosages given above.
2. Repeat only once at 5-min interval if needed.
3. Supplement with acetaminophen elixir.
4. Contact a member of the anesthesiology department if pain is not relieved.

In 100 consecutive patients aged 2 to 7 years who underwent T&A surgery at our ambulatory surgery center, fentanyl was given during administration of the anesthetic (in addition to inhalation anesthesia) and was repeated by our nursing staff in the PACU according to postoperative pain policy. Supplemental oral acetaminophen was added at the discretion of the nurse. No patient who followed this routine required any additional physician examination or order for the relief of pain during their 3-hour PACU stay.[113]

Establishing a PACU policy for pain management eliminates the problems that may occur when each physician orders different postoperative pain medication for his or her patients. Without a standard policy, surgeons and anesthesiologists who are used to working in an inpatient environment would order morphine or meperidine in substantial intramuscular dosages for postoperative pain. One must be careful that this does not happen because of the long-acting effects of these drugs.

Oral analgesics ordered by the surgeon as take-home medications can also be used in the PACU once the patient has taken fluids and shows no signs of nausea or vomiting.

Nausea and Vomiting

Nausea (30%) and emesis (20%) are the most common complications occurring in the PACU at the Phoenix Surgicenter.[31] Contributing factors are pain, narcotic analgesic drugs, sudden movement or position changes, history of motion sickness, hypotension, and obesity. Emesis was the most common single complication in the PACU following ambulatory surgery in 977 pediatric patients and was of sufficient severity in 1.7% of the patients to require overnight hospitalization.[3] We have found that ambulatory surgery patients who experienced emesis at some point in their postoperative recovery tended to be heavier than those who experienced no emetic symptoms.[63]

Anderson and Crohg established a relationship between postoperative pain and the frequency of nausea in the early postsurgical period.[8] Although the study was not done on an ambulatory surgery population, its implications are significant for the outpatient. Complete pain relief without simultaneous relief of nausea was unusual. Patients who had inadequate pain relief and continued nausea after the first analgesic injection (50% of the subjects) were relieved of both complaints after a supplementary dose of an opiate. Only 10% of patients complained of postoperative nausea without accompanying pain. Nausea often accompanies pain in the postoperative period and can be relieved in 80% of cases when pain relief is achieved by the intravenous use of opiates.

A major problem following ambulatory surgery anesthesia is nausea and vomiting. Admission to the hospital can result not only from uncontrolled nausea and vomiting, but also from prolonged somnolence following treatment with potent antiemetics. A history of motion sickness or nausea and vomiting following prior anesthetics obtained during the preanesthesia interview should alert the anesthesiologist to use an antiemetic intraoperatively.

Emetecone, tigan, compazine, and metoclopramide have all been tried for the control of postanesthetic nausea and vomiting with limited success.[26,28] For patients with a prior history of nausea and vomiting associated with anesthesia, Natof* has found the intra-anesthetic administration of 1.25 mg droperidol given intravenously to be effective in lessening these distressing postanesthetic symptoms. Cohen et al compared the effects of droperidol and metoclopramide on postoperative nausea and vomiting in outpatients who received the drugs intravenously 2 to 10 minutes before induction of anesthesia.[26] A trend toward a lower incidence of nausea and vomiting in the droperidol patients was not statistically significant. The droperidol patients had a higher incidence of complaint of dizziness at home than the metoclopramide and the placebo group. There were no differences among the groups with regard to postdischarge nausea, vomiting, or other symptoms. Although a lack of antiemetic effect was noted from metoclopramide, patients seemed to benefit by being able to sit, walk, and be ready for discharge earlier than other patients.

At the Children's Hospital of Philadelphia, Transderm-V scopolamine (Alza Corp., Palo Alto, California) has been tried to control nausea and vomiting. Researchers have not found the results statistically significant, but they have noted an increased incidence of psychological side-effects (visual hallucinations) once their patients have gone home.†

Vomiting is the major limiting factor delaying discharge from the hospital in ambulatory surgery patients undergoing strabismus corrective surgery. In two separate studies, droperidol was given intravenously 30 minutes prior to the termination of surgery.[1,2] A dose of 50 μg/kg reduced the incidence of vomiting by 25% and patients who received this treatment were discharged 38 minutes earlier than the placebo group. The reduction was not statistically significant. A second study was undertaken using a dose of 75 μg/kg, and the incidence of vomiting was significantly reduced following droperidol (43%) compared to the control group (85%). In the second study there was no

*Natof HE: Personal communication, 1984
†Betts EK: Personal communication, 1984

statistically significant difference in PACU length of stay in either the control group (360.7 ±13.1 min) or the droperidol treated group (347.9 ±21.4 min). Ten patients in the control group had vomiting of such severity that they required treatment with droperidol in the PACU. When giving doses of 75 μg/kg, be prepared for a lengthy PACU stay. At the Children's Medical Center in Dallas* and at our own institution, we have been able to decrease nausea and vomiting using 20 to 25 μg/kg of droperidol administered as a single bolus immediately following intubation without significant prolongation of recovery (personal observation, not evaluated by study).

There is a significantly higher incidence of postoperative nausea and vomiting in the pediatric patient who undergoes strabismus or orchiopexy surgery. Following orchiopexy, up to 5% of patients may have to be admitted because of drowsiness, nausea and vomiting, or more extensive surgery than planned.[20]

A recovery time of 4 to 6 hours after surgery would be considered prolonged in children following myringotomy or herniotomy, but, because of nausea and vomiting, is not an unusual length of stay after strabismus or orchiopexy surgery.[1,2] Intraoperative droperidol is recommended in these patients.

We studied the effects of low-dose droperidol on postoperative nausea and vomiting and length of PACU stay.[114] Three hundred laparoscopic tubal patients were divided into three equal groups. Group 1, the control, received no treatment for nausea and vomiting; group 2 patients received droperidol, 0.625 mg to 1.25 mg, intravenously immediately following intubation; group 3 patients received no antiemetic medication intra-anesthetically, but were treated for nausea and vomiting in the PACU according to established policy, which allows our nursing staff to institute early treatment of nausea and vomiting without requiring specific physician's orders (see next page). In our study, the patients who received droperidol during anesthesia had a lower incidence of nausea and vomiting in the PACU, resulting in a shorter length of stay than either of the other two groups.

Shelly and Brown found droperidol to be an effective antiemetic in doses as low as 0.25 mg intravenously in a group of ambulatory surgery D&C patients.[95]

Droperidol can potentiate drowsiness and, if administered during the final phases of recovery care, may increase the patient's length of stay. In an ambulatory surgery setting, the maximum effective antiemetic dose of droperidol should not exceed 2.5 mg; as the dose is increased above 1.25 mg, drowsiness becomes more noticeable.

When nothing seems to help, the situation should be explained to both the patient and the family member in attendance, and the option of spending a night in the hospital should be considered. Almost all patients will elect to recover at home. Patients should be instructed, if nausea and vomiting does not improve following rest at home, to call the facility, their physician, or the emergency room if they feel it necessary to return to the hospital and be admitted. Patients usually stop vomiting on arrival home; only one of our patients returned to the hospital because of vomiting.

*Morris R: Personal communication, 1983

☐ *PACU Policy for Control of Nausea or Vomiting at the Methodist Ambulatory Surgery Center*

Droperidol IV for persistent nausea or after second emesis.

ADULT PATIENT (12 YR AND OVER 80 LB)

Droperidol, 0.625 mg, IV (0.25 ml). If no improvement in 15 min, repeat once only.

CHILDREN (2–12 YR)

WEIGHT (LB)	DOSAGE
20–25	0.25 mg (0.1 ml)
26–50	0.375 mg (0.15 ml)
51–75	0.50 mg (0.2 ml)
76–100	0.625 mg (0.25 ml)

A repeat dose of droperidol in pediatric patients requires examination and written order by department anesthesiologist. A department anesthesiologist should be contacted in all cases where nausea or vomiting persist.

Postintubation Croup

Ambulatory surgery lends itself to managing the pediatric patient. The most serious immediate postintubation complication in the young child is laryngeal edema or tracheitis evidenced by hoarseness, croupy cough, and stridor. If not treated early and appropriately, the condition has the potential to progress to the point at which the child becomes restless, uses accessory muscles of respiration, and develops intercostal retraction. Tachypnea and fatigue set in, and the stage is set for a major problem. With improvement in technique and equipment, the incidence of postintubation croup appears to be decreasing from earlier reports of 6% to more recent reports of 1% of patients.[51,65,67,86] The overall incidence of croup (1%) in 7875 children intubated during a 2-year period at the Children's Hospital Medical Center in Boston, could be attributed to no single factor as a chief cause, but several—patient's age, intubation trauma, and length of surgery—were strongly related to the incidence of this complication.[67]

Mechanical trauma is related to a considerable extent to the anesthesiologist's experience with pediatric patients. The infantile larynx resembles a funnel; the narrowest point is situated at the lower border of the cricoid cartilage. The anesthesiologist may easily insert an endotracheal tube between the vocal cords, only to find that it is too large to pass the cricoid constriction. A tube left in this position may produce subglottic swelling, whereas if the tube is forced through the cricoid narrowing, it may cause ischemia of the laryngeal mucosa followed by edema after extubation.[40] In spite of all precautions and use of flawless technique, subglottic edema may still occur.

By understanding the potential causes of postintubation croup, anesthesiologists may be able to lessen the incidence of occurrence (Fig. 7-4).

Contributing factors in the development of postintubation croup are[67]

1. Age of patient: Children between 1 and 4 years of age are more likely to develop this complication.

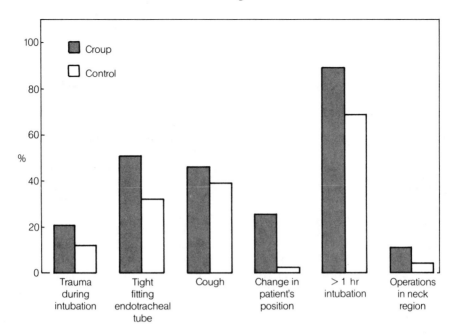

FIG. 7-4 Contributing factors in the development of postintubation croup. All the factors shown increased trauma to the larynx. (Koka BV, Jeon IS, Andre JM et al: Postintubation croup in children. Anesth Analg 56(4):501, 1977)

2. Trauma related to intubation: Repeated attempts at intubation result in a higher incidence of postintubation croup.
3. Size of endotracheal tube: In patients in whom there was no leak around the endotracheal tube when positive pressure of approximately 25 cm H_2O was exerted on the breathing bag, postintubation croup was more prevalent.
4. Coughing with endotracheal tube in place: There was a positive correlation between the development of croup and active coughing or straining by children at any time while the endotracheal tube was in place.
5. Changing patient's position: A higher incidence of croup occurred in patients whose head changed position during surgery.
6. Duration of intubation: Longer periods of intubation were followed by more airway irritation.
7. Position of the patient: Operations performed in positions other than supine had a higher incidence of croup.
8. Site of operation: Croup occurred more frequently following operations around the neck.

Symptom onset varies from immediately after extubation to a maximum of 3 hours. Epstein feels that in the pediatric outpatient population, symptoms that will require treatment will become evident within the first hour in the PACU.*

*Epstein BS: Personal communication, 1983

There is no universal agreement as to the effectiveness of prophylactic regimens. Children treated prophylactically with 2% lidocaine (2 mg/kg) injected intravenously 1 minute prior to extubation had no laryngospasm, compared to a 20% occurrence in a nontreated group.[11] Subsequent intravenous injection of lidocaine (2 mg/kg) in the nontreated group, controlled the spasm within 30 to 90 seconds. Moderate bradycardia was observed in one child and transient respiratory depression occurred in two children. The study group (20 patients) was too small to evaluate the effectiveness of intravenous lidocaine in preventing hoarseness or croupy cough. Subjects given dexamethasone, 0.3 mg/kg, and lidocaine, 1 mg/kg, intravenously, separately and in combination, had a smaller incidence of postintubation croup than a control group.[88] Dexamethasone appeared to be more effective than lidocaine.

When treatment of the early symptoms of laryngeal complications did not prove effective and signs of layngeal obstruction became more evident, Deming and Oech combined intravenous diphenhydramine chloride, 0.25 mg/kg to 2.5 mg/kg, with dexamethasone (a single dose of 4 mg for infants under 1 year of age and 8 mg for older children).[32] Definite improvement was noted in 10 patients from 20 to 40 minutes after the administration of this combination of drugs.

Jordan et al treated postintubation croup with cool-mist inhalation alone and cool mist plus dexamethasone, 4 mg to 8 mg, intravenously.[65] Fewer of the dexamethasone patients required additional treatment (intermittent positive-pressure breathing with epinephrine).

By the very nature of surgical procedures performed in an ambulatory setting, the severity of symptoms and percentage of patients experiencing postintubation croup are less than in an inpatient population. However, in view of the large number of ambulatory surgery pediatric patients, anesthesiologists should be aware of a simple, inexpensive, and effective means of handling postintubation croup. Racemic epinephrine will quickly and effectively manage this problem with minimal recurrence. Dilute 0.5 ml 2.25% racemic epinephrine (Vaponefrin, Fisons Corp., Bedford, Massachusetts) with 3 ml sterile saline or water and deliver this through a face mask and nebulizer. This is easily accomplished with the patient seated in a parent's lap. By making a game of it, one usually encounters no resistance; we let the patient know he or she can take the disposable face mask ("space mask") home. When patients receive racemic epinephrine, they should be observed in the PACU for a minimum of 2 hours in case of symptom recurrence. Additional factors to be considered are

1. The patient's age (a determinant of airway diameter)
2. The severity of the croup and how it responds to treatment
3. The reliability of the parents for home care
4. How far the family lives from the facility
5. Once home, how much time would elapse before the parents could access emergency care

The answers may influence the anesthesiologist's decision to discharge to home care or admit for observation.

Postanesthetic Delirium

Emergence from anesthesia may be accompanied by restlessness, disorientation, crying, moaning, or irrational speech. In its extreme form, excitement can be referred to as emergence delirium, in which the patient will scream, shout, and thrash wildly about.

Emergence delirium is prevalent among children and common in healthy adult patients, but as age increases the incidence decreases. Among the more common factors contributing to delirium are pain, stress, anxiety, hypoxia, anticholinergic drugs, phenothiazines, barbiturates, ketamine, varying inhalation anesthetics, and distended urinary bladder. It is important to assess restlessness and delirium accurately in the postanesthetic patient and to treat the potential causes appropriately.[48] Appropriate treatment may be simply medication for pain or reversing muscle relaxants or narcotic agents.

Longo first used the term *anticholinergic syndrome* in describing the central nervous system manifestations of toxicity from belladonna alkaloids and related compounds.[75] The symptom complex includes confusion, restlessness, agitation, dizziness, delirium, visual and auditory disturbances, stupor, and coma. In addition to belladonna alkaloids, phenothiazines and tricyclic antidepressants may also have a central anticholinergic action.

Physostigmine has been used successfully in treating the central anticholinergic syndrome. Sedation and delirium following diazepam and lorazepam, as well as sedation following the use of hydroxyzine and droperidol have been reported to be completely relieved by the administration of physostigmine, 1 mg to 2 mg, slowly intravenously.[16, 72, 93] Spaulding et al noted an apparent increase in awareness following physostigmine administration, but concluded that the accompanying ventilatory drive decrease may contraindicate its use in patients with diazepam-induced ventilatory depression.[100] The mechanism by which physostigmine reverses the effects of benzodiazepines is yet to be explained. Garber et al were unable to speed the recovery process or improve psychomotor function in a group of outpatients undergoing dental extraction under intravenous diazepam sedation with a mixture of physostigmine and atropine.[50] The anticholinergic effects exerted by atropine may be the reason results differed from prior studies when physostigmine was used alone. Intravenous physostigmine, 2.0 mg, administered intravenously 10 minutes after induction with 1.5 mg/kg ketamine resulted in significantly reduced PACU nystagmus, blurred vision, and length of stay, but a higher incidence of nausea and vomiting.[109]

Although physostigmine's ability to reverse somnolence induced by anticholinergic drugs represents a specific antagonistic action, its reported ability to reverse postoperative somnolence induced by other depressant agents probably represents a nonspecific arousal response. Hannallah et al administered physostigmine, 60 μg/kg, intravenously over a period of 60 seconds in the PACU to pediatric outpatients who had received rectal methohexital induction for bilateral myringotomy. There was no improvement in recovery score for the patients who received physostigmine compared to a control group. There was no slowing of the heart rate from physostigmine, and atropine was not used in any patient.[54]

Side-effects of physostigmine that occur infrequently are bradycardia, ventricular arrhythmia, abdominal cramping, nausea, and increased bronchial secretions. Atropine will counteract these muscarinic effects.

Syncope

Symptoms of dizziness, drowsiness, weakness, and hypotension singly or in combination and of sufficient severity to prevent home readiness fall into my classification of syncope. Patients are not able to ambulate without support.

At the Phoenix Surgicenter, postoperative hypotension occurs in 16% of patients.[31] Usual causes are positional changes, pain, a full bladder, analgesic or antiemetic drugs. Always rule out more serious possibilities including hypoxia or mycardial problems. All of our adult ambulatory surgery patients having services of the anesthesia department receive 1000 ml of intravenous fluids during operation and in the immediate recovery period. The intravenous line is maintained until patients retain oral fluids and ambulate. Depending on the severity of postoperative hypotension, one can treat the cause, administer oxygen, put the patient in a supine position, continue intravenous fluids, and if necessary, give a vasopresser drug (i.e., ephedrine).

Orthostatic hypotension has not been a major problem in our facility. We attribute this to a two-phase recovery room and particularly to the use of reclining chairs in our second phase. By slowly being brought into an upright seated position, our patients are able to tolerate sitting and ambulating with minimal occurrence of hypotension. Patients who have had spinal or epidural anesthesia should be closely observed because their sympathetic block may outlast sensory and motor blocks. If you plan to use spinal or epidural anesthesia in your facility, be sure that an adequate explanation is provided for the postanesthesia care staff.

If narcotic drug administration is considered the cause of excessive drowsiness and an inability to ambulate, reversal can be accomplished with the use of naloxone. In clinical dosages, naloxone does not produce respiratory depression, even when used in the absence of narcosis. By titrating naloxone intravenously in repeated doses of 0.1 mg, one may be able to provide reversal of sedation and ventilatory depression without affecting pain control. In addition, depressed blood pressure may rise. There is potential for return to the narcotized state, particularly if long-acting narcotic drugs have been used.

Doxapram provides pure respiratory stimulation without a change in the patients' narcotized state. Minute volume is affected by first increasing the depth of ventilation, and then the rate. Robertson et al administered 80 mg of doxapram intravenously to a group of ambulatory surgery patients who had received methohexital, nitrous oxide, and halothane.[91] This was associated with a significantly more rapid recovery from anesthesia. In a single dose of 1 to 1.5 mg/kg, doxapram effectively antagonized respiratory depression induced by morphine without affecting analgesic action.[53] Diazepam sedation during endoscopy, biopsy procedures, and minor surgery was effectively and safely reversed without any potentially serious side-effects.[7] Stephen and Talton administered single intravenous doses of 1.5 mg/kg or a sustained administration of 300 mg over a period of 30 minutes by intravenous drip and found the drug predictable, controllable, and therapeutically safe in patients who received inhalation anesthetics.[102] Although oxygen consumption increases moderately after doxapram administration, there is a concomitant increase in oxygen availability such that the extraction ratio does not change, and there is no evidence of peripheral hypoxia.[66] Janis administered 1.0 to 1.5 mg/kg by slow intravenous push at the conclusion of the procedure, followed by a 0.1% infusion drip (5 mg/min) to hasten arousal in ambulatory surgery patients.[62] In healthy patients there were minimal effects on blood pressure and pulse rate and few complicating arrhythmias. Caution should be exercised in elderly patients with severe hypertension, irritable ventricular arrhythmias, or seizure disorders.

Thompson et al reported one case of reactive hypoglycemia as the cause of prolonged recovery in an outpatient. Although exceedingly rare, this condition can be treated easily if suspected.[108] Apparently, there is wide variation in what constitutes a clinically significant level of hypoglycemia. Certain patients develop headache, weakness, vertigo, palpitations, and nausea. Other people with similar blood glucose levels may be completely asymptomatic. In most instances, there is little physiologic rationale to support the diagnosis, but if a low blood glucose value is obtained, treatment of symptoms by the administration of intravenous dextrose will be simple and effective.

Arrhythmias

While arrhythmias may develop in healthy individuals, they occur more often in patients who have a history of an abnormal rhythm or some preexisting cardiac disease. In the healthy ambulatory surgery patient, sinus tachycardia and bradycardia and premature atrial and ventricular contractions are the arrhythmias most frequently encountered. The more common causative factors in the ambulatory surgery population are respiration inadequacy related to obstruction or depression and hyperactivity of the sympathetic nervous system associated with pain.

Postoperative Hypertension

In the relatively healthy ambulatory surgery population, it is more likely that hypotension, rather than hypertension, will be a problem following surgery. Hypertension, if it occurs, is usually due to pain, anxiety, stressful emergence from anesthesia, hypoxia, hypercarbia, distention of urinary bladder, or previous hypertension in which the patient was denied antihypertensive medications. All patients on hypertensive therapy should take their medication the morning of surgery with a sip of water.

Significant hypertension (mean 130 mm Hg) not relieved by appropriate treatment of the cause will respond to a short-acting peripheral vasodilator. Hydralazine, 2.5 to 5 mg, by slow intravenous bolus up to a total dose of 20 mg will usually control a transient hypertensive episode. Using a peripheral vasodilator to treat hypertension caused by hypoxia may cause a serious and profound drop in blood pressure as it counteracts compensatory vasoconstriction.[43] A single 10-mg dose of nifedipine given sublingually in the immediate postanesthetic period is effective and safe for the management of hypertension.[98] Its onset of action is fast (2–15 min), its duration is long (3–5 hr), and blood pressure level remains stable during its use. Hypertension, which may accompany emergence delirium, will respond to physostigmine.

Length of Stay in the Postanesthesia Care Unit

According to Reed,[89] heavy, long-lasting premedication, an additional 100 mg to 200 mg of barbiturate, or extra depth with an inhalation agent may cause no deleterious effect in the healthy patient. The resulting increase in recovery time, however, will have an unfavorable impact on the surgical outpatient who would otherwise safely ambulate; it could even create an 'anesthetic inpatient' out of what was meant to be an outpatient surgical procedure.

Many anesthesiologists feel that using inhalation anesthesia is superior to intravenous anesthesia for ambulatory surgery because the patient recovers more rapidly and is discharged from the facility more promptly. White feels that intravenous anesthetics would be more controllable, and hence more like the volatile anesthetics, if administered by continuous infusion rather than by intermittent injection.[115] By using a continuous infusion, the anesthesiologist minimizes the "peaks and valleys" of drug concentrations, the amount of drug administered is less, and recovery time is shortened. In comparing fentanyl and ketamine, given by continuous infusion to intermittent bolus, as intravenous adjuvants to nitrous oxide for maintenance of general anesthesia following thiopental induction, the amount of drug decreased approximately 45%, and time to awakening decreased approximately 60% with infusion techniques. Trieger scores were consistent with a more rapid recovery in the infusion groups; the incidence of common postoperative side-effects did not differ significantly between bolus and infusion groups.

Azar et al assessed the neurologic state and psychomotor function of ambulatory surgery patients recovering from isoflurane, enflurane, and fentanyl balanced anesthesia.[10] Arousal scores at 20 minutes were highest in the fentanyl group, but at 40 minutes scores were similar in all three groups. Psychomotor function was depressed equally in all groups 1 hour after anesthesia, but returned to normal at 2 hours. The return of psychomotor test scores to preanesthesia values suggested sufficient recovery of mentation and coordination for safe discharge 2 hours after anesthesia under the care of an accompanying responsible person.

Ideally, the ambulatory surgery patient should receive an agent capable of a rapid induction of surgical anesthesia and swift emergence followed by a rapid return to normal activity and appetite with no side-effects. In comparing the three major inhalational agents (halothane, enflurane, isoflurane) following a short anesthetic (<30 min), no single agent stands out as being superior to any of the others in getting the patient home in a timely manner.

In 300 pediatric patients, there was very little difference in recovery at 15 minutes and 30 minutes, following a variety of ambulatory surgical procedures.[56] Incidence of recovery delirium in the isoflurane group (19%) was more than twice that in the halothane group (8%); nausea, vomiting, headache, and bad dreams were identical in all groups. There was a higher incidence of coughing and laryngospasm following extubation with the enflurane group. Steward compared recovery from enflurane and halothane in pediatric outpatients.[106] During the early recovery period, postanesthesia scores for the enflurane group were higher on admission to the postanesthesia care unit, but this was not statistically significant, and there was no difference in scores after 15 minutes and at the time of discharge. Examination of returned questionnaires showed that the majority of patients in both groups rapidly returned to a normal status and were considered by their parents to be bright and alert and to have a normal appetite. A higher incidence of bad dreams previously reported after enflurane in children[56] was not demonstrated by Steward. Headache and muscle pains, however, seem to have occurred with somewhat greater frequency in the enflurane group. In comparing isoflurane with halothane and enflurane, the rate of postoperative recovery was comparable with any of the three agents; return to normal status at home occurred somewhat more rapidly with isoflurane than with either of the other agents. Late complications (nausea, vomiting, lack of appetite) occurring at home were seen less frequently with isoflurane than with halothane or enflurane. Steward feels that halothane remains the potent inhalation agent of choice for pediatric patients in preference to enflurane. However, except for a slower induction time, isoflurane compares favorably with halothane. Although variation in PACU length of stay is present among the three major inhalational agents, initial studies did not establish one agent as being superior for the ambulatory surgery patient.[60,83] Korttila found that the longer the duration of enflurane anesthesia, the longer it took the patient to recover.[116] This was not the case with isoflurane. Korttila concluded from this and prior studies[71] that, of the three major inhaled anesthetics, isoflurane should be preferred in ambulatory anesthesia because of faster recovery following its usage.

Dundee, in comparing ultra-short-acting barbiturates for ambulatory surgery, felt that only methohexital appeared to be an improvement over thiopental because of a more rapid return of consciousness.[39] In the real world of anesthesia, assuming a single intravenous bolus induction, there is very little difference in PACU length of stay between these two agents. Fragen and Caldwell evaluated awakening times following thiopental or etomidate induction in 40 women scheduled for gynecologic ambulatory surgery procedures.[46] Awakening times were similar for both induction agents (Table 7-8), but the incidence of nausea was higher after etomidate (55%) than after thiopental (15%). In studying only early recovery from anesthesia, Horrigan et al found no difference in time or quality of recovery between etomidate-induced and thiopental-induced patients.[57] There was a threefold increase in nausea and vomiting in the etomidate group. Fentanyl supplementation of anesthesia significantly shortened the time before patients opened their eyes and were able to follow commands in both groups.

The measurement of extraocular muscle balance (Maddox-Wing test) has been used as a clinical test of rate of recovery following anesthesia.[49,55] More rapid recovery was noted in patients given only nitrous oxide, oxygen, and halothane than in those induced with methohexital, thiopental, or propanidid. Thiopental recovery was slightly longer than that of methohexital or propanidid, but there was a higher incidence of retching and vomiting in the

---

☐ **Table 7-8 Awakening Times Following Etomidate Vs. Thiopental**

Measurement	Etomidate Patients		Thiopental Patients	
	Mean	Range	Mean	Range
Open eyes to command (min)	2.8	1–13	3.4	1–17
Normal Bender test (min)	23.3	15–60	23.5	15–45
Normal Trieger test (min)	31.5	15–75	39.8	15–75

(Fragen RJ, Caldwell N: Comparison of a new formulation of etomidate with thiopental side-effects and awakening times. Anesthesiology 50:242, 1979)

early postoperative period after propanidid. When compared directly in equipotent induction dosages, recovery from methohexital appears to be faster than recovery from thiopental.[111]

Propanidid, alphathesin, and diprivan have all been used in the United Kingdom as induction agents for ambulatory surgery patients. These drugs are all formulated in Cremophor EL and all have been implicated in hypersensitivity reactions. Although there may be small advantages to using these induction agents because of a more rapid awakening time, the disadvantages of potential hypersensitivity reactions far outweigh them.

Length of stay in the postanesthesia care unit not only depends on our choice of anesthetic agents, but also varies with the length of procedure, the criteria the facility uses to evaluate the patient for discharge, and other factors such as pain, nausea, vomiting, drowsiness, and dizziness.

It is difficult to determine with great accuracy when patients can safely be allowed home, and the clinical judgment of the anesthesiologist must be the final determinant. Studies of postanesthesia care unit length of stay have produced differing results even with the same agents, because dosage, length of surgery, and time spans between testings have all varied. Temporary arousal of patients to complete testing may allow them to score well even though certain areas of coordination are still impaired. If anesthetic agents that are appropriate for the ambulatory surgery patient are used, then anesthesia will not play a major role in increasing patients' length of stay in the PACU.[44] The Phoenix Surgicenter reports patients are usually ready for discharge within 4 hours. At George Washington University Hospital, the usual stay in the PACU is 2 to 4 hours and at our own institution, The Methodist Medical Center of Illinois, ambulatory surgery recovery stay averages 2 hours. Of our general anesthesia patients, 31% are children (who are subject to a shorter length of stay), and this affects our overall average. Length of stay in the PACU is probably related more to the skill and experience of the anesthesiologist administering the agents than to the specific agents used.

"What's the hurry?" said the tortoise to the hare.* Ambulatory surgery facilities are not competing for record discharge times. Whether a patient is discharged in 2 or 4 hours following their procedure should not be the most important consideration. However, facilities cannot lose site of the fact that time spent by patients and their families in the ambulatory facility can influence their level of satisfaction. To meet the goal of discharging satisfied patients on the same day as their surgery, anesthesiologists and surgeons must be willing to modify techniques; facilities should regularly evaluate their discharge criteria, and physicians and staff should regularly discuss problem areas that affect length of stay.

When to Feed, What to Feed

Patients should be able to tolerate oral fluids without nausea and vomiting prior to discharge. Berry feels the patient's perception of hunger is one of the most helpful clinical signs in determining whether he or she is able to tolerate fluids.[14] When they are able, his pediatric patients are given oral fluids slowly (1 oz every

*Tortoise T: Personal communication, 1984

20 minutes for an hour) in the PACU, advancing their diet intake as tolerated. In our two-phase PACU, pediatric patients are transferred into phase two immediately upon reaching a postanesthesia recovery score of 10. Infants and small children who are alert and fussing are given water or a nippled bottle containing a solution of dextrose and water upon entry into the second phase of recovery. We find that quickly giving clear oral fluids has a calming influence and makes for a smoother postoperative course. Infants who were not intubated during anesthesia and tolerate dextrose in water will quickly progress to milk, formula, or mother's milk. For those infants who had been intubated during anesthesia, even though we allow sips of water or dextrose and water, we do not allow milk products until 1 hour has elapsed from extubation. Our older pediatric patients are usually given water 1 half-hour after the conclusion of anesthesia.

For our adult patients in phase one recovery who complain of a severe dry mouth, we have had no problem allowing them to rinse their mouth with water if they are alert, have progressed to the point that they can rest comfortably with the head of the cart elevated, and have no complaints of nausea. In phase two they receive water; if this is tolerated without nausea, they quickly progress to cola and 7-Up. All fluids given in our recovery room are served at room temperature; we stay away from iced fluids and ice chips.

Patients are also given soda crackers to eat. If a patient insists on having tea or coffee, this is provided as long as nausea is minimal or absent. Patients are not given oral pain medications until they have tolerated liquids and soda crackers. Pain medications taken orally, on an empty stomach, are more likely to cause nausea and vomiting. At home, patients are instructed to take liquids and soda crackers prior to any oral pain medications.

When Can a Patient Drive?

Clinically, we consider the patient recovered from anesthesia when he or she is capable of responding to commands in the PACU and performing other simple tasks, whereas from the patient's standpoint, recovery often signifies return to normal function in a familiar environment. As anesthesiologists, we are interested in patients meeting specific criteria for discharge home; patients are more interested in when can they drive a car and go back to work.

Korttila assigned certain tests as specific indicators of return of particular functions in patient recovery from anesthesia (Table 7-9).[68] The less complex the test, the less sensitive it is in evaluating complete psychomotor recovery. Driving simulators,[52,70,71] reaction timers, and complex psychodiagnostic testing are of value, providing reasonably reliable and objective information about the duration of effects of anesthetic agents. The recommended minimal times for length of hospital stay and ability to drive a car (Table 7-10) can serve as points of reference for a facility when establishing discharge criteria.

A member of the legal profession in the United Kingdom, writing about anesthetics and driving stated, "after most general anaesthetics it is safer to advise against driving for 48 hours."[58] Members of the Anaesthetic Sub-committee of the Association of Anaesthetists immediately challenged the statement. The 48-hour rule was refuted with the conclusion that a patient who has had a good night's sleep after an anesthetic should be able to drive the

☐ **Table 7-9 Stages of Recovery from Anesthesia and Tests Valid for Their Evaluation**

Stage of recovery	Tests of recovery
Awakening	Opening eyes Answering
Immediate clinical recovery	Sitting steady Negative Romberg and other clinical tests
Fit to go home* (hospital stay)	Maddox-Wing test Paper and pencil tests Single reaction time tests Single coordination or attention tests Flicker fusion
"Street fitness"*	Flicker fusion Psychomotor test batteries EEG
Complete psychomotor recovery* (fit to drive)	Carefully selected psychomotor test batteries Driving simulators

*More than a single test is needed.
(Korttila K: Minor outpatient anaesthesia and driving. Mod Probl Pharmacopsychiatry 11:91, 1976)

following day.[12] Herbert et al monitored ambulatory surgery patients for 2 days following hernia surgery with a choice reaction time test.[59] Reaction times gradually returned to baseline values during the first 24 hours, but there was a slowing during the second postoperative day. This occurred in patients who had been breathing spontaneously during surgery but not in those whose breathing was assisted. The authors feel it is wise to extend the warning not to drive to at least 48 hours postoperatively.

There is an obvious difficulty in establishing firm conclusions from data provided by heterogeneous groups administered varying doses of different anesthetic agents and tested in different ways. Until such time as results conform and definite conclusions can be drawn, a period of 24 hours before resuming driving is a reasonable time to recommend following most of the commonly used ambulatory surgery anesthestic agents.[29]

EEG readings following barbiturate induction returned to normal within 30 minutes, but 2½ and 3½ hours later, drowsiness appeared. At 4½ hours, a transitory sleep stage ensued, and this persisted for up to 12 hours.[38] These results provide substance to recommendations that, following anesthesia, patients should be accompanied by a responsible person, refrain from activities in which a decrease in alertness might be a hazard (driving a car, making crucial business decisions), and abstain from alcohol for 12 to 24 hours.

Discharge Criteria

Ambulatory surgery facilities go to great length to develop criteria for patient selection; it is of equal importance to have criteria for patient discharge.

Although the varying psychomotor tests can provide us with information that is usable in developing criteria, the majority of tests are too complex, time-consuming, and cumbersome to be used in a clinical setting. Practical discharge criteria must be tailored to the particular facility, size of the PACU, and number of postanesthesia care nurses and must not compromise patient safety.

Patients should be informed before being discharged home that they may experience pain, headache, nausea, vomiting, dizziness, and muscle aches and pains not related to the incision for at least 24 hours following surgery and anesthesia. Fahy and Marshall found that women are more likely to be affected than men, that the incidence of postanesthesia morbidity among patients

☐ **Table 7-10 Recommended Minimal Values for Length of Hospital Stay and the Length of Time Patients Should Be Advised against Driving**

Treatment	Hospital stay (hr)	No driving (hr)
Dental local anaesthesia dose variable	Unnecessary	1
Plain lidocaine, 200 mg, IM	1	1–1.5
Lidocaine, 500 mg, with adrenaline IM	0.5	No limitations
Plain bupivacaine, 1.3 mg/kg, IM	2	2–4
Plain etidocaine, 2.6 mg/kg, IM	2	2–4
Diazepam, 10 mg, IM	1	7
Pethidine, 75 mg, IM or IV*	2–3	24
Fentanyl, 0.1 mg, IV	1–2	2
Fentanyl, 0.2 mg, IV	2	8
Diazepam, IV		
0.15 mg/kg	2	8
0.30 mg/kg†	2–3	10
0.45 mg/kg‡	3–4	10
Diazepam, 0.15 mg/kg plus*		
Pethidine, 1 mg/kg, IV	2–3	10–24
Flunitrazepam, 0.01 mg/kg, IV	2	8
Flunitrazepam, 0.02–0.03 mg/kg, IV*	3–4	24
Flunitrazepam, 0.015 mg/kg plus*		
Pethidine 1 mg/kg, IV	3	24
Droperidol, 5 mg, IV*	4–6	24
Droperidol, 5 mg, plus†		
Fentanyl, 0.2 mg, IV	4–6	24
Thiopentone, 6 mg/kg, IV‡	3	24
Methohexitone, 2 mg/kg, IV‡	2	24
Propanidid, 6.6 mg/kg, IV	1–2	3–4
Alphadione, 85 μl/kg, IV	2	8
Halothane–N_2O–O_2 (5–10 min)	2	7
Enflurane–N_2O–O_2 (5–10 min)	2	7

*Treatment should be avoided in outpatient practice.
†Recurrence of impaired performance should be taken into consideration if food is eaten within less than 5 hr.
‡Other treatment is preferable in outpatient practice.
(Korttila K: Minor outpatient anaesthesia and driving. Mod Probl in Pharmacopsychiatry 11:91, 1976)

undergoing anesthesia for the first time (49.1%), was higher than that of patients who had a previous anesthetic experience (29.4%), and that increasing the length of surgery over 20 minutes was associated with both the occurrence and severity of symptoms.[44] When halothane is a part of the anesthetic technique, a higher incidence of headache within the first 24 hours has been reported.[110]

In 100 consecutive outpatients who were provided no written instructions at discharge, Ogg found 31% of patients went home unaccompanied by a responsible adult; 73% of car owners drove within 24 hours of surgery, with 30% driving within 12 hours; 9% of patients drove themselves home, and a bus driver returned to work on the same day, driving a busload of passengers a distance of 95 miles.[81] Patients in this study reported postoperative symptoms of headache (27%), drowsiness (26%), nausea (22%), and dizziness (11%). Fifty percent of medical outpatients do not follow physicians' instructions, but the addition of written and verbal education techniques at discharge has a marked impact on improving compliance.[15]

Malins studied compliance following ambulatory surgery.[76] Generalized written instructions on admission to the outpatient area were given to a group of patients without any discussion or explanation. A second group was given instructions on admission specific to the patient's postanesthetic activities, and these instructions were read to the patient, who was asked to retain the form and take it home on discharge. Between 77% and 95% of the patients in the first group did not remember getting any instructions as to postanesthetic activities, and they consequently drove cars, operated machinery, and drank alcoholic beverages in less than 24 hours. The group who kept the written instructions that had been read to them were in compliance 88% to 96% of the time. Only 1 of 30 patients failed to remember being told not to drive for 24 hours, whereas 22 of 30 patients in the first group claimed they did not remember this instruction. Another problem area that surfaced during this study was the number of patients undergoing general anesthesia who did not understand or speak any English. In areas with high immigrant populations, consent forms, procedural explanations, and discharge information may have to be written in appropriate languages, and the services of an interpreter provided. Case Report 12, in Chapter 8 provides an excellent example of how an unrecognized language barrier created a problem.

Simple general anesthetic techniques affect patient memory retention in the immediate postoperative period.[82] Inhalation and narcotic techniques cause impairment of recall of new material at 1 hour postanesthesia, even though patients appear clinically fit for discharge. At 3 hours postanesthesia, recall of new material in all patients returns to normal.

Hippocrates said, "keep an eye on the faults of your patients; they often lie about what medicines they are taking." Two thousand years later, we can still say that patient compliance is less than perfect. In the medicolegal climate of today, providing patients with written discharge instructions should be part of every facility's discharge policy.

Following discharge, patients should continue their recovery at home in bed. The discharge examination does not determine the patient's readiness to return to normal activities, but establishes whether he or she can safely be released for a trip home. The Phoenix Surgicenter prefers the term *home readiness* to *street fitness*.[90] To be ready for the ride home, Surgicenter patients, in addition to a responsible person, must have[89]

1. Stable vital signs for at least 1 half-hour
2. No new signs or symptoms postoperatively that may threaten a safe recovery (for example, the patient with mild shoulder pain following laparoscopy will be released home, but a patient with more than mild abdominal pain following a diagnostic D&C will be detained for further observation)
3. Cessation of oozing or bleeding when bleeding was a feature of the operation
4. No nausea or emesis for 1 half-hour or evidence that it is waning
5. Good circulation in, and return of sensation to, the operated extremity when a tourniquet has been used
6. No evidence of swelling or impaired circulation in an extremity when a cast has been applied
7. Voided clear urine following cystoscopy
8. The ability to recognize time and place
9. Little or no dizziness after changing clothes and sitting for 10 minutes
10. No pain not subject to control by oral analgesics

After a state of home readiness has been established, the responsible nurse notifies the anesthesiologist, and together they make sure that the applicable requirements of the Surgicenter's postoperative checklist are satisfied. This is known as *informed discharge*.[89]

1. Dietary instructions are given. Clear liquids until stomach is settled, then progress to regular feedings. No alcohol should be taken (unless by physician's order) for at least 12 hours.
2. Pain is provided for. Medication appropriate to the need.
3. Prescriptions are checked. The patient or responsible person has prescriptions for all medications ordered by the surgeon.
4. Surgeon's instructions are reviewed. Limitation of activity, elevation of operated extremity, when to return to office, anticipated complications, whom to call in event of unanticipated complications.
5. Anesthesiologist's instructions are given:
   a. "You may feel sleepy and somewhat sluggish for several hours." "Don't drive until tomorrow." "Postpone important decisions until tomorrow."
   b. "You may have a sore throat for a few hours" (if patient was intubated). Instruct patient in use of salt-water gargles, humidifying devices, aspirin, or acetaminophen, and advise to call if soreness persists more than a day.
   c. "You may have some muscular soreness for a day or two" (soreness, which follows the use of succinylcholine, may be more pronounced than any other discomfort). It is often, but not always, relieved by the medication prescribed for relief of pain at the operative site. Aspirin is recommended for the relief of this soreness, and a warm bath is suggested if not contraindicated by the surgical procedure.
6. Return dentures, valuables, and clothes.
7. The patient is reassured that he has behaved properly. The patient should be informed that dreaming often occurs, and an opportunity should be afforded for the patient to discuss any dream that may be remembered.

8. The patient is informed that a follow-up call is routine and is to be expected.

Patients often expect to drive, travel, return to work, and participate in a variety of activities following what they assume to be a short procedure carrying with it very little morbidity. It is important they be made aware of how they may feel within the first 24 to 48 hours following their procedure. At the Virginia Mason Hospital, Seattle, Washington, guidelines include the following points:[108]

1. The first night after surgery must be within 1 hour traveling time from hospital.
2. A responsible adult should accompany the patient home.
3. A staff anesthesiologist should discuss at least the following five Ds prior to discharge.
   a. Do not drive.
   b. Do not drink.
   c. Beware of dizziness.
   d. Don't make critical decisions.
   e. Discuss any questions or problems with us (call or come in).

Hospital staff evaluate the patient's ability to walk prior to discharge, and this, plus the anesthesiologist's interview, form the basis for their discharge criteria.

Fragen and Shanks use additional discharge criteria for ambulatory surgery patients who have received nondepolarizing muscle relaxants (see below).[47] The degree of recovery following muscle relaxant use can be assessed clinically, but this requires cooperation by the patient (i.e., head lift, negative inspiratory force, grip strength, and evidence of diplopia). Use of a peripheral nerve stimulator with a T4/T1 greater than 70% usually correlates with a clinical impression of adequate reversal. Patients should be watched closely and treated immediately if residual curarization is suspected.

☐ ***Discharge Criteria for Patients Who Have Received Nondepolarizing Muscle Relaxants***

---

1. A minimum of 1 half-hour must elapse past full recovery of grip strength.
2. A minimum of 2½ hours must elapse after the end of surgery and anesthesia.
3. Vital signs must be stable.
4. If unusual muscle weakness or adverse effects unrelated to muscle relaxant administration occurs, patients will be kept in the hospital until the adverse reaction is controlled or reversed.
5. The patient must be able to tolerate all fluids, void, and walk without assistance.
6. No other complications must be present.

(Fragen RJ, Shanks CA: Neuromuscular recovery after laparoscopy. Anesth & Analg 63:51, 1984)

In addition to achieving a postanesthesia recovery score of 10, our patients must meet other discharge criteria (Fig. 7-5), which are incorporated into our phase two PACU record:

MASC
Phase II

The Methodist Medical Center
of Illinois

Date_____ Time in_____ Time out_____

Operation_____

Anesthesia   General   ☐
             Regional   ☐
             Local with
             sedation   ☐
             Local   ☐
             ET   ☐

Time	
BP V A	240 220 200 180 160
Pulse ●	140 120 100
Resp. ○	80 60 40 20 0
Temp.	

Discharge Criteria

☐ Vital signs stable

☐ Swallow, cough, and gag reflex present

☐ Able to ambulate

☐ Dressings checked   ☐ Take home medication   ☐ Nausea, vomiting, dizziness minimal

☐ Voided   ☐ Authorization signed   ☐ Absence of respiratory distress

☐ Patient given discharge instruction sheet   ☐ Alert and oriented

☐ Responsible adult present to escort patient home   ☐ Postanesthesia recovery score 10

Medications	Nurses Notes

Name

_____ R.N.
Signature of RN discharging patient

_____ M.D.
Signature of physician discharging patient

FIG. 7-5   Discharge criteria, Methodist Ambulatory Surgery Center.

1. Vital signs stable: This includes temperature, pulse, respiration, and blood pressure when appropriate. Vital signs should remain stable (i.e., blood pressure ±20 mm Hg) for a period of not less than 1 half-hour and be consistent with patient's age and preanesthesia levels.
2. Swallow, cough, and gag reflex present: The patient must demonstrate ability to swallow fluids and either be able to cough or demonstrate a gag reflex.
3. Able to ambulate: The patient demonstrates ability to perform movement consistent with age and development level (sit, stand, walk).
4. Nausea, vomiting, dizziness minimal:
    a. Minimal nausea: Absence of nausea or, if nausea is present, patient can still swallow and retain some fluids.
    b. Minimal vomiting: Vomiting is either absent or, if present, does not require treatment. Following vomiting that requires treatment, patient should be able to swallow and retain fluids.
    c. Minimal dizziness: Dizziness is either absent or present only upon sitting, and patient is still able to perform movement consistent with age.
5. Absence of respiratory distress: The patient exhibits no signs of snoring, obstructed respiration, stridor, retractions, or croupy cough.
6. Alert and oriented: The patient is aware of surroundings and what has taken place and is interested in returning home.

Patients have their dressings checked and are walked to the bathroom to void. Patients receiving spinal or epidural anesthesia must void before leaving the facility. Nursing staff reviews the authorization form (Fig. 7-6) completed prior to the procedure and the surgeon's postoperative orders (preprinted for specific procedures by our facility on a copy of their office letterhead) with the patient and responsible person. These orders are reviewed annually by the surgeon according to recommendations of the Joint Commission on Accreditation of Hospitals (JCAH). Specific discharge instructions are given to patients who have had services of the anesthesia department (Fig. 7-7), and additional instructions are included for patients who have had spinal or epidural anesthesia.

Our postspinal patients are instructed to rest in bed for 24 hours. They may be propped up on pillows, sit up to eat and have bathroom privileges, but we prefer they wait until the next day before resuming appropriate normal activities. They are instructed to call if they develop a headache not relieved by acetaminophen, a stiff neck, or elevated temperature. Similar instructions are given to epidural patients, but we are more liberal in allowing them to be up and out of bed.

Complete bed rest (flat in bed) for 24 hours to prevent postdural puncture headache was first recommended in 1902 by Sicard and is a ritual still followed without question by many physicians.[96] Jones, in studying the effects of recumbency for 4 to 12 hours following spinal anesthesia with 20- to 25-gauge needles in 1134 hospitalized patients, found there was not a predictable pattern relating the time spent recumbent to the occurrence of postdural puncture headache.[64] As soon as motor function permits, he sees no reason to delay ambulation and feels this approach would also result in better patient acceptance of spinal anesthesia. Carbaat and van Crevel performed diagnostic

THE METHODIST MEDICAL CENTER OF ILLINOIS
Ambulatory Surgery Center

PATIENT AUTHORIZATION

* 1. I have read and fully understand the Patient Instructions and have arranged for a responsible person to accompany me to and from the hospital after discharge.

   2. I certify that the information on the Preanesthesia/Surgery Questionnaire is correct to the best of my knowledge.

* 3. I certify that I have had nothing by mouth (this includes water) since 12:00 midnight.

   4. I will notify my doctor immediately if any unusual bleeding, respiratory problems or acute pain occurs after my discharge from the hospital.

* 5. I do understand that driving a car, operating any machinery or power tools less than twenty-four (24) hours after general anesthesia or sedation is *prohibited.*

* 6. I do understand that ingestion of alcohol less than twenty-four (24) hours after general anesthesia or sedation is prohibited.

   7. I also understand that if a condition arises during my surgery and the doctor feels that admission to the hospital is best for my recovery, then he or she shall admit me as an inpatient following my surgery.

* NA   Not applicable for no or local anesthesia patients.

_____
(Patient)

_____
(Witness)

_____
(Responsible Party)

_____
(Date)

_____
(Relationship)

FIG. 7-6   Patient authorization, Methodist Ambulatory Surgery Center.

lumbar punctures with 18-gauge needles in 50 patients who were kept ambulant and 50 patients who were kept on 24-hour bed rest following the procedure. The average incidence of postdural puncture headache (37%) was the same on 7-day follow-up in both groups.[21]

Does recumbency have some rationale? Coombs and Porter performed 17 spinal taps—single punctures with 25-gauge needles—at L3–4 on 10 female and 7 male volunteers ages 24–35, all members of an anesthesia health care team, for radioimmunoassay studies. All taps were done between 6:30 A.M. and 7:45 A.M., and all volunteers then worked a full day. Classic spinal headaches occurred in 9 of 17, including the two authors. Epidural blood patch was required in two cases.[27] A point is made for recumbency.

THE METHODIST MEDICAL CENTER OF ILLINOIS
Ambulatory Surgery Center

DISCHARGE INSTRUCTIONS

For patients who have had: ☐ Local Anesthesia with Sedation

☐ General Anesthesia

1. The medicine which was used for sedation or to put you to sleep will be acting in your body for the next 24 hours; you might feel a little sleepy when you get home. This feeling will slowly wear off. For the next 24 hours the adult patient should not:

    a. Drive a car, operate machinery or power tools

    b. Drink any alcoholic drinks (not even beer), or

    c. Make any important decision, such as to sign important papers.

    Children should rest at home, but may be up and about according to doctor's instructions.

2. The patient may have some pain. A prescription for pain may be given by the doctor. This should be taken as directed; if it does not improve the pain, *contact your doctor.* If the doctor prescribes nothing for pain, the patient may take a non-prescription, non-aspirin pain medication, which can be purchased at the drugstore. Please follow the directions on the label.

3. The patient may eat anything, but it is better to start with liquids; such as soft drinks (soda), then soup and crackers, and gradually work up to solid foods. Babies can be fed their milk as soon as they are hungry for it.

4. The patient is not expected to have any fever; but if he/she does feel warm after today, take his/her temperature. If temperature is 101 degrees, or higher, *call your doctor.*

5. We strongly suggest that a responsible adult be with the patient for the rest of the day and also during the night for the patient's protection and safety.

6. If any questions arise, call your doctor. If unable to reach your doctor, please feel free to call the Ambulatory Surgery Center. During the day (7:00 a.m. to 5:00 p.m.), Monday through Friday, you may phone 672-5935. At night or on weekends, phone the Emergency Room at 672-5500.

7. The patient has an appointment with Dr._____

    Date_____ Time_____

    Call Doctor_____ for an appointment:

    Date_____ Telephone Number_____

FOR TONSIL AND ADENOID PATIENTS: If the patient continually spits up bright red blood after leaving the hospital, contact your doctor. If you cannot reach your doctor, contact the unit immediately, Monday through Friday (7:00 a.m. to 5:00 p.m.) at 672-5935. At all other times, call the Emergency Room, 672-5500.

FIG. 7-7 Discharge instructions, Methodist Ambulatory Surgery Center.

Spinal or epidural anesthesia should not be defined the ambulatory surgery patient based only on his or her intention to go home on the day of the procedure. Burke considers spinal anesthesia with a 26-gauge needle for laparoscopy to be safe and satisfactory and to provide excellent relaxation with significant freedom from morbidity and mortality.[19] In his study, pain during the procedure was minimal and limited to transient mild neck or shoulder discomfort. Of 1063 cases, 240 were discharged on the day of surgery. There was an overall headache incidence of 1.3%. When laparoscopy anesthesia is either spinal or epidural, approximately 40% of patients complain during the procedure of mild shoulder or neck discomfort that is readily relieved by intravenous administration of a short-acting narcotic (fentanyl). Explaining this to the patient prior to the procedure will dispel fears that the anesthesia is wearing off, and this mild discomfort will be well tolerated when appropriately treated.

When is it safe to permit patients to ambulate following spinal or epidural anesthesia? The sequence of return of function generally accepted is motor, then sensory, and finally sympathetic. Several studies examining the sequence of return of function have found recovery of sympathetic activity occurring prior to complete regression of the subarachnoid block.[30,87,92] Pflug et al consider the ability to urinate a final indication of reversal of sympathetic paralysis, since an intact functioning sympathetic nerve supply to bladder and urethra is necessary for this function.

In our facility, patients who have received spinal or epidural anesthesia are transferred from our phase one recovery (patient on stretcher) to our phase two recovery (patient on recliner) after return of sensation and motor strength. As with our other patients, they are gradually brought into an upright seated position prior to ambulation. Suitable criteria for ambulation after spinal anesthesia include normal perianal (S4–5) pinprick sensation, plantar flexion of the foot, and proprioception of the big toe.

At the Day Surgery Unit of the Brigham and Women's Hospital, discharge criteria after spinal anesthesia include return of normal sensation, ability to ambulate (return of strength and proprioception), and ability to urinate (return of sympathetic nervous function).* Their patients are encouraged to "take it easy" for the remainder of the operative day, as are their other patients, and to maintain good fluid intake. They are told not to lift heavy objects or strain, but ambulation, activity, and position are not otherwise limited. Patients are encouraged to call the unit if any postoperative problem occurs, such as headache. Discharge after epidural anesthesia is evaluated by the same three criteria.

Postspinal ambulatory surgery patients at the Virginia Mason Hospital are instructed to resume normal but quiet activity (no dancing, no weightlifting), and there are no bed rest restrictions.†

Following a major peripheral nerve block, discharge criteria should include return of normal sensation and motion. Variations are acceptable, and each ambulatory surgery facility should establish criteria they consider practical and medically appropriate. Is there a difference if residual, sensory or motor block involves the upper or lower extremity? What if there is only a patch of numbness after a minor peripheral block? These are the questions that should be asked and answered before patients are discharged.

Philip does not think it prudent to discharge a patient with residual sensory or motor block of the lower extremity.** There is the possibility of injury after a fall, which may be due to a patient's overestimation of return of function or to a lack of experience with crutches. However, patients are discharged with residual sensorimotor impairment after an upper-extremity major nerve block.

*Philip BK: Personal communication, 1984
†Thompson G: Personal communication, 1984
**Philip BK: Personal communication, 1984

Even when appropriate agents are used, the duration of action is sometimes exceptionally long. Patients are discharged with the extremity in a sling. They are reminded that the normal sensation that would protect the extremity against injury is absent and are cautioned particularly not to smoke cigarettes or cook. Patients are given the name and telephone number of an anesthesiologist or the Day Surgery Unit written on their discharge instruction sheet and told to call the next day. Instructions and precautions are documented in the chart. Patients are reassured that nothing has "gone wrong"; a block *does* sometimes persist for a long time, and sensation and motion are expected to return shortly. A patch of numbness after a minor peripheral nerve block often does not warrant a sling, but requires similar precautionary instructions against injury and use of fire. At George Washington University In and Out Surgery, patients who have received regional anesthesia must have complete return of sensory and motor function in the affected extremity.* However, criteria for discharge may be modified at the discretion of the anesthesiologist. As each facility attempts to establish its own policies, the question must be asked, "Is the use of crutches to go home considered more acceptable following arthroscopic surgery than following prolonged sensorimotor anesthesia (major block)?" Specific discharge criteria will depend on how this question is answered by the physicians in the individual ambulatory facility.

Nursing staff should assess the adult who will take the patient home to determine whether the individual is in fact a responsible person. We have on two occasions had "responsible" persons who appeared intoxicated. We did not question the ability of this person to take care of the patient at home, but we made certain that another adult was present to drive the patient home and stay with him or her during the early recovery period. The term *responsible* is defined in Chapter 2 of this book as someone physically and intellectually capable of taking care of the patient at home. There is an additional precaution ambulatory surgery facilities might consider: have both the patient and responsible person sign the medical record signifying that they have both understood and received verbal and written discharge instruction.

At our facility, additional considerations are as follows:

1. Patients whose anesthetic management has included endotracheal intubation remain for a minimum of 1½ hours following extubation.
2. Patients receiving depressant medication for relief of pain, nausea, or vomiting must be observed for a minimum of 1 hour.

Patients are told they will receive a telephone call the next day from one of our postanesthesia care nurses to find out how they are recovering from their surgery and anesthesia. Some facilities give patients a follow-up postcard with instructions to fill in comments on recovery and return it within 1 or 2 weeks. Patients appreciate the facility that cares enough to follow up.

When all discharge criteria have been met, an anesthesiologist is called to examine the patient and sign the PACU record to indicate that the patient is home ready. Patients should never leave with the impression they are being rushed out of the facility. This is avoided by having postanesthesia room personnel who are sympathetic, understanding, and compassionate, as well as *upbeat* in caring for the patient. In the words of Francis Weld Peabody, "The secret of the care of the patient is in caring for the patient."[85]

*Levy M-L: Personal communication, 1984

References

1. Abramowitz MD, Oh TH, Epstein BS et al: The antiemetic effect of droperidol following outpatient strabismus surgery in children. Anesthesiology 59:579, 1983
2. Abramowitz MD, Epstein BS, Friendly DS et al: The effect of droperidol in reducing vomiting in pediatric strabismic outpatient surgery. Anesthesiology 55(3):A329, 1981
3. Ahlgren EW, Bennett EJ, Stephen CR: Outpatient pediatric anesthesiology: A case series. Anesth Analg 50(3):402, 1971
4. Aldrete JA: Are intramuscular injections obsolete in the recovery room? Current Reviews for Recovery Room Nurses 5(18):147, 1983
5. Aldrete JA, Kroulik D: A postanesthetic recovery score. Anesth Analg 49(6):924, 1970
6. Alexander CD, Wetchler BV, Thompson RE: Infiltration of the mesosalpinx with bupivacaine 0.5% effectively relieves pain following laparoscopic tubal sterilization. Third Annual Symposium on Anesthesia for Ambulatory Surgery, Williamsburg, Virginia, 1985
7. Allen CJ, Gough KR: Effect of doxapram on heavy sedation produced by intravenous diazepam. Br Med J 286:1181, 1983
8. Anderson R, Crohg K: Pain as a major cause of postoperative nausea. Can Anaesth Soc J 23(4):366, 1976
9. Apgar V: A proposal for a new method of evaluation of the newborn infant. Anesth Analg 32:260, 1953
10. Azar I, Karambelkar DJ, Lear E: Neurological state and psychomotor function following anesthesia for ambulatory surgery. Anesth 60(4):347, 1984
11. Baraka A: Intravenous lidocaine controls extubation laryngospasm in children. Anesth Analg 57:506, 1978
12. Baskett P, Vickers M: Driving after anaesthetics. Br Med J 1:686, 1979
13. Batra MS, Driscoll JJ, Coburn WA et al: Evanescent nitrous oxide pneumothorax after laparoscopy. Anesth Analg 62:1121, 1983
14. Berry FA: Pediatric outpatient anesthesia. ASA Regional Refresher Courses in Anesthesiology 10(2):17, 1982
15. Blackwell B: Treatment adherence. Br J Psychiatry 129:510, 1976
16. Blitt CD, Petty WC: Reversal of lorazepam delirium by physostigmine. Anesth Analg 54(5):607, 1975
17. Boas RA, Newson AJ, Taylor KM: Comparison of midazolam with thiopentone for outpatient anaesthesia. NZ Med J 96(728):210, 1983
18. Brody DC: Criteria for patient care. Current Reviews for Recovery Room Nurses 19:155, 1983
19. Burke RK: Spinal anesthesia for laparoscopy: A review of 1,063 cases. J Reprod Med 21:59, 1978
20. Caldamone AA, Rabinowitz R: Outpatient orchiopexy. J Urol 127:286, 1982
21. Carbaat PAT, van Crevel H: Lumbar puncture headache: Controlled study on the preventative effect of 24 hours' bed rest. Lancet 2:1133, 1981
22. Carignan G, Kerri-Szanto M, Lavelle JP: Post-anesthetic scoring system. Anesthesiology 25:396, 1964
23. Clark AJM, Hurtig JB: Premedication with meperidine with atropine does not prolong recovery to street fitness after outpatient surgery. Can Anaesth Soc J 28:390, 1982
24. Coakley CS, Levy ML: Anesthesia for ambulatory surgery. J Arkansas Med Soc 68:101, 1971
25. Cohen RL, MacKenzie AI: Anaesthesia and cognitive functioning. Anaesthesia 37:47, 1982
26. Cohen SE, Woods WA, Wyner J: Antiemetic efficacy of droperidol and metoclopramide. Anesthesiology 60:67, 1984
27. Coombs DW, Porter JG: Lumbar puncture headache. Lancet 2:87, 1981
28. Craig J, Cooper Gm, Sear JW: Recovery from day-case anaesthesia. Comparison between methohexitone, althesin and etomidate. Br J Anaesth 54:447, 1982
29. Cundy JM: Medical aspects of fitness to drive. Anaesthesia 34:1056, 1979
30. Daos FG, Virtue RW: Sympathetic block persistence after spinal or epidural analgesia. JAMA 183:285, 1963
31. Dawson B, Reed WA: Anaesthesia for day-care surgery: A symposium. III. Anaesthesia for adult surgical outpatients. Can Anaesth Soc J 27(4):409, 1980

32. Deming MV, Oech SR: Steroid and antihistamine therapy for post-intubation subglottic edema in infants and children. Anesthesiology 22:933, 1961
33. Denis R, Letourneau JE, Londorf D: Reliability and validity of psychomotor test as measures of recovery from isoflurane or enflurane anesthesia in a day-care surgery unit. Anesth Analg 63:653, 1984
34. Dhamee MS, Gandhi SK, Kalbfleisch JH et al: Morbidity after outpatient anesthesia—a comparison of different endotracheal anesthetic techniques for laparoscopy. Anesthesiology 57(3):A375, 1982
35. Doctor NH, Hussain Z: Bilateral pneumothorax associated with laparoscopy. Anaesthesia 28:75, 1973
36. Doenicke A, Gurtner T, Kugler J et al: experimentelle unterschungen uber das ultrakurznarkotikum propanidid mit serumcholinesterase-bestimmungen, EEG, psychodiagnostischen tests und kreislaufanalysen. Horatzk K, Frey R, Kindler M (eds): Anaesthesiology and Resuscitation 4th ed. Berlin, Springer Verlag, 1965
37. Doenicke A, Kugler J, Schellenberger A et al: The use of electroencephalography to measure recovery time after intravenous anaesthesia. Br J Anaesth 38:580, 1966
38. Doenicke A, Kugler J, Laub M: Evaluation of recovery and "street fitness" by EEG and psychodiagnostic tests after anaesthesia. Can Anaesth Soc J 14(6):567, 1967
39. Dundee JW: Ultrashort-acting barbiturates for outpatients. Acta Anaesth Scand (Suppl)17:17, 1965
40. Eckenhoff JE: Some anatomic considerations of infant larynx influencing endotracheal anesthesia. Anesthesiology 12:405, 1951
41. Epstein BS: Outpatient anesthesia. ASA Refresher Courses in Anesthesiology 2:81, 1974
42. Epstein BS, Levy ML, Thein MH et al: Evaluation of fentanyl as an adjunct to thiopental–nitrous oxide–oxygen anesthesia for short surgical procedures. Anesthesiol Rev 2(3):24, 1975
43. Estafanous FG: Postoperative hypertension: incidence and management. Current Reviews for Recovery Room Nurses 5:11, 1983
44. Fahy A, Marshall M: Post-anaesthetic morbidity in outpatients. Br J Anaesth 41:433, 1969
45. Figueroa M: The post-anesthesia recovery score: A second look. South Med J 65:791, 1972
46. Fragen RJ, Caldwell N: Comparison of a new formulation of etomidate with thiopental-side effects and awakening times. Anesthesiology 50:242, 1979
47. Fragen RJ, Shanks CA: Neuromuscular recovery after laparoscopy. Anesth Analg 63:51, 1984
48. Fraulini KE: Post-anesthetic delirium—a conceptual approach. Current Reviews for Recovery Room Nurses 4(20):155, 1982
49. Gale GD: Recovery from methohexitone, halothane and diazepam. Br J Anaesth 48:691, 1976
50. Garber JG, Ominsky AJ, Orkin FK et al: Physostigmine-atropine solution fails to reverse diazepam sedation. Anesth Analg 59:58, 1980
51. Goddard JE, Phillips OC, Marcy JH: Betamethasone for prophylaxis of postintubation inflammation: A double blind study. Anaesth Analg 16:348, 1967
52. Green R, Long HA, Elliot CJR et al: A method of studying recovery after anaesthesia. Anaesthesia 8:189, 1963
53. Gupta PK, Dundee JW: Post-operative pain relief with morphine combined with doxapram and naloxone. Anaesthesia 29:33, 1974
54. Hannallah RS, Abarmowitz MD, McGill WA et al: Physostigmine does not speed recovery following rectal methohexital induction in pediatric outpatients. Anesthesiology 57(3):A412, 1982
55. Hannington-Kiff JG: Measurement of recovery from outpatient general anesthesia with a simple ocular test. Br Med J 3:132, 1970
56. Horne JA, Ahlgren EW: Halothane and isoflurane for outpatient surgery: A pediatric case series. Abstracts, American Society of Anesthesiologists Meeting 269, 1973
57. Horrigan RW, Moyers JR, Johnson BH et al: Etomidate vs. thiopental with and without fentanyl—a comparative study of awakening in man. Anesthesiology 52:362, 1980
58. Harvard JA: Medical Aspects of Fitness to Drive. London, Medical Commission on Accident Prevention, 1976

59. Herbert M, Healy EGJ, Bourke JB et al: Profile of recovery after general anaesthesia. Br Med J 286:1539, 1983
60. Hoyal RHA, Prys-Roberts C, Simpson PJ: Enflurane in outpatient paediatric dental anaesthesia. Br J Anaesth 52:219, 1980
61. Hunt TM, Plantevin OM, Gilbert JR: Morbidity in gynecological day-case surgery: A comparison of two anaesthetic techniques. Br J Anaesth 51:785, 1979
62. Janis KM: Outpatient anesthesia in geriatric setting. Int Anesthesiol Clin 20:87, 1982
63. Jensen S, Wetchler BV: The obese patient: An acceptable candidate for outpatient anesthesia. J Am Assoc Nurse Anesthetists 50:369, 1982
64. Jones RJ: The role of recumbency in the prevention and treatment of postspinal headache. Anesth Analg 53:788, 1974
65. Jordan WS, Graves CL, Elwin RA: New therapy for postintubation laryngeal edema and tracheitis in children. JAMA 212:585, 1970
66. Kim SI, Winnie AP, Carey JS et al: Use of doxapram in the critically ill patient: Does increased oxygen consumption reflect an oxygen dividend or an oxygen debt? Crit Care Med 1:252, 1973
67. Koka BV, Jeon IS, Andre JM et al: Postintubation croup in children. Anesth Analg 56(4):501, 1977
68. Korttila K: Minor outpatient anaesthesia and driving. Mod Probl Pharmacopsychiatry 11:91, 1976
69. Korttila K: Recovery after intravenous sedation. A comparison of clinical and paper and pencil tests used in assessing later effects of diazepam. Anaesthesia 31:724, 1976
70. Korttila K, Linnoila M, Ertama P et al: Recovery and simulated driving after intravenous anesthesia with thiopental, methohexital, propanidid or alphadione. Anesthesiology 43:291, 1975
71. Korttila K, Tammisto T, Ertama P et al: Recovery, psychomotor skills and simulated driving after brief inhalational anesthesia with halothane or enflurane combined with nitrous oxide and oxygen. Anesthesiology 46:20, 1977
72. Larson GF, Hurlbert BJ, Wingard D: Physostigmine reversal of diazepam-induced depression. Anesth Analg 56(3):348, 1977
73. Levy ML, Coakley CS: Organization and experience with outpatient anesthesia in a large university hospital. Int Anesthesiol Clin 14(2):131, 1976
74. Levy ML, Coakley CS: Survey of in and out surgery, first year. South Med J 61:995, 1968
75. Longo VG: Behavioral and electroencephalographic effects of atropine and related compounds. Pharmacol Rev 18:965, 1966
76. Malins AF: Do they do as they are instructed? A review of out-patient anaesthesia. Anaesthesia 33:832, 1978
77. McGlinchey J, McLean P, Walsh A: Day case penile surgery with penile block for post-operative pain relief. Ir Med J 76(7):319, 1983
78. Meridy HW: Criteria for selection of ambulatory surgical patients and guidelines for anesthetic management: A retrospective study of 1,553 cases. Analg Anesth 61(1):921, 1982
79. Nagel EL, Forster RK, Jones D et al: Outpatient anesthesia for pediatric ophthalmology. Anesth Analg 52:558, 1973
80. Newman MG, Trieger N, Miller JC: Measuring recovery from anesthesia—a simple test. Anesth Analg 48(1):136, 1969
81. Ogg TW: An assessment of post-operative outpatient cases. Br Med J 4:573, 1972
82. Ogg TW: Fischer HBJ, Bethune DW et al: Day case anaesthesia and memory. Anaesthesia 34:784, 1979
83. Padfield A, Mullins SRC: Recovery comparison between enflurane and halothane techniques. A study of outpatients undergoing cystocopy. Anesthesia 35:508, 1980
84. Patterson JF, Bechtoldt AA, Levin KJ: Ambulatory surgery in a university setting. JAMA 235(3):266, 1976
85. Peabody FW: The care of the patient. JAMA 88:877, 1927
86. Pender JW: Endotracheal anesthesia in children: Advantages and disadvantages. Anesthesiology 15:495, 1954
87. Pflug AE, Aasheim GM, Foster C: Sequence of return of neurological function and criteria for

safe ambulation following subarachnoid block (spinal anaesthesic) Can Anaesth Soc J 25:133, 1978

88. Phillalamarri ED, Tadoori PR, Abadir AR: Prophylactic effect of dexamethasone and/or lidocaine on post extubation croup in children. Anesthesiology 57(3):A429, 1982

89. Reed WA: Recovery from anesthesia and discharge. In Shultz R (ed): Outpatient Surgery, p 45. Philadelphia, Lea & Febiger, 1979

90. Reed WA, Ford JL: The surgicenter: An ambulatory surgical facility. Clin Obstet Gynecol 17(3):17, 1974

91. Robertson GS, MacGregor DM, Jones CJ: Evaluation of doxapram for arousal from general anaesthesia in outpatients. Br J Anaesth 49:133, 1977

92. Roe CF, Cohn FL: Sympathetic blockade during spinal anesthesia. Surg Gynecol Obstet 136:265, 1973

93. Rosenberg H: Letter to the editor: Physostigmine reversal of sedative drugs. JAMA 229:1168, 1974

94. Shandling B, Steward D: Regional analgesia for post-operative pain in pediatric outpatient surgery. J Pediatr Surg 15(4):477, 1980

95. Shelley ES, Brown HA: Antiemetic effect of ultralow dose droperidol. Abstract, American Society of Anesthesiologists Annual Meeting, 1978

96. Sicard JA: Leliquide Cephalo-rachidien, p 55. Paris, Mason & Gauthier-Villars, 1902

97. Soderstrom RM, Butler JC: A critical evaluation of complications in laparoscopy. J Reprod Med 10:245, 1973

98. Sodeyama O, Ikeda K, Matsuda I et al: Nifedipine for control of post operative hypertension. Anesthesiology 59(3):A18, 1983

99. Soni V, Burney R: Anesthetic techniques for laparoscopic tubal ligation. Anesthesiology 55(3):A145, 1981

100. Spaulding BC, Choi SD, Gross JB et al: The effect of physostigmine on diazepam-induced ventilatory depression: A double-blind study. Anesthesiology 61:551, 1984

101. Staertow C: Recliners are advantageous in the recovery. Same Day Surg 7(11):141, 1983

102. Stephen CR, Talton I: Investigation of doxapram as a post-anesthetic respiratory stimulant. Anesth Analg 43:628

103. Steward DJ: Experiences with an outpatient anesthesia service for children. Anesth Analg 52:877, 1973

104. Steward DJ: Anaesthesia for day care surgery: A symposium. IV: Anaesthesia for paediatric out-patients. Can Anaesth Soc J 27:412, 1980

105. Steward DJ: A simplified scoring system for the post operative recovery room. Can Anaesth Soc J 22(1):111, 1975

106. Steward DJ: A trial of enflurane for paediatric outpatient anaesthesia. Can Anaesth Soc J 24(5):603, 1977

107. Steward DJ, Volgyesi G: Stabilometry: A new tool for the measurement of recovery following general anaesthesia for outpatients. Can Anaesth Soc J 25(1):4, 1978

108. Thompson GE, Remington JM, Millman BS et al: Experiences with outpatient anesthesia. Anesth Analg 52(6):881, 1973

109. Toro-Matos A, Rendon-Platas AM, Avil-Valez E et al: Physostigmine antagonizes ketamine. Anesth Analg 59:764, 1980

110. Tyrrell MF, Feldman SA: Headache following halothane anaesthesia. Br J Anaesth 40:99, 1968

111. Vickers MD: The measurement of recovery from anaesthesia. Br J Anaesth 37:296, 1965

112. Wetchler BV: Anesthesia for outpatients. In Mauldin BC (ed): Ambulatory Surgery: A Guide to Perioperative Nursing Care. New York, Grune & Stratton, 1983

113. Wetchler BV: Pain management for outpatient T&A surgery. Presented at Same-Day Surgery Conference, San Francisco, 1981

114. Wetchler BV, Collins IS, Jacob L: Antiemetic effects of droperidol on the ambulatory surgery patient. Anesthesiology Rev 9(5):23, 1982

115. White PF: Use of continuous infusion versus intermittent bolus administration of fentanyl or ketamine during outpatient anesthesia. Anesthesiology 59:294, 1983

116. Korttila K, Valanne J: Recovery after outpatient isoflurane and enflurane anesthesia. Anesth Analg 64:185, 1985

8

Complications

Herbert E. Natof, M.D.

Complications: There is probably no subject in medicine in which the search for pure truth is as evasive. Complications highlight our failures, betray our ignorance, and reaffirm that the mastery of our skills has limitations. And yet, as practitioners of medicine we must have a realistic understanding of the potential dangers of ambulatory surgery if we are to establish preventive measures and be prepared for prompt and effective treatment.

This chapter focuses not only on anesthesia complications but on the full range of complications associated with the ambulatory surgical setting. The role of the anesthesiologist in both the hospital-affiliated and freestanding center frequently assumes many of the characteristics of a primary-care physician. The anesthesiologist serves a central and crucial role in the preoperative screening process and plays a significant and broad role in the postoperative phase of care. Emphasizing this point, Brown states, "Never has the role of anesthesiologist been more challenged than in outpatient evaluation."[5]

It is essential from the onset to formulate a simple and uniform definition of the term *complication*. One of the pervasive pitfalls of any discussion of complications is the lack of a uniform definition, and the practicing physician finds himself or herself trying to evaluate information based on different ideas and concepts. In 1981, the Freestanding Ambulatory Surgery Association (FASA) established the following definition of a complication for the purposes of collecting data: an untoward response or abnormal condition resulting from treatment and care associated with ambulatory surgery.

A *major complication* is defined as an untoward response or abnormal condition *having the potential for serious harm*. Major complications include hemorrhage, infection, serious anesthetic complications, any medical problem requiring hospitalization, and other potentially harmful occurrences. A *minor complication* is an untoward response with minimal or no potential for serious harm and includes transient episodes of nausea and vomiting, weakness, headache, muscle aching, sore throat, and dizziness.

It is evident that any simple definition of a concept as complex as complications will have many gray areas in spite of our best efforts to seek uniformity. The reader may consider these examples:

1. The patient who complains of unusual pain postoperatively but heals normally
2. The patient who manifests premature ventricular contractions during the course of anesthesia but requires no specific therapy and has no sequelae
3. The patient who has an apparent sterilizing procedure but becomes pregnant 1 year later
4. The patient who develops a benign episode of laryngospasm that relents without specific therapy
5. The patient whose bunionectomy heals in an overcorrected position

Should any or all of these patients be classified as a complication case? There is no clear and authoritative answer, and the decision ultimately must be based on the individual evaluation of each case and a consensus of established criteria. In general, I would not classify as a complication an anesthetic or surgical event that was a relatively common deviation from the norm and required no special treatment or action on the part of the surgeon or anesthesiologist and presented no substantive danger to the patient. In addition, I would not classify as a complication a less-than-satisfactory surgical result unless it posed an increased risk to the general health of the patient. The vast majority of complications, however, are clearly identified by this definition and need not be subjected to arbitrary interpretation.

After collecting and studying ambulatory surgery complication data for the past 10 years, there are certain general concepts that emerge from our search for truth in this area.

■ GENERAL CONCEPT NO. 1

The incidence of many major complications is related to specific surgical procedures such as tonsillectomy or adenoidectomy, laparoscopy, arthroscopy of the knee, augmentation mammoplasty, and other plastic and reconstructive operations. This does not mean that the same complications would be less likely to occur in the inpatient setting, nor does it mean that major complications cannot occur in association with other surgical procedures. It does mean that one can predict with reasonable confidence that certain major complications are more likely to occur in patients scheduled for certain specific operative procedures.

A corollary to this concept is that the types and incidence of major complications are generally related to the incidence of the specific surgical procedures being performed in an ambulatory surgery center. Each center has its own profile that will influence the occurrence of complications.

■ **GENERAL CONCEPT NO. 2**

Given any specific surgical procedure or anesthetic experience, there is the potential for the same complications whether the patients are inpatients in a hospital or outpatients in an ambulatory surgery facility.

There are several identifiable exceptions to this concept. First, there is considerable evidence that the incidence of infection is substantially less among ambulatory surgery patients. This is an important and unique advantage to patients whose surgery is performed in the ambulatory surgery setting. Second, there is circumstantial evidence, based on many case reports, that complications resulting from errors in patient identification such as "wrong surgery performed," medication errors, and incorrect entry of laboratory results rarely occur in the ambulatory surgery setting.

The diminished infection rate is probably due to the separation of ambulatory patients from the reservoir of nosocomial infections prevalent within the general hospital population. The paucity of identification errors is most likely due to the overall simplicity of the routine admission and preparation process of the ambulatory surgery setting. In addition, most ambulatory surgery patients do not receive preoperative sedative medications and are quite aware of what is happening until the anesthetic is begun.

Furthermore, there is some evidence that certain surgical procedures have fewer complications when performed in the ambulatory surgery setting. Williamson has performed over 3000 outpatient cataract procedures and has stated that the ambulatory patient has less chance of experiencing pneumonia, cross-infection, and pulmonary embolism.[35] Nabatoff and Aufses have reported on 2000 patients who had varicose-vein surgery using general anesthesia in the ambulatory setting.[22] The authors reported wound healing that seemed better than usual, no significant hematomas, and no wound infections. Importantly, there were no instances of phlebitis or embolism.

■ **GENERAL CONCEPT NO. 3**

If something can go wrong—given a sufficient number of patients over a sufficient period of time—it will. This adaptation of Murphy's famous law is all too familiar to experienced physicians who have seen unfortunate and tragic events occur in spite of prudent precautions and care.

A recently opened ambulatory surgery center experienced the death of two apparently healthy patients within a 5-week period in 1983. Examination of one of the two anesthesia machines used to administer inhalation anesthesia revealed a malfunctioning vaporizer valve. Information released by the center's administrator implied that a similar malfunction in the other anesthesia machine may have been implicated in the other death.

Looking at Complications from Different Perspectives

Complications in the ambulatory surgery setting may be viewed in an instructive fashion from many perspectives. We will consider three: the major complication compared to the minor complication, the relationship of complications to the phase of patient care, and the general etiology of complications.

Magnitude of Complication

MINOR COMPLICATIONS

There appears to be little difference in the incidence of minor complications within the inpatient and the ambulatory settings when similar surgical procedures are compared. Minor complications may cause discomfort and anxiety but do not pose a threat to the life or limb of the patient. However, the ambulatory patient and his or her family should be well informed about potential minor complications prior to discharge.

The hospitalized patient who experiences an episode of nausea, muscle aching or sore throat at two o'clock in the morning may be reassured by a concerned nurse. The uninformed ambulatory surgery patient may suffer unnecessary anxiety and sleeplessness at home. Ambulatory surgery patients should be told about the potential for minor complications such as muscle aching after the use of succinylcholine, the shoulder discomfort associated with laparoscopy, the sore throat following intubation, the frequent occurrence of nausea and vomiting after eye-muscle surgery, and the feeling of generalized weakness after a particularly long anesthetic. The basic key to dealing with minor complications in ambulatory surgery patients is predischarge reassurance and information. These brief case reports illustrate.

■ CASE REPORT NO. 1

A 30-year-old woman called her surgeon early on the first postoperative day after an ambulatory diagnostic laparoscopy. With "tears in her voice," she reported that she had not slept because of a "gnawing" sore throat that became more painful and more frightening during the course of the night. She was sure that something "dreadful" had happened. The surgeon explained that the sore throat was due to a tube that was inserted by the anesthesiologist and necessary for safe anesthesia. Clearly, a few words of explanation by either the anesthesiologist or one of the postanesthesia care unit (PACU) nurses would have prevented the patient's anxiety.

■ CASE REPORT NO. 2

In contrast to the case described above, a 7-year-old child was scheduled for a myringotomy and adenoidectomy. The patient vomited once in the PACU but manifested no other problems. The PACU nurses informed the parents prior to discharge that their daughter might have some additional nausea and vomiting. The parents were instructed to call their surgeon if there was persistent vomiting or bleeding. They were reassured that an occasional bout of vomiting after surgery and anesthesia was not unusual or cause for concern. The following day, one of the PACU nurses called the mother to check on the patient's condition (an excellent routine practiced in many ambulatory surgery centers). The mother reported that the child vomited once after the car ride home and once several hours later, but was now drinking fluids without any problem. The mother commented that "the excellent instructions and reassurance made them very comfortable, and they had not been overly concerned about the two bouts of vomiting."

MAJOR COMPLICATIONS

Major complications associated with ambulatory surgery have several unique aspects. First, the adjective *major*, as it has been defined for the ambulatory setting, has certain quantitative implications that need emphasis. Within the framework of hospital inpatient surgery, we tend to think of major complications as catastrophic or imminently life-threatening occurrences such as massive hemorrhage, septicemia, pulmonary emboli, or myocardial infarction. Although these critical complications may rarely occur among ambulatory surgery patients, a major complication in the ambulatory setting is much more likely to be a postoperative hematoma, localized wound infection, or persistent nausea and vomiting. Hence the term *major complication* must be viewed within the context of its definition—an untoward response with the potential for serious harm.

Second, the majority of major ambulatory complications occur after the patient has been discharged from the ambulatory surgery center. This fact emphasizes once again the importance of precise, clear postoperative instructions and the availability and cooperation of the surgeon.

■ CASE REPORT NO. 3

A 2-month-old infant was scheduled for a bilateral inguinal hernia under general anesthesia. The operating room and PACU phases of care went well. The infant was hospitalized at 1:30 A.M. on the first postoperative day because of a fever of 104°F rectally and purulent drainage from the left incisional area. The patient was treated with intravenous antibiotics and fluids. In view of the rapidity and virulence of the infection, it was assumed that the organism was beta-hemolytic *Streptococcus*. All personnel who participated in the surgery had nose and throat cultures performed. No pathogens were discovered. Culture of the wound drainage of the patient grew *Staphylococcus aureus*. In spite of antibiotic therapy, the patient developed drainage from the right inguinal incision several days later. After 1 week of treatment in the hospital, the patient made a complete recovery, and there was no disruption of the hernia repair.

■ CASE REPORT NO. 4

A 34-year-old woman was scheduled for a laparoscopic tubal sterilization. The surgeon observed at the time of surgery that there were multiple adhesions in the right lower quadrant of the abdomen, and the right tube was freed and grasped with difficulty. The remainder of the surgery was uneventful, and the patient did well in the PACU. She manifested abdominal distention and discomfort on the first postoperative day and was subsequently hospitalized by her surgeon. She was observed in the hospital for several days, and on the fourth postoperative day the abdomen was explored, revealing a segment of inflamed small bowel that had become entrapped in the right lower quadrant adhesions. The bowel was released, and some of the adhesions excised. The patient made a prompt and uneventful recovery.

Postoperative instructions given by an ambulatory surgery center should include a warning that the patient should contact his or her attending surgeon promptly in the event of unusual pain, bleeding, or other unexpected symptoms. Many ambulatory surgery centers have qualified personnel call each patient on the first postoperative day and provide valuable patient follow-up. The patient described above wisely called her doctor when she experienced increasing distention of her abdomen, and her problem was prudently managed.

Phase of Patient Care

We can also view complications from the perspective of the phase of patient care: complications may occur in the operating room, in the PACU, and after discharge.

Many of the most serious and life-threatening complications happen while the patient is in the operating room. Therefore the anesthesiologist, surgeon, and nursing staff should be prepared to respond promptly and offer effective treatment.

COMPLICATIONS IN THE OPERATING ROOM

■ CASE REPORT NO. 5

An 11-month-old girl who appeared poorly developed and who manifested poor muscle tone was scheduled for bilateral myringotomy. The anesthesiologist noted that the child also had a history of a poor weight gain and had been followed by the neurology department of a large university hospital. The child was scheduled for bilateral myringotomy and had been cleared by her neurologist. Approximately one minute into a nitrous oxide, oxygen, halothane inhalation induction (the halothane concentration was set at 1.5%), the child manifested marked bradycardia and suddenly stopped breathing. The anesthesiologist was unable to properly ventilate the infant even after insertion of an oropharyngeal airway. She was immediately intubated and respiration was supported by the administration of only oxygen. The pulse returned to a normal rhythm in approximately 30 seconds, but spontaneous respiration did not return for approximately 10 minutes. The myringotomy was performed, and the patient recovered in the PACU without further difficulty. Since the initial experience, this patient has returned for three additional myringotomies without any further problems.

■ CASE REPORT NO. 6

A 32-year-old woman was scheduled for a laparoscopic tubal coagulation on an ambulatory basis. Upon insertion of the primary trocar, massive bleeding emerged through the trocar cannula. An emergency laparotomy was immediately performed. The hemorrhage, which originated at the hypogastric artery, was partially controlled using direct pressure while proximal and distal control of the artery was secured using clamps. A vascular surgeon was called and arrived approximately 45 minutes later and performed a primary closure of the laceration.

The blood volume was maintained using plasma expanders and the subsequent administration of 5 units of whole blood. The patient made a complete recovery after a 2½-week period of hospitalization.

■ CASE REPORT NO. 7

A 39-year-old woman was scheduled for a laparoscopic tubal cautery using general anesthesia. The procedure was performed without difficulty, but fresh bleeding was observed within the abdominal cavity. The site of bleeding could not be identified through the laparoscope, and an emergency laparotomy was performed. A large retroperitoneal hematoma was discovered, the abdomen was closed, and the patient was transferred to a hospital immediately. In spite of the prompt transfer and a second laparotomy performed at the hospital, the patient died 7 hours later. Postmortem examination revealed massive retroperitoneal hemorrhage and a diffuse bleeding diathesis.

■ CASE REPORT NO. 8

A 7-year-old girl was scheduled for a bilateral myringotomy and adenoidectomy using nitrous oxide, oxygen, halothane anesthesia. There was copious bleeding from the adenoid bed following the use of the adenotome and subsequent curettement. The bleeding was partially controlled with direct pressure. A preoperative partial prothrombin time (PPT) was normal, and the screening medical history revealed no family history of bleeding or clotting problems. Several conservative measures were used to control the bleeding including electrofulguration and persistent pressure. The adenoid bed continued to ooze, and after 75 minutes the surgeon inserted a posterior pack. There was no further evidence of bleeding, and the patient had a smooth and stable course in the PACU.

She was transferred directly to a hospital for skilled observation. The posterior pack was removed the next day, and she was discharged from the hospital. There were no further problems, and the child had a normal recovery at home.

COMPLICATIONS IN THE PACU

Of all the phases of patient care in the ambulatory setting, the PACU phase requires a nursing staff that is alert, knowledgeable about potential complications, and endowed with superior communication skills and an abundant capacity for reassuring both patient and family.

■ CASE REPORT NO. 9

A 5½-year-old boy was scheduled for a rectal biopsy under general anesthesia. There was no unusual bleeding during the course of surgery, and the patient emerged satisfactorily in the PACU. Although the patient's vital signs remained stable, the PACU nurses expressed concern about his malaise and pallor. There was no evidence of external bleeding. The surgeon was requested to return to the center and examine the patient. Gentle but thorough examination by the surgeon revealed a large quantity of blood concealed in the bowel above the level of the surgery. The patient was transferred to a hospital for observation and blood replacement. He was discharged 3 days later in excellent condition.

■ CASE REPORT NO. 10

A 41-year-old woman was scheduled for a right capsulotomy under general anesthesia. The surgery and the initial postoperative period in the PACU were normal. Approximately 1 hour after surgery, the patient complained of increasing pain in the right breast. The PACU nurses followed the patient carefully and observed an increase in the breast size. The surgeon was notified and returned to the center. Removal of the dressings revealed a very large hematoma. The patient consented to a second anesthetic and surgery for evacuation of the hematoma and control of the bleeding. The second procedure went well, and the patient's vital signs remained remarkably stable in spite of a blood loss of approximately 1200 ml. The patient requested that she be allowed to go home rather than to a hospital for observation. The surgeon allowed the patient to be discharged home, and she was followed carefully by the surgeon during the next 48 hours. She made an excellent recovery without any further problems.

■ CASE REPORT NO. 11

A 12-year-old girl underwent a tonsillectomy and adenoidectomy under general anesthesia. The anesthetic and operative phases of care were uneventful. The tonsil and adenoid beds were dry when the procedure was completed, and the pharynx was cleared of mucus and blood before and after the removal of the endotracheal tube. Upon arrival in the PACU, the patient was not awake. She had a clear airway, good ventilation, and stable vital signs. Approximately 10 minutes after her arrival in the PACU, the patient coughed once or twice, manifested severe laryngospasm, and became cyanotic. The PACU nurses who were at her cart side (since she had not emerged from the anesthetic) immediately called for the anesthesiologist and administered oxygen using a portable ventilator and intermittent positive pressure. The PACU emergency cart, which was equipped with a full range of intubation equipment, was brought to the area. Her color was deeply cyanotic, and her pulse slowed to approximately 40 beats per minute. The anesthesiologist was just about to administer succinylcholine when the spasm relented, and the patient's color and pulse rapidly returned to normal. After the patient awoke, the pharynx was cleansed with gentle suction, revealing a small amount of bloody mucus. The laryngospasm was probably triggered by the mucus in an emerging patient still in a state of "light" anesthesia. Although laryngospasm is usually a benign problem when managed properly, failure to observe and care for this patient properly could possibly have resulted in serious damage.

POSTDISCHARGE COMPLICATIONS

Every ambulatory patient should clearly understand who to call in the event of a complication or problem. The patient should also be aware of the common complications associated with the surgery performed. It is the experience of most ambulatory surgery centers that the three most common major complications in the postdischarge period are bleeding, infection, and persistent nausea and vomiting.

The risk of bleeding can, in general, be predicted based upon the surgical procedure. Tonsillectomy and adenoidectomy patients usually do not bleed after discharge for the first 24 hours. The incidence of bleeding in these patients increases during the first week, peaking between the 7th and 10th days. These patients rarely bleed after the 12th day. In contrast, patients who undergo circumcision, submucous resection, rhinoplasty, face lift, and blepharoplasty, if they are going to bleed, usually do so during the first 48 hours. Cervical conization patients are most likely to have bleeding problems between the 7th and 12th postoperative days. Patients who have an augmentation mammoplasty or capsulotomy will usually bleed with hematoma formation during the first 4 postoperative days. Patients scheduled for arthroscopy of the knee (particularly with lateral release surgery) will usually bleed during the first 48 hours, resulting in hemarthrosis.

■ CASE REPORT NO. 12

A 6-year-old Chinese boy was scheduled for a tonsillectomy and adenoidectomy. The parents seemed to understand the admission questions, the preoperative interview with the anesthesiologist, and conversations with the nurses in the PACU. The child did well while in the center, and the parents were given the usual explicit postoperative instructions. Everyone was sure the parents comprehended the instructions. The nurses at the ambulatory surgery center subsequently found out that the child bled seriously on the sixth postoperative day, but the parents ignored the problem. The child was finally brought to an emergency room of a hospital when he became extremely pale and poorly responsive. It was then discovered that the parents understood very little English, did not comprehend the discharge information, and had "faked out" the surgeon, anesthesiologist, and nursing staff by shaking their heads appropriately and using several English words.

This case illustrates the vital importance of communication in the ambulatory setting. The patient or a responsible relative, friend, or companion must fully understand the postoperative instructions and be able to assist during the preoperative interview. A lapse in communication due to language, diminished mental function, or physical disability may cause serious problems.

■ CASE REPORT NO. 13

A 5-year-old boy was scheduled for eye-muscle surgery. The patient's surgical procedure went smoothly under nitrous oxide, oxygen, halothane anesthesia. The patient received only atropine as a premedicant. He did well in the PACU except for one episode of vomiting. The follow-up telephone call on the first postoperative day revealed that the patient had vomited three or four times during the night and was not drinking fluids. The mother was instructed to call the surgeon later in the day if the vomiting did not subside. By 4:00 P.M., the child was febrile, with a rectal temperature of 104°F, and lethargic, and had continued to vomit. He was hospitalized by his surgeon and treated with intravenous fluids. The child was discharged after 2 days in the hospital, and there were no further problems.

■ CASE REPORT NO. 14

A 19-year-old woman was scheduled for a diagnostic dilatation and curettage (D&C) because of irregular menses. The patient was anesthetized using thiopental and nitrous oxide, oxygen, halothane. She had a normal operative and anesthetic course. After awakening in the PACU, the patient wept continuously and complained of severe abdominal cramping. She received only modest relief from oral acetaminophen. The following day, the patient's mother called the surgeon and reported that her daughter had profound generalized weakness, bordering on paralysis, and could not walk. The patient was hospitalized, and a neurologist was called as consultant. No organic disease was discerned, and the patient was seen by a psychiatrist. She was discharged in good condition after 1 week in the hospital with the diagnosis of anxiety reaction.

General Etiology

Complications may also be viewed from the perspective of general etiology: the complication may be due to anesthetic drugs or the conduct of anesthesia, the conduct of the surgery, preexisting disease, fortuitous occurrences, or a combination of several factors.

ETIOLOGY RELATED TO ANESTHESIA

I have noted 17 deaths occurring in ambulatory surgery patients since 1970. These deaths have occurred in freestanding, hospital-affiliated, and office-based ambulatory facilities. The conduct of anesthesia was the most likely cause of the catastrophe in 11 of these cases. This fact reinforces the old cliche that there are no "minor anesthetics."

The most common anesthetic problem resulting in serious morbidity and mortality appears to be violation of the fundamental principles of proper ventilation and clear airway. The two clinical situations that pose recurrent problems in the ambulatory setting are laparoscopy performed with general anesthesia and the use of the intravenous analgesia technique, particularly for nasal and facial surgery.

Although I believe routine endotracheal intubation is not essential for the conduct of safe anesthesia for laparoscopy, the anesthesiologist must exercise constant attention to ventilation and be prepared to intubate the patient at the first indication of inadequate ventilation. I recommend routine intubation if the surgeon requires excessive degrees of Trendelenburg position (usually more than 5-10 degrees) or uses larger than normal volumes of gas (resulting in intra-abdominal pressures exceeding 15-20 mm Hg), and for patients with special problems such as obesity, cardiac or pulmonary disease, or other serious preexisting problems.

The intravenous analgesia technique has many advantages for ambulatory surgery patients such as prompt emergence, a low incidence of nausea and vomiting, and usually a rapid return to clear mental function and general vitality. However, this technique, which is used in association with local anesthesia administered by the surgeon, involves potent respiratory depressants such as narcotics, barbiturates, and tranquilizers. The safety of this technique depends upon the constant observation of ventilation and the respiratory airway. These guidelines are especially crucial when the technique is used for nasal and facial surgery: the anesthesiologist must ensure that the oropharyngeal airway is clear of blood and that there is no glossopharyngeal obstruction. The anesthesiologist must exercise constant vigilance with this valuable but potentially hazardous technique.

One would suspect that a serious and recurring problem among ambulatory surgery patients would be aspiration of gastric contents, including partially digested food, due to the limitations of control in the preoperative period. Prior to 1983 I had found only one reference to an episode of vomiting and aspiration. During the past 12 months, I have discovered three additional cases of vomiting and aspiration that have occurred recently in ambulatory surgical patients. (Clustering of complications is not unusual: a center or group of centers may render service to a large patient population without a particular complication and then experience several within a relatively short period of time.) However, in spite of the newly discovered cases, the incidence of vomiting and aspiration is relatively low. This favorable result may well be due to the special emphasis of preoperative instructions and the thorough questioning of patients about ingestion of food and liquids upon arrival at the ambulatory surgery center. This potentially serious complication, however, is an ever-present danger in the ambulatory setting.

Another remarkable aspect of anesthetic complications in the ambulatory setting has been the relative absence through 1982 of reported cases of malignant hyperthermia. There is certainly nothing unique about outpatient anesthesia, particularly with regard to the pediatric population, that would confer some type of immunity to ambulatory surgery patients. Either these patients are being screened out of the ambulatory setting (a doubtful achievement, even with the most thorough review of family history and consideration of other potential risk factors) or there has been a highly biased complication reporting, or all of us have been incredibly lucky. If the extremely low incidence is due to good fortune, then every ambulatory surgery center should gird themselves for a rash of malignant hyperthermia episodes. In 1983 (with 60 centers reporting) I identified three episodes of malignant hyperthermia occurring in the ambulatory setting, two suspected and one confirmed. Of 40 centers reporting in 1984, three additional episodes were identified, two confirmed and one suspected. We may be seeing the phenomenon of clustering.

There are three pertinent areas of patient care relative to the prevention and treatment of malignant hyperthermia:

1. Screening of every patient's family anesthetic history (blood relatives) and recognition of increased risk factors such as the presence of neuromuscular disease
2. Awareness of the early signs of a malignant hyperthermic crisis under anesthesia such as tachycardia, muscular rigidity, and arrhythmias
3. Preparation of the anesthesiologist and the nursing staff to initiate prompt therapy, which could include the administration of dantrolene, sodium bicarbonate, and methods for cooling the patient

In the ambulatory surgery center geographically separate from a hospital, the objective of treatment should be reversal of the metabolic crisis so the patient can be transferred to a hospital in stable condition for further observation and treatment.

The final topic of complications directly related to anesthesia is reactions to local anesthetic drugs. Based on information voluntarily submitted to FASA in 1982, over 15,000 patients had surgery performed using local anesthesia in 31 ambulatory surgery centers. This figure does not include the use of local anesthetic drugs in other patients who were classified under intravenous analgesia. If these data are extrapolated to encompass the experiences of ambulatory surgery centers throughout the United States, it is evident that an enormous number of patients are administered local anesthetic drugs.

In most cases, the volume, concentration, and rapidity of injection of the drugs are well within safe criteria, and the surgical procedure is limited to excision of small, superficial lesions. However, there is a large number of patients scheduled for surgery such as augmentation mammoplasty, rhinoplasty, submucous resection, rhytidectomy, and multiple podiatric procedures who are receiving marginally safe or unsafe amounts of local anesthetic drugs usually injected over a brief period of time, and often injected into potentially vascular areas where rapid absorption or inadvertent intravascular entry may occur.

The monitoring of patients having surgery with local anesthesia varies considerably among ambulatory surgery centers. The extremes of patient care range from a policy requiring trained anesthesia personnel to attend every patient to only casual observation of the patient undergoing extensive surgery. A common-sense approach based on the pharmacology of the local anesthetic drugs and the data gathered over the years about complications would suggest that patients receiving large volumes and concentrations of local anesthetic drugs, particularly if they are injected over a relatively short period of time or into potentially vascular areas, should be carefully observed and their vital signs monitored by trained personnel during and after surgery.

■ CASE REPORT NO. 15

A 29-year-old woman was scheduled for multiple corrective procedures of both feet. The surgeon injected a total of 83 ml of a mixture of equal parts of 2% lidocaine and 0.5% bupivacaine into the operative sites of both feet. The patient was sedated by an anesthesiologist using the intravenous analgesia technique. The surgery was performed by two surgeons, each working independently on one of the patient's feet and each using a tourniquet above the ankle. The operating room phase of care went well without any hint of a problem. Upon arrival in the PACU, however, the patient manifested grossly jerky movements of the upper extremities, difficulty in swallowing, and inability to talk clearly. The anesthesiologist remained with the patient, administered oxygen and assisted ventilation, and carefully monitored her vital signs. During the next 45 minutes the symptoms gradually abated, and the patient returned to a normal state. This patient received amounts of local anesthetic drugs in excess of recommended safe doses. It is very likely that very high levels of lidocaine reached the systemic circulation when the ankle tourniquets were released.

■ **CASE REPORT NO. 16**
A 19-year-old man was scheduled for a rhinoplasty on an ambulatory basis. The surgery was performed with local anesthesia administered by the surgeon and intravenous sedation administered by an anesthesiologist. The amounts of the narcotic and barbiturate are unknown. Approximately 30 minutes after the onset of surgery, the surgeon commented that the blood looked very dark. The anesthesiologist checked the patient and discovered that he was both apneic and pulseless. In spite of all attempts to resuscitate the patient, he was pronounced dead some 40 minutes later. This case is typical of several similar cases involving the intravenous analgesia technique. It is very likely that death resulted from one or a combination of these factors: central depression of respiration, glossopharyneal obstruction, or blood in the pharynx or trachea and a diminished or absent cough reflex. This patient was not properly monitored, and the case illustrates the crucial importance of constant observation of ventilation and airway when this technique is used.

■ **CASE REPORT NO. 17**
A 28-year-old woman was scheduled for a laparoscopic tubal sterilization under general anesthesia. The patient was anesthetized with sodium thiopental followed by a nitrous oxide, oxygen, halothane routine. No endotracheal tube was used. The anesthetist thought she had a good airway, but admitted later that she could not clearly see "any chest movement." The surgeon noted that the patient appeared pale and dusky as the drapes were removed at the end of the procedure. Examination of the patient revealed no palpable pulse or other vital signs. Attempts to resuscitate the patient were futile. This case illustrates what can happen when the anesthetist is either unaware or unsure of proper ventilation during laparoscopic surgery. The anesthetist should not hesitate for one second to intubate the laparoscopy patient if there is any question about adequate ventilation. If the anesthetist is not skilled in managing these patients without an endotracheal tube, then each of these patients should be routinely intubated.

■ **CASE REPORT NO. 18**
A 21-year-old man was scheduled for a submucous resection under only local anesthesia (the type and concentration were not reported). Packs soaked in a 10% cocaine solution were inserted into both nostrils prior to the injection of local anesthesia. Approximately 5 minutes after the local had been injected and the cocaine packs removed, the patient became unresponsive and pulseless. The surgeon called for help and attempts were made to restore a normal heartbeat. The patient was finally pronounced dead some 45 minutes after the discovery of the arrest.

■ **CASE REPORT NO. 19**
A 69-year-old woman in good general health but with a history of hiatal hernia was scheduled for dental extractions. The anesthetic was a barbiturate, narcotic, muscle relaxant technique. When the anesthesiologist performed

laryngoscopy prior to intubation, it was noted that a large amount of clear gastric contents was in the posterior pharynx. This was suctioned and an endotracheal tube inserted. The surgery was completed in 20 minutes, but the anesthesiologist had ventilation problems because of bronchospasm. Immediately upon the patient's entry into the PACU, a chest film was obtained and a preliminary diagnosis made of aspiration pneumonitis. The patient was admitted into the hospital and placed in the care of a pulmonary specialist. She received aggressive treatment for the problem. She did not require any further intubation or ventilatory support, and was discharged in satisfactory condition 1 week following her procedure.

Although most catastrophic ambulatory surgery complications resulting in death appear to be related to anesthetic drugs and the conduct of anesthesia, the overall majority of major complications are related to the surgery.

ETIOLOGY RELATED TO SURGERY

The single most prevalent surgical complication is hemorrhage. For the purposes of definition, hemorrhage in ambulatory surgical patients is defined as bleeding of sufficient quantity to require special attention and treatment. The volume of the blood loss is not the primary criterion, since it can rarely be accurately measured. The definition of hemorrhage should include adenoidectomy patients requiring a posterior pack; patients who must return to an operating room, emergency room, or physician's office for additional suturing, cautery, packing, or pressure dressings; patients with postoperative hematoma requiring evacuation; and patients requiring laparotomy for intra-abdominal bleeding.

Approximately 1% to 4% of all tonsillectomy and adenoidectomy (T&A) patients bleed sufficiently to require special treatment during either the operating room, PACU, or postdischarge phase of care. Most of the bleeding episodes will occur after discharge from the ambulatory surgery center.

The most urgent and serious episodes of hemorrhage are associated with laparoscopy. The laceration of a major intra-abdominal blood vessel upon insertion of the primary trocar creates one of the most critical situations in the ambulatory surgery facility, as well as in the hospital inpatient setting. Every ambulatory surgery center must have a plan for immediate response to this potentially fatal complication. A sterile laparotomy tray, as well as plasma expander fluids, should be immediately available. The abdomen should be entered without delay and the hemorrhage controlled by any and all means until a primary repair of the laceration can be performed. The center's plan for obtaining blood should be initiated as soon as a blood sample can be drawn for type and crossmatch. In some cases, the use of noncross-matched O negative blood may be life saving. Probably the single most important aspect of treatment is having the center's professional nursing staff well informed about their duties in the event of this complication.

Less serious episodes of bleeding associated with laparoscopy may occur within the abdominal wall owing to the introduction of the secondary trocar or may occur intra-abdominally as a result of the freeing of preexisting adhesions.

The laparoscopy procedure is associated with other serious major complications such as bowel burn, laceration of the bowel or other hollow viscus, bowel obstruction secondary to perforation or adhesions, and peritonitis secondary to unrecognized bowel perforation. Since the introduction of the bipolar coagulation technique, bowel burns have been virtually eliminated.

Two cases of intra-abdominal explosion following the use of nitrous oxide as the filling gas have been reported in the literature.[29] However, I cannot find a single case of explosion reported in the United States in spite of the fact that nitrous oxide has been used extensively in this country. It is very likely that other factors besides the use of nitrous oxide were responsible for the explosions in the reported cases.

Although the incidence of wound infection is low among ambulatory surgery patients, several cases of fulminating streptococcal septicemia have occurred in women who had undergone augmentation mammoplasty. It is not clear why such infections may take such a rampant course in these patients; however, the virulence of these rare infections has prompted some plastic surgeons to use prophylactic antibiotics in their breast augmentation patients.

■ CASE REPORT NO. 20

A 64-year-old man was scheduled for excision of multiple bilateral nasal polyps under general endotracheal anesthesia. There was generous bleeding during the performance of the procedure, which lasted almost 105 minutes. Upon arrival in the PACU the patient bled through the nasal packs, and blood clots were suctioned from his oropharyngeal area. The patient was restless but cooperative. In view of his persistent bleeding, the patient was transferred directly to a hospital for observation. Upon arrival at the hospital, the patient removed his packs and was subsequently scheduled for emergency surgery under general anesthesia to reinsert them. When the patient arrived in the hospital PACU following the second operation, blood continued to soak the newly inserted nasal packing. He was again returned to the operating room for further packing. The patient never awakened from the second anesthetic and died 4 days later. Postmortem examination revealed an iatrogenic defect in the cribriform plate with a laceration of the brain.

■ CASE REPORT NO. 21

A 39-year-old woman was scheduled for a laparoscopic tubal sterilization and D&C. The surgeon accidentally perforated the dome of the bladder during the insertion of the primary trocar. The perforation was observed upon insertion of the laparoscope. A urologist was called and performed a cystoscopy in order to assess the damage. A laparotomy was subsequently performed and the perforation repaired. An open tubal ligation was performed at the same time. The patient was transferred to a hospital for postoperative care after stable emergence in the ambulatory surgery center PACU.

■ CASE REPORT NO. 22

A 39-year-old woman underwent a bilateral augmentation mammoplasty under local anesthesia. The surgery went smoothly and the patient was discharged in good condition. The following day the patient called her surgeon and complained of fever, chills, and generalized weakness. The patient was hospitalized later on the same day. The patient was treated with intravenous antibiotics, and drainage material from the right breast was cultured. Despite intensive antibiotic therapy, the patient died on the third postoperative day. Culture of the breast drainage material grew beta-hemolytic streptococci.

ETIOLOGY RELATED TO PREEXISTING CONDITIONS

The variations of complications that may arise as a result of preexisting disease are limitless and may include such diverse complications and disease entities (which have actually occurred) as subglottic edema in a child with congenital tracheal stenosis, a fulminating episode of bronchospasm in a patient with extrinsic asthma, an arrhythmia in a patient with prolapse of the mitral valve resulting in cardiac arrest, uncontrolled bleeding in a patient with a familial coagulation disturbance, and severe postoperative psychoneurotic behavior in a patient with a history of serious emotional problems.

This discussion focuses on three significant problem areas associated with preexisting conditions that may be present in ambulatory patients: intra-operative or postoperative myocardial infarction, disruption of metabolic control in insulin-dependent patients with diabetes mellitus, and certain complications occurring in pregnant patients (pregnancy is not a preexisting disease, but it is a preexisting condition that presents some unique complications in the ambulatory setting).

Myocardial Infarction. Tinker studied the relationship of myocardial infarction to the surgical and anesthetic experiences.[32] His review and cogent observations were presented at the refresher course lectures at the annual meeting of the American Society of Anesthesiologists in 1982, and his comments are generously referred to in this discussion. Many of the important aspects of his review are as appropriate for ambulatory patients as for hospital inpatients.

Tarhan et al reported that the overall risk of perioperative infarction was 6% in patients who had a history of a previous myocardial infarction.[30] However, if the myocardial infarction had occurred within 3 months prior to the surgical and anesthetic experience, the risk for a recurrent myocardial infarction increased to 37%. The risk diminished to 16% if the interlude between the first myocardial infarction and the surgical experience was between 3 and 6 months. The mortality rate as a result of repeat myocardial infarction in Tarhan's study was 50%!

Tinker also reported on Mahar's review of surgical patients who had survived previous coronary bypass surgery. Mahar et al studied 99 postbypass patients who underwent a total of 168 subsequent noncardiac operations without a single perioperative myocardial infarction.[20] Tinker also presented data gathered by Backer et al and Lang et al.[3,32] Backer and his group studied over 10,000 patients who underwent ophthalmic surgery using local or retrobulbar block anesthesia. Of the patients in his group, 195 had a documented previous myocardial infarction; almost one-half of these patients had more than one surgical procedure. Not a single perioperative reinfarction occurred. Lang et al reported very similar results in patients who had eye surgery under general anesthesia. Tinker commented, "This implies that the magnitude of the surgery, not the type of anesthesia is responsible for these good results." He further observed, "The other relevant point for anesthesiologists is that these seemingly very fragile patients, many of whom are quite elderly with many other medical problems, scheduled for ophthalmic surgery, are in fact not at great risk of peri-operative myocardial infarction."

Tinker's observations may become significantly important as recent changes in the Medicare law may shift older patients scheduled for eye surgery and other less complex surgical procedures to the ambulatory setting.

Diabetes Mellitus. During the past 10 years, over 100 insulin-dependent patients have had surgery at Northwest Surgicare. Our experience has been very favorable, suggesting that the ambulatory setting is ideal for many diabetic patients scheduled for certain types of surgical procedures. Diabetes mellitus is a common disease, and there is a large population of insulin-dependent patients. I have devoted considerable space to this subject in view of many ambulatory surgical centers being reluctant to accept these patients because the traditional methods of diabetic management appear to work less satisfactorily in the ambulatory setting. The method we use works remarkably well, and we have experienced no complications related to insulin management.

The primary objective is to restore the diabetic patient's insulin balance as smoothly as possible to the preoperative state. We have observed that the sooner these patients return to their own environment, accustomed diet, and activity, the less severe will be the disturbance to their insulin balance and associated changes in their metabolism.

There is substantial variation among the individual response of diabetic patients receiving insulin ranging from relative stability on a day-to-day basis to marked "brittleness," manifested by episodes of hypoglycemia (insulin reactions) and periods of high blood glucose. In general, diabetic children and young adults are more likely to fall into the latter group. If the patient has a history of poor or complicated insulin control, the case should be thoroughly discussed with the patient's physician. The patient may not be a candidate for ambulatory surgery.

The traditional methods of managing the insulin-dependent diabetic patient for surgery within the hospital setting are predicated on the administration of fractional doses of the patient's normal insulin requirements (usually one-third to one-half) and the continuous administration of an intravenous glucose infusion. The patient's balance is fine-tuned by obtaining frequent blood sugar determinations and using supplemental regular insulin as needed. If everyone involved in the patient's care (laboratory personnel, nurses, and physicians) work together diligently, the method works reasonably well.

When the traditional method is applied to the ambulatory setting, there are obvious problems. The question of how much insulin to administer and when to administer it is difficult to coordinate with the patient's physician. One frequently used management routine is to administer one-half of the patient's normal insulin requirement on the morning of surgery. This dose may be too much or too little depending on the specific metabolic characteristics of the patient, the type and quantity of intravenous fluids, the length and stress of the surgery, and other factors. In the hospital setting, medical personnel can provide proper attention, making the necessary adjustments with supplemental insulin and regulating the intravenous fluids. Not only is this method difficult in the ambulatory surgery setting, but it also creates many problems for the patient after discharge from the center. The diabetic ambulatory surgery patient will usually resume almost normal meals after returning home, frequently resulting in high blood sugars for the remainder of the day of surgery. The presence of hyperglycemia during this period may increase the incidence of infection.

We often use a different management approach for the insulin-dependent patient that has worked very well in the ambulatory setting. The method is relatively simple and effective, and we call it *moving the sun in the sky.* Each of these patients has a baseline fasting blood sugar preoperatively and may have one or more repeat blood sugar tests performed in the PACU using one of the "home-type" colorimetric techniques. The ultimate success of the process depends on the absence of persistent vomiting. We have been very fortunate and have not had a single patient who experienced recurrent vomiting in the postoperative period. It is axiomatic that vomiting mandates hospitalization and intravenous support until the patient can return to a normal diet and insulin balance. If the patient is scheduled for local anesthesia only, he or she is instructed to take a usual insulin dose and have meals at the accustomed intervals.

If the patient is scheduled for surgery under general or intravenous analgesia, we attempt to assign an early time for surgery. These patients are instructed to omit their normal morning injection and bring their insulin with them. They are instructed to arrive at the center as early as possible in order to manage a possible hypoglycemic episode due to the absence of a normal breakfast. We allow these patients to remain in the reception area; however, they are told to notify our personnel immediately if they perceive an impending insulin reaction. If this happens preoperatively, the patient is moved promptly to the PACU, and the hypoglycemia is reversed by means of an intravenous glucose infusion. The patient's status can be monitored with blood sugar tests if necessary.

After the completion of surgery, the intravenous infusion is maintained until the patient is almost ready to go home. The blood sugar test is repeated at least once in the postoperative period. Barring nausea and vomiting, the patient is instructed to pretend that he or she has just awakened and to take the usual and normal dose of insulin and have normal meals with the usual time intervals between meals—hence the name moving the sun in the sky. The insulin dose may be increased or decreased if the last blood sugar test results were substantially high or low, and the dose may be moderately increased if the patient's activity is to be markedly restricted at home.

For example, if the patient is moved into the PACU at 9:30 A.M. and is ready to be discharged at 11:00 A.M., the patient may take insulin prior to leaving the facility (if he or she lives close to the center) or immediately upon arrival at home. The patient is instructed to have a normal breakfast 20 minutes after the insulin injection, lunch 4 hours later, and dinner approximately 5 hours after lunch (which in this example would be between 8:30 and 9:00 P.M.). The following day the patient takes a normal dose of insulin and has normal meals spaced at a normal interval. All we have done is artificially "move the sun in the sky." The later the insulin is administered on the day of surgery, the greater will be the risk of an insulin reaction the next morning after the normal dose of insulin is taken at the customary time. Therefore, these patients should be cautioned that they may be more vulnerable to an insulin reaction on the first postoperative morning and may require additional carbohydrate at breakfast time.

Pregnancy. The pregnant patient poses at least two potentially serious complications. The first problem may have both a medical and legal component.[25] The anesthesiologist may or may not be aware that the patient is pregnant at the time of the ambulatory surgery (not all ambulatory surgery facilities perform pregnancy testing prior to administering anesthesia). At some point in the future, the patient may allege or blame a miscarriage or a retarded or deformed child on the anesthetic experience at the ambulatory surgery facility. It is prudent to ask every female patient of child-bearing age if she is pregnant before administering anesthesia or performing surgery. Northwest Surgicare has incorporated this specific question into its preoperative medical screening process. If the patient is pregnant or suspects that she is pregnant, have a forthright and informative discussion with the patient about the potential hazards to the fetus. Do not hesitate to cancel the procedure if there is any reluctance on the part of the patient to go ahead, particularly if the surgery could be postponed without any difficulty. Obviously, if the patient elects to proceed, avoid suspected teratogenic drugs such as certain antiemetics and tranquilizers, and carefully document all of this information on the chart.

The second complication associated with the pregnant patient may have even more serious consequences. A very large number of pregnant women come to ambulatory facilities for termination of the pregnancy. It is one of the most common ambulatory surgical procedures performed in the United States. It is essential that the tissue removed be examined by a trained pathologist, and the results of the examination reported to the surgeon as soon as possible. There have been several catastrophic cases of ruptured ectopic pregnancy following an abortion procedure. This complication may be due to failure of the surgeon to request examination of the tissue, failure to promptly inform the surgeon of the results of the examination, or failure of the surgeon to respond properly to the pathology results. The absence of chorionic villi or other conception tissue in the specimen material should immediately alert the surgeon to the potential of an undiagnosed ectopic pregnancy.

■ CASE REPORT NO. 23

A 53-year-old man was scheduled for a minor podiatric procedure using local anesthesia plus intravenous analgesia administered by an anesthesiologist. The patient was moderately obese and had a 20-year history of cigarette smoking. The operating room and PACU phases of care went well without any problems. Approximately 48 hours after discharge, the patient was hospitalized because of chest pain. He spent several days in the coronary care unit of a hospital with a diagnosis of myocardial infarction. The patient had a benign hospital course. No bypass surgery was recommended after a cardiac workup that included a coronary angiogram. During his hospitalization, the patient told his internist that he had experienced occasional chest pain for several weeks prior to his surgery but had told no one.

■ CASE REPORT NO. 24

A 27-year-old woman visited an abortion clinic and consented to the termination of an apparent first trimester pregnancy. The procedure was performed without any unusual problems. The patient returned to her apartment after the surgery. She was found dead several days later by a neighbor. Postmortem examination revealed a ruptured ectopic tubal pregnancy with exsanguination within the abdominal cavity. Material removed from the patient at the time of the abortion had never been examined by a pathologist.

■ CASE REPORT NO. 25

A 36-year-old woman was scheduled for a diagnostic laparoscopy. She had a 15-year history of asthma related to allergic and emotional factors. The patient was administered a nitrous oxide, oxygen, halothane anesthetic following thiopental induction. There were no problems during the operating room phase of care. Approximately 1 half-hour after the patient awakened in the PACU, she began to wheeze and manifested labored respiration. Auscultation of the chest revealed bilateral, diffuse wheezing breath sounds. The asthmatic episode was promptly treated with intravenous aminophylline administered by drip infusion. The wheezing and dyspnea gradually abated over the next hour. She had normal breath sounds prior to discharge, and follow-up revealed that she had no further problems.

ETIOLOGY RELATED TO FORTUITOUS OCCURRENCES

Rarely, there are complications that occur without any rhyme or reason. These complications reflect no deficiency in medical care and seem only to corroborate that there is a capricious nature to life that defies our best efforts to practice safe and knowledgeable medicine.

■ CASE REPORT NO. 26

A 25-year-old man had a vasectomy performed on an ambulatory surgery basis under local anesthesia. Following the procedure, he rested in the reception area before starting on his way home. Approximately 15 minutes later the police pulled his body from his wrecked automobile. He had apparently lost control of the car and crashed into a building. Postmortem examination of the patient revealed a ruptured intracranial aneurysm with massive bleeding. There had been no history of any previous problems in this young man.

■ CASE REPORT NO. 27

A healthy 39-year-old woman elected to have a diagnostic D&C performed under local anesthesia. Her temperature and vital signs were normal on the day of surgery. She had no other complaints or symptoms at the time. On the first postoperative day, she became acutely ill with a cough, fever, and chills. She was seen by her family doctor and chest radiography revealed viral pneumonia.

■ CASE REPORT NO. 28

A 25-year-old man was scheduled for an arthroscopy and arthrotomy of the right ankle under local anesthesia and intravenous analgesia administered by an anesthesiologist. There were no problems during the operative or the PACU phases of care. On the second postoperative day, the patient complained of severe abdominal pain and was hospitalized by his family doctor. The patient was admitted to the hospital with a diagnosis of an "acute abdomen." He spent one week in the hospital and was discharged with a diagnosis of acute gastritis.

ETIOLOGY RELATED TO MULTIPLE FACTORS

There are complications in which the general etiology may be attributed to more than one factor. It may be difficult or impossible to apportion the significance of each individual factor properly, but one cannot rule out that each factor bears a relationship and contributes to the etiology of the complication.

■ CASE REPORT NO. 29

A 58-year-old man with a history of hypertension was scheduled for a hair transplant under local anesthesia and intravenous analgesia administered by an anesthesiologist. The surgeon had intended to implant 100 plugs, but the surgery was abandoned after the placement of 25 plugs because of uncontrolled bleeding. The patient required two 500-ml units of plasma expander and was transferred to a general hospital for observation. A hematologic workup established the diagnosis of von Willebrand's disease. This case report implicates multiple factors, including the history of hypertension, the decision to perform the cosmetic surgery in the first place, and the undiagnosed coagulation disease.

■ CASE REPORT NO. 30

A thin, frail 72-year-old woman was scheduled for cataract surgery under local anesthesia. According to her family, she had lost a significant amount of weight during the past year without any plausible explanation. In addition, she had a history of angina pectoris and coronary artery disease. The ophthalmologic surgeon instructed the circulating nurse to administer 5 mg of diazepam in a single dose intravenously. Approximately 5 to 10 minutes later, the circulating nurse noted that the patient's hands and nail beds appeared blue. The drapes were removed and no respiration or heartbeat could be discerned. Despite closed-chest cardiac massage, the patient's heart action was never restored. This case implicates many factors, including failure to investigate the patient's weight loss and prepare the patient properly for surgery, inadequate monitoring of the vital signs during the procedure in view of her fragile general condition, and the rapid administration of a respiratory depressant drug without proper observation.

■ CASE REPORT NO. 31

A 39-year-old woman was scheduled for multiple podiatric procedures under general anesthesia. In spite of a past history of six episodes of thrombophlebitis, the surgeon elected to use a pneumatic thigh cuff inflated to 450 mm Hg for a period of 100 minutes. The patient had no problems during either the operating room or PACU phases of her care. She was discharged in good condition but developed signs and symptoms of thrombophlebitis on the fourth postoperative day. She was hospitalized for 11 days while receiving anticoagulant therapy. She made a satisfactory recovery without any further problems. However, a potentially serious complication might have been prevented if some other method for the management of bleeding had been used. It is also possible that this patient was not a candidate for ambulatory surgery and should have had preoperative and postoperative anticoagulant treatment.

■ **CASE REPORT NO. 32**

A 59-year-old man was scheduled for excision of redundant gingival tissue. The patient had a long history of alcoholism, recent onset of mild hypertension, and a morbid fear of doctors. He had refused to have the surgery performed under local anesthesia in the oral surgeon's office. Shortly after the onset of surgery using general, endotracheal anesthesia (nitrous oxide, oxygen, halothane), he manifested an irregular pulse followed by ventricular fibrillation. Closed-chest cardiac compression was started promptly, and the patient's color improved almost immediately. The patient was electrically defibrillated without difficulty, and a normal sinus rhythm ensued. Spontaneous respiration returned shortly thereafter, and there were no blood pressure problems. The anesthesiologist felt certain that satisfactory circulation had been restored within a safe period of time. However, the patient did not regain consciousness for several days and was left with diminished cerebral function.

Complication Statistics and Data: Trying to Find the Truth

There are three general modes for the gathering of complication data: the information may be submitted on a voluntary basis to a medical organization or society and subsequently reported or published; it may be extracted from the records of one or more centers in a retrospective fashion and reported or published; or it may be gathered through a planned, ongoing, prospective process and reported or published. The data gathered by each method tell us something. The question is, how close does it come to our search for pure truth? Complication data gathered through voluntary submission to an organization frequently lacks uniformity, and an individual center may choose to avoid participation if it feels its results are "poor." Therefore, the data may be highly biased and incomplete.

Data obtained by reviewing records retrospectively are subject to many problems. Complications are easily overlooked, and vital information that is not recorded is usually lost forever.

The process of establishing an ongoing, prospective complication study requires time, hard work, and dedication on the part of the facility and its personnel. On the positive side, the data obtained are substantially uniform and inclusive. However, there is a drawback because the information usually reflects the experience of *one* center. Each ambulatory surgery center has its own unique characteristics such as the types of surgery performed, the distribution of anesthetic techniques, patient age and physical state, and the experience and training of its staff.

The search that takes us closest to pure truth would require a uniform prospective study involving and combining the experiences of many ambulatory surgery centers. FASA is presently conducting a prospective study that involves the participation of over 40 ambulatory surgery centers throughout the United States. When this project is completed and the data are properly analyzed, we will have a broad spectrum of valuable information.

Data about Minor Complications

Complications that generally fall within the parameters of our definition of minor complications have been studied and published in several earlier articles.

Fahy and Marshall studied postanesthetic morbidity in 408 outpatients selected at random and interviewed at a later date.[13] The authors observed that almost 45% of the patients interviewed manifested some symptoms attributable to the anesthetic. The commonest complaints were drowsiness, headache, malaise, dizziness, nausea, and vomiting. When this group of patients was interviewed, less than 4% reported symptoms that persisted for more than 24 hours. The authors noted that "the disability produced, however, was transient and trivial."

Brindle and Soliman investigated anesthetic complications in 500 ASA physical status 1 female patients who underwent outpatient laparoscopic tubal coagulation.[4] Information was obtained from a questionnaire sent to the patients 1 week to 4 months postoperatively. Of the group, 418 patients returned the questionnaires. The most common complications mentioned were muscle pain (45%) and sore throat (28%). In addition, their patients also reported headache, nausea and vomiting, and cough. There was a high incidence of mild dizziness, and, interestingly, 30% of the patients experienced inability to concentrate that, in one-half of the patients, lasted more than 2 days. Perhaps the most significant finding was that 81% of the patients indicated that in spite of these symptoms, they would submit to the procedure again.

Urbach and Edelist studied 250 patients scheduled for D&C or therapeutic abortion and 100 patients for dental procedures.[33] The authors reported one episode each of hypertension, arrhythmia, and hypotension and 10 episodes of delayed arousal in the PACU. Many of the patients reported minor complications such as nausea and vomiting, dizziness, headache, sore throat, muscle weakness or pain, and other complaints after discharge. Significantly, more than 95% of the patients felt it was safe for them to return to their home after the surgery and anesthesia.

Ahlgren et al reviewed their experiences with pediatric ambulatory surgery at a hospital-based day surgery program in 1969.[2] Outpatient anesthesia was given to 977 pediatric patients. A questionnaire was mailed to the family of each patient postoperatively, and approximately 33% responded. The analysis of minor complications was based on the first 300 questionnaires returned. The authors reported that 4% of the children manifested "considerable" upset stomach, sore throat, and loss of appetite; 1% of the patients complained of considerable dizziness, headache, and 2% of the children suffered considerable hoarseness and bad dreams. Over 80% of the parents indicated that "under similar circumstances they would be happy to again participate in the program."

Based on these reports and my own experience over a 10 year period, several fundamental conclusions may be drawn about minor complications.

It is unlikely that the surgical team will ever be able to render their services in any setting without encountering many minor complications that produce some degree of discomfort or displeasure in the patient. The incidence and types of these complications are closely related to the anesthetic technique and the surgical procedure.

The incidence of nausea, vomiting, sore throat, and delayed arousal is significantly less in our patients whose surgery is performed under intravenous analgesia and virtually absent under only local anesthesia. When the surgery is relatively brief, there is less prolonged drowsiness, delayed emergence, and malaise. The incidence and degree of shoulder pain after laparoscopy is substantially less when nitrous oxide is used as the filling gas. There is a definite relationship between the overall ambulatory anesthesia skills of the anesthesiologist and the occurrence and degree of minor anesthesia-related complications. Many minor complications such as headache and nausea are related to the patient's previous experiences and expectations. And finally, the significance and perception on the part of the patient will be substantially modified by providing sound preoperative information and generous reassurance.

Data about Major Complications

In 1980, I published the results of our initial, comprehensive, prospective study of major complications in the ambulatory setting covering the first $4\frac{1}{2}$ years of experience at Northwest Surgicare and encompassing 13,433 patients.[23] 99.8% of our patient population had been followed through their operating room and PACU phases of care and through the first 2 weeks of the postoperative period. We have continued this program of prospectively documenting major complications; our experience now includes over 32,000 patients and spans almost a 10-year period.

We have documented 253 major complications in our review of 32,001 ambulatory surgery patients (Table 8-1). The most prevalent complication was hemorrhage, which occurred in 138 patients. Of these episodes, 108 occurred after the patient's discharge from the ambulatory surgery center. Table 8-2 illustrates the time relationship of the occurrence of bleeding in these patients.

Perhaps the most surprising aspect of our initial study was the extremely low incidence of infection. At this writing, there has been a total of 24 wound infections in approximately 32,000 patients! Almost all of these infections were well localized and treated without difficulty. There were 26 additional miscellaneous infections including postoperative upper respiratory infections, viral pneumonias, endometritis, flare-up of preexisting pelvic inflammatory disease, cystitis, and other miscellaneous infections.

In 1981, the Centers for Disease Control reported that approximately 5% of all hospital patients contract infections while in the hospital, and about 20,000 of these patients die each year. Many of these patients are nonsurgical, and there are many factors that influence the incidence of infection among surgical inpatients, including the complexity of the surgery and general condition of the patient. It would therefore be a serious distortion simply to compare the general incidence of infection in the surgical inpatient and the outpatient. However, when comparable procedures in similar patients are studied, the significance of hospital nosocomial infections cannot be ignored. Table 8-3 summarizes this information.

Direct-vision laparoscopy has become an increasingly useful diagnostic

☐ **Table 8-1   Major Complications among 32,001 Patients at Northwest Surgicare, April 17, 1974, to January 5, 1984**

Complication	No. of Patients
Hemorrhage	138
Wound infection	24
Other infections	26
Persistent vomiting	11
Other complications (in alphabetical order)	
Abdominal distention (cause unknown)	1
Bowel burn	2
Bowel obstruction	1
Bronchospasm	1
Conjunctivitis (chemical)	1
Corneal ulcer	1
Dehiscence of wound	1
Dehydration (nonvomiting)	3
Delayed emergence from anesthesia	2
Drug allergy (urticaria)	3
Drug reaction—local anesthetic	2
Edema of tongue (severe)	1
Electric burn	2
Hypertensive episode in PACU	1
Hypotensive episode in PACU	1
Laryngospasm (severe)	5
Myocardial infarction (preoperative occurrence with postoperative diagnosis)	1
Pain, severe, unexplained, resulting in hospitalization	2
Perforation of bladder	1
Perforation of bowel	1
Perforation of uterus	2
Phlebitis	8
Psychosomatic reactions	4
Respiratory arrest in the operating room	1
Rigid chest syndrome, anesthesia	1
Subglottic edema	1
Syncopal episodes	2
Ventricular fibrillation (cause unknown)	1
Vertigo (severe)	1

tool, and laparoscopy with tubal disruption has become the most common choice of sterilization technique in women. Both of these procedures are frequently performed in the ambulatory setting.

The most common complications associated with laparoscopy are hemorrhage, perforation of an intra-abdominal viscus, bowel burn, and serious anesthesia-related problems. Hemorrhage may result from the insertion of the trocars or from vascular damage caused by electrofulguration. The incidence of bowel burn and bleeding due to electrofulguration has been reduced dramatically since the widespread use of the bipolar technique has replaced the monopolar technique during the past 5 or 6 years.

☐ **Table 8-2   Relationship of Hemorrhage to Time of Occurrence and Surgical Procedure among 32,001 Patients at Northwest Surgicare**

Time of Occurrence	Tonsillec-tomy or Adenoidec-tomy (4127 Patients)	Augmen-tation Mammo-plasty or Capsulo-tomy (641 Patients)	Submucous Resec-tion or Rhino-plasty (882 Patients)	Cervical Coniza-tion (252 Patients)	All Other Surgical Procedures (26,099 Patients)	Totals
Intraoperative	4	0	1	0	6	11
PACU	10	3	0	0	6	19
Day of surgery after discharge	2	2	4	0	5	13
Postoperative day 1	5	3	2	0	5	15
2	2	3	2	0	1	8
3	1	4	0	0	2	7
4	1	1	1	0	0	3
5	12	0	0	0	2	14
6	7	0	0	0	0	7
7	13	1	1	1	3	19
8	5	0	0	1	1	7
9	2	0	0	0	1	3
10	5	0	0	0	1	6
After the 10th postoperative day	4	1	0	1	0	6
Totals	73	18	11	3	33	138

Table 8-4 summarizes published data relating to laparoscopy complications. Most of the statistics predate the common use of the bipolar method. The data from Northwest Surgicare is current and covers the period 1974 to 1983, including the periods before and after the change from monopolar to the bipolar technique.

One of the most interesting reports originates from the Complication Committee of the American Association of Gynecological Laparoscopists and was published in 1973.[15] Reporting on data voluntarily submitted, the study documents morbidity and mortality associated with 12,000 laparoscopies, including approximately 7,000 tubal sterilization cases.

Their data showed the following results:

Complication	*No. of Cases*
Bowel laceration requiring repair	6
Mesosalpingeal bleeding requiring laparotomy	23
Laceration of major blood vessels	3
Abdominal wall hemorrhage	3
Bowel burn recognized and repaired at time of surgery	6
Bowel obstruction from unrecognized intestinal perforation	9
Cystitis or flare-up of pelvic inflammatory disease	10

☐ Table 8-3 Infection and Ambulatory Surgery

Reference	Relevant Aspects of Study	Results: Incidence of Infection
Othersen and Clatworthy[26]	Comparison of infections in pediatric inpatients and outpatients scheduled for hernia repair	50%–70% reduction in outpatients
Kornhall and Olsson[18]	Comparison of wound infections in adult inpatients and outpatients scheduled for hernia repair	Inpatients 2% Outpatients 0%
Caridis[8]	Wound sepsis in adult inpatients and outpatients scheduled for vein stripping	Inpatients 12% Outpatients 0%
Nabatoff and Aufses[22]	Wound sepsis in 2000 outpatients scheduled for varicose vein surgery	Outpatients 0%
Brownstein and Owsley[6]	Postoperative infection in 227 inpatients scheduled for augmentation mammoplasty	Inpatients 2.6%
Natof	Postoperative infection in 641 outpatients scheduled for augmentation mammoplasty	Outpatients 0.62%
Davis[11]	Infection in surgical outpatients	0.2%
Natof	Prospective study of postoperative infection (all types) in 32,001 outpatients	Overall 0.16% Wound infection 0.075% Nonwound infection 0.081%

There were five episodes of cardiac arrest and three deaths, attributed to air embolism, peritonitis after bowel perforation, and delayed treatment of a lacerated common iliac artery.

Jensen and Wetchler studied over 2100 patients scheduled for laparoscopic ambulatory surgery with particular reference to obesity.[16] They concluded that obesity per se was not a contraindication to ambulatory surgery and anesthesia. However, they noted an increase in surgical complications associated with the

☐ Table 8-4 Complications Associated with Laparoscopy

Source of Data	Tubal Hemorrhage	Bowel Burn	Perforated Viscus	Bowel Obstruction	Cardiac Arrest
American Association of Gynecologic Laparoscopists: 12,000 patients. Mixture diagnostic and sterilization procedures[15]	0.19%	0.25%	0.05%	0	0.04%
Thompson and Wheeless[31]: 231 outpatients	3.9%	0.86%	0.86%	0	0
Hughes and Liston[14]: 1910 inpatients	0.37%	0.1%	0	0.05%	0.05%
Natof: 2620 outpatients	0.038%	0.076%	0.076%	0.038%	0

laparoscopy procedure. The more obese patients (based on the body mass index) had a higher percentage of minilaparotomies as a result of the inability of the surgeon to perform a laparoscopy. The increased numbers of minilaparotomies resulted in a parallel increase in the number of direct hospital admissions.

A review published in the American Journal of Obstetrics and Gynecology in 1983 studied deaths attributable to tubal sterilization in the United States during the years 1977 to 1981.[28] This review included both sterilization by laparotomy and laparoscopy, and it is not specified whether any of the patients involved were operated on in the ambulatory setting. However, the data provide further confirmation of the potential dangers associated with laparoscopy. The authors discovered 29 deaths and identified the following causes: 11 deaths due to general anesthesia, 7 due to sepsis, 4 due to hemorrhage, 3 due to myocardial infarction, and 4 due to other causes. Among the 11 fatalities believed due to anesthesia, hypoventilation was deemed the most probable cause in 6 patients.

The role of anesthetic drugs and the conduct of anesthesia in laparoscopy cases resulting in cardiac arrest may at best be speculative, but usually the crucial issue is adequate ventilation and a clear airway. The indisputable fact is that distending the abdomen with a filling gas and placing the patient in the Trendelenburg (head-down) position impinge on the normal ability to perform ventilation and gas exchange.

There are anesthesiologists who have dogmatically stated that intubation of the trachea is mandatory for laparoscopy patients. Other anesthesiologists maintain that intubation should not be *routinely* performed but used selectively (e.g., for obese patients, patients with a history of possible adhesions, patients with special medical problems). Obviously, surgeons who depend on steep Trendelenburg position and high intra-abdominal filling pressures shift the decision to intubate and provide the anesthesiologist no other safe choice.

My personal experience is that routine intubation is not mandatory for the safe conduct of anesthesia. The intubation technique, even in the most skilled hands, has a morbidity of its own. I believe it is essential to make several points crystal clear: there are many patients scheduled for laparoscopy that should be intubated for good and proper reasons; the anesthesiologist must always have the proper equipment and be prepared to intubate in every case; and most importantly, the patient must be constantly observed to ensure that there is a clear airway and satisfactory ventilation. In the event there is any question whatsoever about proper ventilation, the surgery should be interrupted and the patient intubated.

One other point should be emphasized about episodes of cardiac arrest that are not apparently related to the conduct of surgery or some other obvious cause. There seems to be a widely accepted doctrine that if one cannot provide a simple and clear explanation for a death associated with an anesthetic, then the burden of proof must rest on the anesthesiologist to show that he or she did not commit some error that caused the critical episode. Keats has correctly addressed and commented upon this unscientific and dangerous approach. "Analyses of death continue to focus on 'errors' that are barely described and that are the consequence of a judgement that the investigators do not believe requires documentation."[17]

It is interesting to speculate how many anesthesiologists would have suffered the consequence of litigation and the faulty judgment of their medical peers if the syndrome of malignant hyperthermia had not been identified and elucidated until 1984. Our search for pure truth in the experimental laboratory may frequently come too late for those who work in the "clinical trenches." These comments are not meant to be an excuse for careless anesthetic care, but only a recognition that our medical knowledge is less than perfect.

From 1975 to 1980, Bruns devoted substantial time and energy collecting and tabulating data voluntarily submitted to FASA.* The information requested varied during the years of his tenure, but his pioneering labors have left us with a better overview of many aspects of freestanding ambulatory surgical care. The data associated with 458,000 patients was collected by Bruns from 1975 to 1980. Only one death was reported during this period.

The uniformity of the questionnaires in 1978, 1979, and 1980 make some particularly valuable data sufficiently uniform for review. During this 3-year period, a total of 254,605 patients became part of the study. Of these patients, 75.36% were administered either general anesthesia or intravenous analgesia. The incidence of unanticipated direct hospital transfer was 0.094%. This included all patients who were admitted to a hospital for the treatment and care of complications or were directly transferred for nonmedical reasons. The incidence of direct hospital transfer made under dire circumstances was 0.0078%. This included all patients who were transferred to a hospital under life-threatening or medically urgent conditions. The incidence of blood transfusion within the ambulatory surgical center was 0.01%. In spite of the voluntary nature of his data, Bruns's efforts provided substantive information and a broad foundation upon which others could build in the years to come.

The Direct Hospital Transfer

The annual questionnaires submitted by Bruns under the auspices of FASA focused attention on a nagging and pertinent question with medical, economic, and political overtones. Many hospital-affiliated ambulatory surgery services report high incidences of hospitalization of their ambulatory patients. Cohen and Dillon[10] reported an incidence of 4.1%, Ahlgren[1] 1%, Coakley and Levy[9] 1%, Davis[11] 1.2%, Meridy[21] 2.44%, Lieberman et al[19] 1.1%, Caldamone and Rabinowitz[7] 5%, and Patterson et al[27] 1.54%. Wetchler has reviewed direct hospital admissions at his hospital-affiliated center covering over 45,000 ambulatory patients and has documented an incidence of 0.6%.[34]

If a significant number of ambulatory surgery patients require direct hospitalization, the ambulatory concept has an intrinsically weak link, and the freestanding surgery center is particularly vulnerable to this shortcoming.

Northwest Surgicare has kept prospective records of all direct hospital transfers since its very first day of service. As of this writing, there have been 35 direct patient transfers in a population in excess of 32,000 patients—an incidence of 0.11%. Our experience is similar to other freestanding ambulatory surgery centers, as the Bruns data demonstrated over a 3-year period.

Analyses of our own transfer data during the past 10-year period has confirmed certain significant factors. Only 3 of the 35 transfers were characterized as urgent. The remaining patients were transported to a hospital in a controlled but relaxed fashion. Two-thirds of the patients were hospitalized

*Bruns K: Personal communication, 1984.

for the purpose of observation and were discharged within 48 hours after admission. Table 8-5 summarizes the etiologic factors associated with these 35 direct hospital transfers.

Patients may be discharged from an ambulatory surgery center and directly hospitalized for three general reasons. First, the patient may be hospitalized in order to provide continuity of medical care. For example, a diagnostic laparoscopy may reveal an ectopic pregnancy requiring that the patient be transferred for definitive surgery. In many freestanding and hospital-affiliated centers, the surgeon may elect to perform the definitive surgery while the patient is anesthetized within the ambulatory setting and transfer the patient to the hospital for inpatient postoperative care.

Second, the patient may require skilled observation or further treatment of a complication. The child who has a posterior pack inserted in order to control persistent adenoid bed bleeding would illustrate this group.

Third, the transfer may be effected for completely nonmedical reasons such as the peace of mind of the patient, family, or physician. Two of our patients expressed extreme fear and apprehension after their surgery. In spite of reassurances, the patient requested to be hospitalized.

The substantial difference in incidence of direct hospitalization between hospital-affiliated and freestanding ambulatory surgery centers remains an enigma. I personally suspect the underlying reason may simply be that the transfer from the hospital-affiliated ambulatory surgery service can be exercised with such ease that many transfers are initiated for less than compelling reasons. The freestanding ambulatory surgery centers appear to be

☐ **Table 8-5   Etiology of Direct Hospital Transfers among 32,001 Patients at Northwest Surgicare from April 17, 1974 to January 5, 1984**

Problem	No. of Patients
Hemorrhage	
Hemorrhage in OR, no active bleeding in PACU	4
Posterior pack inserted in OR	7
Hematoma formation	3
Active bleeding in PACU	5
Persistent nausea and vomiting	1
Bronchospasm in OR, possible aspiration	1
Delayed emergence from general anesthesia	2
Perforation of uterus	2
Perforation of bowel	1
Perforation of bladder	1
Severe vertigo (local anesthesia)	1
Febrile episode (acute mastitis)	1
Postresuscitation ventricular fibrillation	1
Unexplained symptoms in PACU	3
No medical problem, patient request	2
Total	35

dedicated to the concept that in the absence of serious problems, the patient will fare just as well at home. Where there is the potential for a serious problem, it is better to err on the conservative side and hospitalize the patient.

Preexisting Medical Problems and Complications

The medical literature is almost silent regarding evidence and information about the significance of preexisting medical problems in ambulatory surgery patients. I have seen statements in government, insurance, and quasimedical literature and have heard statements made at medical meetings that dogmatically single out one or more groups of patients with medical problems as unsuitable for ambulatory surgery. On many occasions, I have tried to seek out the medical or scientific basis for these statements. In each case, the originator of the statement could provide no evidence but only personal opinion.

In 1980, I initiated a comprehensive review of the relationship of patients with preexisting medical problems to complications in the ambulatory surgery setting.[24] The review covered all 17,968 patients who had received service at Northwest Surgicare from its opening on April 17, 1974 to December 31, 1979.

Each of these patients had been followed through their operating room, PACU, and 2-week postoperative phase of care in a prospective fashion, and all major complications (as defined in the first section of this chapter) had been recorded at the time of the occurrence. The presence of a preexisting medical problem was established by reviewing the screening medical history completed by each patient, the surgeon's history and physical examination, and the anesthesiologist's medical review. The complication data was then integrated with the presence or absence of preexisting medical problems.

The study revealed that 1984 patients in our surgical population of almost 18,000 patients had a preexisting systemic disease. Of this group, 560 patients reported hypertension, 373 patients asthma, 229 patients some form of heart disease, 83 patients chronic pulmonary disease, 107 patients diabetes mellitus, and 180 patients some form of central nervous system disease. The remaining patients had a history of preexisting renal, hepatic, gastrointestinal, endocrine, hematologic, allergic, and other disease states. Four hundred and sixty patients had more than one preexisting medical problem.

There was no statistical difference in the incidence of either major or minor complications between the patients who had no preexisting medical problems and the patients with medical problems (Table 8-6).

There were 23 major complications in the group of patients with preexisting medical problems, but there was a direct cause-and-effect relationship between the medical problem and the complication in only 3 cases. This means that 20 of the 23 major complications occurring in patients with medical problems would just as likely have occcurred in normal healthy patients. There was no instance of cardiovascular collapse (cardiac arrest or ventricular fibrillation).

The study also provided some valuable information about the problems of preoperative drug therapy in the ambulatory setting. Of the 1984 patients with preexisting medical problems, 918 were taking specific drugs for their disease at the time of surgery. Of the patients with a history of hypertension, 432 were

☐ **Table 8-6   Major Complications among 17,968 Patients at Northwest Surgicare**

History	No. of Patients	Major Complications
No preexisting disease	15,984	1.12%
Preexisting disease	1,984	1.16%

Fisher exact test, p> .05. No statistical difference between the two groups.

receiving one or more antihypertensive drugs; 97 of the 229 patients with heart disease were taking one or more drugs including beta blockers, cardiac glycosides, diuretics, antiarrhythmics, vasodilators, and anticoagulants; 47 of the 107 patients with diabetes mellitus were insulin dependent; and 226 of the 373 patients with a history of asthma were being treated at the time with asthma-ameliorating drugs.

Information about drug therapy is obtained in four stages:

1. The ambulatory surgery center requests every surgeon to call one of the anesthesiologists if there is any special medical problem, including any unusual medications.
2. One of our secretaries calls each patient the day before surgery and confirms the time of arrival, reiterates the preoperative instructions, and inquires about current medications.
3. Upon arrival at the center, the patient answers a screening medical questionnaire inquiring about current medications.
4. The anesthesiologist interviews every patient scheduled for general anesthesia or intravenous analgesia.

The questions associated with preoperative drug therapy usually fall into one of two categories: (1) should you stop the drug prior to surgery or continue administering it up to the time of surgery? and (2) do you need special laboratory tests, such as serum potassium level in patients taking diuretics?

Patients are instructed to bring their prescription drugs with them on the day of surgery. Patients taking cardiac glycosides, beta blockers, and other antiarrhythmics are told to take their usual medications with a small amount of water upon awakening on the morning of surgery.

There was no complication in this study that was related to any aspect of preoperative drug therapy. During the time span of this review, no serum potassium levels were determined in patients receiving diuretic drugs. Since 1982, the laboratory providing service to the ambulatory surgery center has obtained instrumentation that performs a potassium level within a few minutes. The anesthesiologists now request this test for all patients who take diuretic drugs on a long-term basis. We have identified several patients with low serum potassium levels, and these patients have been cancelled and referred back to their physicians.

There were only four major complications in the 642 ASA physical status 3 patients, and there was no evidence that the presence of serious disease in our population increased the incidence or gravity of complications.

Dawson and Reed reported in 1980 that their overall hospital transfer rate of 0.2% increased to 0.59% for patients over the age of 64 and increased to 1.41% for ASA physical status 3 patients.[12] The experiences of Northwest Surgicare do not corroborate their data. Of 629 patients in our population who were 60 years old or older, 262 had preexisting medical problems. This was the highest incidence, as anticipated, of any age group and included the largest numbers of physical status 3 patients. There were five major complications and one direct hospital transfer in this age group, which was the lowest incidence of any age group of our surgical population.

Since the completion of this study 4 years ago, we have continued to monitor the correlation of complications to patients with medical problems. There has been one episode of ventricular fibrillation (see Case Report No. 32), which occurred subsequent to the 1974–1980 study. Our experience with more than 32,000 patients continues to support the general findings of this study.

Wetchler* reviewed patients 60 years old and older receiving ambulatory surgical care at The Methodist Medical Center of Illinois in Peoria, Illinois, during the years 1981 to 1983.* There was a total of 2951 patients:

Ages	No. of Patients
60–69	1449
70–79	1126
80–89	335
90+	41

Of the total number of 2951 patients over the age of 60, 23 patients were admitted to the hospital on an inpatient basis. This was an admission rate of 0.8%, which is slightly higher than the incidence of direct hospital inpatient admission rate for all ambulatory patients. Twenty-three patients were admitted; 7 (of 2451 patients) had received only local anesthesia, whereas 16 (of 500 patients) had some form of anesthesia or care rendered by the anesthesia department. The reasons for admission to the hospital are summarized in Table 8-7.

There is a parallel between these results and Tinker's observations on the occurrence of myocardial infarction in surgical patients referred to earlier. It would appear that the surgical procedures performed in the ambulatory setting and the overall complexity of the anesthesia required do not usually impose serious degrees of stress and other critical problems. Perhaps one might say we are not pushing these patients to the physiologic "breaking point." In general, major complications associated with the ambulatory surgery setting are much more likely to be related to the specific type of surgery rather than the physical state of the patient or the presence of many preexisting medical problems.

It is essential to emphasize the importance of the screening process. There are many patients with medical problems who are not suitable candidates for surgery in the ambulatory setting. It may be the specific nature of the medical problem (e.g., a history of malignant hyperthermia or a coagulation disturbance), the severity of the medical problem (e.g., poorly controlled diabetes or poorly controlled angina pectoris), the need for hospital-based support systems (as in anemia or marginal renal function), or the need for special preoperative testing

*Wetchler BV: Personal communication, 1984.

☐ **Table 8-7   Etiology of Direct Hospital Admissions among Patients 60 Yr Old and Older at The Methodist Medical Center of Illinois, 1981 to 1983**

Problem	No. of Patients
No responsible person for postoperative care	4
More extensive surgery	6
Positive biopsy results	3
Hemorrhage	3
Reaction to IVP dye	1
PACU arrhythmias	2
Syncope and weakness	1
Nausea and vomiting	1
Chest pain	1
Hypertension in PACU	1
Total	23

or postoperative care. The decision to accept a patient should be based on a review of all factors, including the nature of the proposed surgery, the anesthesia required, preexisting medical problems and their degree of severity, the need for special preoperative or postoperative care, and the perceived ability of the patient to manage in the home environment.

Prevention of Complications

There are, of course, endless admonitions one might make about complications. A list of do's and don'ts could easily fill an entire book. It is very likely that much of the advice could be challenged (and in some instances for good scientific reasons). The subject of prevention should be addressed from three general points of view: a sound quality assurance program, the impaired physician, and the gathering of valid and useful complication data.

Quality Assurance

Every ambulatory surgery center is encouraged to have an ongoing, organized, peer-based quality assurance program. The basic mission of quality assurance is to achieve improvement. The fundamental process is to identify substantive problems and establish criteria for solving them. The methodology of accomplishing these goals may vary from one center to another, but the basic principles of quality assurance remain essentially the same.

During the past 7 years, Northwest Surgicare has conducted an ongoing, comprehensive quality assurance program. The process involves all aspects of patient care and service. We have made many enlightened discoveries and have identified many substantive problems. The quality assurance process has provided us with an opportunity to develop thoughtful and constructive solutions. It is always difficult to measure the "problem" you have prevented. Complications that do occur are relatively easy to measure. We can only speculate about the problem that has been prevented and the complication that never occurs.

The Impaired Physician

The issue of the impaired physician is a potential problem for every aspect of patient care. The doctor (or nurse) whose judgment and skills have been compromised by diminished mental or physical capacity due to age, disease, or drugs is a serious problem. I know of several catastrophes that have been associated with impaired physicians. It is a problem that demands prompt action on the part of the administration and governing body of any hospital-affiliated or freestanding health care facility. The worst possible response is to ignore the problem and hope it will go away.

Gathering Complication Data

The third area of preventive medical care in the ambulatory surgery setting is the need for valid, uniform, and honest complication information. We can learn to practice preventive medicine only when we know the areas of potential danger. Every ambulatory surgery center is urged to expend the time and energy necessary to collect and study its complications. This information will help both the medical and nursing staffs to more effectively avoid critical errors and provide safer patient care. Ignorance provides only a false sense of security.

References

1. Ahlgren EW: Pediatric outpatient anesthesia. Am J Dis Child 126:36, 1973
2. Ahlgren EW, Bennett EJ, Stephen CR: Outpatient pediatric anesthesiology. Anesth Analg 50:402, 1971
3. Backer CL, Tinker JH, Robertson DM et al: Myocardial reinfarction following local anesthesia for ophthalmic surgery. Anesth Analg 59:257, 1980
4. Brindle GF, Soliman MG: Anesthetic complications in surgical outpatients. Can Anaesth Soc J 22:613, 1975
5. Brown BR Jr: Outpatient Anesthesia. Philadelphia, FA Davis, 1978
6. Brownstein ML, Owsley JQ Jr: Augmentation mammoplasty: A survey of major complications. In Owsley JQ Jr, Peterson RA (eds): Symposium on Aesthetic Surgery of the Breast. St. Louis, CV Mosby, 1978
7. Caldamone AA, Rabinowitz R: Outpatient orchiopexy. J Urol 127:286, 1982
8. Caridis DT, Matheson NA: Outpatient surgery: A reassessment. Lancet 2:1387, 1964
9. Coakley CS, Levy M: Anesthesia for ambulatory surgery. J Ark Med Soc 68:101, 1971
10. Cohen DD, Dillon JB: Anesthesia for outpatient surgery. JAMA 196:1114, 1966
11. Davis JE: Ambulatory surgical care: Basic concept and review of 1000 patients. Surgery 73:483, 1973

12. Dawson B, Reed WA: Anaesthesia for adult surgical outpatients. Can Anaesth Soc J 27:409, 1980

13. Fahy A, Marshall M: Postanaesthetic morbidity in outpatients. Br J Anesth 41:433, 1969

14. Hughes G, Liston WA: Comparison between laparoscopic sterilization and tubal ligation. Br Med J 3:637, 1975

15. Hulka JF, Soderstrom RM, Corson SL et al: Complications Committee of the American Association of Gynecological Laparoscopists: First annual report. J Reprod Med 10:301, 1973

16. Jensen S, Wetchler BV: The obese patient: An acceptable candidate for outpatient anesthesia. J Am Assoc Nurs Anesth 50:369, 1982

17. Keats AS: Role of anesthesia in surgical mortality. In Orkin FK, Cooperman LH (eds): Complications in Anesthesiology, Philadelphia, JB Lippincott, 1983

18. Kornhall S, Olsson AM: Ambulatory inguinal hernia repair compared with short stay surgery. Am J Surg 132:32, 1976

19. Lieberman SL, Giacoia EB, Fedak M: Hospital-based outpatient surgery. NY State J Med 75:437, 1975

20. Mahar LJ, Steen PA, Tinker JH et al: Perioperative myocardial infarction in patients with coronary artery disease with and without aorta-coronary artery bypass grafts. J Thorac Cardiovasc Surg 26:533, 1978

21. Meridy HW: Criteria for selection of ambulatory surgical patients and guidelines for anesthetic management: A retrospective study of 1553 cases. Anesth Analg 61:921, 1982

22. Nabatoff RA, Aufses AH: Ambulatory surgery: Experience with 2000 patients. Mt Sinai J Med 46:354, 1979

23. Natof HE: Complications associated with ambulatory surgery. JAMA 244:1116, 1980

24. Natof HE: Ambulatory surgery: Patients with pre-existing medical problems. Ill Med J 166(2): 101, 1984

25. Olson MD: Legal issues. Same Day Surg 8:26, 1984

26. Othersen HB Jr, Clatworthy HW Jr: Outpatient herniorrhaphy for infants. Am J Dis Child 116:78, 1968

27. Patterson JF, Bechtoldt AA, Levin KJ: Ambulatory surgery in a university setting. JAMA 235:266, 1976

28. Peterson HB, DeStefano F, Rubin GL et al: Deaths attributable to tubal sterilization in the United States, 1977–1981. Am J Obstet Gynecol 146:131, 1983

29. Robinson JS, Thompson JM, Wood AW: Fire and explosion hazards in operating theatres: A reply and new evidence. Br J Anaesth 51:908, 1979

30. Tarhan S, Moffitt EA, Taylor WF et al: Myocardial infarction after general anesthesia. JAMA 239:2566, 1978

31. Thompson B, Wheeless RC: Outpatient sterilization by laparoscopy. Obstet Gynecol 38:912, 1971

32. Tinker JH: Assessment of peri-operative risk in patients with myocardial ischemia. 1982 American Society of Anesthesiologists Annual Refresher Course Lectures. Las Vegas, NV, October 22–26, 1982

33. Urbach GM, Edelist G: An evaluation of the anaesthetic techniques used in an outpatient unit. Can Anaesth Soc J 24:401, 1977

34. Wetchler BV: Problem free patient recovery and discharge. Third Annual Conference on Ambulatory Surgical Care, Williamsburg, VA, 1985

35. Williamson DE: The cataract patient: The postoperative regimen. In Brockhurst RJ, Boruchoff SA, Hutchinson BT et al (eds): Controversy in Ophthalmology. Philadelphia, WB Saunders, 1977

9

In the Real World

Harry C. Wong, M.D.

Cynthia Alexander Nkana, M.D.

The patients discussed in this chapter are actual cases that have been seen in ambulatory surgery facilities in the United States. The discussion and responses are not meant to establish standards of care, but rather to present individual methods of management. In certain case presentations the opinions of the discussant and the respondent may differ. These differences may involve anesthetic management or the question of whether the patient is an acceptable candidate for an ambulatory surgery procedure. We are not attempting to establish a correct approach; we are hoping our readers will consider these cases in the light of how they might apply to their own local setting. In addition, this chapter highlights some of the different approaches required by ambulatory surgery patients, many of which may necessitate changes in our practice patterns.

Of the ten most common surgical procedures performed in the United States in 1981, only three—cesarean sections, hysterectomies, and cholecystectomies—are not performed on an ambulatory basis. Oophorectomy, the tenth most common operation, is performed in some ambulatory surgery facilities. The other six—biopsies, dilatation and curettage (D&C), excision of skin lesions, tubal occlusions, cataract surgeries, and hernia repairs—represent 20% of all surgical procedures performed in 1981. In 1981 nearly 50% of all D&C patients were hospitalized for 3.3 days, 91% of all inguinal hernia patients for 4.7 days, and 95% of all cataract patients for 3.3 days. In the future, the majority of these procedures will be moved to ambulatory surgery care facilities.

The convenience and luxury of having patients hospitalized the night before surgery will become a rarity. Anesthesiologists must become more actively involved in preanesthetic preparation, evaluation, and communication with all surgical patients. This not only involves communication with conscious patients and their families, but also surgeons, internists, pediatricians, and other primary care physicians.

We must become more active physician consultants to enhance our role and our specialty in the real world.

■ CASE NO. 1

The patient is a 25 lb 2-year-old girl scheduled for a hernia repair. The mother relates a very interesting family history. Approximately 20 years ago the child's grandfather died while under anesthesia for a reportedly minor procedure. At that time his temperature increased to 104°F. There is also a history of the mother's father having a "near death" under anesthesia with a temperature rise during the anesthetic procedure. Neither parent has been exposed to an anesthetic agent. The child has no history of orthopedic problems and the hemoglobin, hematocrit, and creatinine phosphokinase (CPK) levels are within normal ranges.

Discussant

Frederic A. Berry, M.D.
Professor of Anesthesiology and Pediatrics, Childrens' Medical Center of the University of Virginia, Charlottesville, Virginia

This 2-year-old infant is at risk for inheriting a susceptibility to developing malignant hyperthermia (MH) under anesthesia. MH is usually inherited in an autosomal dominant fashion with variable expressivity. The degree of expression of the disease may vary from generation to generation. The family history is very significant in that both of the infant's grandfathers had a major anesthetic problem with a hyperthermic state that resulted in one death and one near miss. This infant must be treated as a patient who is susceptible to MH. Preoperative tests can be performed on the parents and the child. One screening test that is valuable when positive is the CPK. However, it has been reported that a significant number of patients with MH will have a normal CPK on all determinations. Another preoperative test is muscle biopsy. In general, a muscle biopsy is not recommended in young children because of the number of false-negative results. Muscle biopsy of the parents would be helpful if positive but would not remove the infant from the at-risk group if negative because of the number of false-negative tests. Unfortunately, this is available in only a few centers.

The major preoperative planning in all at-risk patients needs to be directed to three main requirements:

1. The presence of dantrolene in the surgical suite. The lyophilized powder need not be prepared but would need to be available along with adequate personnel to help prepare it.
2. Clinical laboratory support to do blood gases on an immediate basis, ideally within 3–5 minutes because every minute is important.
3. The capability of treating an episode of MH in the postanesthesia care unit (PACU) and the ability to monitor the patient carefully in the postoperative period for 12–24 hours.

Several cases have now been recorded in which there was an apparent recurrence of this syndrome after an initial successful treatment. Patients at risk cannot be treated as ambulatory surgery patients.

Dantrolene has revolutionized the treatment of MH. Before dantrolene, the mortality rate approached 50%. We are still in the early clinical development of guidelines for dantrolene use. Clearly, dantrolene should be immediately available (within 15–30 min) wherever anesthetics are administered. This includes ambulatory surgery clinics. This infant should be admitted to the hospital and receive 4 mg/kg of oral dantrolene in the 24-hour period before surgery. A neuroleptic technique should be used after either rectal methohexital, 30 mg/kg, or intravenous barbiturate induction. Intubation can be accomplished with a mixture of curare, 0.15 mg/kg, and pancuronium, 0.03 mg/kg. Pancuronium can cause a tachycardia and confuse the picture. The most common early signs of MH are tachycardia and tachypnea. The latter may be masked by muscle relaxants. Early findings are metabolic and respiratory acidosis. Usually a late finding is hyperthermia, but temperature monitoring should be carried out and vigorous cooling instituted if the temperature increases. Hyperthermia is an indication for more dantrolene. The occurrence of tachycardia in this child should be considered MH until proven otherwise. A blood gas should be obtained. If metabolic acidosis is present, i.e., a base deficit of greater than 4 to 5 mEq/L, then treatment should be started with intravenous dantrolene in a dose of 1 mg/kg. If the patient has not been pretreated, then the dose should be 3 mg/kg. The surgery should be terminated as soon as possible and an arterial line inserted to follow arterial blood gases. The keystone of therapy is dantrolene. The major side-effect of this drug is that it is a muscle relaxant and may cause weakness. The major complications of MH are myoglobinuria, renal failure, hyperkalemia, non-cardiogenic pulmonary edema, consumption coagulopathy, and neurologic residual.

In summary, infants and children at risk for MH need to be treated as inpatients, with dantrolene and blood gas values available immediately and the personnel and facilities readily available for intensive monitoring if the syndrome should develop.

Response

Dantrolene has revolutionized our treatment of the patient who is at risk for MH. The mortality has decreased from 70% to 75% in 1970 to 15% to 17% in 1984. With this patient's family history, she should be considered MH susceptible and should be pretreated with dantrolene. Can prophylactic dantrolene be safely administered on an outpatient basis? At our ambulatory center, pretreatment with dantrolene as an outpatient is acceptable. The overall reliability and understanding of the parents would be the major consideration with regard to this question. Wingard* uses outpatient dantrolene pretreatment, 2.2 mg/kg, in two equally divided dosages. The medication should be administered 8 hours before the scheduled procedure (1.1 mg/kg), with a second dose (1.1 mg/kg) 4 hours prior to the scheduled surgical procedure. It is important that dantrolene be given on an 8- and 4-hour preoperative schedule. There have been failures reported with dantrolene, usually related to inadequate blood levels.[1,2] Dantrolene is not without side-effects. Severe nausea

---

*Wingard, DW: Personal communication, 1984

and vomiting secondary to a gastritis, weakness, and dizziness have been reported.

Care of the MH susceptible patient requires careful planning and careful monitoring by the anesthesiologist. Postsurgical observation in a hospital setting is mandatory.

References

1. Dolan PF: Dantrolene and malignant hyperthermia. Anesthesiology 57:246, 1982
2. Fitzgibbons DC: Malignant hyperthermia following preoperative oral administration of dantrolene. Anesthesiology 54:73, 1981

■ CASE NO. 2

A 17-year-old male Down's syndrome patient who lives at home with protective parents needs extensive dental restorations and excision of impacted wisdom teeth. The patient has constant upper respiratory infections (URIs) and has had a heart murmur since birth. Examination reveals rhinorrhea, a clear chest, normal temperature, and a grade III/IV systolic murmur.

Discussant

Linda C. Stehling, M.D.
Professor of Anesthesiology and Pediatrics, University of New York Upstate Medical Center, Syracuse, New York

The first question to be answered is whether the patient is a suitable candidate for surgery. As the case is presented, insufficient data are available to make a decision about the safety of performing the procedure on an inpatient or outpatient basis. The benefits of decreased parental separation and lessened exposure to nosocomial infection would appear significant in this patient. The presence of a compensated intracardiac defect does not preclude ambulatory surgery. The nature of the cardiac defect as well as the patient's normal level of activity should be ascertained through consultation with the patient's cardiologist and parents. Was definitive cardiac surgery declined or unnecessary, or is the lesion inoperable? Laboratory studies may offer a clue to the severity of the cardiac disease: a high hematocrit is usually associated with cyanotic congenital heart disease. If the patient is taking digitalis or diuretics, a serum potassium should be determined.

If on the basis of the physical examination and consultation with the cardiologist it is deemed appropriate to perform the procedure on an ambulatory basis, the next concern is appropriate timing of the operation relative to the patient's chronic upper respiratory infection. Although patients with Down's syndrome, especially those who have congenital heart disease, are prone to recurrent URIs, every effort must be made to differentiate an infectious process from vasomotor or allergic rhinitis. The latter do not contraindicate anesthesia and surgery. However, elective operative procedures should be postponed for approximately 4 weeks following apparent resolution of a URI whenever possible. Although the vast majority of URIs are due to viral agents, they are often accompanied by secondary bacterial infection. In addition to laryngospasm, patients with URIs are prone to bronchospasm. Mechanical irritation from an oropharyngeal airway or endotracheal tube, excess secretions, infection, and edema contribute to a hyperreactive response of the bronchiolar musculature, precipitating a marked increase in airway resistance.[2] Both obstructive and restrictive lung disease can be demonstrated for as long as 6 weeks after uncomplicated influenza.[1,3] The history is extremely important in determining the etiology of the rhinorrhea. The parents should be questioned about any alteration in the patient's behavior suggestive of systemic illness. The anesthesiologist must explain, in simple terms, the importance of differentiating an infectious process from other causes of a "runny nose." He or she must also be alert to the fact that parents may deny symptoms if they know the procedure will be cancelled.

Once it is determined that the patient does not have a URI and there is no evidence of cardiac decompensation, the parents should be given instructions about preoperative medication. Presumably, antibiotic prophylaxis is indicated. The drug, dosage, and route of administration should be specified by the cardiologist and the medication administered at an appropriate time prior to induction of anesthesia. Cardioactive drugs are continued. If the patient is hyperactive, oral diazepam, administered approximately 1 half-hour before the patient leaves home, may be beneficial. The importance of supervising the patient closely to ensure that he is NPO must be stressed.

If the parents prefer, and if the anesthesiologist agrees, a parent may remain with the patient until anesthesia is induced. An intravenous induction with thiopental is preferable to an inhalation induction in a patient of this age. Following administration of succinylcholine, a nasotracheal tube is passed under direct vision. Halothane or another potent inhalation agent is suitable for maintenance of anesthesia. The patient should be observed in the PACU until he is awake and able to take liquids.

References

1. Collier AM, Pimmel RL, Hasselblad V et al: Spirometric changes in normal children with upper respiratory infections. Am Rev Respir Dis 117:47–53, 1978
2. Empey DW, Laitnen LA, Jacobs L et al: Mechanisms of bronchial hyperactivity in otherwise normal subjects with upper respiratory tract infections. Clin Res 23:346A, 1975
3. Johanson DG, Pierce AK, Sanford JP: Pulmonary function in uncomplicated influenza. Am Rev Respir Dis 100:141–146, 1969

Response

Dr. Stehling's discussion of the Down's syndrome patient can be applied to any handicapped patient. Her emphasis on thorough preoperative preparation, evaluation, and consultation with the cardiologist and pediatrician are paramount for safe ambulatory anesthesia care. The anesthesiologist's approach should be positive, and concerns should be shared with the parents in a straightforward manner. The commonly used threat to cancel surgery should never be used, because it often prompts parents and patients to deny signs or symptoms. Patients and parents interviewed in this fashion will be more likely to give honest answers. An important part of safe anesthesia care is the appropriate preparation of both the parents and the patient. Whenever possible, handicapped patients should have their procedures performed on an ambulatory surgery basis; they respond better when quickly returned to a familiar environment.

■ **CASE NO. 3**

The patient is a 35-year-old ASA physical status 1 female vocalist scheduled for a laparoscopic tubal ligation. One of her major concerns is the potential voice changes following endotracheal intubation. How would this patient be managed at the Surgicenter?

Discussant

Wallace A. Reed, M.D.

Medical Director, Surgicenter; Chairman of Board for AlternaCare, Phoenix, Arizona

The same screening procedures will be applied to this vocalist as to every other person presenting for an ambulatory surgery procedure. We must be able to answer "yes" to the question, "Is it safe for this person to undergo the procedure for which she is scheduled?"

Although different institutions vary their screening procedures, all are concerned with the state of the cardiac and respiratory systems. All provide as a minimum for a physical examination the use of one's eyes and a stethoscope. In addition to a pertinent history and physical examination, required laboratory tests are completed and results should be within acceptable limits.

Although this female vocalist will undoubtedly be able to open her mouth widely, she should also be able to demonstrate mobility of her cervical spine, since intubation may be necessary. Any tendency to obesity will influence our selection of an anesthetic technique.

Local anesthesia has been described by Pennfield and Wheeles; Bridenbaugh at the Virginia Mason Hospital subscribes to an epidural approach.[1,3,4] At the Surgicenter, in Phoenix, we prefer a light general anesthesia for laparoscopic tubal procedures. Following barbiturate induction anesthesia is maintained with nitrous oxide, oxygen, and enflurane. A succinylcholine drip (1 mg/ml) is used for any needed muscle relaxation. Fentanyl, 0.025 to 0.05 mg, is given intravenously during the induction. If the surgeon is one whose work we are familiar with, and if maintenance of the patient's airway does not present a problem, no endotracheal tube is used; if, on the other hand, the surgeon is relatively inexperienced or length of surgery unpredictable, or if the maintenance of an adequate airway is identified as a problem even before induction of anesthesia, endotracheal intubation will become part of the anesthetic technique.

During a 14-year period (1970–1984) we have performed more than 15,000 laparoscopic procedures. The average duration of the entire procedure is less than 30 minutes. We have found endotracheal intubation is unnecessary in 97.5% of our patients.

Our choice of anesthesia for this vocalist would be light general anesthesia without endotracheal intubation. It is important for the success of this technique that all of the patient's fears and forebodings be addressed during the preoperative interviews. In the case of this vocalist, a special effort should be made to explain the importance of airway management, emphasizing that endotracheal intubation might be necessary, and outlining the minimal risk to the cords if intubation is required. My policy is to use a lubricant such as KY rather than an analgesic ointment or jelly. I agree with Loeser and Stanley that lidocaine lubricants contain preservatives that are irritating to the trachea.[2]

I do not recommend this technique for anesthesiologists who have not learned to manage an airway without using an endotracheal tube. For those who are unfamiliar with a mask technique, it is a very easy matter to inflate the patient's stomach and provide a tempting target for the Verres needle.

At our institution the anesthesiologists are thoroughly familiar with the mask technique. They can maintain an excellent airway and a good exchange without inflating the patient's stomach. Based on our series of 15,000 cases without a serious upper airway problem, this patient would have every reason to expect an uneventful anesthetic course for her laparoscopic tubal surgery under light general anesthesia without endotracheal intubation.

References

1. Bridenbaugh LD: Manpower shortage—fact or fancy? South Med J 64:1221–1226, 1971
2. Loeser EA, Stanley TH, Jordon W et al: Postoperative sore throat: Influence of tracheal tubes lubrication versus cuff design. Can Anaesth Soc J 27:156–158, 1980
3. Penfield AJ: Laparoscopic sterilization under local anesthesia. Am J Obstet Gynecol 119:733–736, 1974
4. Wheeless CR Jr: Outpatient laparoscope sterilization under local anesthesia. Obstet Gynecol 39:767–770, 1972

Response

In contrast to the experience of Reed, 97% of the approximately 7000 patients (1977–1984) at our ambulatory surgery unit that have been scheduled for laparoscopic procedures have been intubated.

Factors influencing the decision to intubate the patient are

1. Increased intra-abdominal pressure from CO_2 insufflation
2. Relaxed gastroesophageal junction
3. Obtunded laryngeal reflexes from the use of muscle relaxants
4. Lithotomy Trendelenburg position
5. The potential for silent regurgitation

This patient is understandably concerned about possible voice changes associated with her anesthetic. She should be reassured in the preoperative anesthesia visit that the risk of permanent vocal cord damage with intubation is minimal. The first obligation to the patient is safe intraoperative management of the airway. If the endotracheal tube better protects the patient against aspiration or hypoventilation during the surgical procedure it should be used without hesitation. Statistics from the Centers for Disease Control (1977–1981) reported six deaths attributed to hypoventilation during laparoscopic tubal sterilization.[1]

At the Methodist Ambulatory Surgery Center this patient's anesthetic was satisfactorily managed with a spinal. The patient and anesthesiologist reviewed all alternatives several weeks before surgery. Having had a prior spinal for an oophorectomy, the patient opted for another spinal anesthetic. On the morning of surgery she was very relaxed and approached the procedure with a sense of calm confidence and left the facility following surgery with a sense of complete satisfaction.

Reference

1. Centers for Disease Control: Annual summary 1981: Reported morbidity and mortality in the United States. MMWR 30(54):126, 1982

■ CASE NO. 4

A 24-year-old woman, ASA physical status 1, was admitted to the ambulatory surgery unit for a McDonald's cerclage to be performed under epidural anesthesia. When the epidural block was performed, the anesthesiologist punctured the dura. The 17-gauge Tuohy needle was withdrawn and a satisfactory epidural was performed one interspace higher. What are the advantages and disadvantages of various anesthetic choices for a McDonald's cerclage procedure?

Discussant

Michael F. Mulroy, M.D.
Staff Anesthesiologist, Mason Clinic, Seattle, Washington

The anesthetic challenge "to do no harm" is magnified in the pregnant patient. In addition to the ordinary risk of anesthesia, three potential hazards are added by the presence of the fetus: the possibility of teratogenicity, the risk of hypoxic fetal injury, and the chance of precipitating premature labor. Despite these potential hazards, a review of anesthetic experience by Shnider[1] has shown that anesthesia can be performed with reasonable safety in the pregnant patient and is often unavoidable, as in the case of this patient.

In considering the risk, there are no data that substantiate actual teratogenic damage from anesthetic agents in humans, although most have been implicated in laboratory animal studies. In this regard, it seems best to use the fewest different drugs and the smallest quantity of each that are possible. Likewise, fetal damage was not directly seen in Shnider's series, though again, it seems prudent to avoid hypoxia, hypotension, or any intervention such as hyperventilation (which might decrease uterine blood flow and fetal oxygen delivery). Premature labor was the most common complication of surgery, but seems more related to the surgical procedure (pelvic or vaginal) than to the anesthetic technique employed. The cerclage operation carried the highest risk, and the highest incidence of premature labor. For this reason, some obstetricians are reluctant to perform this procedure on an ambulatory surgery basis.

Guidelines for choosing a specific anesthetic are sparse. It seems prudent to minimize the quantity of drug exposure, yet to provide adequate anesthesia to reduce the chance of uterine stimulation. General endotracheal anesthesia can be employed to meet these ends, and inhalation agents such as halothane may even be beneficial in reducing uterine tone and reactivity. Care must be taken, however, to preserve maternal blood flow (left lateral tilt), to avoid hypoxia in the face of a diminished functional residual capacity, and to reduce the chance of pulmonary aspiration. This latter consideration would favor the use of preoperative antacids and rapid-sequence endotracheal intubation for anesthesia administered after the beginning of the second trimester.

Regional anesthesia can forestall some of these problems. Lumbar epidural or subarachnoid anesthesia can produce adequate anesthesia. It may provide more rapid recovery in the ambulatory surgery patient. Since epidural anesthesia involves approximately ten times the total dose of local anesthetic agent as a spinal, we have tended to employ the hyperbaric lidocaine spinal anesthetic technique for the cerclage operation. The incidence of headache with a 26-g needle puncture of the dura is less than 0.5%, and 50 mg of hyperbaric lidocaine will provide adequate anesthesia without serious hypotension. The risk of unanticipated hypotension can be further minimized by infusion of Ringer's lactate prior to the performance of the block, as well as by performing the subarachnoid injection with the head of the table slightly elevated and then relying on changes in table position to move the hyperbaric solution cephalad to the appropriate level. Usually no sedation other than the personal attention of the anesthesiologist is required, although occasionally a small dose of intravenous short-acting narcotic is given.

Reference

1. Shnider SM: Anesthesia for Obstetrics. Baltimore, Williams & Wilkins, 1979

Response

General and regional anesthesia are appropriate for the pregnant patient. The majority of cerclage procedures done at the Methodist Ambulatory Surgery Center are performed under either spinal or epidural anesthesia. In this patient we have a dural puncture performed with a 17-gauge Tuohy needle. Harris and Harmel demonstrated that a dural puncture with an 18-gauge or larger needle had an overall incidence of postdural puncture headache of approximately 24%.[1] A 16-gauge needle increases the incidence to approximately 80%. There is no advantage to a prophylactic epidural saline injection or blood patch. At Brigham and Women's Hospital, headache developed in 33% of the patients following dural puncture with a 17-gauge needle. Only 6.7% did not respond to conservative therapy and required an epidural blood patch. Treatment therefore starts with "watchful waiting."

If a headache develops in this patient we would use appropriate conservative therapy. Recent data suggest that placing the patient in a prone position for several hours immediately following puncture may increase pressure in the epidural space, thus decreasing the leakage of cerebrospinal fluid (CSF).[2] The patient should limit activities such as bending or lifting; take minor analgesics as needed; and maintain an adequate fluid intake. If a headache develops that does not respond to conservative therapy, depending on its severity, an epidural blood patch can be performed on an outpatient basis. Once an epidural blood patch is performed the patient should continue limiting activity for 48 hours.

References

1. Harris LM, Harmel MH: The comparative incidence of postlumbar puncture headache following spinal anesthesia administered through 20 and 24 gauge needles. Anesthesiology 14:390, 1953
2. Shnider SM: Anesthesia for Obstetrics. Baltimore, Williams & Wilkins, 1979

■ CASE NO. 5

A nonpremature male infant, 10 months of age, with a hemoglobin of 7 g is scheduled for a myringotomy and ear tube insertion. Would you proceed with the anesthesia and surgery for this patient? Would your criteria be different if the patient were scheduled for an inguinal hernia repair?

Discussant
John S. Hattox, M.D.
Medical Director, Pomerado Outpatient Surgical Center, Polway, California

In considering a 10-month-old term infant with a hemoglobin of 7 g as a candidate for myringotomy and ear tube insertion one should recall that the mean hemoglobin in this age population is between 11 g and 12 g. Therefore, the degree of hemoglobin reduction is less striking if one accepts a hemoglobin of 9 or above as normal. In the absence of a history of blood loss, such as severe nose bleeding, this anemia is most likely a nutritional one. Other rare anemias to be considered are those associated with sickle-cell anemia and thalassemia.

The risk of proceeding with anesthesia in this patient would seem to be only minimally increased, if at all, provided cardiac output is not unduly depressed. If only minimal levels of anesthesia are achieved for this short procedure, any one of the three commonly used vapors—halothane, enflurane, or isoflurane—should be satisfactory, isoflurane appearing to be the agent that would least affect the various cardiac parameters. An intravenous line should be established in order to have the capability of immediate management of laryngospasm with subsequent hypoxia.

Monitoring of any anesthetized patient should consist of some form of constant evaluation of cardiac activity. The precordial stethoscope and electrocardiogram (ECG) would fulfill these requirements.

Pediatric surgeons feel strongly that hernias in infants should be repaired as soon as it is feasible to do so. It should be emphasized, however, in the strongest possible terms that a total clinical evaluation of the infant must be made prior to making a decision about proceeding.

It is of interest to note that at least three large, nationally recognized ambulatory surgery centers have discontinued routine preoperative laboratory determinations of hemoglobin unless it is indicated.

Response

The question to proceed with this short procedure should depend primarily on the guidelines that have been adopted by the individual ambulatory surgery unit. Most ambulatory units have a listing of minimum acceptable laboratory requirements. These requirements should not be neglected or abandoned because of peer pressure and certainly not without thorough patient evaluation and documentation. Ideally, childhood anemia should be evaluated by the pediatrician prior to scheduling an elective procedure. However, the complete blood count (CBC) required in an ambulatory surgery center may be the only screen that an infant would have after birth. A gradual drop in the hemoglobin normally occurs approximately 10 to 12 weeks after birth. This physiologic anemia in which the hemoglobin can decrease to 10 g to 12 g is usually corrected by 8 months of age.[1]

At our facility we would postpone this patient's procedure until the anemia was appropriately investigated. Although 90+% of anemias at this age are nutritional, one must still rule out other causes (thalassemia, sickle cell, spherocytosis). If nutrition is deemed the cause, a change in diet plus supplemental iron can raise the hemoglobin to an acceptable level in as short a time as 2 to 3 weeks. A postponement of 1 month in a child of this age should not pose a major problem for either the patient or the otolaryngologist.

Reference

1. Nathan DG, Oski FA: Hematology of Infancy and Childhood. Philadelphia, WB Saunders, 1981

■ CASE NO. 6

A 4-month-old infant is scheduled in your ambulatory surgery unit for an inguinal hernia repair. The child weighs only 10 lb, 2 oz. The history from the mother reveals the child was 6 weeks premature and spent 3 weeks in the newborn intensive care unit and suffered periodic apnea. The child has continued with an apnea monitor at home.

Discussant

David J. Steward, M.B., F.R.C.P.(C)
Anaesthetist-in-Chief, British Columbia Children's Hospital, Vancouver, British Columbia, Canada; Formerly, Anaesthetist-in-Chief, The Hospital for Sick Children, Toronto, Ontario, Canada

It has become recognized that infants who were born prematurely are at increased risk of potentially serious complications in the perioperative period, even when the surgical procedure is relatively minor.[1,3,5] The most common complication is apnea, which may occur as late as 18 hours after the surgical procedure. It may appear in infants who have never demonstrated apnea previously[5] or who have exhibited no episodes of apnea for several weeks preoperatively. Studies suggest that the infants most at risk are those who are still less than 3000 g body weight, less than 3 months' postnatal age,[5] or less than 41 weeks' postconceptual age (conceptual age equals gestational plus postnatal age).[3] The preterm infant is also at increased risk of suffering the sudden infant death syndrome (SIDS), and this condition may occur up to the postnatal age of 12 months.[4] These facts are alarming to the anesthesiologist, and must demand that he or she prepare an appropriate plan of management for these patients.

Should the preterm infant who is still at risk of these complications be operated on for inguinal hernia in the ambulatory surgery unit? Most authorities would suggest not, certainly if the patient is still less than 45 weeks' postconceptual age. Such infants should rather be admitted to a hospital that has a neonatal service and has facilities to provide for close postoperative monitoring and any necessary respiratory care.[2]

The case for discussion is a child of 4 months' postnatal age and 50 weeks' postconceptual age. The child now weighs 4.5 kg and has been cared for by the mother, using an apnea monitor in the home. Is this infant, then, a suitable patient for ambulatory surgery? When all factors are considered, this child should still preferably be admitted to a hospital with a pediatric unit and facilities to monitor him closely throughout the perioperative period. The child with a history of repeated apnea that has demanded the use of an apnea monitor in the home must be considered at increased risk of postoperative apnea. This child is still underweight for his age, and still is at an age when SIDS is a potential danger. In-home apnea monitoring is now widely practiced, but the effectiveness of such programs is as yet unproven.

Ambulatory surgery for infants and children has proven to be a real advance in surgical therapy. However, it is essential that the few infants who might be at an uncertain but possibly increased risk of serious perioperative complications should be identified. We can then ensure that they be provided with the additional monitoring and treatment facilities of the hospital environment for the postoperative period. We will also avoid the possibility that an ambulatory surgery program may suffer an unnecessary setback if a patient suffers serious postoperative complications, which might be considered to have been predictable.

References

1. Gregory GA: Outpatient Anesthesia. In Miller RD (ed): Anesthesia, p 1329. New York, Churchill Livingstone, 1981
2. Gregory GA, Steward DJ: Life-threatening perioperative apnea in the ex-"premie". Anesthesiology 59:495–498, 1983
3. Liu LMP, Coté CJ, Goudsouzian NG et al: Life-threatening apnea in infants recovering from anesthesia. Anesthesiology 57:506–510, 1983
4. Naeye RL: Origins of the sudden infant death syndrome. In Tilden JT, Roeder LM, Steinschneider A (eds.): Sudden Infant Death Syndrome, pp 77–83. New York, Academic Press, 1983
5. Steward DJ: Preterm infants are more prone to complications following minor surgery than are term infants. Anesthesiology 56:304–306, 1982

Response

Anesthesiologists should take careful note of Dr. Steward's case discussion and become familiar with the references he has listed. It is extremely important to know the expremature infant's birth weight, gestational term, and post-conceptual age before providing anesthesia. Additional information should be obtained before any decision is reached: a current history of apnea, potential aspiration with feeding, or chronic lung infections. Although postconceptual age provides a point of reference, we had one patient scheduled in our ambulatory surgery facility who at 14 months was still on an apnea monitor at home. This patient was monitored in a hospital setting postsurgery.

Ambulatory surgery is uniquely suited for pediatric surgery. Only by careful screening will we limit complications.

■ CASE NO. 7

A 50-year-old woman is scheduled for a facelift and augmentation mammoplasty by her plastic surgeon. The surgeon estimates 6 hours for the surgical procedure. Would you handle this case in an ambulatory surgery unit?

Discussant

Herbert E. Natof, M.D.
Medical Director, Northwest Surgicare, Medical Care International, Arlington Heights, Illinois

The first step in evaluating this case is to focus on some practical considerations. We will assume that this patient is in good general health, is emotionally stable, and has no serious medical problems that would contraindicate elective cosmetic surgery.

Each of the proposed procedures has a well-established incidence of bleeding with hematoma formation. Hemorrhage in bilateral augmentation mammoplasty ranges from 2% to over 10%.[1,2,3,4] The combination of operative procedures would increase the probable chance of hemorrhage to an even higher range of occurrence. The bleeding associated with both mammoplasty and facelift surgery is most likely to occur during the first 72 hours postoperatively.

It would be very difficult to perform both of these procedures using only local anesthesia. In addition to the discomfort associated with multiple injections of local anesthesia, 6 hours is a very long time for a patient to lie on an operating table! I am a staunch believer in the many advantages of an intravenous analgesic technique, but 6 hours of analgesia is pushing the technique beyond its limits in most patients.

If this patient receives a general anesthetic, she will require intubation. In my experience, there is a high correlation between many minor complications and the length of procedure. All of our statistics show that the incidence of nausea, vomiting, slow emergence, generalized weakness, and sore throat increases when the operative procedure exceeds approximately 2 hours of general anesthesia.

In view of all these factors, I would not recommend discharging this patient to a home environment unless there was appropriate nursing care available for the first 48 to 72 hours.

There are centers that have arrangements with nursing homes or hospitals for providing skilled postoperative observation and care for patients such as this one. My concerns would be greatly lessened if the patient was transferred directly to such a facility. In summary, I would not accept this surgical case in our ambulatory surgical center. My primary area of concern would be the post-operative phase of care.

I am reluctant to recommend that each center establish maximum time limits for surgical procedures. Every rule provides another constriction and another potential medicolegal pitfall. I strongly encourage that each patient and surgical procedure be evaluated on an individual basis.

References

1. Brownstein ML, Owsley JQ Jr: Augmentation mammoplasty: A survey of major complications. In Owsley JQ Jr, Peterson RA (eds): Symposium on Aesthetic Surgery of the Breast. St Louis, CV Mosby Company, 1978
2. Cronin TD, Persoff MM, Upton J: Augmentation mammoplasty: Complications and etiology. In Owsley JQ Jr, Peterson RA (eds): Symposium on Aesthetic Surgery of the Breast. St Louis, CV Mosby Company, 1978
3. Natof HE: Complications associated with ambulatory surgery. JAMA 244:1116, 1980
4. Williams JE: Experiences with a large series of silastic breast implants. Plast Reconstr Surg 49:253, 1972

Response

Each procedure and each patient must be considered on an individual basis. Even in a patient who is in general good health, ASA physical status 1 or 2, emotionally stable, and willing and able to follow instructions, and who has a responsible person available to stay with her during the first 24 hours, there are times when the extent of the surgical procedure itself may preclude its being performed on an ambulatory surgery basis. Augmentation mammoplasties and facelifts do have the risk of bleeding in the perioperative period. Blood loss from 2% to 10% has been reported, usually secondary to hematoma formation.[2]

Local anesthetics for augmentation mammoplasties and facelifts have been used successfully for many years. However, the surgeon must be knowledgeable about the local anesthetic agent used and its acceptable total dosage. At the 1984 International Anesthesia Research Society meeting, a technique was presented that used local anesthesia, lidocaine, 0.26%, with 1:1,666,666 epinephrine and supplemental sedation with secobarbital, diazepam, oxymorphone, and ketamine.[1] The total dose of lidocaine used for infiltration was approximately 1.5 to 2.5 times the recommended dose. There is little excuse for administration of significant toxic levels of local anesthetic to any patient given by the surgeon or the anesthesiologist.

Dr. Natof's approach to the "real world case" is a very sound approach. ASA physical status 1 and 2 patients should be capable of having this procedure under general anesthesia with a minimum of complications. However, because of the length of the case and the potential associated problems in the perioperative period, a prudent approach would include an overnight hospital stay following surgery.

References

1. Glauber DT, Buffington CW, Hornbein TF: High dose lidocaine, ultra dilute epinephrine and intravenous sedation for major plastic surgery (abstr). Anesth Analg 63:A219, 1984
2. Grabb WC, Smith JW: Plastic Surgery, 3rd ed. Boston, Little, Brown & Company, 1979

■ CASE NO. 8

A 63-year-old man underwent a two-vessel coronary artery bypass graft 9 years ago. Since that time he has done extremely well and denies any angina or shortness of breath. He is on no antihypertensive or cardiac medications at the present time. He had a left inguinal herniorrhaphy 3 years ago in an ambulatory surgery facility with subsequent admission to the intensive care unit of the hospital because of angina. He denies any history of angina other than after his last hernia repair. At that time, a cardiologist felt the patient had a "vagal reaction with bradycardia, hypertension and angina secondary to his response to pain." He is now scheduled for a right inguinal hernia repair and has voiced concerns for his well-being in the immediate postoperative period.

Discussant

Bernard V. Wetchler, M.D.
Director, Department of Anesthesiology, Medical Director, Ambulatory Surgery Center, The Methodist Medical Center of Illinois; Clinical Professor of Anesthesia, University of Illinois College of Medicine at Peoria, Peoria, Illinois

There appears to be no medical contraindication to this man having his hernia repaired. Whether he has it repaired as an inpatient or an ambulatory surgery patient may well depend on the amount of advance preparation the anesthesiologist is willing to undertake.

Before meeting with the patient, question his cardiologist as follows: Is his cardiovascular status stable? Is he taking any cardiac medications? (Patients don't always remember or at times conveniently forget.) Do you foresee any problem with our proceeding with surgery and anesthesia? Do you concur with my feeling that this patient can be managed in an ambulatory surgery facility?

From the surgeon, you need the answers to these questions: Is this the usual 30- to 40-minute procedure? Do you foresee any technical problems? Can you do the procedure with local anesthesia? Depending on the final choice of anesthesia, will you infiltrate the ilioinguinal and iliohypogastric nerves with local anesthesia at the conclusion of the procedure? Are you comfortable with this patient being managed in ambulatory surgery?

Once all the physicians are in agreement and a game plan is established, then the anesthesiologist should initiate an interview with the patient at least 1 week prior to the scheduled day of surgery. The responsible person who is to take care of him at home should also be present. Is the responsible person capable of managing the patient postoperatively? This may influence the final decision as to where the procedure is performed. Everyone must understand that if there is any recurrence of the patient's anginal pain postoperatively he would be admitted into the hospital for observation.

Let the patient know you are concerned and that you want to respond to his concerns. He will need reassurance that there is no greater risk associated with having the procedure performed as an ambulatory patient than with having it done as an inpatient. It is important that the patient be made aware of the types of anesthesia available and the reasons why one may be preferable to another. He should understand that anesthesia management would be the same whether his procedure was done on an inpatient or ambulatory basis.

My choices of anesthesia would be local, major regional (epidural or spinal), and last, an intravenous induction inhalation technique. He should know that if the procedure is done with local or major regional anesthesia, he will have better control over his environment. If pain comes on in the early postoperative period, he will be alert enough to let our nursing staff know; they have pain medication available to treat it quickly and appropriately. An informed patient is a more cooperative patient.

Pain can be controlled in the postoperative period in the following ways:

1. Use of short-acting narcotic analgesics intraoperatively
2. Use of short-acting narcotic analgesics intravenously at the first sign of pain in the postanesthesia care unit
3. Local infiltration of the ilioinguinal and the iliohypogastric nerves intraoperatively with 0.25% bupivacaine
4. Use of a transcutaneous nerve stimulator for the first 48 hours postsurgery
5. Cryoanalgesia (freezing) of the ilioinguinal nerve during inguinal herniorrhaphy (this provides several days of postoperative analgesia)[1]
6. Oral postoperative narcotic analgesics for home use

The pain control options you have available should be discussed with the patient.

This discussion cannot take place on the morning of surgery. The patient has to realize well in advance of surgery that his anesthesiologist is concerned about his past problem and is interested in providing him with an operative and postoperative course that is both safe and as pain free as possible.

After being fully informed, the patient (and the responsible person) must show a willingness to have the procedure performed on an ambulatory surgery basis. If at this time he is unwilling to have it done as an outpatient, then no further convincing should be attempted and arrangements should be made to have the procedure performed on an inpatient basis. I feel this patient could be safely managed as an ambulatory surgery patient.

Reference

1. Wood GJ, Lloyd JW, Bullingham RES et al: Postoperative analgesia for day-case herniorrhaphy patients: A comparison of cryoanalgesia, paravertebral blockade and oral analgesia. Anaesthesia 36:603, 1981

Response

The key to this patient's management involves thorough and open communication with the patient, responsible person, cardiologist, and surgeon. Remembrances and anxiety over a past painful experience is not the ideal situation for any patient and certainly not one with a history of ischemic heart disease. Options for a "safe" and "comfortable" perioperative course should be thoroughly explained to the patient.

There is a group of ambulatory surgery patients that need more than a preanesthesia visit on the morning of surgery. This could be because of ongoing medical problems, medications being taken, or patient concerns. When necessary, the anesthesiologist must be available to meet with patients in advance of their procedure. Problems can be handled at that time, allowing the patient to arrive better prepared on the day of surgery.

■ CASE NO. 9

A 42-year-old woman is scheduled for an incisional ventral hernia repair. The hernia developed following a hysterectomy that was done approximately 1 year ago. The patient revealed she has been taking furosemide regularly for fluid retention and has noted fatigue, occasional lightheadedness, and palpitations. A stat potassium level was 2.9 mEq/L.

Discussant

K.C. Wong, M.D., Ph.D.
Professor of Anesthesiology and Pharmacology, Chairman, Department of Anesthesiology, University of Utah School of Medicine, Salt Lake City, Utah

The magnitude of hypokalemia presenting in this patient is not unusual for someone who has been taking furosemide regularly without oral potassium supplementation. Since this is a chronic loss of body potassium, it can be assumed that the intracellular loss of potassium is proportional to the extracellular loss. The patient is not having persistent cardiac arrhythmias. Nevertheless, the ability of her myocardium to resist the development of arrhythmias could be reduced.

Although it has been traditionally taught that elective surgery should not be performed in patients whose serum potassium is below 3 mEq/L or in digitalized patients whose serum potassium is below 3.5 mEq/L, there are no hard data to substantiate these recommendations. There are only anecdotal case reports to suggest that these recommendations are intuitively "reasonable." Having been interested in this clinical problem for many years, I have not been able to substantiate in animal models that hypokalemia increases the incidence of arrhythmias during anesthesia.[3] However, asphyxia[2] or epinephrine overdose[3] has produced significant cardiovascular compromise in the hypokalemic dog. I am convinced that hypokalemia can contribute to cardiovascular difficulties in patients who are subjected to severe physiologic trespasses, for example, hypoxia, hypotension, surgical manipulation that can inhibit cardiopulmonary function.

The rate of potassium loss appears to be more important; hypokalemia occurring over hours or days may be more ominous than hypokalemia occurring over weeks or months. Although no hard data are available, it is also reasonable to conclude that hypokalemia can also contribute to cardiovascular instability in the presence of cardiovascular disease and cardiovascular depressant drugs. Optimal preparation of a hypokalemic patient is *not* based on hypokalemia alone but on all of the above factors.

Finally, should the hypokalemic patient receive intravenous potassium to replace lost body potassium? Replacement of cellular potassium loss cannot be accomplished overnight. Potassium administration is not innocuous. As many as 1 in 200 patients receiving potassium may suffer a morbid or fatal episode of hyperkalemia.[1]

With the above discussion in mind, I would use a routine general anesthesia that will allow quick recovery and would pay special attention to maintaining normal acid-base balance intraoperatively. When the environment is conducive to a regional anesthetic, a spinal or epidural could be done with equal safety. At the time of discharge I would encourage the patient to eat more bananas!

References

1. Burke GR, Gulyassy PF: Surgery in patients with renal disease and related electrolyte disorders. Med Clin North Am 63:1191, 1979
2. Wong KC, Port JD, Steffins J: Cardiovascular responses to asphyxial challenge in chronically hypokalemic dogs. Anesth Analg 62:991, 1983
3. Wong KC, Tseng KC, Puerto BA et al: Chronic hypokalemia on epinephrine induced dysrthymias during halothane, enflurane, or methoxyflurane with nitrous oxide anesthesia in dogs. Anaesth Sinica 21:139, 1983

Response

The problem of hypokalemia in a patient scheduled for elective surgery is faced by anesthesiologists on a daily basis. Personal experience indicates that hypokalemia with a potassium level of 3.0 mEq/L in nondigitalized patients has produced cardiac arrhythmias. Though Dr. K.C. Wong has been able to produce arrhythmias in hypokalemia animal models only with hypoxia or epinephrine challenge, the very apprehensive hypokalemic patient may have sufficient circulating epinephrine to develop arrhythmias with the induction of anesthesia.

The most important issue in this case is the need for each ambulatory surgery facility to establish its own acceptable guidelines for safe patient care and then *live by these guidelines.* We must remain ever cognizant of the medicolegal cloud that hangs over our practices and feel comfortable defending in a court of law actions that are taken in providing patient care.

Ambulatory surgery is elective, and at our facility a minimum limit for serum potassium is 3 mEq/L in a nondigitalized patient. This patient's surgery would be cancelled and deferred to a later date after the patient receives potassium supplementation (we also like bananas). A repeat serum potassium would also be drawn to assess the effectiveness of therapy.

■ CASE NO. 10

A 22-month-old infant presents to the ambulatory surgery unit for bilateral myringotomy and tube insertion. He has an axillary temperature of 37.9°C (100.2°F), and the mother states that he has had a runny nose and cough over the last 2 days. There has been no history of fever or chills at home, and the mother states that his cough has not awakened him at night and his cough has improved over the last 24 hours. After auscultation of the child's chest, which reveals no rhonchi or wheezes, and examination of the mouth, which demonstrates minimal pharyngeal erythema, the anesthesiologist must decide whether to pursue the surgical procedure.

Discussant

Eugene K. Betts, M.D.
Director of Operating Room Services, Senior Anesthesiologist, The Childrens' Hospital of Philadelphia; Assistant Professor of Anesthesiology, University of Pennsylvania, Philadelphia, Pennsylvania

There are a number of factors that should be taken into consideration in deciding whether or not to anesthetize a child who presents for a short surgical procedure but has a fever and a history of a cough. Among these factors are the magnitude of the temperature elevation, the presence or absence of a URI, whether the symptoms are increasing or diminishing, and the interval since the child last had a URI.

The range of normal axillary and rectal temperatures is 36.5°C to 37.5°C (97.7°F–99.5°F).[1] Mild dehydration, agitation, crying, and teething may induce temperature elevations of as much as 0.5°C (0.9°F). Temperatures above 38°C (100.4°F) are abnormal and usually indicate the presence of an infectious process.

Each year American children between the ages of 1 and 5 years can be expected to suffer from two to four episodes of viral nasopharyngitis (URIs). Secondary bacterial infections frequently prolong the disease beyond its usual 4-day course.[6] Children with any two of the following have a URI:

1. Mild sore or scratchy throat
2. Mild malaise
3. Sneezing
4. Rhinorrhea
5. Congestion or "stuffiness" of the head
6. Nonproductive cough
7. Mild fever

Combinations 1 and 2, 3 and 4, and 5 and 6 require an additional symptom to make the diagnosis of URI.[8] The patient's mother is frequently a good judge of the presence or absence of a URI in her child. However, the signs and symptoms of a URI may be the prodromata of an exanthem or of Reye's syndrome.

In a retrospective study at the C.S. Mott Children's Hospital in Ann Arbor, Michigan, Tait et al reported the following data:[7]

Group	No. of Patients	Patients Symptomatic for URI on Day of Anesthesia	Asymptomatic Patients Who Had URI Within Two Weeks Preceding Anesthesia	Respiratory Complications (%)	Intubated Patients Who Developed Respiratory Complications (%)
I	3350	0	0	1.60	66
II	122	122	0	1.64	100
III	113	0	113	5.31	83

Perioperative complications occurred in 1.65% of the 3585 patients. Included were laryngospasm (1.26%), bronchospasm (0.17%), respiratory stridor (0.08%), and breath holding (0.14%). The total incidence of respiratory complications was significantly different ($p < 0.05$) only between groups I and III. Children less than 9 years old had a higher incidence of complications and the incidence in males was twice that in females.

Earlier, McGill et al reported an experience similar to Tait's group III: over a 13-month period intraoperative anesthetic complications occurred in 11 asymptomatic patients who had a history of a URI during the 4 weeks preceding an anesthetic.[5] All of the children had been intubated. However, Koka et al reported a lack of correlation between a history, or even the presence, of a URI, and the development of postintubation laryngeal edema (croup) in 7875 children less than 17 years old. Nor did they find a correlation between the incidence of postintubation croup and the patient's sex.[4]

McGill and Tait both reported an increased incidence of perianesthetic complications in patients who had experienced a URI less than 2 to 4 weeks earlier.[5,7] At the time of an uncomplicated URI in children 2.5 to 7 years old, a significant reduction in vital capacity and peak expiratory flow rate has been observed.[2] Abnormal pulmonary mechanics have been reported in adults 5 weeks after a viral URI[3] and impaired clearance of mucus from the trachea for at least a week after the disappearance of URI symptoms.[9]

These data suggest it may be ideal to wait 6 to 8 weeks after a URI has cleared to anesthetize a patient for elective surgery. However, many children are not asymptomatic for that long between URIs. In the Department of Anesthesia and Critical Care at The Children's Hospital of Philadelphia we prefer to wait 10 to 14 days after a patient becomes asymptomatic before proceeding with purely elective anesthesia and operation. The relative risks of anesthesia must be weighed against probable morbidity in patients with urgent but not emergency conditions requiring general anesthesia for surgery.

In the case presented above, the child is afebrile (temp. $>38°C$ [100.4°F] is febrile at our institution) but has a URI evident from rhinorrhea and a nonproductive cough. Thus, we would recommend postponement of anesthesia and surgery for at least 2 weeks, but preferably 4 to 6 weeks. If the child were older and his serious otitis media were producing a hearing loss that interfered with his schoolwork, it might be reasonable to proceed sooner, since the anesthetic could probably be safely administered by mask (Tait group III).

References

1. Braun AW, Cefalo RC: Guidelines for Perinatal Care. Evanston, IL, AAP/ACOG, 1983
2. Collier AM, Pimmel RL, Hasselblad V: Spirometric changes in normal children with upper respiratory infections. Am Rev Respir Dis 117:47, 1978
3. Hall WJ, Douglas RG, Hyde RW et al: Pulmonary mechanics after uncomplicated influenza A infections. Am Rev Respir Dis 113:141, 1976
4. Koka BV, Jeon IS, Andre JM et al: Postintubation croup in children. Anesth Analg 56:501, 1977
5. McGill WA, Coveloer LA, Epstein BS: Subacute upper respiratory infection in small children. Anesth Analg 58:331, 1979
6. Silver HK, Kempe CA, Bruyn HB: Handbook of Pediatrics, 6th ed. Los Altos, CA, Lange Medical Publications, 1965
7. Tait AR, Ketcham TR, Klein MJ et al: Perioperative respiratory complications in patients with upper respiratory tract infections (abstr). Anesthesiology 59:A433, 1983
8. Tait AR, Nahrwold ML, LaBond VA et al: Anesthesia and upper respiratory viral infections (abstr). Anesthesiology 57:A450, 1982
9. Wong JW, Keens TG, Wannamaker EM et al: Effects of gravity on tracheal mucus transport rates in normal subjects and in patients with cystic fibrosis. Pediatrics 60:146, 1977

Response

The child who presents with a fever, a history of cough, and rhinorrhea must be thoroughly evaluated. By separation of symptoms into two major categories, noninfectious and infectious, the physician can be helped in reaching a decision about the acceptability of this child as a candidate for surgery and anesthesia at this time. (The differential diagnosis of runny nose is found in Chap. 4, Special Problems.)

A history from the parents, usually the child's mother, can be invaluable in helping you determine whether this is a chronic or an acute change for the child. The simple question, "Are these new symptoms for this child?" can provide you with information that can influence your judgment. In the face of an obvious acute URI we would not proceed with an elective surgical procedure.

■ CASE NO. 11

On the day of surgery a 3-year-old child's mother presents the anesthesiologist with a letter stating she had a low pseudocholinesterase level. She had a cesarean section approximately 4 months ago and required postoperative ventilation. Her child is scheduled to have an ambulatory surgery hernia repair.

Discussant

Andrew A. Jeon, M.D.
Instructor in Anaesthesia, Harvard Medical School; Medical Director, Ambulatory Surgery Unit, The Children's Hospital, Boston, Massachusetts

Pseudocholinesterase (plasma cholinesterase) is an enzyme formed in the liver that is responsible for the hydrolysis of succinylcholine. Located in the liver, brain, pancreas, and plasma, it affects the duration of action of succinylcholine by regulating the amount of drug that eventually reaches the motor end-plate. Low pseudocholinesterase levels may be due to a number of causes (echothiophate, liver disease, burns, organophosphate poisoning, and pregnancy). Fortunately, there is a wide margin of safety between the amount of enzyme available and the amount necessary to hydrolyze a normal dose of succinylcholine (1 mg/kg). Foldes et al, in 1956, discovered that when severe liver disease reduced pseudocholinesterase to 20% of normal, the duration of apnea after succinylcholine administration was increased from a normal period of 3 minutes to almost 9 minutes.[1] The average reduction in pseudocholinesterase activity associated with pregnancy is approximately 25%.[3] This degree of reduction in pseudocholinesterase levels is not sufficient to cause a clinically significant increase in the duration of action of succinylcholine.

The differential diagnosis for a patient with a prolonged period of recovery from succinycholine must include the consideration of the presence of an atypical *plasma cholinesterase*. This variant is genetically determined by an autosomal codominant mode of inheritance and reflects a qualitative rather than quantitative characteristic of the enzyme. Although various alleles of this gene exist, many are extremely rare. The most common can be determined by comparing the relative inhibition of activity of normal and abnormal pseudocholinesterase by dibucaine, a local anesthetic. Dibucaine was found to inhibit the activity of normal pseudocholinesterase more than that of abnormal pseudocholinesterase.[2] A low dibucaine number represents an atypical plasma cholinesterase that will not hydrolyze succinylcholine to the extent that typical plasma cholinesterase will.

A family history of unexpected postanesthetic complications should alert the anesthesiologist to a potential problem in the patient. In this case, the reason for postoperative respiratory support in the patient's mother is not clear. Postoperative ventilation might have been necessary for reasons other than a prolonged recovery from succinylcholine, for example, relative overdose of respiratory depressant drugs or muscle relaxants, metabolic acidosis, or hypocapnia. The diagnosis of prolonged neuromuscular blockade secondary to succinylcholine can be made only with a peripheral nerve stimulator demonstrating a phase II block. The discovery of a low pseudocholinesterase level in the patient's mother may therefore have been an incidental finding.

The likelihood of this child having an abnormally low level of pseudocholinesterase is very small, but the child should still be considered at risk if succinylcholine is used. Appropriate preliminary tests for the child and parent should include a screen for the atypical variant of pseudocholinesterase.

Anesthesia for hernia repair in a 3-year-old can safely be performed without the use of succinylcholine. An induction with rectal methohexital followed by maintenance anesthesia of halothane, nitrous oxide, and oxygen by mask should provide a smooth anesthetic and adequate surgical conditions for hernia repair. If a situation arises in which succinylcholine is needed (e.g., laryngospasm), then the possibility of a prolonged apnea exists.

A patient with a pseudocholinesterase deficiency may safely be administered anesthesia in an ambulatory surgery setting as long as the facility can provide postoperative ventilatory support and has ready access to more intensive medical care should additional problems occur.

References

1. Foldes FF, Rendell-Baker L, Birch JH: Causes and prevention of prolonged apnea with succinylcholine. Anesth Analg 35:609, 1956
2. Kalow W, Genest K: A method for the detection of atypical forms of human serum cholinesterase: Determination of dibucaine numbers. Can J Biochem 35:339, 1957
3. Pantuck EJ, Pantuck CB: Cholinesterases and anticholinesterases. In Katz RL (ed): Muscle Relaxants. Amsterdam, Excerpta Medica, 1975

Response

The family history of the mother having a low pseudocholinesterase level with pregnancy does not give the entire picture. In order for a patient to receive complete testing of plasma cholinesterase level, quantity as well as quality "dibucaine testing" must be done. Although testing for the dibucaine number is not immediately available in most hospitals, it is a test that is "necessary" for evaluation of a suspected plasma cholinesterase deficiency.

The neuromuscular blockade with succinylcholine in a patient with a pseudocholinesterase deficiency is a reversible phenomenon. With ventilatory support and "tincture of time" it, too, shall pass.

In this case we are faced with two acceptable options. Postpone the procedure and have tests done prior to surgery or proceed with the surgery (which we did), drawing blood samples for pseudocholinesterase level and dibucaine numbers. Appropriate testing of the child's parents could be done at any time.

■ CASE NO. 12

A grossly obese 31-year-old woman arrives at your ambulatory surgery unit scheduled for an umbilical hernia repair. She is 5 feet, 3 inches tall and 289 lb. The patient has a history of asthma and takes theophylline-SR, 250 mg, twice a day. Her most recent asthmatic attack was 6 months ago and required hospitalization and intravenous aminophylline therapy. She has been followed by her internist, and her theophylline levels have been in the therapeutic range.

Discussant

Monte Lichtiger, M.D.
Vice Chairman, Department of Anesthesia, Mt. Sinai Medical Center, Miami Beach, Florida; Clinical Professor, Department of Anesthesia, University of Miami School of Medicine, Miami, Florida

There are three factors that must be considered in discussing this case: (1) the pathophysiology of the obese patient, (2) the patient's asthma, and (3) the changes related to anesthesia and surgery. Consideration of these factors and how they interact may prevent us from managing this case in the ambulatory surgery unit.

The basic problem in the obese patient is an increased metabolic rate that is proportional to the increased tissue mass. This leads to a greater requirement for oxygen and an increased production of carbon dioxide. Chest and abdominal fat also reduce the ability of the chest to expand and lead to decreases in tidal volume, vital capacity, and total compliance. Inspiratory capacity and functional residual capacity are markedly decreased. Increases in cardiac output and blood volume develop early in the disease whereas a late change is an increase in pulmonary vascular resistance.[1,2,3]

The patient with morbid obesity may also present some other problems to the practicing anesthesiologist. For example, obese patients have a larger volume of gastric juice and more gastric acid than their thinner counterparts.[4] This, coupled with an increased incidence of hiatal hernia, predisposes to aspiration. It may also be difficult to ventilate these patients with a face mask and to perform endotracheal intubation. In fact, awake intubation may be indicated in some obese patients. Furthermore, thromboembolic complications are more common, and it may be more difficult for these patients to be mobilized after surgery. If minidose heparin is considered, it may be advisable to admit the patient to ensure its efficacy.

From the preanesthetic evaluation, the anesthesiologist should be able to classify the obese patient into one of four types:

Type A. A well-compensated patient with no known medical problems. Intubation should not be difficult.

Type B. A well-compensated patient with no known medical problems. However, further evaluation of the airway may be required.

Type C. A decompensated patient requiring further evaluation and therapy. Airway considerations must remain secondary until medical evaluation and therapy are begun.

Type D. A patient who is decompensated despite medical therapy. There is very little physiologic reserve. The patient requires meticulous care for survival.

Type A and B patients may be candidates for ambulatory surgery. However, type C and D patients are best managed as inpatients. These patients have a marked decrease in physiologic reserve that may require more postoperative care. For example, the anesthesiologist may decide to keep the patient intubated in the recovery room and to extubate only when the patient is fully awake and able to maintain her own airway. On the other hand, he or she may decide to support the patient's ventilation in an intensive care unit and to extubate only when the patient shows she can maintain adequate gas exchange.

Obese patients do have a higher incidence of postoperative pulmonary complications. After abdominal operations, their already compromised pulmonary reserves are challenged further. Postoperative pain limits their ability to cough and deep breathe. In cases of long-standing hernia, there may be an increase in intra-abdominal pressure once the hernia is reduced, which can add to the ventilatory problem.

Our patient with morbid obesity also has bronchial asthma (she is a type C patient) which has required hospitalization in the recent past. This adds to the potential for postoperative respiratory problems. However, it leaves the anesthesiologist with yet another dilemma. He or she may wish to leave the patient intubated as discussed above, but the endotracheal tube may provoke bronchospasm. Our asthmatic patient is also receiving theophylline. This drug can interact with some anesthetic agents to produce dysrhythmias and hypotension. With the patient's potential for postoperative problems, ambulatory surgery is not advisable.

References

1. Bendixen HH: Morbid obesity. ASA Refresher Course 6:1, 1975
2. Brown BR: Anesthesia and the obese patient. Contemporary anesthesia practice. Philadelphia, FA Davis, 1982
3. Gelman S: Anesthesia for the morbidly obese. Curr Rev Clin Anesth 4:103, 1983
4. Vaughn RW, Bauer S, Wise L: Volume and pH of gastric juices in obese patients. Anesthesiology 43:686, 1975

Response

The morbidly obese patient presents many challenges to the anesthesiologist, and Dr. Lichtiger has done a fine job in his discussion. We agree with his conclusion for this particular patient. However, we have found that well-motivated, grossly obese patients can have procedures performed in an ambulatory surgery facility if exclusive of their obesity they can be classified as ASA physical status 1 or 2.[1] Obese patients scheduled for ambulatory surgery must be aware that hospital admission may be necessary if any problems arise. If this patient were not an asthmatic, the factors we would take into consideration before deciding whether to discharge home or hospitalize would be the size of the hernia, length of surgery, and the patient's response in the postanesthesia care unit (pain tolerance, ventilatory status). Local anesthesia supplement during surgery would be an important addition to this patient's management (limiting pain in the early postoperative period).

Reference

1. Jensen S, Wetchler BV: The obese patient: An acceptable candidate for outpatient anesthesia. J Am Assoc Nurse Anesth 50:369, 1982

■ CASE NO. 13

A 20-year-old woman, ASA physical status 1, presents to the ambulatory surgery unit for a laparoscopic tubal ligation scheduled for 10:00 A.M. The patient has been asked to arrive at the ambulatory surgery unit at 8:30 A.M., but does not arrive until 9:00 A.M. At that time she admits to having a glass of juice (approximately 4 oz) at 7:00 A.M. This young woman has failed to appear for her two previous surgery dates. The obstetrician states this woman is unreliable, but since she is here today and will probably be intubated anyway, he would like to proceed with the laparoscopic tubal ligation.

Discussant

Karl J. Kassity, M.D.
Medical Director, Outpatient Surgery, Cottage Hospital, Santa Barbara, California

There are several possible answers to the question of whether to proceed. In the "ideal world," since this is an elective surgical procedure and the patient has not been NPO for the required amount of time, this case would likely be cancelled and rescheduled for a later date.[1] It is difficult to argue with this approach, especially given the type of surgical procedure, and the patient's previous demonstrations of unreliability.

Another approach to this question of the elective ambulatory surgery patient who has not been NPO would be to offer the patient a later time slot on the operating room schedule. What the patient has ingested may influence the decision to postpone or cancel surgery (coffee, juice, milk, solids). In this case, I would feel that a 6-hour delay between the last ingestion of fluids and the commencement of elective surgery would be acceptable. At our facility, if the patient elected to have her surgery later in the day, she would be kept in the ambulatory surgery unit and observed. We would feel comfortable administering a general anesthetic to this patient any time after 1:00 P.M. Many of our patients, and all of our laparoscopic patients, receive 30 ml of sodium citrate or 300 mg of cimetidine orally 60 to 90 minutes preoperatively to increase the gastric pH and decrease the gastric volume.[2] If this patient were not obese and presented with no airway management problems, and the surgeon required minimal or no Trendelenburg position, she might not be intubated. If the patient was intubated, some of the anesthesiologists at our institution would pass an oral gastric tube and aspirate the stomach while the patient was asleep.[3]

Our patient information brochure emphasizes the NPO status in the preoperative instructions read by every patient. In addition, at the Cottage Hospital in Santa Barbara every patient is contacted the day before surgery by telephone to remind them of the date of surgery and when they are to arrive in the ambulatory facilities.

Of course, if this patient had solid food or a full breakfast we would cancel the case for that day. Our objective is not to take undue risks or to be cavalier in our approach to patients' safety, but to use sound judgment after all the facts of a particular case are known and to involve the patient in the decision-making process. Good cooperation is therefore required, as are understanding and compliance on the part of the patient to successfully be involved in ambulatory surgery under general anesthesia and to return home that day. This patient demonstrates a lack of responsibility in this area.

References

1. Fabian LW, Benson DW, Caldwell CB et al: The experts' opinion on the prevention and treatment of pulmonary aspiration of gastric contents. Surv Anesth 27:388, 1983
2. Manchikanti L, Roush JR: Effects of preanesthesia glycopyrrolate and cimetidine on gastric fluid pH and volume in out patients. Anesth Analg 63:40, 1984
3. Ong B, Palakniuk RL, Cumming M: Gastric volume and pH in out patients. Can Anaesth Soc J 25:36, 1978

Response

On more than one occasion this young woman has demonstrated that she is unreliable. On the day of surgery she arrived at the ambulatory facility later than scheduled and also ignored her NPO instructions. Will she follow postoperative instructions? Although we have little control over the patients once they leave the ambulatory surgery unit, it is our responsibility to adhere to basic preoperative management. At The Methodist Medical Center of Illinois, unless there are medications that need to be taken with a sip of water on the morning of surgery, our adult patients are required to remain NPO after midnight.

I agree with Dr. Kassity that the patient could have her procedure performed 6 hours after drinking 4 oz of juice with a very minimal risk to her. However, if aspiration occurs either during anesthesia or in the immediate postoperative period, what would the risk be to the facility and to the anesthesiologist in view of the facility's standard of care being "NPO after midnight"? With this patient's history of unreliability and her not following basic preoperative instructions, we would reschedule her surgical procedure for a later date and even consider managing her as an inpatient.

■ CASE NO. 14

A 20-year-old aphasic hemiplegic man is scheduled for reconstructive facial plastic surgery. One year ago, following an automobile accident, he sustained massive head and chest trauma including a bilateral hemopneumothorax. He was hospitalized for 4 months; unconscious for the first 4 weeks, and in the intensive care unit for 8 weeks. Though he remains hemiplegic and aphasic, he has sufficient central nervous system recovery to understand conversation. He has residual chest deformity and reduced pulmonary function, though blood gases are normal when the patient is at rest and breathing room air. His vital capacity is only two times his tidal volume. The patient and family desire no more hospitalization if at all possible.

Discussants

Jeffrey L. Apfelbaum, M.D.
Assistant Professor of Anesthesia, Division of Day Surgery, Hospital of the University of Pennsylvania, Philadelphia, Pennsylvania
John H. Lecky, M.D.
Associate Professor of Anesthesia, Division of Day Surgery, Hospital of the University of Pennsylvania, Philadelphia, Pennsylvania

There are a number of specific considerations in determining the appropriateness of caring for this patient in an ambulatory surgery setting. These include

A. The physical location and the organization of the unit, which determine how readily the patient can be admitted to a hospital postoperatively, should the need arise
B. The family's capability to monitor the patient and to care effectively for him postoperatively
C. The availability of a recovery room and sufficient nursing personnel capable of monitoring such a patient in a "high-turnover" setting without compromising the care of other patients
D. The anesthetic requirements for the surgical procedure. Is a general anesthetic required, or can a local or regional technique be employed?
E. The specific anesthetic concerns:
  1. The airway management; is there trauma-induced mechanical compromise of the upper airway, or is a tracheostomy present, making control of the airway an easy matter?
  2. The degree and type of pulmonary compromise
  3. The central nervous system derangement:
    a. Can one communicate with the patient?
    b. Can the patient cooperate or is he combative?
    c. How recent or stable is the myoneural pathology, i.e., is the use of succinylcholine appropriate?

At best, failure to address carefully any one of these technical, administrative, or medical issues will impair function of the unit and can compromise the patient's care. At the worst, it will produce a potentially life-threatening postoperative situation. The successful treatment of this patient in the ambulatory surgery setting, then, is dependent on the satisfactory evaluation and resolution of each of these considerations *prior* to the patient's arrival in the unit.

Although this patient is hemiplegic and aphasic, he apparently has sufficient central nervous system function to understand and to be cooperative. From the outset, the medical staff should make every effort to establish and maintain effective two-way communication with the patient and his family. If the patient is unable to cooperate or easily becomes combative, he represents a major disruption and management problem in the waiting area, in the operating room, and in the recovery room. In addition, any unwillingness or inability to cooperate on the part of the patient would mitigate against the possible use of local anesthesia. Such behavioral problems, then, would pose a significant challenge in the ambulatory surgery setting and would probably make inpatient care with preoperative sedation and general anesthesia necessary.

Preoperative evaluation of this patient's diminished pulmonary reserve is also essential. Theoretically, a vital capacity in excess of 15 ml/kg should provide a ventilatory reserve adequate to allow for postoperative deep breathing and coughing in a cooperative patient. Although elective upper abdominal and thoracic procedures generally result in a 60% to 75% decrease in preoperative vital capacity, elective peripheral procedures usually produce minimal compromise of vital capacity.

Because of the location of the surgical procedure, general endotracheal intubation may be required. Evaluation of the upper airway is essential because of the previous facial trauma, and, should intubation be required, awake oral or nasal intubation (with or without fiberoptic endoscopy) may be indicated. If a muscle relaxant is to be used, succinylcholine should, in theory, be avoided because of its association with massive potassium release in patients with significant muscle wasting. In an emergency, it can probably be used safely in this patient because of the age of the myoneural damage (1 year). Alternatively, short-acting, nondepolarizing muscle relaxants, such as atracurium or vecuronium are excellent substitutes.

In case general anesthesia is required, extubation and the postoperative recovery period are critical points in this patient's management. Because of this patient's severely diminished vital capacity, arterial blood gases and pulmonary function should be monitored during the perioperative period. The decision to extubate depends on the state of consciousness, circulatory stability, $AaDO_2$, vital capacity, and minute ventilation required to maintain the $PACO_2$ at a normal level.

Although elective nonthoracoabdominal procedures usually produce only minor decreases in postoperative vital capacity, residual inhalational anesthetic and narcotic effects can be variable. The treatment of postoperative pain with its attendant risk of respiratory depression further complicates the situation. Since decreases in vital capacity in the postsurgical patient can be seen up to 18 hours postoperatively, this patient's severely diminished pulmonary function renders the margin of safety minimal at the time of potential discharge. This patient, then, is hardly a suitable candidate for general anesthesia in an ambulatory care center unless a prolonged period of postoperative observation is possible and adequate means of respiratory evaluation are present. If, however, the patient is willing and the surgeon feels that the procedure can be adequately performed under local infiltration or major nerve block, this procedure can be safely performed in an ambulatory surgery setting.

Response

When caring for surgical patients who have pulmonary dysfunction, one must emphasize good preoperative evaluation *prior* to patient arrival at the ambulatory surgery facility.

This patient had two operative procedures completed on an ambulatory basis without complications. Before the first procedure, the anesthesiologist had discussed the patient's medical problems with the neurologist, the pulmonologist, the surgeon and the patient's family. All agreed that it would be desirable if it could be done in the ambulatory surgery unit as the patient and family requested. It was understood by the patient and family that if any problems developed or concerns arose on the part of any attending physician the patient would be admitted to the hospital.

Because of the patient's anxiety and the extent of facial surgery, he was not a candidate for local anesthesia. A general endotracheal anesthesia was used without preoperative medication or succinylcholine for intubation. The surgeon supplemented the general anesthesia with local bupivacaine, allowing for a "light" inhalation anesthesia. The patient awakened pain free in the operating room and was able to move himself from the operating room table to the recovery stretcher. Careful evaluation of the patient's pulmonary function in the recovery period revealed no adverse changes, and the patient was discharged home. He also had uneventful subsequent surgery on an ambulatory basis.

Cooperative surgeons who will infiltrate local anesthesia in the wound, allowing ambulatory surgery patients to awaken comfortably, add to the success of ambulatory surgery care.

■ CASE NO. 15

A 3-year-old child with a history of chronic hypertrophic tonsillitis is scheduled for a T&A. The child's mother says the patient has had two traumatic experiences in the past with anesthesia and surgery. This child is very apprehensive.

Discussant

Richard A. Elwyn, M.D.
Anesthesiologist, Primary Children's Medical Center; Clinical Professor of Anesthesia, University of Utah School of Medicine, Salt Lake City, Utah

The key question here is "Is it possible to anesthetize any child without some personal trauma being inflicted on that child?" Although one must be as kind and considerate as possible, the interrelationship between anesthesiologist and child cannot be accurately predicted in advance. The relationship of mother to child is important, as is that between the mother and the anesthesiologist in the preoperative interview. A calm, reassuring, and cooperative mother can go a long way in preparing her child for surgery and anesthesia.

It is necessary to determine just what problems were associated with the previous surgical procedures based on the information from the mother and the old chart. The anesthesiologist who relates well with children is indispensable here. "Perhaps the greatest failure to date has been the lack of individualization in preoperative management of children."[1]

The 3-year-old is quite often difficult to deal with. Communication skills are not developed, and thus parental separation is a primary fear. Obviously, parental separation is unavoidable but is its briefest in the ambulatory surgery setting. Even with the limited time available in the ambulatory surgery unit, adequate time should be taken to gain a rapport with the child; find out the child's likes and dislikes in a friendly and nonthreatening manner. Then describe what will happen to the child (not only for the child's benefit but for the mother's as well) in simple terms.

I have the child sit on my lap (if 50 lb or less) during induction, and we conduct a charade together. He or she has a choice of flavors to apply to the anesthesia mask. I find that bubble gum, root bear, banana, orange, and chocolate flavorings are very popular. I tell the child he or she is a helicopter pilot. As the chosen flavored mask is applied and the nitrous oxide and oxygen turned on, the child is shown the controls (the anesthesia machine, its knobs, and alarms). As the child "gives it the gas" the halothane vaporizer is turned on and away we go down the runway. It must be emphasized that the operating room and anesthesia machine must be 100% ready to go *before* the child enters. This is no time for fumbling, looking for tape, applying the blood pressure cuff, and so forth. In healthy children, apply the monitors after the anesthetic induction; keep the child's attention on the diversion and yours on the induction.

If you evaluate the child's fears as irrational and unresponsive to your personal touch, another path may be pursued. Preoperative medication has little use in an ambulatory surgery unit. Short procedures, the possibility of a delayed discharge, and the fact that 2 and 3 year olds are very unpredictable in their response to premedication are the reasons for my opinion. As long as the mother is present the child will be reasonably content and will not need premedicants. Sequester mother and child in a separate room if you have one, until the time for surgery. At this time options that are available include ketamine and methohexital intramuscularly or an intravenous induction. Obviously, if you have the temperament and space available, the mother may accompany the child to the operating room while you induce anesthesia.

Whatever approach you choose, communicate it to the mother and child.

Reference

1. Smith RM: Anesthesia for Infants and Children, 4th ed, pp 87–108, 152–163. CV Mosby, 1980

Response

The most important factors to be considered when anesthetizing a child who has had a "bad experience" with anesthesia include open communication with the child and communication with the parents. The latter is often the key to a smooth trip to the operating room and a tearless induction. It is also necessary to thoroughly investigate what is meant by a "traumatic experience." The experience may have been more traumatic for the parent. Hopefully, this could be lessened by a good preoperative visit from the anesthesiologist. The need for preoperative sedation should be evaluated on an individual basis. In our ambulatory surgery unit we have a policy that children having T&As are kept a minimum of 3 hours in the PACU. This gives us the option of using oral premedication if we feel it is necessary. The availability of "short-stay" hospital beds may also influence your premedication decision. Our approach for this patient would be a "steal technique" using either ketamine or methohexital intramuscularly. A variety of induction techniques with appropriate dosages are discussed in detail in Chapter 4.

■ **CASE NO. 16**

A 33-year-old diabetic woman who takes 30 units of NPH insulin and 10 units of regular insulin on a daily basis is scheduled for elective sterilization. The patient is intelligent and has been a well-controlled diabetic.

Discussant

Cynthia Alexander Nkana, M.D.
Associate Medical Director, Methodist Ambulatory Surgery Center, The Methodist Medical Center of Illinois, Peoria, Illinois

The insulin-dependent diabetic presents an interesting problem for the anesthesiologist. There are ambulatory centers that do not schedule insulin-dependent diabetics for ambulatory surgery. Perhaps this approach should be abandoned as we are realizing that patients with medical problems that traditionally have eliminated their having surgery in an ambulatory unit can now be safely done. This case presents an intelligent young woman who we should assume has managed her diabetes with good control. The patient should be scheduled within 1 week of her surgery for a thorough history review and preadmission testing. The questions that should be asked during the initial preadmission testing are[1]

How long have you been a diabetic?
How long have you been on your present insulin dose?
Have you ever been hospitalized for episodes of hyperglycemia or hypoglycemia?
Do you monitor your urine glucose or blood glucose on a daily basis?

With the availability of glucose meters for home use and Dextrostix, the conscientious diabetic can keep glucose levels within a normal range.[2] Of course, the anesthesiologist must be aware of the patient's insulin dose, dosage schedule, and normal meal pattern. Appropriate laboratory studies including a fasting blood sugar should be obtained on the day of surgery.

It is difficult to set absolute values for glucose levels, but a fasting blood sugar greater than 250 mg/dl should alert the physician that the patient may not be as well controlled as she appears.[3] The patient should be scheduled for surgery as early as possible; an 8:00 A.M. surgery time would be most appropriate. This will enable the patient to quickly resume her normal insulin and meal schedule.[4] Upon the patient's arrival at the ambulatory surgery unit a fasting blood sugar should be obtained, an intravenous line containing a dextrose solution such as D₅LR should be started, and one-half of the patient's usual long-acting NPH insulin dose should be given. On the day of surgery insulin should be given only after the patient has arrived in the ambulatory surgery unit and an intravenous is started. This minimizes the chance of hypoglycemia if there is an unavoidable delay in the start of surgery. You should avoid a situation in which the diabetic patient remains NPO overnight for surgery, has taken her insulin at home, arrives at the ambulatory facility to find that surgery is delayed, and receives no glucose solution.

After her surgical procedure has ended and the patient tolerates oral liquids and solids, the intravenous solution can be discontinued. The patient should be instructed to resume her normal diet as soon as possible after she returns home. She should check her urine or blood glucose at approximately 4:00 P.M., and if she is eating and drinking adequately, the remainder of her NPH insulin (15 units) should be administered. If the patient has not been able to tolerate oral liquids or solids, one-third of the 15 units (5 units) should be administered. It is unusual that patients are not capable of eating small amounts of solids and drinking liquids after discharge from the ambulatory facility. Of course, there must also be a responsible adult who is in attendance with the patient. If there are any symptoms suggestive of hypoglycemia or hyperglycemia the patient's physician should be notified immediately. The morning after surgery she should be able to resume her regular full dose of insulin and usual diet intake. At our facility she would receive a follow-up telephone call some time during the first day after surgery.

A second approach to managing the patient who is an insulin-dependent diabetic is that of Dr. H. E. Natof at the Northwest Surgicare. The technique is referred to as *moving the sun in the sky*. The patient presents to the ambulatory surgery unit having been NPO since midnight and brings insulin along. An intravenous line is started. After recovering from surgery, the patient is to begin a regular diet schedule, and receive his or her usual insulin dose. Rarely are patients unable to resume a normal caloric intake. For the remainder of the day they move their meals closer together. Patients are cautioned, however, that they may be slightly hypoglycemic on the morning after surgery. They should compensate for this by increasing their oral intake.

Insulin-dependent diabetics can safely have their surgical procedures done on an ambulatory basis, but they must assume additional responsibility in the postoperative period.

References

1. Miller RD: Anesthesia, p 21. New York, Churchill Livingston, 1981
2. Davidson et al: Perioperative management of diabetes mellitus. Anesthesiology 55:104, 1981
3. Palumbo PJ: Blood and glucose control during surgery. Anesthesiology 55:94, 1981

Response

Most insulin-dependent diabetics are well educated about their health problem and have various devices at home for monitoring glucose levels accurately. Over the last 6 years, at the Salt Lake Surgical Center, patients who are insulin dependent diabetics have had their surgery performed without any known complications in the ambulatory surgery unit. The incidence of nosocomial infections is decreased in ambulatory surgery patients. One could make a strong argument that all diabetic patients should be treated on an ambulatory surgery basis if possible.

At the Salt Lake Surgical Center patients are expected to bring their insulin to the ambulatory surgery unit. In the postoperative period they are given two-thirds of their usual insulin dose and encouraged to return to a normal diet. The key to any successful treatment of the diabetic patient is that the patient be well motivated and well educated and assume the major responsibility for home monitoring and postoperative care.

■ CASE NO. 17

An apprehensive 80-year-old man desires general anesthesia for cataract surgery. Upon arrival at the surgical center his history reveals symptoms of progressive angina and a blood pressure of 190/110. His only medication is nitroglycerin tablets, which he takes prn, approximately twice weekly.

Discussant

Kenneth M. Janis, M.D.
Associate Clinical Professor of Anesthesia, University of California, Irvine, California; San Diego Medical School, San Diego, California; Chief of Anesthesia, Saddleback Community Hospital, Laguna Hills, California

Progressive angina accompanied by hypertension may represent a life-threatening emergency. This patient's problems are of sufficient urgency that the anesthesiologist must act as a primary medical consultant. The patient needs to lie down, have an intravenous infusion started, and be given oxygen and nitroglycerin. An ECG tracing should be obtained. The patient's condition should be discussed with his cardiologist and, if significant abnormalities are noted on the ECG, the cardiologist should come to the facility. The primary concern is stabilization of this patient's cardiac status. Surgery will be postponed for another day.

The anesthesiologist has become familiar with the patient and can now help plan for future surgery. This patient may well return to the ambulatory surgery unit on beta blockers, calcium channel blockers, antihypertensives, and coronary vasodilators.

When the patient returns with a stable blood pressure and is free of angina the anesthesiologist must once again obtain a current history. A current ECG tracing is important, and upon arrival at the ambulatory surgery unit this patient should be automatically attached to an ECG monitor and blood pressure should be taken at regular intervals. Sedation can be initiated with incremental dosages of diazepam, and 50 μg to 100 μg of fentanyl.

At Saddleback Community Hospital and in Laguna Hills, California, approximately 800 cataract operations were performed on an ambulatory surgery basis during 1982. By 1985, it is expected that a combination of freestanding units, physicians' offices, and the hospital-based ambulatory surgery unit will provide services for over 1000 cataract surgeries a year. The predominant form of anesthesia is retrobulbar block with intravenous sedation provided by the anesthesiologist.

After the cataract surgery has been completed the patient is monitored continuously in the PACU. Postoperative hypertension and bradycardia may be prominent findings. In the event of severe hypertension, angina, or critical dysrhythmias, hospital admission would be mandatory.

Response

Geriatric patients with a history of hypertension and vague anginal symptoms are a common problem facing anesthesiologists in ambulatory surgery. Good preoperative preparation and evaluation must be done to provide safe anesthesia care. Most ambulatory surgery is elective. A patient who is ill-prepared for anesthesia should never be accepted. In the present litigious climate it is much wiser to defer surgery and reschedule the patient at a later date after proper evaluation and stabilization of his or her cardiovascular status.

At the time of the surgery minimal intravenous medication should be used for the geriatric patient. At the Salt Lake Surgical Center the use of diazepam has been limited in the geriatric patient because of the duration of its activity and the varied responses seen. Monitoring with a precordial stethoscope in addition to ECG monitoring allows for quicker detection of changes in rhythm and heart tones that reflect changes in blood pressure and cardiac output.

With this patient's hypertension and angina we would use the same prudent approach as Dr. Janis and postpone the patient's surgical procedure until a later time when his cardiovascular status was more stable.

■ CASE NO. 18

A 54-year-old woman is scheduled for a D&C because of menorrhagia. Results of preoperative laboratory studies include a hemoglobin of 8.8 g and hematocrit of 25%. The patient is a Jehovah's Witness and refuses any blood or blood products.

Discussant

Wallace H. Ring, M.D.
Cofounder, Salt Lake Surgical Center; Associate Clinical Professor of Anesthesiology, University of Utah School of Medicine, Salt Lake City, Utah

This patient presents with a significant anemia and the additional problem of a religious conviction that precludes her accepting the administration of blood products. One may assume that the attending surgeon was previously unaware of the anemia and therefore it is likely that the menorrhagia was not so profound as to have compelled the surgeon to order blood work prior to arrival at the ambulatory facility.

Historically, Jehovah's Witnesses who are well informed have accepted the risk of extensive surgery, including open heart surgery, with good results. It would seem that a D&C should be an acceptable operative and anesthetic risk for the Jehovah's Witness who has a low hemoglobin.

Most ambulatory surgery centers have minimum laboratory requirements (hemoglobin, hematocrit), below which surgery is not performed and anesthesia is not administered unless there are unusual clinical circumstances. Uremic patients are routinely anesthetized in many medical centers with hematocrits much lower than that reported for this patient.

The question that needs to be answered is, "What is the risk to the patient, facility, and anesthesiologist if one proceeds with the scheduled procedure?" The risk to the patient is one of decreased oxygen-carrying capacity and myocardial stress related to a compensatory increase in cardiac output. One must always keep in mind that unforeseen complications can occur, even with a D&C (we have all seen unexpected uterine perforation), that may suddenly demand volume expanders or blood transfusions. The patient should be well aware of potential complications.

A risk to the facility would be present if established minimal requirements for hemoglobin and hematocrit were not followed and there were complications during the procedure without documentation on the medical record of the need to have proceeded. The anesthesiologist may well be the one most at risk by proceeding with this case without good reason.

This case history does not reveal whether the patient is bleeding acutely or whether this is a chronic blood loss. For this patient, blood transfusion was not an acceptable alternative. But would it be advisable in a patient who is not a Jehovah's Witness to administer a blood transfusion prior to surgery and then proceed? This question is too often asked to be avoided; the additional risk of an unnecessary blood transfusion is a discussion in itself. If the patient is not at risk and if no other etiology for the patient's anemia is found, iron therapy may be sufficient to restore this patient's hemoglobin and hematocrit to acceptable levels and her D&C could be performed at a later date.

Another issue that should be mentioned in this case is the need for ambulatory surgery facilities to have access to blood in emergency situations. This is not a problem for hospital-affiliated ambulatory surgery units, but may be a problem for freestanding ambulatory surgical facilities. Though the need for transfusions may indeed be rare, accreditation of ambulatory surgery facilities by the JCAH or AAAHC requires access to blood. At the Salt Lake Surgical Center, no blood transfusions have been administered in nearly 50,000 anesthetics. This occurrence is the result of careful preoperative screening. Should the surgeon not wish to postpone this case, it should be referred to a local hospital. This is really not the type of case to be treated in a freestanding surgical facility.

Response

Dr. Ring gives information that should be heeded in caring for the patient with a low hemoglobin. Minimal standards for laboratory studies should be followed. Failure to do so, if problems should arise, would put the ambulatory surgery facility, anesthesiologist, and surgeon in jeopardy. A patient's religious beliefs must not be violated. Discussions about a patient's care must involve the patient before a final decision is reached. The gynecologist must provide input about the patient's overall status: is this an acute bleeding disorder that will be unlikely to stop without the D&C or a chronic blood loss problem that does not pose an immediate threat?

If it is the former, this should be documented and potential risks discussed with the patient before proceeding. If it is the latter, a determination should be made whether it can be postponed until the hemoglobin and hematocrit can be raised to more acceptable levels.

At The Methodist Medical Center of Illinois we determined this to be a chronic problem and the patient was given iron supplements over a 6-week period. She was followed with serial hemoglobin and hematocrit studies every 2 weeks to be sure the hemoglobin was not decreasing and that she was responding to therapy. She returned to the ambulatory unit in 6 weeks with a hemoglobin of 11.3 g and a hematocrit of 33.1%. Her procedure was performed under general anesthesia without any problems.

■ CASE NO. 19

A 25-year-old man is on renal dialysis and needs a new A-V access shunt. His hemoglobin is 8.0 g and his hematocrit is 25%.

Discussant

Surinder K. Kallar, M.D.
Associate Professor and Director, Ambulatory Anesthesia, Virginia Commonwealth University, Medical College of Virginia, Richmond, Virginia

Patients with chronic renal failure on dialysis present several problems to the anesthesiologist, including anemia with a compensating high cardiac output, electrolyte imbalance, acidosis, and hypertension. They are often on antihypertensive medication and have been previously treated with steroids and immunosuppressants. Various psychological factors related to the disease and hemodialysis, especially depression, are also involved. Because erythropoietin production is impaired, it is not uncommon for these patients to have a hemoglobin concentration of 5 g to 8 g. This degree of anemia is well tolerated if the cardiovascular and respiratory systems are normal. Preoperative transfusion is not usually indicated unless the hemoglobin concentration is less than 6 g. When transfusion is indicated, the danger of fluid overload is minimized with the use of erythrocytes rather than whole blood. The decreased oxygen-carrying capacity of blood is normally compensated by increased cardiac output, often to levels twice normal. Therefore, it is important to avoid or minimize cardiac depression during anesthesia. Because uremic patients are acidotic, ventilation that is more than adequate must be provided during anesthesia. Coagulopathies are common and must be remembered in considering a regional anesthetic technique. Hyperkalemia, the most serious electrolyte abnormality, can cause cardiac conduction abnormalities and dysrhythmias. Serum potassium concentration should not be more than 5.5 mEq/L and can be controlled with preoperative dialysis. Hypermagnesemia can potentiate depolarizing and nondepolarizing muscle relaxants. A high blood urea nitrogen (BUN) is accompanied by decreased tolerance to barbiturates; any general anesthetic agents used must be administered in small doses, compared to those administered to patients with a normal BUN, in order to maintain anesthesia.

Regardless of the blood volume status, these patients tend to respond to induction of anesthesia as if they were hypovolemic. This is accentuated if they are on antihypertensive drugs. Drug interactions can be the result of multiple drug therapy, for example,

Corticosteroids causing suprarenal exhaustion and hypotension
Immunosuppressant therapy causing leukopenia
Interaction between digitalis and potassium concentrations
Antibiotics interfering with muscle relaxants

Attention should be paid to the possibility of these drug interactions and steps taken to prevent them. Patients receiving corticosteroids, for instance, should be "prepped" with appropriate increased doses before the operation.

A deficiency of plasma protein, especially gammaglobulin, renders these patients more liable to infection and necessitates meticulous aseptic technique and frequently antibiotic administration. Drugs that are highly protein bound (i.e., thiopental, bupivacaine) may cause prolonged or exaggerated effects. Pseudocholinesterase levels were said in earlier reports to be decreased; this is not a problem with current dialysis membrane materials.

Regarding anesthetic management, patients with chronic renal failure undergoing vascular access procedures can be handled safely on an ambulatory basis. There is no "right" agent or technique; the appropriate choice is based on the patient's psychological and physiological state and the personal skills of the anesthesiologist. Both general and regional techniques have been used successfully. However, some guidelines can be listed.

Ideally, the patient should be dialyzed 1 day prior to surgery. Available laboratory work should include a hemoglobin and electrolytes, including potassium, creatinine, and BUN. An intravenous line should be started with a balanced salt solution and with the use of careful aseptic technique; routine monitoring, including continuous ECG display, is appropriate. General anesthesia may include a slow induction with an ultra-short-acting barbiturate and maintenance with nitrous oxide, fentanyl, and low concentrations of isoflurane or enflurane. Atracurium and *d*-tubocurarine are acceptable in small doses if muscle relaxation is needed. Gallamine and metocurine are dependent on renal excretion and should be avoided. Initial doses of drugs should be reduced at least 50% and subsequent doses determined by the response observed. Small increments at longer intervals should be the expected requirement.

Regional anesthesia with brachial plexus block is ideal in that it abolishes vasospasm and provides optimal surgical conditions by producing maximal vascular dilatation. However, the duration of block produced by local anesthesia is shortened by about 40% in these patients. It is thought that elevated tissue blood flow secondary to increased cardiac output results in a more rapid clearance of the agents from the active site. Mepivacaine 1% or bupivacaine 0.25% have been used successfully. Adequacy of coagulation should be confirmed and the presence of uremic neuropathies excluded before regional anesthesia is considered.

It has been our experience with these patients that the application of simplified techniques for anesthetic management plus careful monitoring has led to a minimum of intraoperative and postoperative complications.

Response

This presentation covers the major physiologic derangements one would encounter with a patient in chronic renal failure. Both general and regional anesthesia can provide adequate analgesia and anesthesia for this group of patients. The anesthesiologist must remember that the patient with chronic renal failure has less physiologic reserve and will respond more quickly and more seriously to hypoxia, hypotension, infection, and myocardial depressant drugs. At our facility the anesthetic of choice would be a brachial plexus block, allowing the patient to maintain his baseline physical status while providing adequate anesthesia for the surgical procedure.

■ CASE NO. 20

A 25-year-old woman is scheduled for a laparoscopic tubal ligation. Well in advance of the date of the procedure the surgeon informs the facility and the anesthesiologist that the patient is a narcotic drug abuser.

Discussant

Fredrick K. Orkin, M.D., M.B.A.
Medical Director, Same Day Surgery, Hahnemann University Hospital; Associate Professor of Anesthesiology, Hahnemann University School of Medicine, Philadelphia, Pennsylvania

Obviously, this is not a patient that can be properly assessed within an hour or two of the procedure, for the assessment will take longer and there must be sufficient time to obtain confirmatory studies. In addition, I would not proceed in the ambulatory setting unless the patient is reasonably healthy. That is, the patient should have a normal exercise tolerance and should not bear *any* stigmata of liver disease (e.g., "spider" angiomata, ecchymoses, ascites, scleral icterus, asterixis). I would request liver enzyme and coagulation studies only to confirm a strong suspicion or a physical sign, because these tests are not cost-effective screening tools. Simply asking the patient whether she feels well is likely to prove more helpful, since malaise accompanies liver dysfunction.

If there is *any* question whether this patient has abused drugs on the day of surgery, I would not proceed on an ambulatory or inpatient basis. In the presence of acute ingestion there is an increased likelihood of acute and clinically important untoward autonomic and cardiovascular responses when one superimposes the administration of anesthetics and other drugs that would act on those systems. Although one can never be certain that a patient is truthful when she denies recent drug use, one must try to obtain a history of illicit drug use that is as complete as possible.

Comfortable that the patient is reasonably healthy and has not abused drugs recently, I would proceed. Starting the intravenous infusion is likely to be a challenge, and the patient should be forewarned that unusual efforts (e.g., internal jugular cannulation) may be necessary. Anesthesia personnel (and all others in the unit) should exercise great care to avoid unprotected exposure to her bodily secretions (blood, saliva, urine), minute fractions of a drop of which can transmit hepatitis virus. For example, gloves ought to be worn when the intravenous infusion is started and when the airway is suctioned. A public health consideration for anesthesia and PACU personnel should be immunization (as a precaution in all cases) against hepatitis B.

Although I generally do not administer premedication to patients having this procedure, once the intravenous has been started in the operating room I usually give an analgesic. A small dose of fentanyl (e.g., 1.5 μg/kg IV) for both mild sedation and supplementation of the general anesthesia would be used. (General anesthesia is chosen over regional in my institution on the basis of time taken to complete the surgery.) I would also exercise great care to avoid administering a partial agonist/antagonist (e.g., butorphanol, nalbuphine) at this time, and throughout the ambulatory experience. These drugs can antagonize residual narcotic effects and precipitate a withdrawal syndrome. The actual general anesthetic would not differ from that which I would give to another equally fit woman. In particular, there is no medical basis for avoiding halogenated agents here, although many would avoid using them for fear of "medicolegal implications," should the patient subsequently develop jaundice. I would opt for a "light" level of isoflurane (1% or less), with 60% nitrous oxide, following atracurium and tracheal intubation. Clearly, in this case (and in many others in the ambulatory setting), the emphasis must be on preoperative assessment and appropriate selection.

Response

Substance abuse has filtered into all groups of our society and we as anesthesiologists may find ourselves involved if there is need for surgery in this patient population. Substance abuse, acutely (within 24 hours of the surgical procedure) or on a long-term basis, must be known to the anesthesiologist. It cannot be overemphasized that careful evaluation of the patient with a history of substance abuse must be done *before* the day of surgery. The extent of drug use and the patient's overall health must be assessed. Appropriate laboratory studies should be obtained and reviewed prior to the day of surgery. All information obtained from this patient should be kept in strict confidence. In Illinois there is no state or local law that requires the physician to report any information about the drug abuser, and the patient should know that all information exchanged with the anesthesiologist will be confidential.

The National Survey on Drug Abuse reports the following figures for drug use in the 18 to 25 age group.[3]

	Ever Used (%)	Used During Past Month (%)
Cocaine	28.3	6.8
Heroin	1.2	1.5
Nonmedical use of analgesics	12.1	1
Stimulants	18	4.7
Tranquilizers	15.1	1.6
Alcohol	94.6	67.9

Although the alcohol-abuse patient is the most common abuser to present to the anesthesiologist, other substance use (cocaine, tranquilizers, narcotics) should be anticipated.

Common problems of drug abusers are[2]

Acute injury or disease
Withdrawal syndrome
Interactions with anesthetics
Interactions with adjuncts
Tolerance
Dependence
Organic changes

Substance abusers are usually not good candidates for regional anesthesia. These individuals often have a very suspicious nature and accompanying psychological problems. General anesthesia with narcotic supplementation is the anesthetic of choice. It is important to recognize that these patients have a higher incidence of hepatitis and frequently have pulmonary lesions that would require higher levels of oxygen. The risk of hepatitis would necessitate increased precautionary measures by hospital personnel:[1]

Gowns, gloves, caps, and plastic overshoes should be worn by anyone in contact with patients.
Disposable materials, such as syringes, sheets, pillows, and tracheal tubes, should be used whenever possible.
All disposable surgical and anesthetic items should be incinerated.
Special caution should be exercised when handling or disposing of contaminated sharp objects.
Surgical specimens should be carefully wrapped and labeled as biohazardous.
Reusable contaminted instruments (e.g., laryngoscopes, airways) and linens should be autoclaved or sterilized with ethylene oxide before washing.
Contaminated surfaces and equipment that cannot be sterilized (e.g., walls, floors, anesthesia machine, ventilator) should be washed with hypochlorite, formalin, or gluteraldehyde.
HBsAg-positive patients should be scheduled last to avoid exposure to other patients.

The anesthesiologist has no responsibility to proceed if this patient appeared to have had a recent ingestion of narcotics—slurred speech, disorientation, respiratory distress. It should be stressed, however, that overzealousness to start detoxification within the perioperative period can lead to increased problems with withdrawal.

This young woman could safely have her procedure performed as an ambulatory surgery patient. The need for *thorough preoperative evaluation* is mandatory, however, and all prescription blanks should be kept under lock.

References

1. Mathieu A, Dienstag JL: The hazard of viral hepatitis to anesthesiologists and other operating room personnel. In Orkin FK, Cooperman LH (eds): Complications in Anesthesiology, p 704. Philadelphia, JB Lippincott, 1983
2. Orkin LR: Anesthetic management of the drug abuse patient: avoiding the pitfalls. Clin Trends Anesth 6(1), 1976
3. U.S. Department of Health and Human Services: Main Findings 1982: National Survey on Drug Abuse.

10

A Successful
Facility

A successful ambulatory surgery facility begins with sound planning. Planning encompasses all aspects of the program—from determining need, to understanding program functions, to marketing the program, to successfully operating the program. Development of an ambulatory surgery program without proper planning is similar to taking a long driving trip without a road map. You may go someplace, but is it the right direction?

A successful program influences the anesthesiologist's caseload and income. Hence, our road map to a successful ambulatory surgery facility is a strategic planning route to our destination. The strategic planning process enables us to determine where we are today, where we want to be in the future, and how we will get there.

This chapter consists of three sections. The first section, which deals with facility planning, focuses on need and demand analysis; the functional/space programming process; and a step-by-step "how to" of planning and developing an ambulatory surgery program and facility. The second section discusses marketing as a responsibility of all managers. The last section considers fundamental operational and management issues.

Facility Planning

Leslie K. Leider, M.H.A.   *Peter M. Mannix, M.H.A.*

Why Is Planning Necessary?

A well-designed and efficiently staffed surgical facility greatly contributes to the success of an ambulatory surgery program. A successful facility, however, doesn't happen by itself—it happens with planning. In any facility program, and specifically in planning ambulatory surgery facilities, we must first plan for the program's function, and then determine the form that will permit this functioning. The cardinal rule of facility planning is *form follows function*.

Planning of the physical surgery facility is critical because its design affects so many aspects of the program. For example, staffing, operating costs, convenience, and often the success or failure of the ambulatory surgery program hinges on the physical facilities and design of the unit. Once constructed, the physical facility is the most difficult and expensive part of the ambulatory surgery program to change. Therefore, it is imperative that the facility be well planned in its early stages, so that its design conforms to the desired function.

What Is the Strategic Planning Process?

The strategic planning process is a structured approach used to determine the future direction of the organization. There are a number of steps in the process. Each step is based upon the results of the previous step. The anesthesiologist who is involved in the strategic planning process should become familiar with these steps, as they will apply to most situations, and specifically to ambulatory surgery program planning.

ROLE AND PROGRAM ANALYSIS

Basic to the strategic plan is the need to know the role of the institution and the programs that fulfill this role. Therefore, you need to study a number of demographic factors, such as the following:

SERVICE AREA
An analysis must be done to determine where ambulatory surgery patients have come from in the past and where they might come from in the future. Is our geographic service area small and concentrated or large and spread out? If it is small and concentrated, what can we do to expand it? If it is large and spread out, how can we increase our market share?

POPULATION
Once the geographic service area is defined, the character of its population should be analyzed. Perhaps the most important population variable is the age/sex specific breakdown of the service area. Although a high proportion of elderly patients (65 and over) historically indicated a heavy use of inpatient hospital services, shifting trends suggest that the elderly will become significant

users of ambulatory surgery. Children, adolescents, and females aged 15 to 44 are frequently good candidates for ambulatory surgery. You should identify the population by age and sex categories and compare it with national figures to help determine ambulatory surgery use patterns.

Historical and projected population trends should also be analyzed. A geographic service area that has a growing population center bodes well for future use of ambulatory surgery services. In fact, a rapidly growing geographic area could potentially be a location for development of a freestanding ambulatory surgery facility.

PHYSICIAN PROFILE

Physicians have a great influence on the types of services offered in an ambulatory surgery program. A physician profile should focus on the following:

Specialties. Some specialties are geared more toward the use of ambulatory surgery facilities than others. Obstetric/gynecologic, otolaryngologic, orthopedic, plastic surgery, and ophthalmologic specialists are heavy supporters of ambulatory surgery. A successful program should include a strong component of physicians in these and other specialties.

Age. A balance of younger and older physicians will contribute to the success of an ambulatory surgery program. It is particularly important to be aware of the numbers and specialties of elderly physicians. Physicians age 60 and over are likely to begin slowing their practices.

Practice Patterns. It is important to have a reasonable understanding of the amount of work a given physician is likely to perform in your facility. You need to determine whether ambulatory surgery is conducive to his or her past practice patterns.

Office Location. Location often has a great effect on physician practice patterns. In planning your program, it is important to consider the location of existing physician offices, clinics, and services. A close location encourages use of the facility.

Recruitment Needs. Analysis of the factors listed above may indicate the need to recruit additional physician specialists to optimize use of your facility. If physician age, office location, or specialty representation is not ideal to support your program, the need to add physicians must be recognized early. Plans should be developed to fill gaps in patterns of health care delivery before they arise and adversely affect the ambulatory surgery program.

VOLUMES OF SERVICE

Historical Use Analysis. Volumes of surgery that historically have been handled in your facility should be carefully analyzed to determine trends. What percentage of the volume has been done on an outpatient basis? How does it compare to that of other surgical facilities in the area, across the state, and nationally? Why is it comparatively high or low? Who are your competitors?

What is your percentage of the ambulatory surgery market? How can you increase your market penetration? How can the relationship with health maintenance organizations (HMOs), preferred provider organizations (PPOs), or other alternative delivery systems (ADSs) affect your volume?

Projected Use Analysis. Unfortunately, there is no totally reliable method to project future volumes of service. However, careful analysis and reasonable understanding of the factors listed above will give a high level of confidence in projecting future volumes. Projected volumes provide the base for the financial feasibility study. Hence, projections should be carefully scrutinized because they will affect the bottom line.

FACILITY ANALYSIS: EXISTING AND PROPOSED

Existing buildings must be analyzed to determine what facilities are necessary to accommodate all of the institution's programs (including ambulatory surgery). The sequence of events necessary to locate physical facilities on a site is called a *master site plan*. It is prepared in such a way as to identify major departmental zones and logical sequencing of construction and renovation.

Together, the *role and program plan* and the *facility plan* form the organization's strategic plan.

FUNCTIONAL PROGRAMMING

Once the master plan identifies a specific facility need for ambulatory surgery, that need must be described before architectural drawings are prepared. Functional/space programming is a planning process that clearly describes the need, function, and facilities required for an ambulatory surgery program. It contains a departmental description, workload analysis, staffing requirements, department organization, functional considerations, and space allocations. Simply stated, it delineates the number, size, and type of each room, together with the appropriate narrative to describe this information. This document is a *functional/space program* and, after revisions with staff input, is given to the architect to prepare drawings. It serves as the foundation for all further planning.

SCHEMATIC DESIGN

A *schematic design* is the architect's translation of the functional/space program into drawings. These first drawings roughly show the "scheme" of the departments, hence the title *schematics*. During this important stage of planning, basic layout and design are determined. If earlier planning steps have been completed properly, this step should proceed quickly and smoothly.

CERTIFICATE OF NEED (CON)

A *certificate of need (CON)* is a regulatory process a health care provider must go through to acquire approval of a particular project. You must check with your regulatory experts to determine whether a CON is needed for your project.

Once the schematics have been developed (at least in initial form), more accurate costing can be done. The cost estimates provide the basis, together with future volumes, to conduct a *financial feasibility study*. The long-range plan, schematic plans, financial feasibility study, and other related materials serve as the basis for the CON application.

DESIGN DEVELOPMENT

After the CON is submitted and the schematic design is finalized, the drawings are prepared in more detail, on a larger scale. In effect, the schematic design is developed further, and hence this step of planning is called *design development*.

In the course of design development, consideration is given to the details of the rooms. Major equipment items are identified (*equipment lists*); special mechanical systems (e.g., ventilation needs and special lighting) are listed; specific door locations are noted. A *room detail summary* is prepared, identifying each room and its detail of equipment, finishes, and so forth.

WORKING DRAWINGS AND SPECIFICATIONS

Once the design development drawings and supporting narrative have been developed, very detailed drawings (called *working drawings* or *construction drawings*) are then prepared. These literally show every nut and bolt in the new facility with a narrative (specifications) to explain the drawings.

BIDDING AND CONSTRUCTION

Working drawings and specifications, when complete, are sent to several contractors who prepare bids. The project is awarded to the successful bidder, and the contractor begins to construct the facility.

What Is the Anesthesiologist's Role in the Ambulatory Surgery Planning Process?

The anesthesiologist is a key player on the ambulatory surgery planning team. He or she generally participates in one of two roles: as a representative of the operating room in the hospital planning process or as an owner or representative of a group that is planning to build its own freestanding ambulatory surgery center (FASC). Each role is discussed below.

HOSPITAL-SURGERY REPRESENTATIVE

The anesthesiologist has much to contribute regarding the hospital's role in, and design of, an ambulatory surgery program. His or her views should be collected in personal interviews with the planners, consultants, or whoever is conducting or coordinating the study. The anesthesiologist should discuss the volume of ambulatory surgery that is currently taking place, current and future anesthesia management practice, the potential for growth in volume, types of surgery programs that would be appropriate for the hospital to develop, need for additional physician specialties on staff, and other topics. The anesthesiologist should also comment on the use of existing surgical facilities for ambulatory surgery, specifically the amount of space, department location, and department design. If new facilities are planned or existing facilities renovated, the anesthesiologist should participate in the planning process as it relates to the development of these facilities.

OWNER

The anesthesiologist's role as an owner in the development of a freestanding ambulatory surgery facility is fairly commonplace. Under these circumstances the role of the anesthesiologist will be far greater than that of the hospital-surgery representative. Instead of relying on the hospital to coordinate the organizational planning process, the owners of the freestanding facility must be responsible for the planning function. A number of planning variables must be carefully analyzed to determine the freestanding facility's appropriate role and, just as importantly, its potential profitability. As discussed in the facilities planning portion of this chapter, construction of surgery facilities is very expensive. Construction of a new unit without thorough need and demand analysis could prove hazardous to the financial health of the facility owners.

Who Else Is Involved in the Planning Process?

Generally speaking, the players in the planning process depend on the size of the project. In a major building program at a hospital, for example, the planning team often can be quite large. The planning team for construction of a freestanding ambulatory surgery facility, however, might be smaller. The following team members may be involved.

Planning or building committee: This group represents the owners of the project. They do not need to be aware of the day-to-day events of the project. However, they should meet regularly, such as once a month, with planning team representative(s) to receive project updates. Major decisions and direction should be provided by this group.

Project manager: The committee should select one individual in their employ to be the project manager. The project manager directs all of the other team members. He or she is responsible for the day-to-day activities of the project and should keep the building committee apprised of major events.

Planner/consultant: This individual is responsible for conducting the market analysis of the study. Also, the planner/consultant provides objective input into the program's function and design. The planner/consultant also may provide financial analyses.

Architect/engineer: The architect takes the functional/space program and translates it into drawings. He or she also is responsible for coordinating the many disciplines (such as civil, mechanical, and electrical engineering) necessary to design the physical structure.

Construction manager or general contractor: In many large building projects, the owner employs a construction manager. This company serves as the owner's representative for the project, keeps close watch on materials used and project costs. For smaller projects, general contractors are usually used to coordinate the many construction disciplines.

This information is presented to give the anesthesiologist the basic background necessary to begin and participate in the ambulatory surgery planning process. The next section will describe in more detail some site selection considerations, the development and use of a functional/space program (F/SP), design criteria, and project budget estimate components.

Site Selection: On or Off Campus?

As a primary participant in the planning process, you should become familiar with some of the basic concepts of site and facility planning. Your ability to translate concepts into architectural renderings and finally into an operational unit will aid in the eventual success (or failure) of the unit.

What are the important site selection criteria for an ambulatory surgery facility? A real estate agent will tell you the three most important characteristics of purchasing and owning property are location, location, and location. Whether the ambulatory surgery unit is located inside or outside a hospital facility, its location must afford convenience, flexibility, and marketability.

Ambulatory surgery unit location must be convenient for the consumer, family, physician, and staff. It should be convenient to find, access, and circulate through. It should be reasonably accessible for support services (matériels receipt and distribution, trash disposal, etc.) and amenable to operational systems (admitting, business, patient records, etc.). Physical constraints resulting from poor location will cause inconveniences and, most likely, create inefficiencies.

Location must promote flexibility in ambulatory surgery unit design, expansion, and, if necessary, alternative uses. Ideally, the unit's design should not be compromised by its location. Within an existing building, structural constraints or immediate "neighbors" may inhibit design. On a hospital campus or land with existing structures, the placement of the new ambulatory surgery unit may be dictated by predetermined site use plans (the master site plan) or situated in an area that limits design alternatives. Whatever the location, the building (and surrounding support zones, such as parking) should be expandable in such a way as to promote maximum integrity of the original or updated design. Also, the facility's location should not limit alternative uses of the site and buildings if the mix of services changes or if the ambulatory surgery program fails. You want to be sure that the site and buildings are attractive to other investors if you need to sell.

Finally, location should promote the marketability of the ambulatory surgery unit. Its visibility and image to the community, consumers, and physicians is important to its success. The concept of marketing is discussed in the second section of this chapter.

SITE SELECTION

What are the key site characteristics to consider when evaluating site options? What type of professionals can assist you in the selection of a site?

Once you've determined a general location for the ambulatory surgery facility through the use of marketing data or other sources, a real estate agent can point you in the direction of usable properties. However, you must be sure that the property is, or can be, zoned for use as an ambulatory surgery facility. In many cities and counties, an ambulatory surgery facility can be operated under zoning codes for health-related or medically related facilities. There are a number of areas, however, that do not have any zoning provisions for these facilities. Therefore, check with your real estate agent, lawyer, and local zoning authority for zoning provisions.

Next, you may want to conduct a general (nonscientific) survey of the "neighborhood." Who are your neighbors? Are they (or you) compatible with one another? Will they detract from the ambulatory surgery program's marketability? In other words, you don't want to locate your facility in a heavy industrial area or a "bad part of town."

As you select the site, visualize the access and egress to the site. Is it logical and convenient? Will it cause congestion off the main streets? Will it serve to enhance the visibility and image of the site and buildings? Usually, you will need the assistance of the architect and city planners to determine site access and egress patterns accurately.

The city authorities can also provide you with information regarding setbacks, right of ways, easements, and building height restrictions. Setbacks are the distances from streets or sidewalks that buildings are located; right of ways and easements are portions of the property that are reserved for future use by city authorities or utility companies; and building height restrictions vary depending on local codes (although most freestanding ambulatory surgery facilities are single-story structures). Be sure to assess the impact of these items on both current building plans and plans for future site/building development.

Also, be sure the soil conditions of the site do not preclude desirable development or that it requires different and more costly foundations for the buildings. Your architect will inform you of soil implications following test borings by a soils sample specialist.

SITE DEVELOPMENT

Once you have selected the site, there are three major criteria to consider in developing it.

LOCATION OF SITE ELEMENTS

Typically, you should master plan the total site before beginning specific drawings for the ambulatory surgery unit. *Master planning* describes the conceptual process one takes in considering all the potential programs, services, and facilities to be offered on the site for the next 5 to 10 years. Once these items are identified, the physical facilities required for them should be estimated (in terms of size) and situated on the site. This will provide you with a development plan for the future. It allows for orderly development of buildings and facilities.

Ideally, the site should be developed by using one-third for buildings, one-third for drives and parking, and one-third for landscaping. Following this general rule of thumb should result in an attractive and functional site.

DRIVES

On-site roadways should logically relate to the buildings and parking zones. Drives are planned to allow for easy and direct access to the site and buildings, especially by patients and visitors. Separation of service and staff traffic from patient and visitor traffic is desirable.

PARKING/ENTRANCES

Parking lots should be positioned to relate closely to various entrances. The key parking-entrance relationships include

Patient and family parking to the main entrance of the building
Physician parking to the physician entrance
Staff parking to the staff entrance
Service-related drives and parking to the receiving dock and service entrance

Functional/Space Programming

A successful planning process begins with a concept. That concept is the foundation of the ultimate program and facility design. To define the concept (ambulatory surgery), a planning team needs to be assembled. Representatives from anesthesiology services, surgical nursing, medical staff (physician users), management, and marketing should be included. To successfully define the concept, differing views must be considered and a consensus reached.

A functional/space program (F/SP) narratively describes the key considerations of the ambulatory surgery concept and program. Why is the F/SP important? It is the planning team's *plan* to coordinate all the different aspects of providing ambulatory surgery. It is the program for physical and operational development.

The F/SP comprises five major sections:

Description: This section describes the proposed functions of the ambulatory surgery program. Obvious activities require only a brief description. Special activities or services require a more complete description. Operational schedules should also be stated because they affect facility requirements.

It is important that this section adequately describe the broad array of ambulatory surgery services to be provided, what types of patients will be served, and unique operational considerations that may affect volumes, staffing, space, and design.

Workload analysis: This section discusses historical and projected volumes of service. Specifically, the number of cases by specialty, average length of time per case, average recovery time, and other pertinent volume-related data should be presented here. These volumes will serve as the basis for projecting staffing requirements and space.

Volumes should be projected for at least a 5-year period. Based on these projected volumes, the number of operating rooms, minor procedure rooms, primary postanesthesia care unit (PACU) stretchers, and secondary stage PACU areas should be listed here.

Staffing levels: Based on workload analysis and the proposed hours of operation, staffing by job category should be provided here. Staffing levels should be projected for a 5-year period. It is also important to estimate the number of staff during the busiest time so that space requirements can be determined accordingly.

Program for design: This section lists the specific design criteria to be used for planning the facility. (Functional areas, relationships, and specific design criteria are discussed later in this section.) Design criteria generally fall into two categories:

Interdepartmental design describes the proposed location of the ambulatory surgery unit and the major factors that influence its location. Such factors usually relate to vertical and horizontal patterns of public, patient, staff, physician, and matériels traffic. For an ambulatory surgery unit within existing hospitals, this section usually describes the relationships between the unit and laboratory, radiology, admitting/business office areas, building entrances, and general circulation. For freestanding units, this section should describe the desirable site and building entrances and exits as well as locations for parking zones.

Intradepartmental design describes the key factors affecting the layout/design of the ambulatory surgery unit. It discusses the flow of patients, family, staff, physicians, and matériels within the area. It also describes the key locational relationships between major room elements. Also, unique design features of particular rooms (such as an operating room for cystoscopy or special ceiling lights) should be stated here.

Space allocation: In this section, ambulatory surgery facility rooms or areas are listed. Proposed net square feet on a room-by-room basis is also presented. Net square feet is defined as the usable space within a room and is usually calculated from the wall-to-wall dimension.

To move into master planning and other design activities, the architect relies heavily on the space allocation and program for design sections of the F/SP. These sections narratively describe the major design guidelines for the architect to follow. Therefore, these two sections require detailed consideration by the planning team.

General Planning Guidelines: Operating Rooms and PACUs

Ambulatory surgery programs should have at least two dedicated operating rooms. This allows for optimal patient throughput. Each ambulatory surgery operating room can accommodate 1300 to 2000 procedures per year, depending on average length of procedure, available hours of surgery per day, number of operating days per week, and the efficiency of operating room turnover. A "lean and mean" program and facility will have high throughput and high profitability.

In addition to the main operating rooms, minor operating rooms should also be considered. These rooms can be used for "lumps and bumps" and minimally time-consuming procedures. This also could be used for specialty services such as ophthalmology (YAG laser use) or endoscopy.

The preoperative holding area is used to prepare the ambulatory patient for surgery. Note the term ambulatory. The patient and family member should have easy access to this area and it should have a nonclinical atmosphere. Because the majority of ambulatory surgery takes place in less than 30 to 40 minutes, there should be a minimum of 1.5 preoperative holding areas per operating room.

The primary recovery area is used for the immediate stage of postanesthesia recovery (regaining consciousness). Stretchers are used in this area. The number of primary recovery stretchers is usually a multiple of the number of operating rooms. Usually, 1.5 primary recovery stretchers to one operating room is sufficient. However, to determine the number of primary recovery stretchers appropriate to your particular situation, consideration must be given to the patient mix, volume per operating room, type of anesthesia used, and expected average length of immediate recovery time.

The second-stage recovery area is for patients who have regained consciousness, require less nursing care, and are being readied to go home. Second-stage recovery times vary between 1 and 6 hours, depending on the surgical procedure, the side-effects of anesthesia, and the patient's general physical and mental state. This area should be comfortably furnished for patients with recliners, chairs, couches, and, if necessary, a stretcher. This is a minimal care area, and hence a relative or friend of the patient should be allowed in this area.

Assembling the Functional/Space Program

The ambulatory surgery planning team needs to carefully consider the major elements an ambulatory surgery program comprises. Not all the major issues can be addressed in this chapter. However, Exhibit 10-1 is provided to familiarize the anesthesiologist with the key issues. It is organized by the key sections of the F/SP. By responding to these issues and others pertinent to your situation, you will develop and refine the F/SP.

Once these issues are addressed, the F/SP can be assembled. Usually, four to five meetings are required to agree upon a F/SP. You should provide ample time between meetings to allow for research and data collection, analysis, and consideration of major issues.

Exhibit 10-2 is an *example* of a completed F/SP. The space allocation is based on the functional requirements of this example program. It cannot be applied to individual situations. Your particular F/SP depends on functional programming requirements and budget considerations for your situation. This F/SP is presented for illustrative purposes only.

Exhibit 10-3 lists the common room elements (and their respective sizes) found in ambulatory surgery facilities. This list provides a range of room sizes. It should serve as a *guideline* when developing the space allocation section of the F/SP.

Room sizes and dimensions, when listed on paper or discussed in concept, are difficult to grasp for most people. When planning room spaces, measure a familiar area or room and use it as a guide for space comparisons. This will raise the comfort level of team members during this space planning phase.

☐ *Exhibit 10-1 Functional Programming: Selected Issues in Ambulatory Surgery*

DEPARTMENT DESCRIPTION

1. What are the goals and objectives of the ambulatory surgery program?
2. What types of surgical procedures and anesthetics will be allowed in the ambulatory surgery program?
3. What should be the maximum length of surgical procedures?
4. Will the ambulatory surgery unit be open 7 days a week?
5. What will be the hours of operation? At what time will the last general anesthesia case begin? The last local anesthesia case?
6. Should the ambulatory surgery program accept known contaminated cases?
7. Should patients selected for surgery be limited to ASA physical status 1 and 2 (ASA physical status 3 with controlled medical problems such as insulin dependent diabetes)?
8. Should an anesthesiologist be present at all times? If so, should the anesthesiologist or the attending physician discharge the patient?
9. Should non-MDs/DOs or others (podiatrists, oral surgeons, etc.) be allowed to use the facility?
10. Will students or residents of teaching or training programs participate in ambulatory surgery activities?
11. Should children under 12 years of age be operated on before 12 noon?
12. What laboratory and radiography diagnostic work will be needed for the patient? Will these services be provided in the ambulatory surgery facility?
13. Should all preregistration (admitting and financial) and preadmission testing (laboratory and radiographic tests as well as history and physical) occur prior to the date of surgery? If so, how many days in advance?
14. Will instrument clean-up, packaging, and processing occur in the ambulatory surgery department?
15. Is there need for an anesthesia induction room?
16. What is the function of the primary PACU? What is the function of the secondary stage PACU? At what time in the postanesthesia recovery process will the patient move from primary recovery to second-stage recovery?

WORKLOAD ANALYSIS

1. What are the projected annual volumes of service—by patient age, sex, and surgical specialty—for the next 5 years?
2. How many operating rooms, preoperative holding areas and PACU beds (both primary and secondary) will be needed to support these projected volumes?

STAFFING

1. How will the ambulatory surgery operating room, preoperative holding areas, and PACUs be staffed?
2. How will the support departments/areas be staffed?

PROGRAM FOR DESIGN (FUNCTIONAL CONSIDERATIONS)

1. How will the internal design of the ambulatory surgery unit
   a. Maximize patient privacy?

*Exhibit 10-1 **Continued***

    b. Minimize the mixing of inpatient and ambulatory surgical patients?

    c. Appropriately separate people, supply, and equipment flow?

    d. Maximize patient visibility?

    e. Provide for separation of functions?

    f. Allow for appropriate circulation linkage from waiting zone to preoperative holding and second-stage recovery zones (for family members)?

    g. *Provide for expansion?*

2. What external factors need to be considered in the location or design of the ambulatory surgery unit?

SPACE ALLOCATION

What physical facilities (including parking) should be made available to support the ambulatory surgery unit?

☐ *Exhibit 10-2 **Ambulatory Surgery Functional Program***

DEPARTMENT/PROGRAM DESCRIPTION

This hospital will provide facilities for scheduled ambulatory surgery. *The ambulatory surgery department will be a separated unit*—located within the hospital but not using inpatient surgical facilities. Existing hospital services will complement the ambulatory surgery department.

1. The ambulatory surgery program allows surgical patients to return home the same day as their surgery. No overnight hospital stay is required.

2. General, regional, and local anesthesia will be used.

3. It is anticipated that ambulatory surgery services will be available Monday through Friday between 7:00 A.M. and 4:00 P.M.

4. The surgery schedule will begin at approximately 7:30 A.M. and the last case will begin at approximately 1:30 P.M. for general anesthesia and 2:00 P.M. for local anesthesia.

5. Typically, surgical procedures of less than 1 hour will be permitted in the ambulatory surgery program. Depending on the surgery schedule, longer procedures may be scheduled if operating room time is available.

6. Any type of surgical procedure will be allowed, providing:

    a. It is not a known contaminated case

    b. Patients selected for surgery will be low risk as defined by ASA 1 and ASA 2 criteria. ASA physical status 3 patients will be accepted if their medical condition is under good control.

    c. It is safe on an ambulatory basis (recovery time less than 4 to 6 hours)

    d. Postoperative care does not require inpatient facilities

    e. A responsible person is available to take the patient home and appropriately monitor the patient's needs during the first postoperative day

    f. It is in accordance with the ambulatory surgical procedure list developed and approved by the medical staff's designated approval body

7. The anesthesiologist will have final authority for patient admission and discharge.

8. Patient scheduling, preoperative test results, history and physical, and registration will be completed in advance of surgery. Selected laboratory tests will be completed not more than 72 hours before surgery.

9. Emergency inpatient admission protocols will be in effect should transfer to inpatient status be necessary.
10. All processing, packaging, and sterilization functions will be performed in the central service department. Flash sterilization equipment will be available in the ambulatory surgery department. A case cart system will not be used.

WORKLOAD ANALYSIS

1. Projected ambulatory surgery:
   a. First year: 3500 procedures
   b. Second year: 4100 procedures
   c. Third year: 4500 procedures
2. Three operating rooms (including a cysto operating room), 5 preoperative holding beds, 5 primary PACU beds, and 12 secondary PACU beds will be needed to support projected volumes of service.
3. There should be 16 parking spaces allocated for ambulatory surgery unit patients and their families.

STAFFING AND ORGANIZATION

It is anticipated that

1. One anesthesiologist will be available and on-site during normal hours of operation.
2. As volumes dictate, three to four anesthesiologists or certified registered nurse anesthetists (CRNAs) will be available to staff the operating rooms.
3. As volumes dictate, three to four circulating nurses or surgery technicians will be available to staff the operating rooms. Scrub nurses will be used as necessary and in a cost-effective manner.
4. Five registered nurses will staff the PACU/holding area.
5. Total staffing, based on an approximate 9-hour working day:
   a. One to four anesthesiologists (or one anesthesiologist and three to four CRNAs if CRNAs are used)
   b. Three to four circulating nurse/surgery technicians
   c. Five PACU/holding area nurses

FUNCTIONAL CONSIDERATIONS

1. Patient flow will be as follows: admission/reception ⟶ waiting ⟶ change area/gowning ⟶ preoperative holding ⟶ operating room ⟶ primary PACU ⟶ second stage PACU ⟶ change area ⟶ discharge
2. Maximum nurse/patient visibility is desirable, allowing for reasonable patient privacy.
3. Family members will be allowed in the secondary recovery area.
4. There will be separate zones for waiting, preoperative and postoperative, and operating room areas.
5. Functions will be combined when feasible from a staffing, space, convenience, and economic viewpoint.
6. There will be minimum conflict of patient, family, staff, supply, and equipment traffic flow patterns.
7. Access to dedicated ambulatory surgery parking areas will be as convenient as possible.
8. Access to other hospital support departments will be as convenient as possible.

Exhibit 10-2 Continued

SPACE ALLOCATION BY DEPARTMENT AND SERVICE ELEMENT

ROOM ELEMENT	NO.	SIZE	TOTAL NSF	COMMENTS
Operating room areas				
General operating room	2	360	720	
Cystoscopic operating room	1		360	
Cysto control	1		40	
Cysto toilet	1		30	
Scrub area	2	24	48	
Stretcher alcove	3	17	51	
Soiled utility room	1		80	
Equipment storage	1		160	
Instrument storage	1		140	
Clean core	1		300	
Flash sterilization				
Solution warmer				
Cart area				
Circulation				
Storage				
Medication				
Linen	—		——	
Subtotal	14		1929	
Central staff support				
Nursing/control station	1		120	
Anesthesiology workroom/ storage	1		140	
Supervisor office (1)/file (1)†	1		100	
Anesthesiology office (1)/ file (1)	1		100	
Waiting room—family (16)	1		280	
Staff lounge (8)	1		160	
Locker—male	1		100	
Toilet/shower	1		60	
Locker—female	1		140	
Toilet/shower	1		80	
Janitor closet	1		30	
Subtotal	11		1310	
Patient holding area				
Change/locker area	4	40	160	
Children's playroom	1		60	
Preoperative holding room	5	70	350	
Primary PACU	5	80	400	
Second-stage PACU	12	70	840	
Clean supply/linen	1		80	
Soiled utility room	1		60	
Patient toilet	2	40	80	Disabled accessible
Janitor closet	1		40	
Subtotal	33		2170	
*Total operating room NSF**	15		1929	
G/N @ 1.6 DGSF				3086

ROOM ELEMENT	NO.	SIZE	TOTAL NSF	COMMENTS
Total central staff support and patient holding areas	44		3480	
G/N @ 1.4 DGSF				4872
Total NSF	59		5409	
Total DGSF				7958

*NSF (net square feet) is usable space within rooms. DGSF is departmental gross square feet. DGSF is NSF plus circulation space, wall thickness, and other nonusable space within departments/areas. DGSF represents the total amount of space needed to support the ambulatory surgery program and is expressed as a multiple of net square feet. If a satellite or freestanding facility is planned, for cost estimating purposes you need to consider the building gross square feet (BGSF). BGSF considers all the space within the perimeter of the structure itself.
†Figures in parentheses refer to capacity of persons or items.

☐ **Exhibit 10-3 Typical Room Elements and Net Square Footage Range**

ROOM ELEMENT	NSF RANGE*	
Operating Room Areas		
General operating room	320–400	
Minor operating room	240–280	
Cystoscopic operating room	280–360	
Cysto control	30–50	
Cysto toilet	30–40	
Scrub area	15–40	
Flash sterilization area	20–40	
Medications/supply storage/linen	60–160	
Equipment storage	120–300	
Instrument storage	60–240	
Soiled utility room	60–140	
Stretcher alcove	17	Per stretcher
Substerile room	80–140	
Control desk	40–80	
Anesthesia workroom/storage	100–180	
Janitor closet	30–60	
Central operating room staff support areas		
Nursing/control station	80–140	
Physician office	80–120	
Supervisor office	80–120	
Anesthesiology office	80–120	
Male staff lounge/locker/toilet	160–300	
Female staff lounge/locker/toilet	180–400	
Staff lounge	140–220	
Scheduling office	60–80	
Patient holding area		
Change/locker area	60–200	
Preoperative holding	60–100	Per patient
PACU (includes charting space)	80–120	Per patient
Second-stage postanesthesia care	70–120	Per patient
Induction room	80–100	Per patient
Examination room	80–100	

Exhibit 10-3   Continued

ROOM ELEMENT	NSF RANGE*	
Patient toilet	40–60	
Supply/storage/linen	80–200	
Soiled utility room	60–120	
Children playroom	60–120	
Pantry	60–100	
Administrative support areas		
Reception/switchboard/cashier/admitting	180–300	
Waiting room	120–500	
	or	
	12–15	Per person
Children's playroom	60–180	
Private consultation room	60–100	
Dining/vending area	100–300	
Public toilet	40–120	
Business office	60–80	Per work station
Medical records	60–80	Per work station
Administration	140–300	
Diagnostic services		
Laboratory	100–300	
Radiology	340–580	
Supportive services		
Central service	120–360	
Housekeeping	160–300	
Maintenance	160–400	
Pharmacy/gift shop	280–500	
Purchasing/storage	260–520	
Educational areas		
Patient/community education	160+	

*Depending on your particular situation, net square footage (NSF) by room element may fall outside of the NSF range.

Another important feature of Exhibit 10-3 is its obvious emphasis on including all the rooms needed to fit most ambulatory surgery programs. Most anesthesiologists and medical personnel are familiar only with the key areas used to support patient care or as individual work zones. It is important to recognize the different support-related rooms that allow patient care activities to occur (such as clean and soiled utility rooms, janitor closets, equipment storage, and offices).

What Are the Major Ambulatory Surgery Facility Design Features?

The space allocation section of the F/SP is organized into four major categories. The "zones" have differing purposes and design needs. They are discussed below.

Operating room (sterile) zone: This zone includes the operating rooms, substerile area, scrub, and operating room support spaces.

Patient holding zone: This area includes preoperative, primary PACU, second-stage PACU, induction room, nurse control, and support areas.

Central staff support zone: This zone includes the offices, locker rooms, equipment/instrument clean-up, and sterilizing areas.

Reception/waiting zone: This zone includes the reception, waiting, medical record, and business office areas.

The key functional relationships between these zones are as follows:

The operating room zone should be in an isolated area, away from major traffic patterns.

The holding areas should be situated between the reception/ waiting zone and the operating room zone and should be conveniently accessible to the latter.

The central staff support zone should be conveniently accessible to the holding areas and the operating room zone.

There should be two major entrances/exits from the ambulatory surgery unit. One is for the public—patients and families. The other is for staff, equipment, and supplies.

Within the individual zones, the following design criteria should be considered:

In the operating room zone:

The substerile room should be situated between the operating rooms. This area provides access to a sterile work zone from the operating rooms.

Scrub areas should be adjacent to, and ideally have visibility into, the operating rooms.

The stretcher alcoves, equipment storage, clean supply room, and sterile instrument room should be situated across the hall from, or adjacent to, the operating rooms.

The soiled utility room should be situated between the operating room zone (relatively close to the operating rooms) and the central support area (to facilitate easy transport of soiled instruments, supplies, linen, and trash).

A janitor closet should be situated conveniently in the operating room zone.

In the patient holding zone:

The primary and secondary PACUs should each have access to a nurse control station and to clean and soiled utility rooms.

Patient toilets accessible to disabled persons should be located within the secondary recovery area.

Family members should be allowed in the preoperative holding and second stage PACU. Therefore, these areas should be conveniently accessible to the family waiting room to minimize family traffic flow throughout the unit. Public toilets should be located nearby.

The induction room, if used, should be adjacent to the operating room zone but accessible to family members.

In the central staff support zone:

Offices should be located near the staff entrance to minimize visitor travel through the unit.

The staff lounge should be conveniently accessible to the PACU and the operating room zone to facilitate breaks between cases.

The soiled utility room should have the following functional relationships:

It should be situated between the operating room zone and the central support zone.

It should be adjacent to the pack make-up/sterilizer room (if part of the program).

The pack make-up/sterilizer room should be reasonably convenient to the sterile instrument room in the operating room zone.

In the reception/waiting zone:

The reception office should be situated between the public entrance and the waiting room (to facilitate visual control).

The waiting room should be situated near the reception office and the second-stage PACU.

The private consultation room should be situated between the waiting room and second-stage PACU.

The most important design feature of all the areas, however, is that they be flexible and easily expandable. Don't let the unit's design limit the opportunity for expansion. Always plan a unit for possible expansion.

Exhibits 10-4, 10-5, and 10-6 display the concepts and design of a freestanding unit. Each exhibit emphasizes a particular feature. Exhibit 10-4 diagrams the major zoning and access/egress patterns of the building. Exhibit 10-5 traces the movement of patients, visitors, staff, and matériels. Note how zoning and circulation minimize the conflict of patient, family, staff, and matériels traffic patterns. When reviewing your ambulatory surgery facility design, evaluate its traffic patterns and zoning. Attempt to maximize zoning and minimize the inappropriate mix of traffics. Exhibit 10-6 is a sample floor plan of a freestanding ambulatory surgery facility.

Interior Design

Only a qualified interior designer can help you make the best interior design decisions. All visual aspects of the ambulatory surgery facility must be pleasing and comfortable and present a nonclinical atmosphere. The colors and textures of floors, walls, and ceilings should exude a reasonable level of informality yet assure the patient that he or she is in a safe environment.

Colors are usually an important factor in soliciting a positive psychological response. Exhibit 10-7 lists general psychological responses by color. In planning your facility interiors, refer to this exhibit when working with your interior designer.

Equipment Planning

In the latter part of schematic design and during design development, the planning team considers the type of equipment to be used in the facility. At first, a generic equipment list is prepared on a room-by-room basis. As the

□ **Exhibit 10-4 Major Zoning and Room Elements of an Ambulatory Surgery Facility by Functional Area**

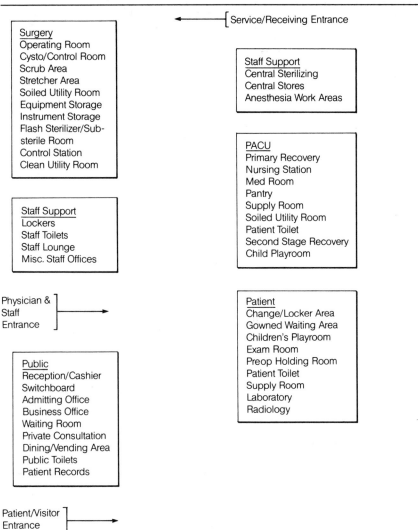

Surgery
Operating Room
Cysto/Control Room
Scrub Area
Stretcher Area
Soiled Utility Room
Equipment Storage
Instrument Storage
Flash Sterilizer/Sub-sterile Room
Control Station
Clean Utility Room

Staff Support
Lockers
Staff Toilets
Staff Lounge
Misc. Staff Offices

Physician &
Staff
Entrance

Public
Reception/Cashier
Switchboard
Admitting Office
Business Office
Waiting Room
Private Consultation
Dining/Vending Area
Public Toilets
Patient Records

Patient/Visitor
Entrance

Service/Receiving Entrance

Staff Support
Central Sterilizing
Central Stores
Anesthesia Work Areas

PACU
Primary Recovery
Nursing Station
Med Room
Pantry
Supply Room
Soiled Utility Room
Patient Toilet
Second Stage Recovery
Child Playroom

Patient
Change/Locker Area
Gowned Waiting Area
Children's Playroom
Exam Room
Preop Holding Room
Patient Toilet
Supply Room
Laboratory
Radiology

Ambulatory Surgery Facility Design (Exhibits 10-4 through 10-6): Space program by Leslie K. Leider, Ernst & Whinney, Minneapolis, Minnesota; Schematic drawing by Robert Stilwell, Flad & Associates, Milwaukee, Wisconsin, 1985

design process continues, specific equipment (by manufacturer and model) is selected.

Equipment is generally categorized into three groupings:

Group 1: This equipment is often referred to as *fixed equipment.* Equipment in this category is permanently affixed to the structure; it is not "plugged

☐   ***Exhibit 10-5   Internal Traffic Patterns of an Ambulatory Surgery Facility***

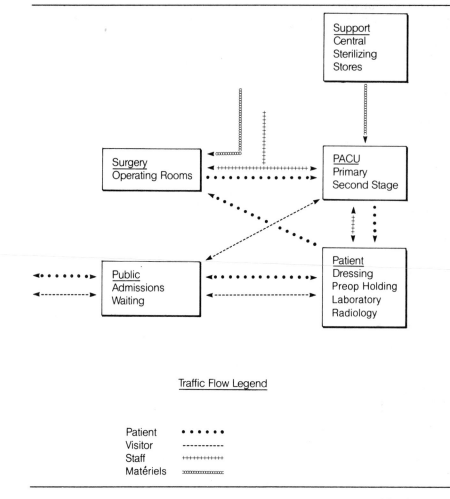

Traffic Flow Legend

Patient	• • • • •
Visitor	-----------
Staff	+++++++++
Matériels	xxxxxxxxxxx

in." Life expectancy is typically 10 years or more. Examples of group 1 items are sterilizers/washers, surgical lights, radiographic systems, communication systems, and built-in cabinetry.

Group 2: This equipment is movable and is usually referred to as *movable equipment*. Life expectancy is typically 5 years or more. Examples of group 2 equipment are stretchers, wheelchairs, surgical tables, laboratory equipment, refrigerators, and furniture.

Group 3: Equipment in this category consists typically of small, durable items, easily transported, and having a life expectancy of 3 years or more. Examples of items in this category are surgical instruments, diagnostic instruments, chart holders, reusable trays, and stainless steel jars and cannisters.

☐ **Exhibit 10-6 Prototype Floor Plan of a Freestanding Ambulatory Surgery Facility**

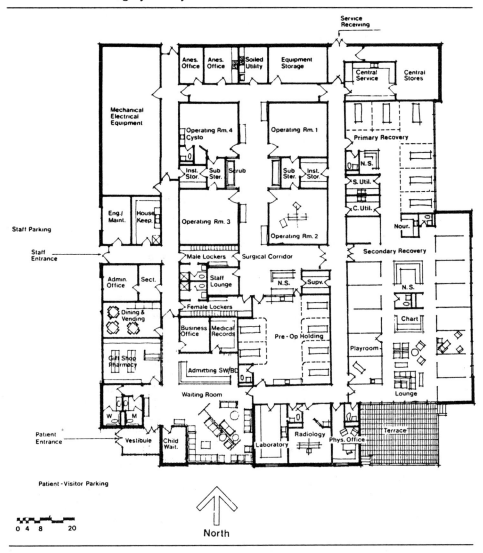

There are nine major steps in equipment planning. Each will be briefly discussed. Your consultant or architect can further detail each step.

  Programming: This is the assessment and documentation of equipment needs for the new facility.

  Inventory and evaluation of existing equipment: Existing equipment should be inventoried and evaluated for possible use in the new facility. Reusable equipment is documented, and a list of equipment to purchase is prepared (called a buy list).

☐ *Exhibit 10-7* **General Psychological Response by Color**

COLOR	GENERAL PSYCHOLOGICAL RESPONSE
Black	Despondent, ominous, powerful, strong
Blue	Peaceful, comfortable, contemplative, restful
Green	Calm, serene, quiet, refreshing
Orange	Lively, energetic, exuberant
Pastel colors	Neutral, nonrespondent, soothing
Purple	Dignified, mournful
Red	Stimulating, hot, active, happy
White	Cool, pure, clean
Yellow	Cheerful, inspiring, vital

Budget estimates: The buy list is priced out. This includes any costs associated with reinstallation of reusable equipment. Equipment budget estimates should be refined throughout the planning process.

Architectural planning and design: During the design development phase, equipment is laid out on the drawings on a room-by-room basis. At this stage, room function, workflow, and equipment use is carefully considered.

Purchased specifications: Buy-list equipment is categorized by who purchases and installs it (contractor or owner). Equipment specifications are developed to be used in asking for bids by vendors.

Bid evaluation and purchasing: Bids are received, reviewed, and awarded. A master equipment list is developed that includes the specific equipment, vendor, and final purchase price.

Coordination and scheduling of medical equipment delivery and installation: An equipment delivery and installation schedule is developed. Delays in equipment delivery and installation will adversely affect the opening and operation of the facility.

Coordination of staff orientation and training: Appropriate facility staff members need to be oriented and trained to use the equipment. This should occur 2 to 4 weeks before the opening of the facility to identify and resolve problem areas, if any exist.

Preventive maintenance programming: A preventive maintenance schedule of group 1 and 2 equipment should be developed. Improper, ill-timed, or avoided preventive equipment maintenance will result in unnecessary "down-time."

Project Cost Components

Most major capital expenditures are long-term commitments and are accompanied by an element of risk. Decisions about capital expenditures are among the most difficult an organization must face, particularly for the renovation or new construction of physical facilities. The project cost budget aids facility planning through identification of capital needs. A well-planned expenditures budget provides assurance that the equipment and facilities needed are available at the proper time, helps to define the risk involved, and facilitates the establishment of priorities for asset acquisition.

Ambulatory surgery facility project costs consist of

Construction: Costs related to the physical structure ("bricks and mortar"), either new construction or renovation, as well as group 1 equipment

Site preparation: Costs related to physically preparing the site for construction, including the cost of roadways and parking areas

Equipment: Group 2 and 3 equipment costs

Professional fees: Fees associated with architectural, consulting, engineering, and other professional services

Contingency: A sum of money dedicated to changes in the project scope or unexpected variations in costs

Financing: The cost of acquiring and using capital dollars during the planning and construction of a facility

Site acquisition: Costs associated with the purchase of land

Administrative: Costs for such items as soil tests, site survey, legal fees, and related expense that the owner is obliged to pay in connection with facility construction

Total project cost is typically 1.5 to 2 times the building cost. Hence, if the facility construction cost is estimated at $1 million, the total project cost may approximate $1.5 million to $2 million. Project costs can be controlled through reasonable and consistent review of all project phases.

Appropriately, most owners tend to concentrate on minimizing construction costs since these costs constitute the greatest portion of the budget. However, the planning team needs to use a *life-cycle cost analysis* when evaluating building design, systems, and equipment. A life-cycle cost analysis considers the capital and *operating* costs of an item over its expected lifetime. Although an item may have a lower capital cost than another similar item, it may be more expensive to operate over its lifetime. Hence, dollars may be saved initially but greater operating expenses may significantly offset the initial capital cost savings.

The quality of the final ambulatory surgery facility design is directly related to the quality of time and effort given to the facility planning process. Each ambulatory surgery program is unique; an existing program cannot be simply transferred to a new situation.

The planning process presented here provides the anesthesiologist with an important concept and approach to planning ambulatory surgery facilities. The next two sections in this chapter discuss key marketing and operational considerations for the ambulatory surgery program.

Suggested Readings

Berkoff MJ: Planning and designing ambulatory surgery facilities for hospitals. J Ambulatory Care Management 4(3):35–51, August 1981

Breen PC: Circular patient flow highlights facility expansion program (interview). Same Day Surg 4(4):49–50, April 1981

Burn JM: Facility design for outpatient surgery and anesthesia. Int Anesthesiol Clin 20(1):135, 1982

Grubb R, Andou G: Planning Ambulatory Surgery Facilities, St. Louis, CV Mosby, 1979

Leider LK, Mannix PM: Facilities planning outline. American Hospital Association Seminar on Ambulatory Surgery, October 1984

Medical Equipment Planning. Promotional brochure. Robert Douglass Associates, 1984

Moser DR: Steps in the Strategic Long Range Planning Process. Unpublished manuscript, Robert Douglass Associates, 1984

Reed WA, Dawson B: The ambulatory surgery facility. In Schultz RC (ed): Outpatient Surgery. Philadelphia, Lea & Febiger, 1979

Surgery/Day Surgery—Evaluation and Space Programming Methodology Series; Chi Systems. Published by Authority of the Minister of National Health and Welfare, November 1978

Tronnes HF: The Building Consultation Process. Unpublished manuscript: Robert Douglass Associates, 1984

Marketing: The Responsibility of All Managers

William A. Flexner, Dr.P.H.

Whether they be owners, medical directors, or simply specialists involved in the delivery of ambulatory surgical services, anesthesiologists have a major impact on the way the service is delivered to customers. Producing customer satisfaction is the key to building demand in a growing and successful ambulatory surgery business—whether this business is organized as an integrated surgical program using the main operating rooms, as a separated service contained within the walls of the hospital, or as a completely freestanding entity run separately from the traditional hospital business. This section focuses on the fundamental issues that should be considered by key decision makers in an ambulatory surgery setting as they attempt to build and maintain the demand for their services.

The rapid growth of ambulatory surgery during the early 1980s comes at a time when many of the factors that influence the delivery of health care services are changing. These factors include the

1. Escalating cost of health care
2. Increasing (or excess) supply of physicians and hospital beds
3. Growth and diversification of health care organizations
4. Changing interaction, even direct competition, between physicians and hospitals
5. The changing relationships among patients, physicians, health care organizations, and the payers of health care services

The purposes of this section are

1. To describe in what ways these factors are market forces shaping the position of the organization in the marketplace

This section is adapted from Flexner WA: Marketing. In Schenke R (ed): The Physician in Management. Falls Church, VA, The American Academy of Medical Directors, 1980

2. To explain how a marketing orientation differs from more traditional approaches to health care management
3. To identify how an anesthesiologist associated with an ambulatory surgery facility can use a marketing orientation to compete more effectively in this dynamic environment

The Changing Health Care Marketplace

A market consists of two or more individuals, each having something the other wants, and each wanting something the other has. A market transaction occurs when these individuals get together and make an exchange. Items that may be exchanged include, among others, goods, services, money, ideas, time, and attention. As long as both parties are satisfied with the transaction, each time they want to make an exchange of similar items, they will return to the marketplace and agree to transact another piece of business.

In the first part of this century, the health care marketplace was structured quite simply. It consisted primarily of solo-practice physicians providing direct services to patients in the physician's office or at the patient's home. When a patient's illness was serious enough, the physician arranged for hospitalization, often in the only hospital in town, but certainly in the hospital where the physician preferred to practice. When a physician felt the patient needed a specialist, the patient was referred along an established network. In response to the knowledge and skill of the physician ministering to their medical needs, patients trusted the physician's judgment and followed the advice that was given. Seldom in any of these transactions was the patient consulted about preferences in anything more than a perfunctory way; nor did the patient expect to be given options, since it was the physician who had the necessary knowledge.

In those days, there were almost always more patients than physicians or hospital beds; demand exceeded supply. Thus, there were few market incentives motivating the physician to be responsive to varying patient preferences. In essence, the physician's tasks in managing exchanges with the marketplace were as simple as the market structure: establish an office practice in primary care or a specialty and provide equal medical treatment for all patients, whether rich or poor (product/service design); affiliate with a hospital and with other specialist physicians (distribution channels); price the services at a usual and customary level—typically near what others were charging since overcharging based on what the market would bear was frowned on (pricing); and let word-of-mouth referrals from physicians and patients build the practice (promotion).

Good interpersonal relations, timeliness in meeting appointment schedules, provision of sufficient information about medical options, and other patient-oriented actions were entered into if the physician so desired; but these were not essentials of the practice. To be sure, physicians varied along a continuum from self-centeredness to patient-centeredness, but this variation had to do with the nature of the physician and not the demands placed on the physician by the marketplace.

For anesthesiologists, the market structure was even less of an issue. Since their work was largely confined to the operating rooms of the hospital, all that was needed were medical staff privileges and in some instances an appropriate contractual arrangement with the hospital. And, although responsiveness to other physicians and to patients was desirable, it was not always a requirement for maintaining either privileges or the contract.

The days of the uncomplicated market structure in health care are largely over. In their place, organizations, professionals, and consumers are all changing in ways that require new knowledge and skills to manage a successful health care program.

ALTERNATIVE SOURCES OF CARE

From the consumer's point of view, the cornerstone of the traditional medical practice was the solo-practice physician. Today, the cornerstone is rapidly becoming the health care organization—an aggregate of physicians, nurses, technicians, and administrators; illness programs; and health maintenance or wellness encounters. As the supply of physicians has increased to near equilibrium with demand in many parts of the United States and as the number of hospital beds has increased to produce a marked underutilization of facilities, the number of alternative organizational and professional sources of care has exploded. Hospitals are competing with each other by adjusting their service mix in terms of market demands; they are competing directly with physicians in the ambulatory care business through emergicenters, satellites, and ambulatory surgical centers. Physicians are competing with each other and with hospitals by joining together in small and large group practices that encompass single and multiple specialties, permit prepayment or fee-for-service reimbursement, and provide remuneration through a fixed salary or through various production-related schemes.

With this explosion of organizations, physicians and consumers have the opportunity to match their own preferences with the capabilities and practice style of the different organizational types. Because the opportunity for choice exists in this new market structure, many providers of care are now competing for a share of the same market. Health care organizations are trying to recruit and retain physicians, and physicians are attempting to attract and retain consumers.

In this context, however, it is neither the organization nor the physician who *decides* whether or not to compete. The simple fact that choices exist in the marketplace means that each provider is competing (maybe entirely passively) to be the source of care that is chosen. Thus, the external forces in the market are making competition among the alternative sources of care absolutely essential to survival and growth. To ignore this risks not responding adequately to the factors that influence these choices, which in turn may have an adverse effect on one's practice patterns and income.

CHANGING PHYSICIANS

One of the reasons health care organizations are changing so rapidly is that physicians are changing. First, there are more of them. It has been predicted that by 1990 there will be enough physicians in the United States for the size of the population. In some places there will be too many. This in itself forces physicians to assess more carefully where and how they want to practice. Furthermore, it permits the health care organization to recruit more carefully the kind of physician that will fit best into its type of business. Although anesthesiology is one specialty in which oversupply does not appear to be an immediate problem, this doesn't mean anesthesiologists can ignore marketing themselves, their specialty, or their practice patterns—where they currently administer (hospital) or will administer anesthesia (freestanding ambulatory facility or doctor's office).

Two other changes in physician behavior seem to be market driven. The trend away from inpatient to outpatient treatment reflects the high cost of inpatient care and the increasing share of that cost borne by the consumer through insurance copayments. It also results from increased coverage of outpatient services by third-party payers. Movement toward multiple hospital affiliations by physicians (and especially surgeons) results from their desire to obtain access to hospital resources when they are needed and from consumer demands for specific hospitals. The increase in the number of surgical procedures performed outside of the hospital (procedures performed in freestanding ambulatory surgery centers and office-based surgery) is one of the major responses to the issue of access for both physicians and consumers. By reducing the congestion around traditional operating room schedules caused by unpredicted complications and a higher concentration of technology, ambulatory surgery facilities can respond more rapidly and more specifically to physician preferences.

SELECTIVE CONSUMERS

The traditional health care consumer in today's market is much like the patient described above who trusts the physician's judgment and follows the advice that is given. Whereas the health care market structure has changed dramatically from the days of solo-practitioner dominance, patient behavior has changed more slowly. Only recently (within the past 10 years or so) has evidence begun to mount that compliant patients are becoming active consumers seeking choices among alternatives based on their own personal preferences. A number of reasons can be given for these changes:

Alternative organizational and professional sources of care provide the opportunity to make choices in the marketplace

High mobility, particularly into areas that have health maintenance organizations (HMOs), has turned some consumers toward health care organizations rather than personal physicians for their health needs

Skepticism toward large institutions, which developed during the Vietnam War (e.g., toward the military-industrial complex) is now spreading to other institutions, including health care providers

Self-care, health promotion, and personal wellness activities are becoming increasingly popular, with the result that many people are looking beyond the traditional, dependent patient-physician relationship for the care that is more in tune with their life-styles.

With consumers taking a more active role in the selection of health care resources, it is becoming important for management and physicians to understand what influences their choices. In addition to the availability of the necessary technology, consumers are also influenced by waiting time, patient procedures, interpersonal relations, costs, the facility ambiance, and important spatial aspects related to location. Although certain of these factors may be outside the control of the manager, others are within existing management responsibilities and resources.

OTHER CHANGES

Two other forces in the health care marketplace have become more active in influencing the nature and directions of the health system: (1) the federal government, through control of reimbursements, has begun to squeeze health care organizations in the areas of cost containment and service or facility expansion; and (2) private industry, through more careful attention to health-related fringe benefits, is stimulating the growth of alternatives to inpatient care and providing employees with incentives to purchase less expensive services. These forces will have a direct effect on how and where anesthesia services are provided.

In both of these cases, the primary motivating factor is cost. For the federal government, Medicare and Medicaid expenditures are consuming ever larger proportions of the federal health dollar. For private industry, the rising cost of health fringe benefits is cutting away at profits. The assumption is that by shifting the incentives for both health care organizations and the public, companies will bring overall costs down. Whether this will happen is not yet known. What is known, however, is that these changes are having an important effect on service diversification and consumer choice in the health care marketplace, and they provide a major opportunity for the entrepreneurial manager (whether anesthesiologist or other) to achieve a significant presence in the marketplace.

The health care system in the United States is changing rapidly. External to health care organizations, physicians, consumers, companies, and government are all paying closer attention to how the system benefits them. Internal to the health care organization, service diversification and physician behavior are having an effect (sometimes positive and sometimes negative) on the nature and direction of the organization. As anesthesiologists become more integrated in the decision making and management of "profit centers" or freestanding units (within or outside of the hospital building or campus) such as ambulatory surgery centers, it is important that they understand the market forces that influence their organizations and the methods that can be used to manage transactions with the environment. Marketing is a management orientation that has been shown in industry to be effective in matching the organization with its environment.

Fundamentals of Marketing

Management can be defined as the process of searching for opportunities and then capitalizing on them. An opportunity in this context is an activity or strategy that should be pursued to achieve the organization's higher purpose, but that is not being performed well at the current time. Managers should be constantly looking for opportunities to better achieve their purpose, whether that purpose is economic, technologic, or social.

In the field of ambulatory surgery, a "higher purpose" might be to provide cost-effective, convenient surgical services with arrival and departure all on the same day. In directing their efforts toward opportunities, managers of ambulatory surgery centers basically have three things to manage: dollar resources (financial management); the people who transform the dollar resources into products or services (human resource management); and the demand for products or services (marketing management).

Historically, health care managers who transformed the dollar resources and people into products or services often did so on the basis of what *they* felt the marketplace needed. Almost everything they produced would be purchased. Excess capacity or "inventory" was seldom seen or talked about. During these times, a production or "factory-out" orientation to management would usually work, since demand typically exceeded supply. However, in the new marketplace, there are greater supplies of beds and physicians than there is demand. Under these circumstances, management must identify and respond to the factors that motivate the demand for services. This is called demand management, and its purpose is to ensure that the manager's brand of ambulatory surgery is chosen over competitive brands. The search for opportunities that will influence the demand for ambulatory surgery services (e.g., "demand management") is called *marketing*. And the responsibility for marketing management is that of all managers in the ambulatory surgery facility. To the extent that anesthesiologists influence the design and delivery of ambulatory surgical services, they will be performing a marketing management function. Thus, it is important to understand what this function entails.

MARKETING IN BUSINESS AND INDUSTRY

In industry, marketing is the matching of a company's capabilities and resources with consumers' needs and wants. Needs and wants are the things that are important to consumers and that underlie their behavior. Because consumers' preferences and expectations vary, companies provide many different products and services. Through marketing, management can foster mutually beneficial exchanges between the organization and specified segments of the consumer population.

Defined in this way, marketing encompasses far more than the narrow activities of advertising or promotion in a traditional business setting. To be successful, a business or any other organization must satisfy various consumer segments by providing appropriately designed products or services. Simultaneously, it must achieve its internal goals and objectives, whether these be profit, market share, health outcomes, or patient compliance. To reach these goals, a business or an organization has to offer the right product or service at the right price and deliver it at the right time and place. When planning is oriented toward the marketplace, effective and efficient exchanges are more likely to take place between the business or organization and its consumers. Such an orientation, however, requires an understanding on the part of management as to how and why consumers choose specific products or services in the marketplace.

ANESTHESIOLOGISTS AS MARKETING MANAGERS

While anesthesiologists' roles may vary, each will be involved to some extent in managing exchanges between the ambulatory surgery center and people outside the center. For example:

> The anesthesiologist in the professional role has direct contact with the patient, the patient's family, and the surgeon on a case-by-case basis.
> The anesthesiologist in the medical director's role manages the policies and procedures that govern how the technical aspects of the services will be delivered.
> The anesthesiologist in the owner's role has an influence on the entire operation of the ambulatory surgery center.

Thus, in the context of their managerial roles, it is important that anesthesiologists understand the things they control in the marketing or exchange process. The concluding section focuses on the organization's marketing mix—the controllable variables the organization combines to satisfy the target market—and on the issues in managing the mix that will be particularly relevant to the anesthesiologist.

The Marketing Mix: Management's Controllable Variables

People respond to products offered in the marketplace on the basis of their perceptions of and preferences for four components of the offering:

1. The product itself
2. Its price
3. The place where the product can be purchased
4. The promotion or information made available about the product

In explaining these four components, one of the most common procedures in the ambulatory surgical setting—lesion excision—will be used as an example.

PRODUCT

The *product* in marketing can be described in two ways. From the organization's point of view, it is the thing that is produced—a specific object, a service, or something as difficult to grasp as an idea. In our example, this point of view would focus on the technical aspects of removing a lesion and the rules and procedures that are required to most efficiently get the consumer through the surgery and on the way home. From the consumer's viewpoint, the product is the benefit that is expected or has been received from having made the purchase—it is what the customer gets in the transaction. In removing a lesion, the consumer not only may expect a reduction in the fear of what the lesion could lead to, but also a satisfying, convenient, hassle-free process that minimizes the disruption in an otherwise healthy life. To get a better sense of the significance of this example, picture yourself in three different settings: a university teaching hospital, a general community hospital (integrated program), and a freestanding ambulatory surgery unit. Although the technical aspects of a lesion excision may all be the same, what the physician and patient actually receive may be entirely different from one setting to another:

Customer	University Hospital	Community Hospital	Freestanding Center
Physician consumer	Second class citizen; many people involved in service delivery	Hospital takes control through rules and procedures	Control of patient returned to physician; practice is enjoyed more
Patient consumer	Enters through clinic program; nonpersonal approach	Mingles with much sicker people; takes on sick role/more passive behavior	Self-image of intact, well human being; service designed for patient convenience

In marketing, the benefits that consumers look for refer to the functional, social, and psychological utilities or values that are received. Health care organizations produce specific services, but people usually only purchase aspects of those services—things as tangible as a prescription for medicine or as intangible as the way the staff both talks and listens to them. Consumers look at health services in very different ways, because they are attempting to derive different benefits from the services. In ambulatory surgery, physicians may be seeking a competent, efficient staff, as well as a location and surgical schedule that is most compatible with their existing practice; patients may be seeking a less threatening environment along with the convenience of going home that day. Increasingly, both physicians and patients are demanding less costly services.

Thus, it is incumbent on the manager (and particularly the anesthesiologist manager) to understand what aspects of the organization's services are being purchased, by whom and why, and then to translate these findings so that the producers of the services can maintain a high level of market responsiveness.

The range of services an organization produces is called the *product mix.* Most health care organizations have the capacity to produce a wide range of services. Whether they should do so is a different and strategically important question. In ambulatory surgery, the mix of specialties that will be invited to use the service should be based on the relative time and equipment needs of the surgeons, the compatibility of the specialties with each other, and the capacity of the facility to absorb the demand that each of the physicians in the specialties will generate.

In essence, the decision to include or eliminate a specialty should be made not only on the basis of what the ambulatory surgery center wants to do, but more importantly on what is feasible given a careful assessment of the potential market demand and the strength of existing ambulatory surgery services in the marketplace. Because the decision to alter the mix of services typically involves physicians, the anesthesiologists who have management responsibilities may be required to play a critical role in mediating the often almost automatic desire to add a new capability. In this rapidly changing environment, a more cautious approach to ensure that the organization's resources are being used as effectively as possible is absolutely essential. (Note: an anesthesiologist who does not have management responsibility would have no greater role in these decisions than other technical staff members; the key in this discussion is that the people who will be held accountable for the demand and profit-related outcomes are the ones who should be involved in making the decisions.)

To control the organization's service offerings, a periodic review of the strengths and weaknesses of each service in relation to competitors should be carried out. Given the physician's strong influence on this review process, anesthesiologists with management responsibilities should again be heavily involved. Translating environmental information into service decisions is not an easy task. Having this done only by nonphysician managers may create severe organizational strain. The addition of an anesthesiologist with management responsibilities may reduce this strain while speeding a change to a more market-oriented control of service offerings throughout the organization.

PRICE

The *price* variable in marketing is what is exchanged for the satisfaction or benefits derived from the purchase—it is what is given up to get what has been purchased. In health care there are at least two conceptually different price variables that management can control. The first is the direct monetary price. From the organization's point of view, the price charged has typically been based on a formula that related total costs to total revenue requirements. Although some differential pricing among services has occurred, this practice is not widespread, nor is it necessarily related to the effect that alternative price structures will have on demand for services. With the advent of DRGs, HMOs, and PPOs, this is changing rapidly, ambulatory surgery services being a major tool to develop strongly competitive prices based on reduced costs.

From the consumer's viewpoint, the monetary price is usually less than the full dollar charge because of insurance coverage. As long as the full price of health services has been buffered by third-party payers, the use of the price variable on a competitive basis has been minimal. This is also changing as patients are being required to pick up a higher percentage of the costs of their health care or to go to preselected sources of care based on packaged prices negotiated with volume purchasers of services. Nowhere is this reflected more clearly than with physicians beginning to demand lower prices in the ambulatory surgery setting in order to retain their own patients. In one midwest hospital, 20 physicians went to management to request lower prices for a number of procedures, including lesion excision. Implicit in their request was the statement that they couldn't compete because of current high prices. With the increased concern being expressed from many quarters about the escalating cost of health care, the managers of health care organizations are finding it necessary to begin using price creatively to cover losses due to underreimbursement and to attract particular segments of the population. In so doing, they are taking a new look at the cost factors of the services and making major changes in the organization, staffing, and incentives in the units.

The second concept of price in health care concerns the indirect costs to the consumer of getting into, through, and out of the health care setting. These costs include time, loss of control and dignity, hassle, opportunity costs, and actual loss of salary. All of these costs can be quite high in poorly managed organizations and can cause considerable resentment on the part of the consumer who expects to be able to transact the medical encounter as smoothly as possible. Consider the difference for the consumer coming to each of the following ambulatory surgical facilities for a lesion excision on the hand:

Center A: The patient is required to come to the ambulatory surgery facility the day before surgery for the same battery of tests required of inpatient surgical cases. On the day of surgery, a 6:30 A.M. arrival is required in order for the patient to be interviewed by the anesthesiologist between 7:00 A.M. and 7:30 A.M. (the only time available before the surgery schedule begins). Before going to the main operating room surgery suite, which is scheduled for 11:00 A.M., the patient is required to remove all clothes and slip on a "brief" and revealing gown. When taken to the operating room, the patient is mixed with more severe cases both in the preoperative holding area and in recovery. In postrecovery, back in the ambulatory surgery unit, the patient has to wait an extra hour for the physician to arrive to authorize discharge.

Center B: The patient comes to the ambulatory surgery center 2 hours before the surgery is scheduled. Any tests required before arrival have been handled through the physician's office. A carefully designed instruction pamphlet has been provided to the patient to describe the steps that will be involved in completing the surgery. Since the surgery is on the hand, the patient is only required to remove the shirt or blouse and slip into a covering gown. The anesthesiologist interviews the patient 30 minutes before the surgery to make certain that the procedure is understood and that the appropriate precautions are being taken based on the patient's history and current condition. Preop, surgery, and recovery are all completed in an atmosphere of relaxed confidence, along with other patients who are basically healthy. Checking out is a routine process that is initiated at the point when the patient is adequately recovered. An anesthesiologist is readily available for examining and discharging the patient.

These two examples place in clear distinction the difference between an ambulatory surgery facility that has been designed to serve the needs of the facility staff and one that has been designed to minimize the direct and indirect costs to the consumer. Whenever possible, the ambulatory surgery center should be designed according to the latter philosophy. In those instances when the direct and indirect costs cannot be minimized and consumers are given less than they want, the organization should have a set of procedures established to advise the consumer why these rules and procedures are necessary.

PLACE

The *place (or distribution channel)* variable focuses attention on the problems, functions, and institutions involved in getting producers and consumers together. From the consumer's point of view, the place variable consists of three dimensions: time, location, and ability to obtain possession of the product or service. Time in this context refers to the ease or difficulty of getting to the site where services are obtained. The importance of time will vary depending on the perceived need for speed (e.g., an emergency) and the value of time to the individual. Location refers to the physical and psychological environment in which the service is delivered. Some people won't go to central city locations because of fear of what might happen to them; others won't go to suburban locations because of the fear of getting lost. Some surgeons have refused to go across a parking lot to a new satellite ambulatory surgery center because it would take them too far away from the inpatient surgical suite and cases they are familiar with performing there. One hospital has considered providing "golf" carts to transport the physicians to the satellite location.[1] Thus, availability of transportation is another component that affects consumer demand for given services. Obtaining possession refers to the number of service providers one might go through to obtain the needed service. The lay and professional referral chains are important components of the distribution channel and ones that are used in very different ways from one consumer segment to another. Ambulatory surgery managers should pay careful attention to where the demand for services will originate. The referral chain should be carefully assessed all the way back to primary care physicians and the employers or payers of the potential patients.

From the organization's point of view, the place variable is typically a one-time, strategically important decision that will affect the kind of clients that will come for services. The reason for this is that the commitment to capital expenditures or long-term leases usually prevents the manager from making major changes in the place variable once the initial decision has been made. Thus, it is important to consider the trade-offs of narrowing the gap between the location of the organization and its physician consumers or its public consumers. Historically, the decision usually favored the physician consumers. More recently, with rapidly changing markets and the increasing supply of physicians, health care organizations are beginning to move toward public consumers. The development of satellite facilities, multiple-site group practices and HMOs, and freestanding ambulatory surgery facilities are examples of recent market-oriented place decisions.

PROMOTION

Promotion is the final variable that management controls in its interactions with the marketplace. Promotion is important since it represents the communication between the organization and its consumers aimed at facilitating exchanges. There are four different types of promotion that an organization can undertake. The most familiar type is *advertising,* which is a paid form of nonpersonal communication. The more commonly understood form of promotion in the health care industry is *publicity,* in which the organization actively seeks to get the attention of the public through news stories and other public service announcements. A third form of promotion that is typically not recognized for its importance is *personal selling*. This form represents all of the interpersonal communication that occurs between members of the organization and consumers. Many promotion programs are not successful because they address only the more visible tactic of advertising while ignoring the impact that personal selling has throughout the organization. Each of the staff members involved in an ambulatory surgery facility (e.g., aides, receptionists, nurses, physicians) should be aware of and practice effective communications skill with customers at all times. This starts with simple courtesy with patients, family and friends, physicians, and the physicians' office staff, whether over the telephone or in person. Simple courtesies are not forgotten by customers and can make a difference in whether the patients or physicians use the facility on a repeat basis.[2] The final type of promotion is *sales promotion*, which consists of the booklets, brochures, newsletters, office displays, and direct mailings that are used to enhance the relationship between the organization and consumers.

Using the example of a lesion excision, in what ways would promotion affect the demand for this procedure? First, direct personal communication (e.g., personal selling) would probably be the most important initial means of contact between the center and the segment of physicians that are most likely to perform this procedure. Letting these physicians and their office staff know how the unit is set up to respond to their needs, what the price will be to use the facility, and how easy it is for the patients to use the facility will all help to establish a positive relationship with the physicians. As noted above, direct personal selling is also an essential component of the job of each member of the staff of the facility whenever a physician, patient, or relatives and friends of patients are present at the center. And finally, a follow-up phone call the next day from the facility to patients to check on how they are doing will communicate an important sense of concern for the patients' well being. To complement the direct personal selling, several brochures and pamphlets (e.g., sales promotion materials) should be developed to explain (1) to the physician's office staff how to schedule the procedure, (2) to the consumer the steps to follow prior to and during the procedure, and (3) to the consumer the process of self-care that will be required after the procedure and how to obtain assistance or clarification of instructions after leaving the ambulatory surgery center. Given the nature of this procedure, there would be little need for either advertising or publicity. These would be appropriate as the center is attempting to build awareness of its existence as an alternative to inpatient surgery among the public and payers of services.

The significance of promotion is that without it consumers may not know the organization has a product on the market. If it is done poorly, consumers may be turned off; if it is done well, strong relationships can be established with consumers, which in turn produce loyalty to the organization and build a positive reputation in the community. As anesthesiologists take on greater management responsibilities, they will recognize the importance of this aspect of marketing and the need to coordinate the communication efforts with other management activities aimed at improving the health care organization's competitive position in the marketplace. Anesthesiologists can rarely stand alone. They and their practices are usually identified with the facility in which they deliver patient care. Therefore, placing an emphasis on the way the facility designs and delivers its services (e.g., marketing the facility) is equally important to the technical aspects of delivering technically correct anesthesiology and surgical services, and can have a positive effect on caseload and profitability.

Competing in the Ambulatory Surgery Market

The key to successfully competing in the ambulatory surgery market is to follow a three-step process: (1) understand your consumers' (e.g., physicians', patients', payers') needs and wants and how they go about deciding where to go for specific services; (2) design your services to respond to the consumers who represent the market segments most likely to use your type of service in the volume that you will need to successfully run the service; and (3) locate, price, and promote the services in such a way as to provide maximum attractiveness to the specific market segments that you are attempting to pull to your center.

If these steps are not followed either formally or at least intuitively, market failures may occur. These failures are likely to be caused by one of four different actions:

1. Treating the market as undifferentiated and assuming that all consumers behave basically the same: all consumers are not the same and they don't want the same thing. The task of the ambulatory surgery manager is to understand how various consumers differ and then to respond effectively to these differences.
2. Developing programs that competitors have without understanding the potential demand remaining in the market: for any product or service, demand is limited. Clearly, there is growth in the ambulatory surgery area. But this does not mean that every organization can successfully enter that marketplace and grow. One must carefully assess the strength of competitors and the potential demand remaining in the market before going head to head with them.
3. Designing programs as you think they should be designed, rather than the way the consumer wants them: because demand has exceeded supply for many years in the health care system, professionals have become accustomed to determining how and what the consumer will get from the organization. With the excess supply in the current marketplace, this will no longer work effectively.
4. Thinking that public relations, communications, and marketing will create demand: if the demand is not there, no amount of communications will get people to come and use your services. The demand has got to be there in one form or another, and it is essential for the ambulatory surgery manager to understand where the demand is and how best to attract it.

References

1. Berkowitz EN: Marketing ambulatory surgery centers: Planning considerations and demand analysis. In Burns LA (ed): Ambulatory Surgery: Developing and Managing Successful Programs. Germantown MD, Aspen Systems Corporation, 1980

2. Winston WJ: "Internal marketing" is important part of SDS unit's overall plan. Same Day Surg 8(5):62, 1984

Suggested Readings

Berkowitz EN, Flexner WA: The marketing audit: A tool for health services organizations. Health Care Management Review 3(4):51–57, 1978
Clarke RN, Shyavitz L: Marketing information and market research—valuable tools for managers. Health Care Management Review 6(1):73–77, 1981
Flexner WA: Effective Marketing Strategies That Work. Successful Management of Ambulatory Surgery Programs. Atlanta, American Health Consultants, 1981
Flexner WA, Berkowitz EN: Marketing research in health services planning: A model. Public Health Rep 94(6):503–513, 1979
Hughes GD: Marketing Management: A Planning Approach. Reading, MA, Addison-Wesley, 1978
Kotler PE, Clarke RN: Marketing for Health Care Organizations. Englewood Cliffs, NJ, Prentice-Hall, 1985

Fundamentals for Success

Anne Frey Dean, R.N., B.S.N.

Organization

Lack of communication is the root of all (or at least most) evil. Poor communication can be the cause of a failed relationship or business venture. An ambulatory surgery facility is not immune to this problem.

Effective communication among team members takes on even more importance in an ambulatory surgery facility than in a traditional hospital setting. The facility is smaller in size, all patients are there for surgery (resulting in higher stress levels), and almost all of the staff makes contact with the patient. Patients of the 1980s want information about their treatment; communicating information effectively among patients, staff, and physician is good practice from the standpoints of health care and marketing.[13]

When interviewed, physician-owners of surgery centers cited many different reasons for leaving the hospital environment. But all these reasons referred back to communications problems. Lack of control over their patients; too much bureaucracy, red tape, and paperwork; lack of follow-through on problems; and lack of interest in the physicians' or ambulatory patients' problems are all complaints centering on defects in communication channels. The hospital's organizational chart must be designed not only to identify but also to simplify channels of communication. Flexibility and quick response is essential to the ambulatory surgery facility if it is to retain satisfied patients and physicians.

ORGANIZATIONAL STRUCTURE

In most hospital-oriented health care facilities the traditional organizational structure is a pyramid with five levels of management hierarchy (Fig. 10-1). The

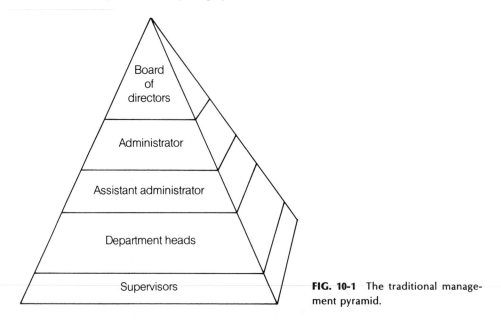

FIG. 10-1 The traditional management pyramid.

top three levels set policies and goals, plan strategy to effect the policies and obtain the goals, and assume the responsibility for implementing the plans. The department director serves as the middle manager who has direct responsibility for the functioning of the unit. Reporting to the department directors are area chiefs (charge nurses) who are responsible for the day-to-day functioning of their areas.[6] Reporting and communication channels assume an upward-downward configuration . . . as weighty as the pyramid design in Figure 10-1, and as cumbersome. In examining this design, one cannot help but notice the distinct divisions depicted much like fences dividing lines of authority. Such fences defeat the team concept of health care delivery, and as they relate to a hospital-affiliated ambulatory surgery facility depict a common but weighty problem.

Regardless of the format used by a facility, the organization's structure should be easy to implement, simple to use, understood by the staff, and able to facilitate the team concept.

Ambulatory surgery organizational charts that duplicate the structure found in hospitals will reflect many of their problems, such as "poor morale, decreased productivity, poor communication, lack of concern, and, ultimately, a lack of progress in creative thinking."[11] In the ambulatory surgery center, it is essential to promote the concept of team management. Organizational charts must be simplified to incorporate this concept. The fewer persons involved, the less cumbersome are communication channels. Don't become management heavy. A football team composed of all captains is not a team.

THE TEAM CONCEPT

Let's look at the ambulatory surgery health care team. The patient would be the captain. He or she has called the plays by electing to have ambulatory surgery and keeping his or her surgical appointment. The anesthesiologist (coach) evaluates the patient and procedure and decides on appropriate anesthesia. The surgeon (quarterback) picks up the ball and runs with it (quickly, we hope) to the goal. The surgery center staff (blocking backs) lead the way by preventing problems (regarding scheduling, interviewing and data collection, equipment and supplies, or staffing) that might interfere with attaining the goal. The field of play is the surgery center. The configuration this team assumes in planning, implementing, and evaluating patient care is the circle of the team huddle.

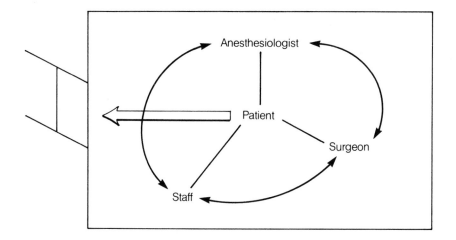

All team members go toward one goal—a satisfactory ambulatory surgery experience.

The area of most concern in a physician-owned or -managed facility is the question of where the duties and responsibilities of the administration and those of the physician-owner or director merge, separate, or diversify? Identifying these roles may be a more difficult political task. Separating them may be an even greater challenge. Enforcing and adhering to the separate role descriptions and responsibilities is essential if the members are to work as a team. To do otherwise creates confusion, reduces morale, and decreases the quality of health care services provided. Ultimately, fewer goals are attained. Frequently, the temptation to call individual plays becomes too much for many physician-owners or medical directors who may attempt to assume the administrator or nurse's role. This temptation may manifest itself in many forms, from counseling a staff nurse, arbitrarily changing policies, or rearranging furniture and equipment. Operational functions such as staffing, counseling, patient flow, and nursing procedures should be left to the persons hired to manage those functions. Problems in these areas should be noted for discussion in future management meetings. Management must appear as a unified team if the facility is to be successful. Theodore Roosevelt once said that the "best executive is one who has sense enough to pick good men for the job and self-restraint enough to keep from meddling while they do it."

THE MEDICAL DIRECTOR
Regardless of any problems the administrator and medical director may discover in defining their relationship, the advantages of having an on-site medical

director far outweigh the disadvantages. In a hospital-affiliated program, the medical director is frequently the chief of anesthesiology services. Since the medical director conducts or supervises the preanesthesia assessment, his or her knowledge and expertise are invaluable in determining the surgeon's compliance to patient selection criteria. He or she frequently will uncover valuable information pertinent to the anesthetic-surgical plan.

As an impartial member of the team, the medical director's professional opinion is most valuable in such areas as meeting selection criteria, rescheduling a patient, or even cancelling the case altogether. The medical director's knowledge of the philosophy and the daily functioning of the facility is valuable in this role as he or she assumes the capacity of advisor over front-line manager.

Who is going to be the medical director of the unit? This person will have the responsibility for:

1. Preoperative risk evaluation, both surgical and anesthetic
2. Dealing with all of the surgical specialties fairly, without being accused of favoring his or her own speciality
3. Examining and signing patients out of the facility
4. Providing continuity of care for patients by being available in the facility until the last patient has been discharged[12]

The medical director's assumption of these duties relieves the executive director from the "policing" role and permits physicians to consult together. An anesthesiologist would easily qualify in all areas. Having an anesthesiologist as medical director is a special bonus; it guarantees the availability of this important specialist. As part of the team, the anesthesiologist will be most eager to identify educational deficiencies and provide inservice education programs. His or her knowledge and experience are immeasureable in assessing patient problems and in performing discharge assessments.

NURSING STAFF

The nursing staff selected for the ambulatory surgery center must have a different orientation from that of traditional hospital-oriented nurses. Staff members must be selected for their people orientation. The person applying for a position in a strongly patient-centered, family-oriented unit who never mentions the patient during the interview would probably be incompatible with the ambulatory work setting.

Frequently, nurses coming from a strong inpatient hospital background have not been oriented to outpatient care. The imbalance between attention given to inpatients and that given to outpatients has forced many surgeons to admit potential ambulatory surgery patients in order for them to receive first-class operating room treatment. In hospitals that are established for inpatient care, staff members tend to place greater emphasis on the sick patient.[5] As a result, the ambulatory surgery patient may suffer from skillful neglect as the staff rushes to meet the acute needs of the sick. In comparison, the needs of a well patient may not seem as important. There has been so much emphasis placed on care of the sick that few staff members are truly knowledgeable about the special needs to be met in caring for the well patient.

THE PATIENT

The ambulatory surgery patient has health range needs that are different from the acutely or chronically ill patient; he or she

1. Is independent, maintains himself or herself well within the community setting, and wishes to do so
2. Desires to return to a social environment in as short a period of time as possible with the least disruption as can be attained
3. Does not view himself or herself as being sick
4. Suffers ambivalency, for by coming to the hospital, the ambulatory surgery patient is inclined to assume the sick role arbitrarily

The hospital environment tends to validate this patient's complaint as an illness. *Sick people do not care for themselves:* rather, they assume a *passive* role. The ambulatory surgical patient is more desirous of maintaining an *active* role in his or her own health care, and thereby maintain control over therapy. These are very basic—but essential—needs.

When planning the care of the sick hospitalized patient, it seems fairly simple to identify needs, for they center on the illness. Even when applying biopsychosocial delineations, the focus remains primarily on the illness. In the ambulatory surgery environment, wellness is promoted. The patient enters as a normal person with a problem. As such, he or she ambulates and in some instances may even continue this activity all the way through the operating room portion of care. The whole philosophy of ambulatory care promotes the patient's self-image as an otherwise healthy, intact, socially active person with special needs. Care is designed around promoting individualized attention, and, as such, flexibility in standing procedures is the rule.

Health care professionals, like all people, tend to develop routines that become carved in stone. These, then, become rigid rituals irrespective of the needs of the individual patients. There seems to be no impetus to change approaches used for years by both physicians and patients. If the approach to patients that was taught in nursing or medical schools has worked, there seems to be a resistance to changing it. The problem, however, is that the approach taught in the last three decades has centered on the sick patient; as a result, when hospital oriented medical persons enter the ambulatory environment, they take the same approach with the patients, to the potential detriment of all concerned. This standard approach can be clearly recognized in the following example:

> Patients enter the ambulatory surgery facility for their surgical appointments as scheduled, and are greeted warmly by the preop nurse. After advising the responsible persons accompanying the patients to remain in the waiting room, the nurse accompanies the *patients* to their assigned changing areas and has them change into a *patient* hospital gown. The nurse has the patient get in bed, starts appropriate intravenous lines, and puts up the side rails on the *stretchers.* Skin preps may be performed at this time, followed by preoperative medication. The patients' responsible persons enter, visit, and *leave* to remain in the *waiting room.* The patients are pushed to the operating room on their stretchers. After surgery, they may be given ice chips before leaving the facility in a wheelchair.

With this approach, the only difference separating the inpatient preoperative routine from the outpatient is that the patient comes into the facility on the morning of surgery and hopefully goes home the same day.

Examine the words used in the example above:

Patients
Waiting room
Hospital gown
Put to bed
Stretcher

They are all connected with and identified with hospitals and sick people. They hardly promote an image of the patients as well people. Yet, in just a few hours these patients will be returned to home care and be responsible for effecting their own transition back to full activity.

Now, examine the approach used when the staff has internalized the ambulatory health care philosophy of promoting wellness:

> The surgical *guests* enter the ambulatory surgery facility and are warmly greeted by the staff. After collecting the necessary last-minute information, the guests and their responsible persons are escorted to the preoperative dressing area where the nurse shows them the *scrub suit or pajamas*, located in the cubicle, that will need to be put on. The nurse remains nearby if assistance in changing is needed. Family members frequently enjoy being of help in this activity. In some instances, changing clothes may not be necessary. This is dependent on the type of procedure and location of the incision site. After determining the guest's readiness, the nurse returns and determines the need for venous access. If such a need is indicated, a prn adapter is started in the hand, covered with a clear plastic adhesive strip (tape covers wounds). The guest's responsible person may stay in attendance. This option is offered prior to the procedure. Since no premedication will be given, the surgical guest relaxes in a comfortable recliner. Skin preps or marking can be accomplished quite comfortably here. With appropriate equipment this area can be used for regional block induction. With no premedication, the guest will ambulate to the operating room accompanied by the circulating nurse. After surgery (depending on type of anesthesia), the guest may ambulate or be transported to the postanesthesia care unit (PACU). At an appropriate time light nourishment will be given while the patient is seated in another recliner. Upon discharge, the nurse will escort the guest and responsible person to their car.

In both models, the patients received "good care." In the second example, however, the nurse promoted the guest's image of wellness while recognizing the role of the responsible person in the guest's health care. In assessing the otherwise healthy patient, the nurse must be able to determine the patient's level of self-sufficiency accurately. This skill comes from learned knowledge and experience.

The temptation to rotate staff from other hospital areas to the ambulatory surgery area is great. Such practices may seem cost effective and efficient initially; however, rotating staff members often do not possess the necessary philosophy, knowledge, or skills to provide quality ambulatory care. Ambulatory surgery nurses are a special breed committed to promoting individualized, quality health care to the outpatient at a reduced cost with the least emotional, psychological and physical trauma possible. The ambulatory nurse team member must be aware of the cost of health care, and stringent cost containment measures should be enforced among staff members.

Ambulatory surgery nurses must be aware of their role in marketing to both the physician and the patient. They promote the image of themselves and their fellow staff members as people pleasers. These members are especially interested in cooperating and assisting at each step of the plan to attain the common goal of a satisfactory ambulatory surgery experience for all involved parties. As such, these nurses approach their jobs as eager agents in data collection, assessment, preparation, and planning. As team members, they recognize the importance of their functions being accomplished promptly in providing consumer satisfaction. Tact and diplomacy are innate characteristics. Surgeons should find their visits to the facility productive and satisfying. Highly skilled, productive staff members should exhibit motivation, initiative, and enthusiasm in a positively spirited environment. Such enthusiasm and positive interest filters down from the top (i.e., the nursing director).

THE NURSING DIRECTOR

In choosing a nursing director, physicians and administrators frequently choose a "good nurse" from among the staff nurses with whom they have worked. In these instances an injustice may be done to the physician, the nurse, and the facility, since being a good nurse implies skill in the technical field and not, necessarily, in management. Often, the director may not be a nurse at all, but a person especially skilled in business, finance, or office management. Whatever the person's background, it should reflect a mixture of all of the above as well as a strong ability and interest in marketing. This skill should cover not only developing advertising copy, brochures, physician letters, flyers, and newsletters, but also the ability to call on doctors' offices and communicate effectively with them and their staffs.

The enthusiasm generated can be felt and appreciated by those fortunate enough to enter its bright circle. It is contagious and may well be among the most positive attributes a manager possesses. Enthusiasm springs from enjoyment. That enjoyment springs from gaining pleasure from one's commitments. The manager who is able to emit enthusiasm for the ambulatory surgery facility as well as the concept of ambulatory health care will find staff and physicians alike responding to that enthusiasm, basking in its pleasure and passing it on to other patients, physicians, staff members, and community representatives.

It is a wise manager who includes staff members in the management of the facility and who becomes involved in it also. This may mean digging in side by side with the staff, working together to set up matériels management programs, develop policies and staffing patterns, or on a particular day even make coffee, escort patients, or provide staff relief. Such occasional involvement will do much to promote a strong sense of comraderie while serving to identify rough spots in the system to the manager. While delegating is important, shared responsibility is a must. However, managers must be aware that their primary function is to manage the facility overall—not to staff it. Sharing staff duties should be reserved for occasional shortages; as a steady diet, it affects the manager's primary responsibility, and by so doing leaves the manager position temporarily vacant.

The key to good management will always lie in effective communication, both overt and covert. The effective manager makes it a point to visit each area of the facility frequently, even if it means donning scrubs to mingle with staff and physicians. Being interested in individual staff members is essential.

Remembering particular aspects of each member's life reflects this concern and interest. Developing thorough orientation and evaluation programs is a part of effective management. Holding frequent staff meetings, promoting open discussion, soliciting opinions and concerns, responding with appropriate explanations or changes, sharing budget restrictions and plans, and soliciting staff participation in every phase of operation promotes mutual interest and satisfaction. Being involved with the staff is essential to the promotion of harmony and participation; however, the wise manager also knows it is essential to keep a certain distance in order to maintain objectivity in evaluating staff and in assessing the large picture. Becoming close friends with individual staff members will cause problems detrimental to the overall functioning of the facility. Wise managers will seek their own counsel while maintaining the confidentiality of those who confide in them. The temptation to become a pal is great, but will lead to graying of the lines of authority. It's essential for management to maintain a professional image in order to be a role model for the staff.

Policies and Procedures

Developing policies and procedures seems to be one of the most overwhelming tasks facing the management team. These written guidelines must be clear, concise, practical, and applicable to the day-to-day functioning of the facility. Do not establish policies you do not or cannot follow. Rewrite them when needed, to reflect what you are doing. Policies must be established for all operational aspects, while goals, objectives, and philosophies must be written in such a manner as to reflect the true spirit desired by the governing body. Policies must cover

    Medical staff credentialing
    Committees required
    Quality assurance programs, safety, and risk management plans
    Infection control measures
    Emergency transfer or admission arrangements
    Consultant use and criteria for selection
    Job descriptions
    Medical/surgical staff privileges
    Anesthesia services
    Pathology services
    Radiology services
    Medical direction
    Hours of operation
    Scheduling procedures
    Preadmission criteria
    Preoperative and postoperative contact with patients
    Distribution of clothing and valuables
    Responsible person requirements
    Acceptable procedures and anesthetic agents
    Laboratory requirements
    Inservice education plans

The explicit guidelines provided by credentialing bodies as well as organizations responsible for developing recommended standards and codes aid greatly in developing policies and procedures for accreditation and daily operations. Such guidelines issue from

The Accreditation Association for Ambulatory Health Care
The Joint Commission on Accreditation of Hospitals
The Association of Operating Room Nurses
The Centers for Disease Control

These groups set optimal, achievable standards designed to provide quality patient care. Developing policies designed to identify and implement these standards of recommended practices will prevent hasty last-minute rewrites prior to credentialing visits. Additional policies designed to meet standards would include

A statement on patients' rights
Governance/organizational structure
Medical records practice and administration
Facility environmental control
A survey process for evaluation of services

Combined with the standards required to meet state licensure codes and certification, these policies do much to ensure that the quality of care rendered at the facility will be optimal, thus providing a safe environment for patients, physicians, and staff members alike.

It is not enough merely to develop an impressive-looking policy and procedure manual. Each staff member, including the medical director, should read the manual prior to assuming active duty. This responsibility should be a routine part of the basic orientation program. Additions or changes should be announced at regular staff meetings. Typewritten copy should be hung on the communication board for at least 2 weeks in order for everyone to become familiar with the new policy. Updating should be an ongoing process. Time should be set aside on a regular basis to review sections of the manual for accuracy and applicability (are you following it? can you follow it?). This will ensure that the manual is an active part of the functioning of the facility. Such a practice also keeps persons knowledgeable about the governing policies while eliminating the formidable task of last-minute review prior to credentialing visits.

Any policy should be open enough to permit growth and individual flexibility in carrying it out while strict enough to provide the necessary governance. Do not try to establish a policy for everything.

Forms and Records

The basic concept of ambulatory health care incorporates the KISS principle (keep it simple, stupid). Implementation of this principle can be easily accomplished through consolidation and streamlining of existing forms. In the hospital environment, this requires educating the medical records committee to the need for redesigning existing forms and omitting others that are specific to inpatients. In the hospital outpatient department it is not uncommon to find at least 22 forms on the patient's chart. This number can effectively be reduced to a reasonable number (5–9) by

> Consolidating and streamlining existing forms
> Eliminating unnecessary forms
> Using preprinted orders and instructions designed with space for additional, individualized notes
> Using both the front and back of forms
> Using dictation stations to replace written records

Nurses may complain of not having enough space to write, but if the forms are well designed, a mere check in the appropriate space will adequately document care.

Physicians enjoy the streamlined chart, since its efficiency saves valuable time. The physician's signature may be required on only a few of the forms. Preprinted instructions and orders can be individually checked for appropriateness and signed.[10] Physicians' preference cards should always be used and should include the preference of individual anesthesiologists on cards stating use of intravenous access and other preferences. An ambulatory surgery facility should reduce paperwork and bureaucratic red tape while promoting nurse initiative.

Equipment

Purchasing equipment can be somewhat like purchasing a surprise gift—unless selected carefully, the equipment can end up in the back of the closet just like last year's Christmas tie.

Equipment lists should be developed from the accepted procedures to be performed at the facility, but individualized to the personal requirements of the physicians in the area. Do not try to second-guess the items that will be needed, the style, or the manufacturer. If the manager or director of nursing is from one of the area hospitals, a common mistake is to assume that the same equipment will be acceptable at the ambulatory facility to all the physicians. Whether this is true or not depends on the scope of the physician draw area. Will the facilities physician staff be composed only of physicians with privileges at that particular hospital, or will other physicians in the area also be using the facility? This must be determined in order to ensure acceptability of selected equipment.

In order to provide knowledgeable data for the physician, collect information about styles, sizes, costs, probable discounts, and service and maintenance agreements. All this information should be considered in selecting equipment as well as the return on investment determined by use and overhead. Solicit a commitment from physicians prior to the purchase. Will the item keep you abreast of hospital activity, or maybe even provide a competitive edge over the other facilities in town? Is it state of the art or is it about to be replaced by something newer and better (and maybe less expensive)?

Before the facility opens, make use of an ad hoc or advisory committee composed of physicians representing all specialities planning to use the facility. This group can assist in effectively choosing between similar items, thus taking the burden of selecting controversial items away from the management—a wise political move.

As equipment comes in, it should be checked and inventoried. Maintenance programs should be planned in the initial phase. Warranties and instruction manuals should be filed in a handy manual accessible to all. One person should assume responsibility for this.

The astute manager will scurry to stay abreast of changing trends in order to determine possible future equipment needs. Being receptive enough to a physician's request for a new item to explore and study the possibility of procurement will gain many friends for the facility. This means faithful scanning of equipment ads and articles in professional journals and a keen interest in progressive new trends—another basic concept of ambulatory surgery centers.

Matériels Management

Matériels management refers to the overall use and control of supplies and equipment within the facility. An active matériels management and inventory control program is the financial backbone of a successful ambulatory surgery program and should be approached with determination and forceful consistency. A lack of understanding results from a lack of education in the financial process of matériels management. Cost containment and cost reduction are essential for the financial survival of ambulatory care. It will work if staff members assume an active role in the budgeting process and are cognizant of line item costs, overhead expenses, profit margins, and procedure fees. Share this information with physician users.

Monthly budget and inventory review meetings enhance compliance and promote enthusiasm for the program among staff members who recognize their important role in making the program financially successful.

Staff members should always be actively involved in the inventory control program, providing valuable input about specific items needed and those best suited to meet the objectives of the facility. One of the staff members should be recognized as the official matériels manager. This person would be responsible for all the ordering and organization of supplies in order to provide a smooth flow of matériels.

Determine a specific ordering day. Identify the primary receiving day (and clerk). Keep shelves stocked, but not overstocked. The phrase "A place for everything, and everything in its place" can effectively be fulfilled with space-saver shelves on tracks, wall-hung bins, and even rectangular laundry baskets to store loose supplies in bulk. Each shelf and bin should be labeled with the item, vendor, and quantity stocked. Frequent stock reviews will identify little-used items that may be omitted in order to add a new one. Keeping inventory low but adequate keeps costs down.

In order to curtail costs, inventory and overhead must be determined. Set realistic goals. Analyze procedure costs. Determine the break-even point and push for it, keeping the original goals in mind. With staff members especially cognizant of these factors, promote cost-containment and reduction ideas— even the smallest. Turn lights and suction off when not in use. Monitor environmental temperatures. Practice stringent use of physician preference cards. Do not overstock rooms or oversupply cases. Do not horde supplies. Do not open supplies unless you are certain of their being used.

Assess staffing needs. Do not overstaff or understaff. Develop a prn pool and an active volunteer program to assist professional staff members. These persons will be of great assistance on especially busy days. Each area should be concisely planned and staffed for the most efficient use. Such organization and planning of duties will go far to decrease overtime and staffing budgets. Part-time pool staff should be selected by the same stringent criteria used for full-time employees. Volunteer and prn services should reflect the personalized, people-oriented philosophy of the facility. These persons should also be motivated enough to stay abreast of policy changes or additions and interested enough to participate in pertinent inservice programs.

Budgeting should, of course, reflect facility use and growth for staffing purposes. The initial budget may be difficult to determine; however, knowledge of area health patterns will provide a guide to facility use. For example, in the Sun Belt, January, February, and March are heavy tourist months for retired persons who may choose to have surgical procedures performed during this time. Hence, use may increase during this period. On the other hand, school vacations usually result in increases in pediatric and adolescent surgery.

Plan your growth rate realistically. Can you add ten cases per month or one to three new physicians per month? What methods will you use to solicit their participation? Will they be effective? To what extent? Is the growth rate dependent on service expansion requiring major or minor equipment purchases? Have these been included in the annual budget? For example, are there plans to expand orthopedics to include arthroscopy and radiology services?

Scheduling

One of the primary advantages of a separated, satellite, or freestanding ambulatory surgery facility is the flexibility afforded in scheduling procedures. This is a prime asset, especially when it comes to marketing, since most physicians list "problems with scheduling" as one of their primary problems with hospital operating rooms. The ambulatory surgery facilities' scheduling staff should exhibit an eagerness to please, cooperate, and accommodate when scheduling procedures through the physician or his or her office staff. Block scheduling should be promoted in the initial phase of the marketing and development program. Such a service becomes highly feasible and profitable if the facility is designed efficiently to incorporate alternate treatment or procedure rooms, and if equipment is designed to be moveable. Developing minor procedure rooms for local lumps and bumps frees up valuable sterile operating room space and increases flexibility. In developing block scheduling policies, determine how this service can be most effective and, especially, how long a block of time will be held for a specific surgeon or group. Resistance in the medical community to the idea may be high initially, if the concept is not currently being practiced in other facilities. Many surgeons feel it is more efficient for them to use two rooms in a hospital operating suite on their surgery day. They perform major procedures in one room and minor in the other, alternating between the two. However, grouping all their outpatient cases on one day in a block at the ambulatory surgery unit will enable them more time for major inpatient procedures while increasing patient satisfaction. The ambulatory surgery staff recognizes a time savings, since changing surgeons increases room turnover time. Surgeons using this concept find they can better schedule their time knowing they have a definite block each week for their ambulatory surgery cases.[2,4]

Equipment and instrument needs also benefit from block scheduling. Instead of having several physicians arguing over the use of a microscope, the facility can stagger the schedule so that on any given day only one physician would be working with a microscope. Block scheduling not only helps to project staffing needs, but also helps staff to project supplies, equipment, and instrument needs.

Keep equipment and staff mobile. Put locking wheels on everything. This practice enhances flexibility and will prove invaluable in handling "add-ons" as well as scheduled blocks. Many physicians prefer using ambulatory surgery centers for minor emergencies presenting to their office (e.g., a child with a dog bite that needs attention, or a young woman suffering a spontaneous abortion). Facilities with limited space can optimize space use by combining examination and procedure rooms and having moveable furniture and equipment. Developing treatment facilities in ancillary areas such as a pain clinic in postanesthesia care or preoperative holding capitalizes on space. Mobility should be promoted even in a dedicated room such as cystoscopy. Tables can be mobile, enabling this specialty space to be used for other radiographic purposes as well as routine procedures.

Quality Assurance

Quality assurance is a term heard repeatedly in all industries. It encompasses all the goals, objectives, standards, and plans formulated to deliver a quality product to the consumer. It involves staff, physician, and management representatives participating together in defining the components of quality care, methods for implementation, and tools for evaluating or measuring the process. Quality assurance is the identification of potential problem areas and the development of policies and procedures to prevent their occurrence.

The development of an active quality assurance program can readily be achieved by organizing a defined committee, consisting of no less than the medical director, the nursing director, a medical records statistician, and a member of the nursing staff.[1]

The committee will

Identify all activities concerned with the delivery of quality care
Recommend additional activities or modification of existing activities
Establish outcome, process, and structure standards and criteria
Develop assessment and evaluation tools designed to identify discrepancies between practices and standards
Recommend corrective action and monitor the results of the change in behavior or performance as it applies to the delivery of quality care

Natof lists six basic components of a quality assurance program:[8]

1. *Identify* problems.
2. *Develop* solutions.
3. *Disseminate* information.

4. *Reassess* at a later date.
5. *Correlate* with educational activities.
6. *Report* activities to responsible parties.

In order to appraise the quality of care as well as the process, periodic formal assessments must be performed with a measuring tool or audit. The audit tool should be developed to reflect the standards of practice. The audit process involves review of documentation such as the operating room or anesthesia records.[7] There are two methods that can be used to identify substantive problems. A *problem-oriented* audit involves a review of a number of charts to look for substantive problems (deviation from the norm); a problem we would be embarrassed to defend with our peers. A *topic-oriented* audit establishes a particular topic for review (e.g., postoperative instructions). There must be a problem-oriented question (e.g., are patients obtaining instructions and do they understand them?). Charts are also reviewed to see if instructions were received and patients can additionally be called to see if they understood them.

Quality assurance is an ongoing, cyclic, nonpunitive process designed to promote excellence in the health care delivery system.

Happiness

Happiness is an essential component of any successful ambulatory surgery program and refers to the happiness of the persons concerned—physicians, guests (patient and responsible person), and staff.

The primary consumer for any surgery center remains the physician. Surveys reveal 98% of patients contacted used a given facility on the recommendation of their physician. With that fact in mind, it is imperative to keep the physician happy by

Being pleasant, obliging, and cooperative
Anticipating needs and problems
Practicing effective problem solving and follow-through
Using updated preference cards
Keeping instrument trays and equipment neat and in good working order
Minimizing room turnover time
Maximizing efficiency
Soliciting ideas

The surgery center guests assume the facility has state-of-the-art technology. The guests' happiness (assuming a satisfactory outcome) will stem from the staff providing psychosocial gratification by

Being pleasant and sincere
Displaying warmth and empathy
Exhibiting a genuine interest in the patients, their problems, and their responsible persons
Providing personalized care to meet their needs
Maintaining a professional attitude, providing patients with a sense of security as to the staff's skills

Holding preoperative and postoperative conferences to impart information and answer questions

Providing extras such as teaching tools or special touches such as toys or extra blankets

Providing written instructions for ready reference by the patient or family member

Promoting the image of wellness

Practicing patient-centered, family-oriented care

The happiness of staff members is essential to maintain the high morale that will provide an ambiance of warmth and relaxation. Flexibility and communication remain at the core of happiness. This is achieved by

Allowing free days and time off when the facility is not busy

Flexibility with hours and breaks

Providing rotation and cross-training within the facility

Distribution of praise and recognition

Open group discussions and participation in the management circle

Development of continuing education

Profit sharing and incentive plans

Conclusion

Physicians, managers, staff, and patients need to be aware of the advantages of ambulatory surgical care. As each group participates in a satisfactory ambulatory surgery experience, each will in its own way promote the advantages to colleagues, friends, co-workers and the community at large—all potential users.

Although providing quality care is an essential ingredient of success, it alone will not ensure a successful facility. In addition to making the facility easily accessible to both physician and patient, Wetchler feels the following are essential components that every facility must incorporate as part of its game plan in order to become or remain successful.[12]

1. *The team concept:* Continually interacting within the facility are three different groups. The physician, the patient, and the staff must work toward a common goal of providing a successful, satisfying ambulatory surgery experience for all involved parties. Each of the three groups are equal in importance, and one group should not attempt to gain importance at the expense of either of the other groups. Professional turf battles must be minimized.

2. *Simplified medical records:* Develop medical records that are easy for the physician and staff to use and are specific for the ambulatory surgery patient and procedure.

3. *Physician convenience:* Develop channels of communication so that information flows freely from the facility to the physician's office in scheduling procedures. Work out block scheduling time. Involve the physician's office in problem solving. Develop standing preoperative and postoperative orders and discharge instructions. Regularly monitor the physicians and their office staff's level of satisfaction with the facility.

4. *VIP (very important patient):* Let the patients know how important they are by preoperative and postoperative phone calls, priority registration, patient education through brochures, an attractive environment, and limited waiting time. Regularly monitor patient satisfaction levels (Fig. 10-2). Keep family members or responsible persons informed about the patient's progress. "The secret of the care of the patient is in caring for the patient."[9]

5. *Careful selection criteria:* Selection involves not only the patient, but also the surgical procedure, as well as physicians and staff who will work in the facility.

6. *Careful discharge criteria:* Discharge criteria should be practical. A responsible person should monitor the patient's care at home. Both the patient and the responsible person should have all discharge information explained and provided to them in writing.

7. *Separate outpatients from inpatients:* Breen feels "patients just entering the in and out surgery unit should never be exposed to post-anesthesia patients returning from the operating or recovery rooms. The psychology of ambulatory surgery is very important in all aspects . . . even the registration and scheduling should be separate, it should be located in the same area as the outpatient surgery."[3] Every effort should be made to have a separate ambulatory surgery PACU.

8. *Medical director:* The medical director must be available, impartial, and knowledgeable in the complete selection process. Direction fairly administered makes it easier for all physicians who wish to schedule procedures in the facility.

9. *Be competitive:* As we continue to have constraints placed on the way we practice and as competition springs up around is, it is essential that we evaluate the way we deliver health care and make every effort to do it
   a. Better
   b. At greater convenience
   c. At a lower price

10. *Market appropriately—everybody sells:* Every member of the staff must be aware of the facility's philosophy, policies, goals, and objectives. We are our own best salespeople when it comes to providing physician, patient, and staff satisfaction.

Ambulatory surgery is a concept whose time has come. However, merely constructing a facility and opening its doors will not guarantee success. This will require the active participation of all parties who are involved in working in the ambulatory surgery facility. Success is multifaceted and depends directly on any and all of the factors mentioned in the preceding pages.

You and your doctor chose the METHODIST AMBULATORY SURGERY CENTER for your surgical care and treatment. We have tried to make your Ambulatory Surgery experience as comfortable and convenient as possible. We are interested in your assessment of our services, personnel, and facilities. Please take a moment to complete this postage paid comment card and return it to us. Your comments and suggestions help us to evaluate our services. Your cooperation is appreciated. Thank you.

CIRCLE ONE:

1. If you came to the hospital for testing several days prior to your surgery:

    (a) Were you treated in a courteous, pleasant and professional manner?   Yes   No

    (b) Did you have laboratory tests?   Yes   No

    (c) Did you have a chest X-ray?   Yes   No

    (d) Did you have an EKG?   Yes   No

    (e) Were your tests carried out smoothly and efficiently?   Yes   No

    (f) Do you feel your visit to the Ambulatory Surgery Center (prior to surgery) was beneficial?   Yes   No

    (g) How long did it take for your testing to be completed?_____(hours)

2. Do you feel your instructions prior to surgery were adequate?   Yes   No

3. Were your personal and informational needs met?   Yes   No

4. Do you feel the Ambulatory Surgery Center personnel were interested in you as a person?   Yes   No

5. Were you comfortable in our facilities regarding lighting, temperature control, and furniture?   Yes   No

6. Were the facilities convenient to use?   Yes   No

7. Do you feel your separation from your family member or friend was minimal?   Yes   No

8. If your child had surgery, as a parent, do you feel you were reunited with your child as soon as possible?   Yes   No

9. Do you feel you have been given adequate post-operative instructions?   Yes   No

10. Were the waiting room facilities adequate for whoever accompanied you the day of your surgery?   Yes   No

11. If you would have this surgery again, would you prefer to be an Ambulatory Surgery Patient?   Yes   No

12. How would you rate your overall surgery experience at the Methodist Ambulatory Surgery Center?

    ☐ Excellent   ☐ Good   ☐ Fair   ☐ Poor

Please list any general comments, suggestions, or employees who provided exceptional service:

_____

_____

_____

_____

DATE OF SURGERY:_____

NAME: (Optional)_____

FIG. 10-2 Patient satisfaction questionnaire used at The Methodist Medical Center of Illinois. This form is given to the patient at the time of discharge from the facility.

References

1. Batalden PB, O'Conner JP: Quality Assurance in Ambulatory Health Care, Germantown, MD, Aspen Systems, 1980
2. Battaglia CJ: New block approach smooths OR scheduling. Same Day Surg 7(7):61, 1983
3. Breen P: Facility design. Same Day Surg 5(4):50, 1981
4. Drier CA, VanWinkle RN, Wetchler BV: Block scheduling contributes to ambulatory surgery center success. AORN J 39(4):673, 1984
5. Ford JL: Outpatient surgery: Present status and future projections. South Med J 5(7):311, 1978
6. Herkimer AG, Jr: Understanding Hospital Financial Management. Germantown, MD, Aspen Systems, 1978
7. Kneedler J: Nursing audit: Challenge to the operating room nurse. University of Texas Health Science Center Teleconference Network Program, San Antonio Texas, June–August 1978
8. Natof H: Managing a successful quality assurance program. Fourth Conference on Same-Day Surgery, Atlanta, 1983
9. Peabody FW: Care of the patient. JAMA 88:877, 1927
10. Perks M: Preprinted discharge instructions save time and trouble. Same Day Surg 5(7):81, July 1981
11. Skagg RL: Programming and design of ambulatory care facilities: Hospitals. JAHA, p 42, July–August 1977
12. Wetchler BV: Development of a successful ambulatory surgery program. In Jackson J, Roach C, Myers M, Norins LC (eds): Development of a Successful Ambulatory Surgery Program, p 67. Atlanta, American Health Consultants, 1981
13. Winston WJ: Proven marketing strategies. Fifth National Conference on Same-Day Surgery, Dallas, 1984

Suggested Readings

Burn J: Facility design for outpatient surgery and anesthesia, In Developing and Managing An Ambulatory Surgery Program, p 135. Boston, Little, Brown & Co, 1981.
Davis JE: Developing the ambulatory surgery unit: The physician's responsibility. J Ambulatory Care Management 4(3):27, 1981
Kirkpatrick KW, Flasck ED: How to implement a quality assurance program, Today's OR Nurse 3:(12):26, 1982

Index

Numbers followed by an *f* indicate a figure; *t* following a page number indicates tabular material.